Imagine What It's Like

A PUBLICATION OF

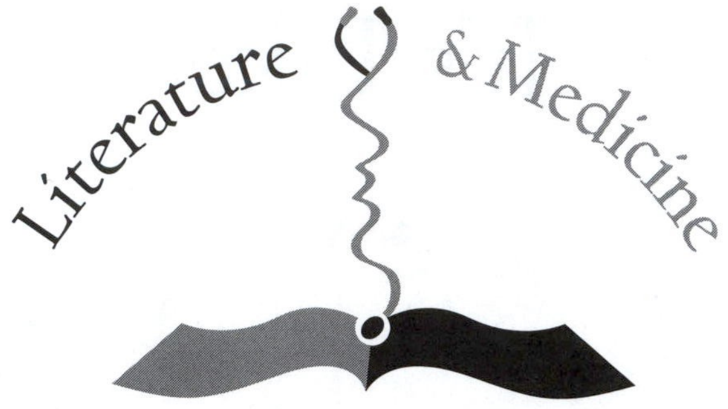

humanities at the heart of health care

A PROGRAM OF THE
MAINE HUMANITIES COUNCIL

PUBLISHED WITH FUNDING FROM

NATIONAL ENDOWMENT FOR THE HUMANITIES
ANTHEM BLUE CROSS AND BLUE SHIELD
MAINE HUMANITIES COUNCIL
MORTON FAMILY FOUNDATION
HAWAI`I COUNCIL FOR THE HUMANITIES

Imagine What It's Like

EDITED BY
RUTH NADELHAFT
WITH VICTORIA BONEBAKKER

A LITERATURE AND MEDICINE ANTHOLOGY

A BIOGRAPHY MONOGRAPH

PUBLISHED FOR THE BIOGRAPHICAL RESEARCH CENTER
BY THE UNIVERSITY OF HAWAI'I PRESS
2008

Printed in the United States of America

13 12 11 10 09 08 6 5 4 3 2 1

Library of Congress Cataloging-in-Publication Data

Imagine what it's like : a literature and medicine anthology / edited by Ruth Nadelhaft, with Victoria Bonebakker.

p. cm.

Includes bibliographical references and index.

ISBN 978-0-8248-3317-6 (pbk. : acid-free paper)

1. Medicine—Literary collections. I. Nadelhaft, Ruth L., 1938– II. Bonebakker, Victoria.

PN6071.M38I43 2008

808.8'03561—dc22

2008011874

University of Hawai'i Press books are printed on acid-free paper and meet the guidelines for permanence and durability of the Council on Library Resources

Designed by Lori Harley
Printed by Edwards Brothers, Inc.

CONTENTS

- SECTION TWO -
BEGINNINGS AND ENDINGS

- SECTION THREE -
TRAUMA AND RECOVERY

- SECTION FOUR -
COMING TO TERMS

- SECTION FIVE -
HEALING COSTS

ACKNOWLEDGMENTS

Since the beginnings of *Literature & Medicine: Humanities at the Heart of Health Care,*® originated by the Maine Humanities Council more than a decade ago, I've had the privilege of working with literally hundreds of medical professionals, humanists of every stripe, and any number of interested and supportive friends and family members. My reading habits, always eclectic (undisciplined is a much better word), have become more focused as well as more meaningful.

This anthology would not have come about had it not been for key members of the Maine Humanities Council board and staff. Former Council Executive Director Dorothy Schwartz and board member Dr. Geoffrey Gratwick ensured that one of three Maine Seminars for Civic Leadership was held at Eastern Maine Medical Center in Bangor, Maine in 1997. That is when I first came on the scene, to co-facilitate with Professor Marli Weiner of the University of Maine the first humanities reading and discussion program for health care professionals. From this pilot offering, the Council's Associate Director Victoria Bonebakker developed the vision for a humanities reading and discussion program focused exclusively on health care professionals, which would be long lived and far reaching. Thanks to major support from the National Endowment for the Humanities, this has now become the national *Literature & Medicine: Humanities at the Heart of Health Care.* Part of NEH's support went to this anthology, which I was asked to edit. Victoria has been an invaluable collaborator throughout the collecting and editing process.

Additional support for the anthology has come from the Maine Humanities Council, Anthem Blue Cross and Blue Shield, The Morton Family Foundation, and the Hawai'i Council for the Humanities. I am particularly grateful to Craig Howes, Professor of English and Director of the Center for Biographical Research at the

University of Hawai'i-Mānoa for his enthusiasm for the anthology and his help in bringing it to life.

I am also grateful to the members of the Planning Committee which met with me early in my work on the anthology. Peter Harris, Professor of English at Colby College, is responsible for the anthology's title. Carole Webber, R.N., who served as the Director of Nursing Education at St. Joseph Hospital in Bangor, was a key supporter of the reading group at that hospital, and a great friend as well.

Finally, I thank my husband, retired Professor of History Jerome Nadelhaft, who found materials for me, opened pathways to data bases and libraries, organized my computer files, and was even willing to read and talk through some of the difficult and challenging selections I chose. We promised to stay faithful to one another many years ago, in sickness and in health, and we are still honoring that promise

Most people who have participated in the *Literature & Medicine* reading and discussion groups say that in some ways their lives are different as a result. Health care professionals have made changes in the way they treat their patients; scholars have redirected their research and teaching; across Maine and other states in hospitals where *Literature & Medicine* has become a part of the culture, notions of hierarchy and hospital customs have been challenged. Not just "medicine" but relationships have been humanized

We hope this anthology will support the continuation and expansion of *Literature and Medicine* and other programs that integrate medicine and the humanities—for the benefit of patients, their friends and families, and those who care for them.

INTRODUCTION

Robertson Davies, the great Canadian writer, asked in an essay derived from a speech he delivered to an audience of medical specialists, "Can a Doctor be a Humanist?" His eventual answer was "Yes," but only, he thought, if the doctor returned to the domain of the *wisdom* of humanities from the world Davies called the *knowledge* of science. Davies spoke and wrote within a long tradition; health care and humanities have long been perceived as vital to one another and yet on different paths. A necessary but still imagined intersection of medicine and the humanities has always been richly populated. Health care workers, including doctors, nurses, and technicians, with philosophers, historians, poets, playwrights, novelists, and short story writers, are among those who have lived and worked at the crossroads, sometimes using their own lives as immediate subject matter. Wisdom, unlike the knowledge of Science, as Davies suggests, involves the realms of feeling and reflection, domains adjacent to the realm of the intellect. Davies urged his listeners to integrate those realms into the living tissue of empathetic practice. This imagined intersection of wisdom and science is the territory of this anthology—ground which is contested, sometimes harrowing, and often ennobling.

The human experience of health care, whether ancient or modern, has always engaged those who practice and those who encounter it in the guise—sometimes temporary, sometimes permanent—of patients. Both those who live with illness of body and mind, and those who live alongside the patients, crave the opportunity to reflect on their experiences. In recent years, practitioners and patients have called attention to a critical moment in our collective experience of medicine. There is a growing awareness of very different cultural expectations around and about the nature and treatment of illness. The intersection is busy. Machinery seems to crowd the space, while human encounters have become brief and often deeply unsatisfying to patients and caregivers alike. Much has been written in recent decades about the crisis in healthcare, from a variety of perspectives. Despite the disparate approaches, from economics to ethics, there is agreement that patients and the world of medicine need more time together, so that illness does not find expression only in the context of the emergency room.

It is as a response to the collective sense of crisis and alienation that anthologies such as this one have been constructed. Inside and outside the health care community many have called for the chance to use the humanities not only as opportunities to reflect on their own experience, but also as a means of improving the experiences of all of us whose lives will be touched by illness and healing, birth and death. Medical schools regularly now include courses based on literature and the arts; later in their careers, members of the health care professions write and read poetry and prose, memoirs and diatribes, about their occupations as professionals, and sometimes from their perspectives as patients who have experienced suffering and noted the inadequacies of their own professions. Paradoxically, while almost every such publication documents the fragmented, interrupted, and even contradictory nature of the medicalized experience, the anthologies bring together short pieces, often excerpted from longer, more coherent meditations. Such anthologies usually attempt to provide diverse readings about illness, health care, and cultural contexts within the restricted compass of short literary forms.

This anthology, too, must rely on short forms, including the occasional selection from the larger context of memoir or collected stories. It differs, however, in attempting to provide some reflection on some long works—some recent, and others from the long accumulation of thoughtful works about health care—whose reading will illuminate the selections which follow. Thus the closing piece, Suggested Longer Readings, touches on significant works from differing regions and cultures which may serve as touchstones—to use the valuable critical reference given to us by Matthew Arnold in the nineteenth century—for thoughtful reading, reflection, and conversation or structured discussion.

SECTION ONE

THE EXPERIENCE OF ILLNESS

INTRODUCTION

Acute illness, pain, the suffering which invades mind and body, take place in what seems an eternal present. Past health and future recovery vanish as the borders of the body disappear. A vast loneliness replaces, apparently forever, the comforting awareness of relationship, community, belonging. It requires supreme imagination and discipline, apparent in the seventeenth chapter of Darcy Wakefield's book chronicling the progress of ALS throughout her body, to remember back to the time before. *I Remember Running,* the title of her book, invokes the past to imagine a future. Where then is literature? And what can literature offer the sufferer or the bystander in the face of the endless formlessness and present tense of the experience of pain and suffering?

Literature offers form, structure, and the illusion of dimension to what was out of control and without limit. Sometimes, in its most practical and approachable mode, literature offers a road map, as in Robert Lipsyte's book, *In the Country of Illness,* whose first chapter testifies to the survival of the author and the implied survival of the reader. Like Lipsyte's work, Jane Lazarre's memoir of her experience with breast cancer provides candor and hope at the same time.

While pain and suffering may seem accidental or gratuitous in their imposition of a miserable new reality, the poem or story or essay is never accidental. Each form has meaning and confers meaning. In Susan Fromberg Schaeffer's short story, "Homage to Isaac Bashevis Singer: A Story," an old woman's meandering and chaotic illness becomes both recognizable and manageable through her vision of the transformative reality Singer took for granted in his stories, written in the Yiddish of a shared youth and culture.

At the conclusion of his remarkable study, *The Noonday Demon: An Atlas of Depression,* an enormous book too large even in excerpted form for an anthology,

Andrew Solomon notes that he has "discovered what I would have to call a soul, a part of myself I could never have imagined until one day, seven years ago, when hell came to pay me a surprise visit. It's a precious discovery" (443).

What people wrest from illness forms the content of this first section of *Imagine What It's Like.* One participant in a *Literature and Medicine* reading group, formed precisely to improve health care professionals' understanding of the world of illness, said earnestly, "I'm not so much interested in illness as in what people make of their illness." These stories, poems, essays, and memoirs are what those who went to the country of illness were able to bring back; these works serve as records, as testimony, as instruction; they are what the writers *made* of their experience.

The creation of empathy and understanding that might make possible the direct apprehension of the writer's experience fuels much of the description of sickness and pain. Across years and cultural differences, those who have "been there" find ways of using the forms of literature to contain and convey the almost formless experiences they have undergone. Sometimes the imaginative writer chooses to depict those experiences, immersing the writer's self in the patient. Often, in recent times, it is those who are trained to be healers who return from their own journeys into illness to report, with some astonishment, how different the world looks from the place within the pain.

Those who know pain directly, as well as those who intuit it and inscribe it into their writing, provide a variety of experiences at which we can marvel even as we begin to integrate them into our own world view. William Cowper's eighteenth-century poem, "The Cast-Away," allows a twenty-first-century reader to apprehend the desperate appeal of suicide to the depressive in a way which is unique to the form of the poem. Cowper's stunning line, "We perish each alone," like Coleridge's more formal ode, "Dejection," engages the reader so thoroughly that the essential loneliness of depression, of a long-persisting and ultimately terminal illness, becomes a shared experience. The reader who survives to the conclusion of these poems knows the depressive's experience as it can perhaps only be known imaginatively. The shape and imagery of the poems allow the illness to penetrate the reader as a clinical account cannot, and perhaps should not.

There has long been discussion among health care practitioners, patients, families, and those who seek to improve medical education and care about the interplay between feelings and care giving. Caregivers fear for their own ability to use their skills if they are overwhelmed by their patients' feelings or their own empathy. Patients complain, as some do in the selections in this section, that they are denied their subjectivity by unfeeling onlookers, some of them the very healers to whom they must entrust themselves. A reading such as "The Cast-Away" serves as a bridge, a living conduit between the sufferer and the outside world, because the poet's ability to give form to his suffering, to contain its immensity in a formal construction on the page, testifies to his strength as well as to the reader's ability to encounter the pain without flinching or losing necessary skills.

From the small, honest voice of Molly Holden's poem, "Hospital," to the more expansive but no less candid account Michel de Montaigne gave to us several hundred years ago, first-person narratives in this first section speak with an immediacy that disarms and engages. Even those written as imaginative works, such as Conrad Aiken's brilliant account of a young boy's descent into schizophrenia, "Silent Snow, Secret Snow," leap the space between illness itself and those who stand beside the bed or outside the door. Using forms as varied as the lyric poem, the journal, the memoir, and the short story, their authors pull readers into the experience of suffering. Form serves as the container for suffering, providing secure dimensions to experiences which might otherwise cause observers to recoil or to shut down their emotional portals.

MUSÉE DES BEAUX ARTS

W. H. AUDEN

About suffering they were never wrong,
The Old Masters: how well they understood
Its human position; how it takes place
While someone else is eating or opening a window or just
  walking dully along;
How, when the aged are reverently, passionately waiting
For the miraculous birth, there always must be
Children who did not specially want it to happen, skating
On a pond at the edge of the wood:
They never forgot
That even the dreadful martyrdom must run its course
Anyhow in a corner, some untidy spot
Where the dogs go on with their doggy life and the
  torturer's horse
Scratches its innocent behind on a tree.

In Brueghel's *Icarus,* for instance: how everything turns away
Quite leisurely from the disaster; the ploughman may
Have heard the splash, the forsaken cry,
But for him it was not an important failure; the sun shone
As it had to on the white legs disappearing into the green
Water; and the expensive delicate ship that must have seen
Something amazing, a boy falling out of the sky,
Had somewhere to get to and sailed calmly on.

OF TRAINING

MICHEL EYQUEM DE MONTAIGNE

It is difficult for reasoning and instruction, even though our belief be readily accorded to them, to be powerful enough to guide us as far as action if we do not, in addition, exercise and train our mind by experience to the course for which we wish to prepare it; otherwise, when it comes to the point of action, it will doubtless be at a loss. This is why those among the philosophers who are ambitious to attain to some greater excellence were not content to await the rigors of Fortune under shelter and in repose, lest she should surprise them inexperienced and new in the combat, but rather sallied out to meet her and purposely threw themselves into the trial of difficulties. Some of them have abandoned riches to exercise themselves in a voluntary poverty; others have sought labor and a painfully austere life to inure themselves to hardships and toil; others have deprived themselves of the most precious parts of the body, such as sight and the organs of generation, lest their too pleasant and too easy use should relax and soften the steadfastness of their souls. But as for dying, which is the greatest task we have to do, practice can give us no assistance. A man may by use and experience fortify himself against pain, shame, want, and other such accidents; but as for death, we can essay it but once: we are all apprentices when we come to it.

In ancient times there were men who were such excellent husbanders of their time that they tried even in death to taste and relish it and strained their minds to see what their passage was; but they have not returned to tell us news of it:

> No man wakes up
> On whom once falls the icy pause of life. (Lucretius)

Canius Julius, a noble Roman of singular virtue and firmness, having been condemned to die by that scoundrel Caligula, besides a number of other wonderful proofs that he gave of his fortitude, as he was about to receive the stroke of the executioner, he was asked by a philosopher, a friend of his: "Well, Canius, in what way

Montaigne wrote "De l'exercitation" in 1573–1574; it forms Chapter 6 of Book 2 of his *Essays*. This translation, by Blanchard Bates, is from Montaigne's *Selected Essays* (New York: Modern Library, 1949).

is your soul now? What is it doing? What are your thoughts?" "I was thinking," he replied, "to keep myself ready and tensed with all my strength in order to see whether in this so short and quick instant of death I shall be able to perceive any sallying forth of the soul, and whether it will have any consciousness of its leave-taking, in order that, if I learn anything, I may hereafter return, if I can, to inform my friends." This man philosophizes not only up to the moment of death, but in death itself. What assurance was this, what intense courage, to desire his death to be a lesson to him, and to be free to turn his thoughts elsewhere in so great a pass!

That mastery of mind he had in death. (Lucan)

And yet I think there is some way of becoming familiarized with it and in some sort of making trial of it. We may have some experience of it, if not complete and perfect, at least such as may not be useless to us, and that may make us stronger and more assured. If we cannot come to grips with it, we can approach it, we can observe it; and if we do not advance as far as its fortress, we shall at least see and try its avenues of approach.

It is not without reason that we are taught to consider our sleep itself for the resemblance it bears to death. How easily we pass from waking to sleeping! With what little concern do we lose consciousness of the light and of ourselves!

Perhaps the faculty of sleep, which deprives us of all action and all feeling, might seem useless and contrary to nature were it not that by its means Nature instructs us that she has shaped us to die as well as to live and presents to us, early in life, the eternal state she reserves for us after it, in order to accustom us to it and to take away our fear of it.

But they who by some violent accident have fallen into a swoon and lost all consciousness have, it seems to me, been very near to seeing its true and natural face. For as to the moment and the point of passing away, there need be no fear that it brings with it any pain or suffering, in as much as we can have no feeling without leisure. Our sufferings require time, which in death is so short and swift that it must necessarily be without feeling. It is the approaches that we have to fear, and these may fall within our experience.

Many things seem greater to us in imagination than they are in fact. I have passed a good part of my life in perfectly sound health; I may say not merely sound, but even sprightly and bubbling over. This state, full of fresh energy and jollity, made the thought of sickness so horrible to me that, when I came to experience it, I found its attacks weak and feeble compared with my fear.

Here is something that I experience daily: if I am warmly sheltered in a good room on a stormy and tempestuous night, I wonder at and feel distressed for those who are then in the open country; if I am there myself, I do not even desire to be anywhere else.

That thought alone, of being always shut up in a room, seemed to me unbearable. I was suddenly trained to be there for a week and a month, beset by agitation, disorder, and weakness; and I have found that when I was in good health I pitied the sick much more than I think myself to be pitied when I am one of them, and that the force of my imagination exaggerated by nearly a half the essence and reality of the thing. I hope that it will turn out the same way for me in the matter of death, and that it is not worth the pains that I take in making so many preparations and in calling in and assembling so many aids to sustain the shock. But at all events we cannot give ourselves too much advantage.

In the time of our third civil war, or the second (I do not well remember which), having gone one day to take the air about a league from my house, which is seated in the hub of all the trouble of the civil wars in France, thinking myself in all security and so near to my home that I stood in need of no better equipage, I had taken a horse of very easy gait, not very strong. On my way back, an occasion having suddenly arisen for me to use this horse in a kind of service that he was not quite used to, one of my men, big and strong, mounted upon a powerful work-horse that had a hopelessly hard mouth, fresh to boot and vigorous, to cut a bold figure and outstrip his fellows, forced his horse full tilt straight into my path, and bore down like a colossus upon the little man and the little horse, and blasted us with his speed and weight, sending us both head over heels; so that there lay the horse prostrate and stunned and I ten or twelve paces beyond; stretched out on my back like a corpse, my face all bruised and skinned, my sword, which I had in my hand, more than ten paces farther on, my belt in pieces, having no more movement or feeling than a log. It was the only swoon I had experienced till that hour. Those who were with me, after having tried all the means they could to bring me to myself, thinking I was dead, took me up in their arms and carried me with much difficulty home to my house, which was about half a French league away. On the way, and after I had been for more than two good hours considered as being dead, I began to move and breathe, for so great an abundance of blood had fallen into my stomach that Nature had need to rouse her forces to discharge it. They put me up on my feet, whereupon I threw up a bucketful of clots of pure blood, and several times on the way I had to do it again. By this means I began to recover a little life, but it was by slow degrees and over so long a stretch of time that my first feelings were much nearer death than life,

For still in doubt of its return to life,
The stricken soul rests unsure of itself. (Tasso, *Jerusalem Delivered*)

This recollection, which is strongly imprinted on my mind, bringing the image and idea of death before me in so nearly natural an aspect, somewhat reconciles me to it. When I began to see, it was with so blurred, so weak, and so dead a sight that I could as yet distinguish nothing but the light,

Like him who opens now, now shuts his eyes,
Lying midway 'twixt sleep and wakefulness. (Tasso, *Jerusalem Delivered*)

As to the functions of the mind, they revived at the same rate as those of the body. I saw I was all bloody, for my doublet was stained all over with the blood I had vomited. The first thought that came to me was that I had been shot in the head by a harquebus; indeed at the same time as the accident several had been fired around us. It seemed to me that my life just hung upon the edge of my lips; I shut my eyes to help, so I thought, to thrust it out, and took a pleasure in languishing and letting myself go. It was an idea that only floated on the surface of my mind, as weak and feeble as all the rest, but, in truth, not only free from distress, but mixed with that pleasant tranquility felt by us when we are gliding into slumber.

I believe it is the same condition those people are in whom we see faint with weakness in the agony of death, and I think that we pity them without cause, supposing that they are agitated with grievous suffering and their minds beset by painful thoughts. It has ever been my belief, contrary to the opinion of many, and even of Etienne de La Boetie, that those whom we see so overwhelmed and stupefied at the approach of their end, or crushed by the length of their sickness, or by an attack of apoplexy or the falling sickness,

> And oft before our eyes someone o'ercome
> By illness topples as by lightning struck,
> And spews forth foam; he twitches and he moans;
> His sinews tense, he drivels, writhes, and gasps,
> And wearies out his limbs with tossing wild. (Lucretius)

or hurt in the head, when we hear them moaning and at times uttering poignant sighs, although we gather from these signs and from some movements we see them make with the body that they still retain some consciousness, I have always believed, I say, that their mind and their body are shrouded and asleep:

> He lives, and is unconscious of his life. (Ovid, *Tristia*)

And I could not believe that in so great a stupefaction of the members and so great a failing of the senses the soul could maintain any force within to be conscious of itself, and that, therefore, they had no power of reflection to torment them and make them feel and measure the wretchedness of their condition, and that consequently they were not much to be pitied.

I can think of no state for me so unbearable and dreadful as to have the soul alive and afflicted without means of expressing itself. As I should say of those who are sent to execution with their tongues cut out, were it not that in this kind of death the most silent seems to me the most becoming if accompanied with a grave and firm countenance, and of those wretched prisoners who fall into the hands of the villainous, inhuman soldiers of this age, by whom they are tortured with every kind of cruelty to compel them to pay some excessive and impossible ransom, kept in the meantime in a condition and place where they have no means of expressing or signifying their thoughts and misery.

The poets have imagined some gods favorable to the deliverance of those who thus drag on a lingering death,

> This offering unto Dis I bear,
> As bid, and from thy body set thee free! (Virgil, *Aeneid*)

And the brief and disconnected words and replies which we extract from them by dint of shouting in their ears and storming at them, or the movements which seem to correspond somewhat to what is asked of them, are, however, no evidence that they are alive, at least fully alive. So it happens to us in the stammering beginnings of sleep, before it has fully seized us, that we perceive, as in a dream, what is done about us and follow the voices with a confused and uncertain hearing which seems but to touch upon the borders of the soul; and to the last words that were spoken to us we give answers that are made up more of chance than of sense.

Now that I have actually tried it, I make no doubt that my judgment of it hitherto has been correct. For in the first place, being fully unconscious, I was laboring with all the strength of my nails to open up my doublet (for I was not in armor), and yet I know that in my mind I was not aware of anything hurting me, for we make many motions that do not start forth from the direction of our will,

> Half-dead, the fingers move and clutch anew the sword. (Virgil, *Aeneid*)

So falling people throw their arms out in front of them by a natural impulse which causes our limbs to lend each other their services and to be moved quite apart from our reason:

> They say that scythe-armed chariots lop off limbs
> So quickly that the part which is cut off
> Is seen to quiver on the earth below,
> While yet the mind and powers of the man
> Can through the rapid blow perceive no pain. (Lucretius)

My stomach was oppressed with the clotted blood, my hands hastened to it of their own accord, as they often do to the part that itches, against the direction of our will. There are many animals, and even men, whose muscles may be seen to contract and move after they are dead. Everyone knows by experience that there are parts which often stir, rise up, and lie down without our leave. Now these feelings which only touch the outward bark of us cannot be said to be ours. To make them ours the whole man must be involved in them; and the pains which are felt by the hand or the foot while we are sleeping are not ours.

As I drew near to my house, where the alarm of my fall had preceded me, and as the members of my family came out to meet me with the outcries usual in such cases, not only did I give some sort of reply to what was asked of me, but they even say that I had the sense to order them to give a horse to my wife, whom I saw stumbling and struggling on the road, which is hilly and rough. It seems that this thoughtfulness must have proceeded from a mind that was awake; yet I was not there at all: they were nothing but idle thoughts in the clouds, they were stirred up by the senses of sight and hearing; they did not come out of myself. I did not know, for all that, whence I was coming, or whither I was going, neither was I able to weigh and consider what was asked of me: those are slight effects that the senses produce by themselves, as if by habit; what the mind contributed was as in a dream, very lightly touched, only licked, as it were, and bedewed by the soft impression of the senses.

Meanwhile my condition was, in truth, very easy and peaceful. I was grieved neither for others, nor for myself; it was a languor and extreme weakness without any pain. I saw my house without recognizing it. When they had put me into bed, I found an inexpressible sweetness in that repose, for I had been wretchedly dragged about by those poor people who had taken the pains to carry me in their arms over a long and very bad road and in doing so had tired themselves out two or three times in relays. They offered me many remedies, none of which I took, holding it for certain that I was mortally wounded in the head. In truth, it would have been a very happy death, for the weakness of my reason prevented me from having any opinions about it, and that of my body from feeling anything. I was letting myself glide away so gently, and in so soft and easy a manner, that I scarcely know any action less burdensome than that was. When I began to revive and to resume my faculties,

> As my lost senses did at last return, (Ovid, *Tristia*)

which was two or three hours later, I felt myself suddenly involved again in pain, my limbs being all pounded and bruised by my fall, and I was so ill for two or three nights after that I thought I was dying once more, but by a more painful death; and I still feel the shock of that crash. I do not want to omit this, that the last thing I could recover was the recollection of this accident, and I had them tell me over and over again whither I was going, whence I was coming, and at what hour that had happened to me, before I could comprehend it. As to the manner of my fall, that was concealed from me for the sake of the man who had been the cause of it, and another story was invented. But a long time after, on the following day, when my memory began to return and picture to me the state I was in at the instant that I perceived this horse bearing down upon me (for I had seen him at my heels and thought I was a goner; but this thought had been so sudden that there was no time for fear to arise), it seemed to me that it was a flash of lightning that struck my mind with a jolt, and that I was returning from the other world.

This story of so unimportant an event is rather pointless were it not for the instruction I have derived from it for my own use; for, in truth, I find that to become familiar with death there is no way except to approach it. Now, as Pliny says, everyone is a very good subject of study to himself, provided he have the capacity to examine himself closely. This is not my teaching, it is my study; and it is not a lesson for others, but for me.

And yet one should not be displeased with me if I communicate it. That which is of use to me may also by chance be useful to another. Besides I spoil nothing, I make use of nothing but my own. And if I play the fool, it is at my own expense and without detriment to anyone. For it is a folly that dies with me and has no consequences. We hear of only two or three ancients who have trod this road, and yet we cannot say whether it was at all in this manner, knowing only their names. No one since has thrown himself on their trail. It is a thorny undertaking, and more so than it seems, to follow so roving a movement as that of our mind, to penetrate the opaque depths of its innermost folds, to choose and arrest so many little emanations of its stirrings. It is a new and extraordinary pastime which withdraws us from the ordinary occupations of the world, yes, and from those most recommended.

For many years my thoughts have had no other aim than myself; and if I study any other thing, it is to apply it at once to myself, or rather in myself. And I do not think it a fault if, as is done in other incomparably less useful sciences, I communicate what I have learned in this one, though I am not very well pleased with the progress I have made in it. There is no description equal in difficulty to the description of oneself, nor certainly in usefulness. Furthermore a man must have his hair well groomed, he must make himself trim and neat to appear in public. Now I am continually decking myself out, for I am continually describing myself. Custom has made it a vice to speak of oneself and obstinately forbids it in hatred of the boasting that seems always to be attached to men's testimony about themselves. Whereas a child's nose should be wiped, that is called pulling it off,

> Fleeing a fault may lead into a vice. (Horace, *Ars Poetica*)

I find more evil than good in this remedy. But even if it were true that to talk to people about ourselves is necessarily presumptuous, I ought not, following out my general plan, to forbear an action that publishes this infirmity, since it is in me; and I ought not to conceal this fault which I not only practice but profess. But to speak my mind freely, it is a wrong custom that condemns wine because some get drunk on it. Only things that are good can be abused. And I believe that this rule concerns only the weakness of the common people. Such rules are bridles for calves with which neither saints, whom we hear speak so highly of themselves, nor philosophers, nor theologians will curb themselves; nor will I, though I am as little the one as the other. If they do not expressly write about themselves, at all events, when the occasion arises, they do not hesitate to put themselves on parade. Of what does Socrates treat more largely than of himself? To what does he more often direct the conversation of his disciples than to speak of themselves, not of the lesson in their book, but of the essence and movement of their soul? We scrupulously confess ourselves to God and our confessor, as our neighbors do to the whole people. But, someone will answer me, we confess only our sins. Then we confess all, for our very virtue is faulty and repentable. My trade and my art is to live. He that forbids me to speak of it according to my own sense, experience, and practice, let him order an architect to speak of buildings not according to his own opinions, but according to his neighbor's, according to another's knowledge, not according to his own. If it is vainglory for a man to proclaim his own worthy traits, why does not Cicero push to the fore the eloquence of Hortensius, and Hortensius that of Cicero?

Perhaps they mean that I should give testimony of myself by works and deeds, not barely by words. I chiefly portray my thoughts, a shapeless subject which cannot be expressed in the productivity of deeds. It is all that I can do to couch it in this airy body of the voice. The wisest and devoutest men have lived shunning all visible actions. The actions would tell more about Fortune than about me. They testify to their rôle, not to mine, unless it be conjecturally and uncertainly: samples showing only certain particular details. I expose myself entire: it is a skeleton on which, at one view, the veins, muscles, and tendons are apparent, each part in its place. The effect of a cough brought into evidence one part of it; the effect of pallor or the beating of the heart another, and that dubiously. It is not my deeds that I write about; it is myself, it is my essence.

I maintain that we must be judicious in forming an estimate of ourselves and equally conscientious in giving an account of it impartially, be it high or low. If I thought myself good and wise, or nearly so, I should sing it forth at the top of my voice. To say less of ourselves than what we are is foolishness, not modesty. And to pay ourselves off with less than we are worth is cowardice and pusillanimity according to Aristotle. No virtue is helped by falsehood; and truth is never a matter of error. To say more of ourselves than is really true is not always presumption, it likewise is often foolishness. To be inordinately pleased with what one is, to fall into an undiscerning self-love, is, in my opinion, the substance of this vice. The supreme remedy for curing it is to do the very opposite of what is prescribed by those who in forbidding us to speak of ourselves consequently forbid us even more to think of ourselves. Pride lies in the thought. The tongue can have only a very slight share in it. It seems to them that to give attention to oneself is to be pleased with oneself, that to frequent and to converse with oneself is to hold oneself too dear. It may be so. But this excess arises only in those who try themselves only on the surface, who look to themselves only after their business, who call it dreaming and idleness to reflect upon themselves, and look upon the building up and the equipping of oneself as building castles in Spain, considering themselves as a third person and a stranger.

If anyone, looking at those beneath him, becomes intoxicated with his knowledge, let him but turn his eye upward towards past ages and he will lower his horns, finding there so many thousands of minds that trample him under foot. If he assume any flattering presumption of his own worth, let him recall the lives of the two Scipios, so many armies, so many nations that leave him so far behind them. No particular quality will make any man proud who will at the same time take account of the many other weak and imperfect qualities that are in him, and, in the end, the nothingness of the state of man.

Because Socrates alone had seriously bitten into that precept of his god, "to know himself," and by that study had come to scorn himself, he alone was considered worthy of the title of Sage. Whoever shall so know himself, let him boldly make himself known by his own mouth.

INNOCENTS ABROAD

ROBERT LIPSYTE

My own journey began with a vague ache in my right testicle, which seemed larger and firmer than usual. I began touching my right testicle so often to check if the swelling had gone away and it became a habit, a tic. In the beginning, I would touch it only when I happened to be in a bathroom, but soon I made visits purely for self-exams. So many journeys to Malady seem to start this way, undramatic distant warnings, a tingle in a joint, shortness of breath, a fleeting chest pain after running for a train.

When I couldn't keep my hands off myself—poking through my pants pocket on the street, at the swim club, at the dinner table—and when I was giving Margie hourly updates, like testicular weather reports, it seemed time to go to our local family doctor, a pleasant technician we usually visited for strep throat cultures. Probably nothing, we agreed.

On my calendar, under June 20, 1978, I wrote the doctor's name and "Balls." It was my first attempt at tumor humor, which would soon become very important.

As it turned out, the doctor was not concerned, so I didn't have to be. Normally, after I'd been standing awhile, blood vessels called varioceles would drop down into my scrotum like strands of linguine and sometimes feel twingey. For twenty years doctors had told me not to worry about it, although I did. This was probably a variation, the doctor said. He called it "an unspecified inflammation" and prescribed tetracycline for two weeks. He told me to take hot baths several times a day and to put my feet up whenever I could so the varioceles could slide back up into my body. It was non-alarming advice, yet proactive; I was doing something to correct a minor problem. I stopped touching myself more than a few times a day. The ache kept nagging for the next two weeks, but at a greater distance. Because I had faith in the doctor's nondiagnosis—you bet I wanted to believe it—the anxious edge that often stimulates pain faded.

(This was the same doctor who prescribed Provera for Margie's painful menstrual periods. Perhaps, she later thought, it was a cause of her own cancer.)

I was feeling physically fit that summer. I was forty years old, a husband, father, suburban householder. My weight, a chronic problem, was down to 174, only five or six pounds more than it should be. I was swimming and playing tennis almost every day. I was traveling to the South Bronx regularly to work on the local political campaign of a friend, and the tough, streety Puerto Ricans I was hanging out with were turning up as characters in a not-very-thrilling thriller I was writing about a fortyish, novel-writing journalist whose life was turned upside down by a female journalism student who challenged him to be better. Based on guess who?

When I went back to the family doctor, he shook his head in puzzlement and sent me up the medical chain to a local urologist, who thought my swelling was "epididymitis," an inflammation of a tiny tube of ducts attached to the testicle. He prescribed ampicillin and Chymoral and longer, hotter sitz baths. This was July 17.

If it's not epididymitis, I asked, what could it be? He shrugged. I asked him one of the three most common dramatic questions (the other two are, "Is he dead?" and "Are you having an affair?"), and he shook his head. At forty, he explained, I was too old for testicular cancer, a disease of men twenty years younger. Come back in two weeks if the swelling doesn't go down, which it should, he said.

Margie remembered those weeks, more poignantly than I do, as my vain attempt to poach the swelling away. She described me sitting in the bathtub, twice a day, with books, music, once even, she said, with a cigar in a show of bravado. I don't remember the cigar, and my calendars never mention baths. But I'm sure she was right. Who wants to remember something so pathetic?

I do remember during those weeks that Fraidy, the little white kitten that my daughter Susannah and I rescued from her Brownie leader's car engine, had to go to the vet, and that my son Sam took two fastballs on the same finger during two different Little League games. The second time, as I remember it, he hit a home run off his finger, but broke it. (Sam remembers that he struck out.) I remember that Margie and I took the kids to camp in the Adirondacks, that we visited them, and sat through the camp production of *Annie,* in which the role of President Roosevelt's Secretary of Labor, Frances Perkins, was played by a boy. Margie talked about that most of the way home. Perkins was the first female Cabinet member! What kind of camp were we entrusting the kids to? I remember that we saw movies, *Coming Home* and *House Calls* and *An Unmarried Woman,* met friends, and almost every afternoon after writing we drove to the local swim club and did laps.

What I didn't remember for a long time was my mounting concern, the rising certainty that something was wrong. Another vignette that Margie remembered and I had erased, or at least buried deep in the hard drive, was the pool party at which I asked my oldest friend, Mark Chapman, a gastroenterologist at Mt. Sinai hospital, to feel my swollen testicle. He lived in the next town, and one night at his house, after the guests went inside for dinner, I made him follow me into his pool house. I pulled down my trunks. Obviously, I was getting scared. He said it was probably nothing to worry about, but of course I should check it out right away.

On the last day of July, I returned to the local urologist. Margie came with me this time, and followed me right into his examining room. This was not routinely done in 1978. She was ahead of her time. Also, she told me years later, she thought I "looked tortured" and was "a basket case," atypically passive and weak. The urologist was surprised by Margie's presence, but probably intimidated. When he tried to at least draw a curtain, she said she had seen me naked before.

After he examined me, he suggested "we take a look-see" at what he now called "a testicular mass." As he explained it, the look-see was a simple operation called an orchiectomy. A slit would be cut in my groin near the hair line, and the testicle lifted out by the long duct cord that connected it to the rest of my body. Dangling like a yo-yo on the end of its string, the testicle would be examined. If it was benign, it would be dropped back into the sac. If it was malignant, the string would be snipped and the testicle would be examined further to determine the next steps.

When I asked why he didn't take the easy route through the sac to the testicle, the same way he would go in for a vasectomy, he explained that should it actually be cancer, malignant cells could spill and spread. He didn't tell me that most testicular masses turn out to be cancerous.

Margie asked, "how many of these do you do a year?" It was her first cancer question, the first of thousands, and it still stands as one of the best. When it comes to any kind of important decision or procedure, it is essential that the doctor be experienced. Never, ever, hesitate to ask about experience and credentials.

The urologist admitted that he and his suburban partners got to see only two or three cases like this a year. We sensed he looked forward to it as a good experience for the team. He never suggested we go to a larger center with more experienced doctors.

We made an appointment to have the operation at a local hospital in a week. (This doctor disappears from the story now, but my memories of him are still warm; months later, he actually called me to find out what had happened and how things had turned out. The fact that he cared enough to follow up, even if it was only professional curiosity, makes him unusual and a good guy in my book.)

I was scared. It was not The Dread, that cloak of catatonia I would feel later when I knew more, but it was enough to dry my mouth and loosen my bowels and leave me staring into the future, unable to make the next move. I crossed my legs just thinking about the orchiectomy. I had always been terrified of a hernia operation, and at the time when vasectomies were becoming popular I rejected having one out of the fear of being cut down there. And here we were about to go to a hospital for what might turn out to be a serious disease. I was, according to Margie, a "whimpering wreck."

She kicked me into gear, ordering me to get advice from some of those pre-meds with whom I'd gone to college. They were now doctors in major teaching centers.

Mark was away on vacation, and so was Arthur Frifkin, a psychiatrist, but Dave Kinne, a leading breast surgeon at the Memorial Sloan-Kettering Cancer Center, was at work. I was lucky, though even more scared now; to an inexperienced patient like myself, that world-famous cancer treatment center conjured up more visions of illness and death than of health and healing. As a sportswriter, I knew that Babe Ruth had died there.

Steady, kindly Dave took my call very seriously. He told me to wait fifteen minutes, so he could call first, then to call Poppy, the secretary of the great Dr. Willet F. Whitmore, Jr., who would give me the first available appointment. That turned out to be for the next morning. I relaxed a little, feeling an expert was on the case now.

I took the kids—Sam was ten, Susannah seven-and-a-half—to see *Grease.* We ate at a local pizza joint. I usually loved such kid-stuff outings, but I was distracted: I kept jostling my testicle during the movie and the meal, expecting the swelling to go down before morning and embarrassing me in front of Dr. Whitmore for making such a fuss.

It was still there when Margie and the kids dropped me off at Memorial on their way to the airport to pick up visiting cousins. After my appointment, I would catch a bus back home in time for the welcoming barbecue.

Dr. Whitmore turned out to be the ur-urologist, the famous surgeon who had treated writer Cornelius Ryan and former Vice President Hubert Humphrey. He was a handsome, middle-aged swashbuckler who swept into the chilly little examining room with his young resident as if they were Batman and Robin. The moment I saw them, my fears vanished; Whitmore managed to create an unreal world in which we were setting off together on an adventure. Terry and the Pirates! Captain Midnight! I had nothing to worry about.

They smiled knowingly as they took my history, cupped and squeezed my testicle as they examined it. No doubt about it. They seemed energized that I would give them another go with the enemy.

Dr. Whitmore said, "Looks suspicious to me; let's go in there. We should do this right away."

I was so caught up in his spirit, I said, "What are you doing this afternoon?"

Surgeon and Robin winked at each other and clapped my shoulders. I was pleased to imagine them thinking what a gamer I was; this boy has come to play! That tendency to want to please our doctors is a dicey matter. When it leads us to become active in our own healing, to take better care of ourselves, it's terrific, but when it makes us passive, too accepting, it's dangerous; a lot depends on the doctor, of course, and a little skepticism on our part never hurts. In this particular case, my wanting to please the doctors was probably helpful. It carried me mindlessly through what would have been anxious hours.

Dr. Whitmore told me to go out and have a second breakfast, as if I'd been able to have a first, buy a toothbrush, then call Poppy, who by then would have made arrangements for my admittance that very day. There would be a day of tests, he said, then the orchiectomy on Friday. I might be able to go home by Sunday. I left the examining room as if it were a locker room—if not overjoyed, at least up for the game.

It was my first professional contact with jock surgeons, who are different from other doctors, more like quarterbacks, test pilots, hot street cops, those give-me-the-ball types who seem to subscribe to the macho creed of If in Doubt, Do Something! The scalpel is a performing tool in a win-lose game, a life-and-death theater, and the surgeon is the star, surrounded by supporting players. Other specialists are often more important than the surgeons, but none can beat them for sheer glamour.

Many surgeons are too quick to cut, true, and their optimism is frequently unjustified. The way they coo over a fresh cut—"That looks so goooood!"—or reverently touch fading surgical scars calls for satire. Unless, of course, those cuts and scars are on your body and the surgeons are leaning over you as if you are the game they'd just finished playing. Not quite so funny. And when things go wrong, surgeons, like athletes, tend to place blame beyond themselves, on the referees, the field conditions, the stubborn refusal of the patient to heal properly. But with the big game on the line, nothing is as encouraging as the hearty confidence of those jock surgeons who think they can carve you to victory. Their confidence is not always well placed, but it is always welcome.

* * * * *

My room, 831, was pleasant and light. The first two nights I shared it with a shrunken, pearl-gray man whose curtain was drawn most of the time. His visitors seemed to be his wife and their grown children. They looked grim, especially during whispery bedside conferences with doctors. In the middle of the second night there was chatter and scuffle—I was tranquilized and I remembered it as a dream—and the next morning the curtain was open and his side of the room was uninhabited. Even the plastic water jug with the bent straw was gone. His mattress was rolled to the foot of the bed. The nurses would not tell me where he had gone. I later found out that a rolled mattress in the morning meant the guest had checked out that night. Permanently.

The first operation, the orchiectomy, less than forty-eight hours after Whitmore first hefted my testicle, was no big deal in retrospect, although the hours around it—my first overnight in a hospital since losing my tonsils at four—were vivid. Everything was freighted with significance, alarming, confusing. I was in-country now.

There was a bewildering, eventually annoying, parade of man-child doctors marching importantly into my room with big steel clipboards and little black notebooks. They were tired because they were overworked and they were defensive because they weren't quite sure what they were doing. The youngest were the worst, hiding their studenthood behind the slightly distracted arrogance then in vogue at better medical schools.

This being early August, many were just rotating into urology, or on urology fellowships that had begun in June. They were practicing their interviewing, chart-scanning, testicle-squeezing. On me. I had no way of reading their "Hmmmmms" and "Ah-hahs." What do you see, I asked, is it bad? They had no information for me because they didn't know much yet, and they had yet to develop the lofty benevolence of their elders. So they hmm'd some more, and left me sweating. Had I known more then, I would have been able to disregard their murmurings, let them poke and move on or even send them packing. It was not likely any of them could help me. The downside of a great teaching hospital is all the eager students.

Meanwhile, the nurses were bucking me up with the false chirpiness of flight attendants in a wind shear. I didn't know how to read that, either. Were they so cheerful because I was in such bad shape?

And then there were the aides, clanging bedpans in the night. Practicing the cymbals for Carnegie Hall? For the Urologists' Ball?

Thank goodness for tumor humor.

We didn't have a name for it yet (the first time I saw that term in print was in a 1980 Young Adult novel, *Waiting for Johnny Miracle,* by Alice Bach), but that Thursday night before the first operation, we had our first experiences with that enormously helpful genre of sick humor.

Tumor humor is not warm and friendly; it does not necessarily release feel-good endorphins. It is not what the writers Joseph Heller and Norman Cousins have prescribed, and it is not the "Laughter Is the Best Medicine" feature my grandfather used to read to me from *Reader's Digest.* Tumor humor is scrappy and sometimes nasty and tasteless, a sort of chemotherapy for the spirit, necessary and never nice. Trash talk. Really sick jokes.

Example: Margie sat on my bed and while we were going over the next morning's procedure for the hundredth time, I suddenly asked, "So if they pull it out and it's cancerous, what do they do with it after they test it? You can't just throw a malignant testicle in the garbage disposal, can you?"

Soon we spun off into a dark fantasy about my diseased testicle floating off into the world. I mean, after all, what *did* they do with the cancerous testicles they threw away? Into the sewer, out to the ocean, adventures on other continents? Did people pick them up, display them as found art?

This probably doesn't seem all that funny to you. As I read it now, it doesn't seem all that funny to me. But I remember how hilarious it seemed then, not because of its intrinsic humor, but because it gave us some release and it also gave us some sense, however false, of control. We might be swept away on this tidal wave, but we still had an oar in the water. We could still crack wise.

Tumor humor is a tough sell until you need it. And then it's a saver. Tumor humor is for the comedian, not the audience. I learned that when a friend of mine, suffering from prostate cancer, had a heart attack. I was taken aback when he said, "See, I told you guys that cancer wasn't going to get me." His recovery might be in part attributable to that attitude, which keeps you positive and aggressive in the pursuit of getting better.

Tumor humor is a form of gallows humor, the brave and edgy, often self-mocking jokes that the oppressed, the minority, the scared silly tell each other to keep from crying.

Two Jews about to be shot by a firing squad. Abe says, "Wait a minute, what about my last request? I want a cigarette." Izzie elbows him and whispers, "Don't make trouble."

Or

Down South in the sixties, Dick Gregory is about to tear into a whole fried chicken when those three brothers Ku, Klux, and Klan walk into the restaurant and say, "Boy, whatever you do to that chicken we'll do to you."

So Gregory kisses the chicken's butt.

Get it?

Cancer has no special claim on tumor humor. It should be practiced by every traveler in Malady. In recent years, some of the best examples of that gallant, life-affirming whistling in the dark have come from AIDS patients. But it is tricky, since it can seem offensive if it comes from people who haven't earned the right to use it—by being a patient or a caregiver—and it shouldn't be used by patients and caregivers to shut out others who might be helpful. No rules here. I just remember how it helped us get through that night before the first operation. We were able to make believe everything was normal. After all, weren't we being our usual smart-alecky selves?

After Margie left, a wiry young man named Edward strutted into the room and shaved my pubic area with entertaining theatrics. He told me he had never lost a patient, and that this was a simple deal. He made me feel good until he said, "Good luck," in the same tone Las Vegas changemakers use when they give you rolls of coins for the slot machines. I didn't know then that everyone says "Good luck"—it means only as much as you want it to mean—but I worried about it until my sleeping pill hit. Actually, I hated to take that pill and stalled as long as I could; it meant letting go, losing control. This, I later found out, is very common. But unless you plan to stay up during the operation and direct it, take the pill. Get your rest.

There was a lot of bustle the next morning. Margie was there as I was wheeled out of my room. I remember saying, "I'm sorry," to her. I really was sorry, anticipating all the anguish and dislocation I was causing her and others. We talked about it later because she was touched that I could have such a feeling at that time. It was probably a good thing, in that I wasn't totally absorbed in my own immediate concerns, but if it led to my becoming depressed over something that was not my fault it would clearly hamper recovery. It's worth keeping in mind.

I think I saw Dr. Whitmore, but everything was mostly dim and pale and chilly. I woke up in Recovery, shivering, one of many slabs of meat on tables lined along a wall. Nurses moved among us. I must have been in better shape than most of the patients coming out of the operating rooms because I looked around, noticed a woman's pretty face, and studied the outline of her body under the sheet.

That I could appreciate the good-looking woman on the next slab, though only theoretically, indicated to me that I was sort of okay. But I was very cold, bone-chilled, and for years I wondered if that was from the shock of the cutting or the anesthesia. Or was it from the temperature of the operating room, presumably kept cold for good medical reasons, perhaps to slow the blood or kill off the bad germs.

It was almost twenty years later that I read an article explaining that operating rooms were routinely kept at about 65 degrees so that the surgeons, heavily gowned and sweating under the bright lights, could perform in comfort. According to the article, a new study had found that patients who were kept warm during an operation, even with something as simple as a blanket, recovered more quickly and had far less risk of infection than those operated on in a cool room. A drop in temperature interferes with the body's defense against germs. Finally, hospitals are turning up the heat.

I was still too groggy to be scared when I was told the next day that I had cancer, and that it looked as though it had broken out of the testicle. One of the doctors said, "It's a bad one," but his tone seemed to indicate that this would be less a danger to me than an exhilarating challenge for him.

Dave Kinne told Margie that it would be several days before "the numbers were in." It sounded like off-track betting to me. There would be more tests, and a second, much more extensive, operation.

I'd be in-country for a while.

APPLICANTS

FELICIA NIMUE ACKERMAN

There were books about job interviews. There were books about college interviews. But for this interview, I was on my own. Of course, I could use some of what I had read.

LOOK YOUR BEST. I had slept with my hair braided, and now it was wavy and soft. My little mirror showed a heart-shaped face (appropriate), large light-blue eyes, skin maybe a trifle pale, but except for the bluish tinge of my lips, I thought I looked almost more like a movie invalid than the real thing. Hard to decide about makeup, though. The books said it should be effective but unobtrusive, but they weren't too specific about what that meant. Probably best to compromise: enough lipstick to give my lips a better color, but no eye-shadow. I tweezed my eyebrows just enough to make the arch look natural. Yes, I liked my reflection. And I had read somewhere that attractive people were rated better on everything, even things you would think had nothing to do with looks.

BE ON TIME OR SLIGHTLY EARLY. No problem there. My interview was coming to me. Where else would that happen? Suppose I were trying to adopt a child. I'd spend hours getting the house ready: sweeping, scrubbing, vacuuming, dusting. Hiding things. My controversial books would go in boxes in a closet, my bearskin rug under my bed in case the interviewer was big on animal rights. I'd put sheet music on the piano, although I hadn't played it in years. Your home reflects you. . . . But I didn't have to worry about that here. This room was cleaner than I could have made it myself, even if I had been able to get out of bed. Walls, linoleum, curtains, chairs: everything was pure, dazzling white. Sterile, institutional, dehumanizing, my sister would have said. I liked it. It meant business. At the hospice where she had wanted me to go (and which took mainly cancer patients, she had added, as if I were being offered a special favor), they had wallpaper with pretty flowers, and you could even bring some of your own furniture, but they wouldn't resuscitate you if you stopped breathing. Forget it, I told her; I'm not that stuck on my night table.

From *Ascent* 10.2 (1985): 2–18, lightly revised. Reprinted by permission of the author.

DRESS IN A WAY THAT IS BECOMING AND APPROPRIATE. I could hardly get more appropriate than a hospital gown. Over it I wore the pink-and-blue quilted bed jacket my sister had sent instead of coming. The blue was almost the shade of my eyes, and my rose quartz ring matched the pink. I pinned my circlet of pearls on the collar; no oversized Middle Eastern pendants or jangly earrings today.

REHEARSE ANSWERS TO THE QUESTIONS YOU ARE LIKELY TO BE ASKED. I had been at that for months, and last week I got Nick started, too. They would interview him separately later. It was like trying to become a corporate executive; your family got checked out as well. You had to have a "supportive family." My sister was useless, my parents were dead, but I had Nick. My supportive family. At a price.

The gold watch that had been my mother's said nine-thirty. Half an hour to go.

There were two of them, and they were ten minutes late. The psychiatric screeners, keepers of the gates of life. Dr. Reynolds and Dr. Garner. One tall and one short, one male and one female, one black and one white. Equal opportunity.

Dr. Garner was my age or maybe a few years older, thirty-five at the most. She had blond hair cut like a helmet, gold-rimmed glasses, and wore a severely tailored charcoal gray skirt and white blouse underneath her open white coat. Nothing like how I would be dressed on the job. I favored heavily embroidered ethnic clothes, and I'd always been proud that I could get ahead without "dressing for success." But now, someone who used words like "supportive" and dressed like a disciple of *The Woman's Dress for Success Book* would decide whether my personality made me fit to live.

Dr. Reynolds was fortyish and heavy-set, with a thick neck and broad shoulders, as though he might have played football in college. How did I feel about the prospect of having a heart transplant? he wanted to know.

I looked at the two of them steadily (MAKE EYE CONTACT) and said I had never wanted anything so much in my life.

Dr. Garner pushed her glasses up the bridge of her nose and asked why. I thought of the woman who had interviewed me for college fifteen years ago.

And why do you want to come to Wellesley, Yvonne?

I like everything I know about it. The curriculum, the campus, the high academic standards.

"It's my only chance," I said now.

Dr. Garner nodded. Was I afraid of the operation?

Somewhere there was bound to be a study showing that patients who were afraid of surgery had a lower survival rate.

"No," I said firmly.

"But you realize the surgery carries a mortality risk?" Dr. Reynolds asked slowly, leaning forward as if he were about to run with the ball.

I assured him that the operation was worth the risk. That I knew I couldn't last more than a few months without a transplant. That I had come here because it was the best transplant center in the world, and I had absolute confidence in the surgical team.

No, it doesn't bother me that there are no men at Wellesley, Dean Morrison. I like the idea of a women's college.

Once more with feeling. That sort of thing had never been my strong point—too hard to keep my voice from coming out sing-song. But this time, I'd practiced again and again.

Dr. Garner shifted her position. Now she was sitting with her legs crossed at the ankles and her hands clasped in her lap. Wasn't that how little girls sat in portraits a century ago? She wore elegant black calf shoes with stacked heels. I had not worn shoes in over a month.

Dr. Reynolds was looking at his hands. Then he glanced up at me again. It struck me that he seemed more hesitant than she did. Maybe he had doubts about what he was doing. So what?

I wondered if he knew what used to be said about blacks: let them earn equal rights.

How did I feel about my illness? he asked finally. It must have been quite a blow to have this happen to me so young and so suddenly.

At least these examiners, like the ones at my Ph.D. oral examination six years ago, were asking nothing I had not anticipated.

"Well, at first, I could hardly believe how sick I was. I knew how sick I felt, but I kept telling myself it would go away, like mono or the flu. And then. . . ." I let my voice trail off.

"Yes?" prompted Dr. Reynolds, as sympathetically as a friend.

As sympathetically as a friend. These days, kindness affected me like music: immediately, automatically, even when I knew the kindness was professional and purposeful. Why couldn't someone invent a vaccine for it? Already I could feel myself wanting to yield, to say, Oh, Dr. Reynolds, I am so scared. Please let me live. Aren't you my friend? I'll say anything you want. Do anything you want. And I'll be so grateful.

My eyes stung. Steady on. The dentist I had gone to during my year in London used to say that, and it always made me furious. Who was he to tell me how to feel? No one likes to be told to calm down. . . . Focus on something neutral. Dr. Reynolds's tie. It was red with a design of little black puppies. Was it a present from one of his children? It didn't look like something an adult would have chosen. It looked silly. But this man would decide whether my personality made me fit to live.

"For a while, I was bitter and resentful, I have to admit," I said carefully. "And I was scared. Why did this have to happen to me? I kept wondering, as if I were the world's first person ever to become critically ill. That stage lasted about two weeks." (Psychiatrists liked stages, didn't they?) "But then. . . ."

"Yes?" said Dr. Garner. They were both nodding now—in agreement? Approval? Were they lapping it up like a pair of sleek cats? Or were they just telling me to continue?

What else could I do, anyway?

"Well, resentment never accomplished anything, did it?" I said.

As if it were supposed to. And anyway, it did. I never would have lost eleven pounds in junior high school if I hadn't resented how popular Kathy McKinley was.

"So, after a while, something in me just got tired of using up my energy that way and started wanting to use it to combat my illness instead."

At least, I hadn't said "use my energy constructively."

"And that made all the difference," I continued. Getting my tone right was the hard part here. The trick was to make the platitudes sound both reasonable and as if I'd originated them. I plowed on through the whole growth-through-adversity speech. The interviewers looked impressed. Of course, they also looked healthy enough to fall for it, and I had all my hesitations and facial expressions down pat. Good thing I'd been so active in college dramatics. It was enough to vindicate that Wellesley dean who was always trumpeting the value of extra-curricular activities.

What time was it? No way I could find out without being obvious. My hands were under the blanket. They were cold. They were always cold now. My heart was too weak to keep them warm. *How long are you going to keep this up, for Christ's sake? I'm tired. I'm deathly ill, remember? Have a heart. Have mine; let's trade.*

Dr. Garner was asking whether I was afraid of death. Easy to guess the right answer. Didn't every healthy person with at least forty years of life ahead know that a truly emotionally mature individual had worked through the fear of death?

Of course, there were no right or wrong answers. The answers that could condemn me to death weren't wrong answers.

Did I have any questions?

I had prepared some innocuous ones just in case.

Now the interviewers were rising to leave. Would my fiance be able to talk with them next Thursday at four?

"Yes, he will. I'll tell him. He'll be there."

* * * * *

"They want to interview you Thursday at four," I said when Nick came into my room two days later.

He kicked the door shut behind him. "I've got a choice?"

"Nick—"

"Yeah, okay." He sat down in the white plastic chair facing me, slouched forward, and started cracking his knuckles—one of his more irritating habits, I had recently decided.

"*American Historical Quarterly* turned down my paper," he said, glaring at the floor. "Did you see that pretentious Hitchens crap they published in October? Yes, if you're at Cornell. No, if you're at Tomlinson State College. What a coincidence. Almost as big a coincidence as that my mother and my father both got married on the same day. Ever occur to you that 'editor' rhymes with 'predator'?"

He transferred the glare to me as if I were one of those creatures myself. His face seemed designed for ineffectual glares. It was tired and heavy-featured, with black hair spilling across his forehead, and chronically red, puffy, irritable-looking eyes. Hardly the most prepossessing supportive family I could have chosen. If I'd had a choice.

I thought, I have got to be the world's only heart-transplant candidate who's expected to get excited about someone's rejected articles. Then again, maybe not. Who knew what went on in the other supportive families?

"You know that's the third place I sent it to? No point in my trying anywhere else now. Might as well wait until—" He cracked another knuckle. "Might as well wait."

I nodded. I knew what he had been about to say. I thought about our conversation in December, the agreement we had made.

* * * * *

I had telephoned him on Friday evening a few weeks before Christmas. It had taken me all afternoon to get up my strength.

"Nick? It's Yvonne."

I had still been at home then, propped up in bed on three pillows. I could no longer breathe lying flat. But it had been one of my better days. I could manage a long phone call.

"Yvonne? Not sure I ought to be talking to you." Over the telephone, Nick's voice had sounded harsher and duller than I'd remembered. "Think I forgot how you ditched me at the convention so you could go off with some Harvard hotshots?"

I'd had an image of Nick in his cracked old leather jacket and black chinos (he didn't dress for success, either), his face bleak and rigid as I hastily ended our conversation when the Harvard people appeared in the hotel lobby. Of course, he hadn't forgotten. But I had. I hadn't anticipated this.

"Nick, I had been corresponding with Peter for months. I explained it to you later, remember?" The following morning at the convention, I had also told Nick about the secret manuscript I was planning to spring upon the world as soon as I was done with the finishing touches. I had loved having a secret manuscript. It was so different from the way other people worked, and it had felt exquisitely private, as I supposed having a clandestine lover might feel. But, of course, Nick had accused me of picking him to hear the secret because I figured he didn't count.

"Yeah, so what's this, your winter slumming trip?" I could hear him breathing roughly into the phone. "You got the right place. Just found out I won't get tenure unless I have what they call a 'vastly improved publication record' next year. Know when my chairman's last publication was? Eight years ago. Well, what are you up to? Tell me how the other half lives."

I had told him.

"Jesus." There'd been a long pause. "Is it hard to get a transplant?"

"Harder than getting tenure. It's not just medical, anyway. It's fantastically expensive, which I can just about manage, and they have to approve of your personality and think you're stable enough. And you've got to have a family. They have some theory that what they call a supportive family is supposed to help you get through all this, so if you haven't got one, the hell with you."

"You're kidding."

"No. You've got to have a family."

"Wages of singleness is death," Nick had said, and I'd told him I had been oversimplifying. They didn't actually require relatives as long as you could prove someone cared about you enough. They had even given a transplant to a lesbian with a long-term, live-in lover, which must have made them feel very liberal.

"You're nobody till somebody loves you," Nick had said. "Yeah, very liberal. How's your family?"

"Dead. Except my sister, who believes in death with dignity. For me. She refused to help me get a transplant."

"Even though you want one?"

"That's right."

"Jesus."

My right had hand become almost numb by this point. The fingertips were startlingly blue. I'd been gripping the receiver like the edge of a raft.

"Jesus can't help me," I had said. "But you can."

"What could I do? I can't be your family."

"No, but you could fake it."

He had been bewildered. Intrigued. But most of all—I could tell—he had been afraid. Afraid of being trapped. He had his own problems; hadn't he just been telling me? And I knew perfectly well how he resented me for having tenure at UCLA and being well-known in our field.

But he was practically the only unattached male friend I had, even if we hadn't seen each other much since graduate school, where I'd found his lack of the usual academic veneer refreshing. And he wouldn't actually have to marry me or live with me, I had assured him. He'd just have to say he would. Let them interview him. Come to visit me three times a week at the Center, so they would know he really cared. Lucky he lived so nearby.

"It's not so nearby. It's an hour away."

"I'll give you anything you want in return. Anything. My BMW, all my family jewelry—"

"Christ! Look, I'd like to help you, even with the crummy way you treated me. I just can't. Don't have that kind of time now, not if I want any chance to keep my lousy job. There's got to be someone else you could get."

"There isn't." He hadn't asked why. Probably he could guess that I'd been too busy being a success to get close to anyone, just as he'd been too busy resenting not being one. One thing I had to say for Nick: at least he didn't think that having no loved ones in your life was a personal defect.

"Nick, without the transplant, I'm going to—*die,* can't you see?" My voice had almost broken, and I hadn't even tried to control it. "Think it over. Please. There must be something I can give you that would make up for what I'm asking."

The next morning Nick had called me back. "Well, I thought of something." His voice had been heavy, gritty, dragging. I'd had an image of a car being pushed uphill. "Pretty crummy, though. You'll hate it. Maybe you can guess already."

* * * * *

That had been two months ago, and now, sitting at my bedside in the white room, Nick was thinking about it again. I could tell by his expression, at once defiant and uncomfortable. He was thinking about the manuscript I'd described at the convention, the manuscript no one else knew about. No one else would ever know about it now, until it appeared under Nick's name with enough revisions to make it look as though it could be his. It would be his, if I got the transplant. Your book or your life. I had chosen my life.

"You could have said no," Nick said suddenly. "At least I gave you a choice. Would I be less of a louse if I'd been like your sister and left you to die?"

I closed my eyes. "Nick, I don't know and I don't care. It's beside the point, anyway. We made a deal." No point in telling him how horribly I minded it.

"I did try to come yesterday." Nick's voice was eerily disembodied in the dark. "They wouldn't let me in. They said you had a bad night and needed to rest."

"Yes." He didn't ask for details. I didn't give them.

"Yeah, I know you think I'm a crumb to want to get ahead off your book," Nick persisted, like a buzzing insect. "I tried it the other way. You teach at a state college, you need something special to get published anywhere decent. Yvonne?"

"What?"

"Don't you think they should have taken my paper?"

He was cracking his knuckles again. It sounded like popping corn. I opened my eyes. The air in the room seemed heavy and close, as though the window had not been opened in days.

"Nick, this is probably going to astonish you, but that isn't the main question on my mind right now." I looked at him. A muscle twitched under his left eye. I looked away. "We've been all through this sort of thing, anyhow. Your papers are good enough to be in good journals, and you're probably right about why they get turned down." I wasn't lying. But I hoped he wouldn't ask me exactly how I thought his work compared with mine.

"Will you bring me more mysteries next time?" I said.

Nick nodded. I began giving him titles to look for and some to avoid. He pulled a brown imitation-leather-covered notebook out of his back pocket and started writing with his bumpy fingers. The knuckles were misshapen and enlarged, and his fingernails were dirty. "Clean fingernails are a mark of a lady," my mother used to say, "but whether you want to be a lady is another matter."

I thought about the time Steffi Gibson in graduate school had told Nick sweetly that in addition to being offensive, cracking his knuckles would probably give him arthritis in later life. Nick had stared, then walked over to her, cracked three knuckles right in her cool Ivy League face, and slammed out of the room. "He's so crude," Steffi had said. "So what?" I had said.

The following year Steffi flunked out of the program. It was the last time I could remember Nick being really happy about anything.

Now he was finishing up my list and muttering to himself. "Anyway," he said loudly, abruptly, when I was running out of names, "I'd never have time to get anything written myself this term. Not when I've got to drive up here to see you three times a week."

* * * * *

Two days later, Nick came back with four detective novels and a Venus flytrap.

"All homey little murders, none of that spy stuff, and I checked the flaps to see that there's nothing about illness," he said, handing me the books.

"Thank you." I had read one of the Christies, and Nick had forgotten how I disliked Sayers for her cloying fascination with the British aristocracy. The other two were titles I had requested.

I had not requested a Venus flytrap. Why did he bring it? I asked.

"Better than flowers. More unusual. Impress the staff."

"Impress them how? Are they supposed to think it's a tender symbol of a beautiful relationship?" I looked at the evil little spines and began to laugh. "Really, Nick, a Venus flytrap!"

His face tightened. "Yeah, well, if you want to know, I went to three places looking for something special," he said slowly. "You don't like it? I'll take it back."

"It's okay," I said. "Are you also going to provide the flies?"

"Doesn't need them." Nick gave me a quick glance, then grinned awkwardly, as if he were out of practice. "Bring you a cactus with lots of spikes next time," he said and sat down with a small thud, slouching and rubbing his eyes with the back of his hand. "I saw one of your rivals in the corridor," he added, cracking a knuckle.

One of my rivals. My room was in a nursing home whose inmates were all candidates for transplants at the Center, but I seldom saw or heard any of the others. It was almost like living here alone. I felt a surge of curiosity as intense as hunger.

"Well?" I said.

"Man in a wheelchair, about fifty, a little overweight. Wore glasses and, you'll be happy to hear, no wedding ring. Maybe he's got no supportive family. Score one for you."

"Lots of married men that age don't wear wedding rings," I said, but I hoped Nick was right. It was like the hope I felt whenever I heard an ambulance siren: maybe that's a heart for me. A common reaction in people awaiting transplants, I had once read in a news magazine, and then, a few weeks later, someone had written in to say heart transplants should be discontinued because waiting for them was so bad for people's character.

"I hate healthy people," I said.

"I know," said Nick, as though he weren't included.

I told him about the article and the letter, and he pulled a bruised apple out of his jacket pocket and bit into it noisily. "Know what that reminds me of?" he said, his mouth full. "Feature I saw in the Tomlinson local paper about this kid who has leukemia and needs blood. It was all about how sweet and patient she was—like if she'd acted like a crabby bitch because she didn't get off on being sick all the time, she wouldn't deserve to have people donate."

Loud crunching and sucking noises were accompanying these remarks. I kept my eyes on my blanket and wished I could avert my ears as well. I had always admired Nick for not being concerned enough about social niceties to bother with polite eating habits, but I preferred to admire this without actually watching him eat. It occurred to me, though, not for the first time, that much as I hated Nick for what he was making me do, I was glad for his visits. At least with Nick, I didn't have to act like the constant epitome of mental hygiene, as if I'd washed my mind out with germicidal soap. With the staff, on the other hand, even orderlies and cleaning women, I kept myself eternally pleasant and cheerful. Nick disliked pleasantness and cheer. I wondered what he did for fun.

I pushed myself up further against the pillows and asked him.

He cracked two knuckles simultaneously. "I like to sleep."

"What?"

"You heard. I can sleep ten, twelve hours a day. Don't have much time for it now. When you sleep, you could be anyone. I have good dreams, better than being awake." He rubbed his puffy eyes longingly and glanced at his watch as if it were nearly bedtime. It was five-fifteen.

For a moment I felt sad. Nick had had a lot of vitality once. But then, so had I.

"Well, don't come out with that at your interview," I said. "Stick to crossword puzzles." I had chosen crossword puzzles as the perfect hobby for an invalid's fiance. He could do them at my bedside. I could participate. Interruptions wouldn't matter.

It also wouldn't matter that Nick in fact hated crossword puzzles and all intellectual games. If I'm thinking that hard, I want to learn something, he had told me.

"For once, give me credit for half a brain, will you?" Nick got up and tapped the top mystery on the night table. *Death Comes As The End.* "Read this one first. It looks good," he said, putting on the beat-up leather jacket I had warned him not to wear to his interview.

"Wait," I said urgently. "We have to go over the stuff for your interview again."

"We've done it a million times already. I know my lines. Don't worry; I'm not going to screw up, for Christ's sake." He turned to leave. "I've got a lot at stake, too, remember?"

* * * * *

I tried to read *Death Comes As The End,* but it annoyed me. The story was set in ancient Egypt, and I preferred mysteries where the murderer was the sort of person I could have known. Ancient Egypt was too remote and peculiar. But even my own field of history, the nineteenth-century American West, seemed remote and peculiar now. My world had shrunk to my heart and this room. Just the sort of thing invalids were always getting criticized for, but I couldn't see why. When I had no idea whether I would be alive next fall, was I supposed to be able to get excited about ante-bellum patterns of westward migration? My department had sent me a new book on the subject, with a note signed by everyone on the faculty. I knew the author slightly. He taught at Yale, and I'd had dinner with him twice at conventions. I liked him. Nick didn't. Nick resented everyone at Yale. But until I had gotten this illness, I had not resented anyone in all my adult life. No reason to. I had been the favored one. Yes, I'd been smug, which was maybe why I had no close friends, but I had never expected this to be a capital offense.

I put the mystery aside and opened the book from my colleagues. I was surprised to discover I could still get drawn into it. But when I came upon some flattering references to the work of Sibley, it was a few moments before I realized the author was talking about me.

* * * * *

The next two days were bad days. There was pain, I couldn't eat, and I slept a lot. I kept dreaming about wandering, thirsty and lost, alone in the Mojave desert. When I reached an oasis, there was a long line of people, like the queues I had seen in England, with everyone patiently waiting for a turn. But when it came to my turn, I was refused water. "You're too unsocial, too odd," I was told. "You weren't even in a sorority in college." "My college didn't have sororities!" I screamed silently, and woke up gasping and sweating.

God, do you have a dumb unconscious, I said to myself when I calmed down. A maladjusted and unwholesome one, too, no doubt. Good thing they couldn't monitor my dreams.

I thought about Nick, with his good dreams. He didn't deserve them.

* * * * *

On the morning of Nick's interview, I woke up refreshed and alert, but uneasy. Nick would remember his lines, I was sure, but he'd turned surlier than usual at some of my other instructions: sit up straight, speak in complete sentences, don't say "yeah" all the time, don't crack your knuckles. Don't be a slob, polish up your image, it all came down to, and I recalled how outraged he had been when his dissertation supervisor made similar suggestions when Nick was on the job market. Nick's moral code permitted plagiarism, but not the deliberate upgrading of his personal style. It had taken me fifteen minutes to persuade him to go along with me on this, and I doubted he'd be much good at it, anyway.

At five-thirty, Nick appeared in my room, wearing wool pants and a sports jacket, as I had insisted. The pants were too blue. The jacket was too tight. Would it matter? Who knew? But fraternities rejected people for less, much less.

"Well?" I demanded as soon as he closed the door.

Nick rubbed his eyes for a long time. He didn't sit down. "I did okay."

"What did they ask?"

"About what you expected."

"Well, sit down and tell me all about it." I gestured toward the white chair, but he just stared at it as though wondering what it was for. He hadn't looked at me once, I realized. This in itself wasn't surprising—we were hardly enough enamored of each other to spend time gazing into each other's eyes—but now he seemed almost to be avoiding me. His glance shifted to the Venus flytrap, then to the window, which faced north, away from the sun.

"Look, I—got to get home. I'm tired. I'll be back in a couple of days." He turned to leave, cracking all his knuckles at once with a sound like a little explosion. From the back he looked worse. The jacket gaped at the slit, making an inverted "V."

"Nick—is anything wrong?"

"No, I did fine. I told you. I'm just tired."

Before I could say anything else, he was gone.

Nothing had gone wrong, I kept telling myself; nothing could have gone wrong. Nick wouldn't lie about having done well. And he certainly wouldn't be having second thoughts at this point, not when I was counting on him. Not when he was counting on me. I've got a lot at stake, too, remember? he had said.

But my mind would not stop. What if something had changed? What if . . . he had been told he wouldn't get tenure in any case? What if he'd decided my book couldn't help him anymore? What if he'd decided no one would believe it was his?

Stop being ridiculous; he would have said something. Steady on. But when I tried to telephone Nick in the evening, there was no answer.

* * * * *

For three days there was no answer. On the morning of the fourth day, Dr. Reynolds came into my room. He was smiling.

"Good morning. I have good news for you."

I had passed. Like the director of admissions at Wellesley, the director of graduate studies at Berkeley, and the chairman of the history department at UCLA, Dr. Reynolds was pleased to be able to tell me that I had been weighed in the balance and found not wanting. My application had been approved. I was in.

"How long—do you think I'll have to wait a long time for the operation?"

Hard to say. But probably not a terribly long time. My blood and tissue typing had shown that I would not be difficult to match. That was one reason I had been accepted. Aside from my psychological stability and supportive family situation, of course.

I smiled. I kept on smiling. And I thanked him over and over.

But there was still no sign of my supportive family situation that afternoon. No answer when I phoned. Where was Nick?

* * * * *

"Where were you?" I asked when Nick walked into my room the following afternoon as if he had never stayed away.

He grunted, sat down in the white chair, and gazed blisteringly at the floor. Even when I told him we had passed the final test, his expression did not change.

"Well, really, Nick, you'll be getting what you want, too, you know. You ought to be happy. . . ."

My voice trailed away as Nick raised his eyes and gave me a look of the most concentrated hostility I had ever seen. He *hates* me, I thought, frantically scanning my memory for all the times when, in spite of everything, we'd had a kind of momentary rapport.

"I don't want your lousy book," he said.

"*What*?" I had imagined this possibility so often during the past few days that it seemed almost as if I were still doing it. Don't be ridiculous, Yvonne; Nick would never pull out. He's got a lot at stake, too, remember. Remember? My face was growing hotter by the second, and in a moment. . . .

"Christ! Take it easy. Jesus." Nick's voice sounded drained, disgusted, and who was he to tell me to take it easy, especially now? "Christ, I didn't say I wouldn't keep on with the supportive family crap. I'll do it. You can just keep your lousy book, like I said."

"What?" I was still faintly panicky. Disoriented.

"I said—"

"I heard what you said. Have you given up on getting tenure? Did you decide you want something else from me instead?"

"Nah."

"Then what happened?"

"I changed my mind."

"Why?"

He cracked several knuckles. "I just did. Look, do we have to talk about it?"

"I want to talk about it."

"You want to." Nick got up and started pacing the floor with tense, awkward movements. "You want to, so of course we have to. Okay, it was because of the shrinks."

"What?"

He was still pacing, not looking at me. "They made me want to puke," he muttered in a tone suggesting I had the same effect. "Especially her. She was so serene, just so goddamn sure of her right to make you bargain for your life by being the kind of person she wanted. I couldn't stand being in the same room with her. Never felt so superior to anyone, except I obviously wasn't; you don't have to tell me about it." He shot me another inflamed look. "So anyway, you don't have to bargain with me anymore."

I gaped at him. He looked about the same. (Puffy-eyed, belligerent, unappealing.) What had I expected?

I said the first thing that came into my mind. "But you knew all along you were making me bargain for my life."

He sat down heavily. "You can know something all along, but it's different when you see it."

It's different when you see it. Nick had finally applied his sense of outrage to somebody's plight besides his own. I opened my mouth to speak, but what came out were small puffs of laughter, over and over with all the breath I could manage, as if I were on a roller coaster or being tickled.

"What the hell's so funny?" Nick's voice took a moment to penetrate.

"It's not funny." I stopped laughing and caught my breath. "I just think everything may turn out all right, after all."

"Sure," said Nick, "for you."

"But it was your decision."

"Christ, don't you know anything?" He began cracking his knuckles again, and maybe I only imagined that the sound was sharper than before. "I spent the whole goddamn weekend trying to make myself take your book, or maybe just drop out of the whole thing. Just because I couldn't do it doesn't mean I didn't want to, for Christ's sake!"

"You actually considered leaving me to die."

"I couldn't possibly do it, so calm down." He rubbed his eyes, which were redder than usual. "Jesus, I didn't even sleep much. Drove over half the state. . . ."

Heaven help half the state. When Nick was upset in graduate school, I suddenly remembered, he used to go off for days at a time, driving over backroads in his ancient Mustang, stopping only when he got worn out, sleeping in his car. He drove viciously but skillfully, like a teenage greaser who practically lived in his hotrod, and he returned from these journeys looking dissolute and exhausted, as if he'd been on a week-long bender.

"I see," I said. "Well, this is very . . . nice of you."

"Nice?" Nick got up so roughly and abruptly that he nearly knocked over the chair. "Jesus. I'm not nice. And I wouldn't pick you to be nice to. You treat me like dirt, you know that? Do this, do that, sit the way I tell you, talk the way I say. . . . You're the last person—"

I would ever want to be nice to, I finished in my mind. I closed my eyes and could see Nick driving furiously along the bumpiest road he could find, snarling at anyone and anything that got in his way, stuffing himself with fistfuls of French fries from the nearest McDonald's, and finally falling asleep, exhausted by the discovery that the pull to do right could be as hard to resist as the pull to do wrong, and you could feel just as terrible when you felt yourself giving in.

"Yes," I said, opening my eyes. "I think maybe I understand now. I just don't know what to say. I could say I'm grateful, only I can't stand sick people being humble and grateful, like the kids on those awful Easter Seal posters. But why don't you go get some sleep, Nick? Have some good dreams."

Nick nodded. He didn't say anything. Didn't smile. Didn't even look at me. But his face seemed to relax ever so slightly, as if maybe he hated me a tiny bit less, or maybe it was just a trick of the light.

THE CAST-AWAY

WILLIAM COWPER

Obscurest night involved the sky,
The Atlantic billows roar'd;
When such a destined wretch as I,
Wash'd headlong from on board,
Of friends, of hope, of all bereft,
His floating home for ever left.

No braver chief could Albion boast
Than he with whom he went,
Nor ever ship left Albion's coast
With warmer wishes sent.
He loved them both, but both in vain,
Nor him beheld, nor her again.

Not long beneath the whelming brine,
Expert to swim, he lay;
Nor soon he felt his strength decline,
Or courage die away;
But waged with death a lasting strife,
Supported by despair of life.

He shouted; nor his friends had fail'd
To check the vessel's course,
But so the furious blast prevail'd,
That, pitiless perforce,
They left their outcast mate behind,
And scudded still before the wind.

Cowper wrote "The Cast-Away" in March 1799; it was published posthumously in 1803. This edition is from *The Norton Anthology of English Literature,* M. H. Abrams, general editor. 5th ed. (New York: Norton, 1986).

Some succour yet they could afford;
And, such as storms allow,
The cask, the coop, the floated cord,
Delay'd not to bestow:
But he (they knew) nor ship nor shore,
Whate'er they gave, should visit more.

Nor, cruel as it seem'd, could he
Their haste himself condemn,
Aware that flight, in such a sea,
Alone could rescue them:
Yet bitter felt it still, to die
Deserted, and his friends so nigh.

He long survives who lives an hour
In ocean, self-upheld:
And so long he, with unspent power,
His destiny repell'd:
And ever, as the minutes flew,
Entreated help, or cried—"Adieu!"

At length, his transient respite past,
His comrades, who before
Had heard his voice in every blast,
Could catch the sound no more:
For then, by toil subdued, he drank
The stifling wave, and then he sank.

No Poet wept him: but the page

That tells his name, his worth, his age,
Is wet with Anson's tear:
And tears by bards or heroes shed,
Alike immortalize the dead.

I therefore purpose not, or dream,
Descanting on his fate,
To give the melancholy theme
A more enduring date:
But misery still delights to trace
Its semblance in another's case.

No voice divine the storm allay'd,
No light propitious shone;
When snatch'd from all effectual aid,
We perish'd, each alone:
But I beneath a rougher sea,
And whelm'd in deeper gulfs than he.

DEJECTION: AN ODE

SAMUEL TAYLOR COLERIDGE

Late, late yestren I saw the new Moon,
With the old Moon in her arms;
And I fear, I fear, my Master dear!
We shall have a deadly storm.

–*Ballad of Sir Patrick Spence*

I

Well! If the Bard was weather-wise, who made
The grand old ballad of Sir Patrick Spence,
This night, so tranquil now, will not go hence
Unroused by winds, that ply a busier trade
Than those which mould yon cloud in lazy flakes,
Or the dull sobbing draft, that moans and rakes
Upon the strings of this Aeolian lute,
Which better far were mute.
For lo! the New-moon winter-bright!
And overspread with phantom light,
(With swimming phantom light o'erspread
But rimmed and circled by a silver thread)
I see the old Moon in her lap, foretelling
The coming-on of rain and squally blast.
And oh! that even now the gust were swelling,
And the slant night-shower driving loud and fast!
Those sounds which oft have raised me, whilst they awed,
And sent my soul abroad,
Might now perhaps their wonted impulse give,
Might startle this dull pain, and make it move and live!

"Dejection: An Ode" was written on April 4, 1802, and is reprinted here from *Selected Poetry and Prose*, by Samuel Taylor Coleridge, edited by Elisabeth Schneider (New York: Rinehart, 1951).

II

A grief without a pang, void, dark, and drear,
 A stifled, drowsy, unimpassioned grief,
 Which finds no natural outlet, no relief,
  In word, or sigh, or tear—
O Lady! in this wan and heartless mood,
To other thoughts by yonder throstle woo'd,
 All this long eve, so balmy and serene,
Have I been gazing on the western sky,
 And its peculiar tint of yellow green.
And still I gaze—and with how blank an eye!
And those thin clouds above, in flakes and bars,
That give away their motion to the stars;
Those stars, that glide behind them or between,
Now sparkling, now bedded, but always seen:
Yon crescent Moon, as fixed as if it grew
In its own cloudless, starless lake of blue;
I see them all so excellently fair,
I see, not feel, how beautiful they are!

III

  My genial spirits fail;
  And what can these avail
To lift the smothering weight from off my breast?
  It were a vain endeavour,
  Though I should gaze for ever
On that green light that lingers in the west:
I may not hope from outward forms to win
The passion and the life, whose fountains are within.

IV

Oh Lady! we receive but what we give,
And in our life alone does Nature live:
Ours is her wedding garment, ours her shroud!
 And would we aught behold, of higher worth,
Than that inanimate cold world allowed
To the poor loveless ever-anxious crowd,
 Ah! from the soul itself must issue forth
A light, a glory, a fair luminous cloud
  Enveloping the Earth—
And from the soul itself must there be sent
 A sweet and potent voice, of its own birth,
Of all sweet sounds the life and element!

V

O pure of heart! thou need'st not ask of me
What this strong music in the soul may be!
What, and wherein it doth exist,
This light, this glory, this fair luminous mist,
This beautiful and beauty-making power.
  Joy, virtuous Lady! Joy that ne'er was given,
Save to the pure, and in their purest hour,
Life, and Life's effluence, cloud at once and shower,
Joy, Lady! is the spirit and the power,
Which wedding Nature to us gives in dower
  A new Earth and new Heaven,
Undreamt of by the sensual and the proud—
Joy is the sweet voice, Joy the luminous cloud—
    We in ourselves rejoice!
And thence flows all that charms or ear or sight,
  All melodies the echoes of that voice,
All colours a suffusion from that light.

VI

There was a time when, though my path was rough,
  This joy within me dallied with distress,
And all misfortunes were but as the stuff
  Whence Fancy made me dreams of happiness:
For hope grew round me, like the twining vine,
And fruits, and foliage, not my own, seemed mine.
But now afflictions bow me down to earth:
Nor care I that they rob me of my mirth;
    But oh! each visitation
Suspends what nature gave me at my birth,
  My shaping spirit of Imagination.
For not to think of what I needs must feel,
  But to be still and patient, all I can;
And haply by abstruse research to steal
  From my own nature all the natural man—
  This was my sole resource, my only plan:
till that which suits a part infects the whole,
And now is almost grown the habit of my soul.

VII

Hence, viper thoughts, that coil around my mind,
Reality's dark dream!
I turn from you, and listen to the wind,
Which long has raved unnoticed. What a scream
Of agony by torture lengthened out
That lute sent forth! Thou Wind, that rav'st without
Bare crag, or mountain-tairn, or blasted tree,
Or pine-grove whither woodman never clomb,
Or lonely house, long held the witches' home,
Methinks were fitter instruments for thee,
Mad Lutanist! who in this month of showers,
Of dark-brown gardens, and of peeping flowers,
Mak'st Devils' yule, with worse than wintry song,
The blossoms, buds, and timorous leaves among.
Thou actor, perfect in all tragic sounds!
Thou mighty Poet, e'en to frenzy bold!
What tell'st thou now about?
'Tis of the rushing of an host in rout,
With groans, of trampled men, with smarting wounds—
At once they groan with pain, and shudder with the cold!
But hush! there is a pause of deepest silence!
And all that noise, as of a rushing crowd,
With groans, and tremulous shudderings—all is over—
It tells another tale, with sounds less deep and loud!
A tale of less affright,
And tempered with delight,
As Otway's self had framed the tender lay,—
'Tis of a little child
Upon a lonesome wild,
Not far from home, but she hath lost her way:
And now moans low in bitter grief and fear,
And now screams loud, and hopes to make her mother hear.

VIII

'Tis midnight, but small thoughts have I of sleep:
Full seldom may my friend such vigils keep!
Visit her, gentle Sleep! with wings of healing,
  And may this storm be but a mountain-birth,
May all the stars hang bright above her dwelling,
  Silent as thought they watched the sleeping Earth!
    With light heart may she rise,
    Gay fancy, cheerful eyes,
Joy lift her spirit, joy attune her voice;
To her may all things live, from pole to pole,
Their life the eddying of her living soul!
  O simple spirit, guided from above,
Dear lady! friend devoutest of my choice,
Thus mayest thou ever, evermore rejoice.

DOCTORS

ANNE SEXTON

They work with herbs
and penicillin.
They work with gentleness
and the scalpel.
They dig out the cancer,
close an incision
and say a prayer
to the poverty of the skin.
They are not Gods
though they would like to be;
they are only a human
trying to fix up a human.
Many humans die.
They die like the tender,
palpitating berries
in November.
But all along the doctors remember:
First do no harm.
They would kiss if it would heal.
It would not heal.

If the doctors cure
then the sun sees it.
If the doctors kill
then the earth hides it.
The doctors should fear arrogance
more than cardiac arrest.

If they are too proud,
and some are,
then they leave home on horseback
but God returns them on foot.

THE WALL

ANNE SEXTON

Nature is full of teeth
that come in one by one, then
decay,
fall out.
In nature nothing is stable,
all is change, bears, dogs, peas, the willow,
all disappear. Only to be reborn.
Rocks crumble, make new forms,
oceans move the continents,
mountains rise up and down like ghosts
yet all is natural, all is change.

As I write this sentence
about one hundred and four generations
since Christ, nothing has changed
except knowledge, the test tube.
Man still falls into the dirt
and is covered.
As I write this sentence one thousand are going
and one thousand are coming.
It is like the well that never dries up.
It is like the sea which is the kitchen of God.

We are all earthworms,
digging into our wrinkles.
We live beneath the ground
and if Christ should come in the form of a plow
and dig a furrow and push us up into the day
we earthworms would be blinded by the sudden light
and writhe in our distress.
As I write this sentence I too writhe.

For all you who are going,
and there are many who are climbing their pain,
many who will be painted out with a black ink
suddenly and before it is time,
for those many I say,
awkwardly, clumsily,
take off your life like trousers,
your shoes, your underwear,
then take off your flesh,
unpick the lock of your bones.
In other words
take off the wall
that separates you from God.

THE POET OF IGNORANCE

ANNE SEXTON

Perhaps the earth is floating,
I do not know.
Perhaps the stars are little paper cutups
made by some giant scissors,
I do not know.
Perhaps the moon is a frozen tear,
I do not know.
Perhaps God is only a deep voice
heard by the deaf,
I do not know.

Perhaps I am no one.
True, I have a body
and I cannot escape from it.
I would like to fly out of my head,
but that is out of the question.
It is written on the tablet of destiny
that I am stuck here in this human form.
That being the case
I would like to call attention to my problem.

There is an animal inside me,
clutching fast to my heart.

The doctors of Boston
have thrown up their hands.
They have tried scalpels,
needles, poison gasses and the like.
The crab remains.
It is a great weight.
I try to forget it, go about my business,
cook the broccoli, open and shut books,
brush my teeth and tie my shoes.
I have tried prayer
but as I pray the crab grips harder
and the pain enlarges.

I had a dream once,
perhaps it was a dream,
that the crab was my ignorance of God.
But who am I to believe in dreams?

CLEANING
Early February 2004

DARCY WAKEFIELD

Before I got ALS, I didn't know what it was. Now, after several months of research, I know more about it than I'd like to know. I know, for example, that ALS is an orphan disease. According to Hope Happens, an organization dedicated to funding research for ALS and other neurological diseases, an orphan disease is any disease that affects fewer than 200,000 people in the United States at any given time. Their Web site also claims that there are 6,000 orphan diseases that affect 25 million Americans, and that pharmaceutical companies and biotechs rarely pursue treatment of these diseases because so few people have them.[1]

In the course of my research, I've also learned that ALS has been around for a while. Indeed, the first mention of ALS was in the 1830s, in French and British medical literature, and in 1874, a French physician, Jean-Martin Charcot, established the clinical and pathological characteristics of ALS and gave it its name. Rumor has it that he once hired a housemaid with ALS so that he could study her.[2]

I've thought often of this maid ever since I read about her. Did she know that she had ALS and that her employer was studying her? I like to think that she did, and that she didn't think too highly of Charcot for not being straight with her. In my fantasy, I see her spitting in Charcot's soup and taking cleaning shortcuts, like not sweeping under beds. She kept working for him, I decided, because she knew he was a brilliant doctor, and she hoped, desperately, that what he learned from her would benefit countless others, and maybe even cure the disease.

I think of Charcot's maid at the oddest times, such as today, as I do laundry at Steve's Colorado home. This home of his, this lovely bungalow, is on the market; in a little over a week, movers will pack up pretty much everything in this house and drive it across the country, to Maine, to our new home. But before that happens, we will have clean laundry.

This is my only household chore. It's self-imposed, too. Other than doing the laundry, there is nothing else for me to do here to be helpful. Steve's house needs very little cleaning; twice a month, his two cleaning ladies come in, and Steve returns home to a shiny teapot and spotless counters. So I leave the cleaning to them, and tackle the laundry, wondering, all the while, how it will be when we move in together in a few weeks, sans cleaning ladies.

Before Steve, I worked full-time as a teacher. When I dated, it was usually in or near my own income bracket, and I always figured that if I was ever in a long-term relationship, we'd find a way to divvy up the household tasks. Sometimes I fantasized about being a stay-at-home mom, raising a bunch of kids while canning, cooking, and cleaning, but as I approached thirty-four, I became increasingly convinced that I was destined to be a single, working parent.

But I'm with Steve now, and he and I weren't in the same income bracket before I stopped working; he is a doctor and I was a teacher. Now the wage gap between us is wider than the Atlantic. And I'm staying home, all right, but I struggle to figure out how I can contribute, how I will find equal footing in a relationship I am entering at a financial disadvantage. Mind you, this is my issue—it doesn't seem to keep Steve up at night—but if I want my contribution to our relationship, in lieu of money, to be household management, and in particular, cleaning, how will I ever do it? I'm not as agile as I used to be, and as it is, cleaning my three-room, first floor apartment takes planning and time. How will I clean a whole house by myself?

Perhaps that is why I'm so fixated on the rumor about Charcot: I want to have my own ALS cleaning lady. I'd like one my age because it would be so nice to have someone female and young to talk with about this ALS stuff, someone who would know where I'm coming from. That's one of the problems, I'm finding, with having an orphan disease: there aren't a lot of you.

So I recently posted a query on an ALS chat line, seeking other young women with ALS. One woman, also in her thirties, responded. She lives in Florida, has children, and used to be physically active. I've received two e-mails from her, and both times, it was like finding a twin I'd been separated from since birth. It's hard being around able-bodied people all the time, people who don't have terminal illnesses. Some days, I feel an aloneness that's bigger, meaner, more all-encompassing than anything I've ever known. I don't ever remember feeling this way before September 15. These days, I find many situations stressful, unless close friends or family are around. I never know when I'll hear an unintentionally hurtful remark. I never know when someone will feel sorry for me, something that irritates me more than an eyelash in a contact lens. I understand that the people who make these comments and behave this way just don't know how to respond to my life changes, but still, their comments or insinuations sting.

My fantasy ALS maid, by contrast, would understand. And you know, I'll bet we could be pretty efficient, even though I imagine we'd talk a lot as we scrubbed floors and vacuumed rugs and cleaned bathrooms. Perhaps we could clean my house one week and hers the next, just the two of us, working together—just like Steve's Colorado cleaning ladies, only different.

There's another reason, I fear, that I'm so fixated on Charcot's supposed maid. There's a nagging worry in my brain that I was she in another life. Maybe that explains why I love dishwashers and the smell of Pine-Sol and Murphy Oil Soap. Maybe that explains why I don't mind doing laundry. And maybe, just maybe, that explains my endless frustration that there is still no cure for this disease—not even after all that cleaning.

NOTES

1. www.alshope.com.
2. Mitsumoto, Hiroshi, and Theodore L. Munsat, M.D., eds. *Amyotrophic Lateral Sclerosis: A Guide for Patients and Families* (New York: Demos Press, 2001): 2.

IN KAFKA'S HOUSE

LEONARD KRIEGEL

Like nightmares, private terrors bind themselves to our sense of the possible. The imagination's violence is inflicted by the mind upon itself. And when that violence is made visible, we stand in dread as terror is transformed into reality.

Ever since I took sick with polio at the age of eleven, I have been terrified of waking up one morning to discover I am once again helpless. I am not talking about the prospect of stroke or heart attack or cancer. No matter how life-threatening, ordinary illness is simply among the risks one takes by having been born and growing older. I am talking about my nightmare of enforced isolation, in which I am held captive by the ability of others to structure the aftereffects of my disease.

One can be imprisoned by the world and yet not stand within it. At the heart of my dread I see a human being begging for the space he occupies and the air he breathes. The vision consumes me, even as fantasy. I cannot rid myself of the belief that a person has the right to hold on to the self he has created.

My idea that I have created a self may simply be another false god I choose to worship. I recognize that. Still, the prospect of being forced to function as others command I function is terrifying. I think I could lie without moving, a sentient vegetable, if only I still believed I could maintain allegiance to my idea of who I was and what I had made of my life. I know, of course, that every man and woman desires a strong sense of the self. But the prospect of discovering that one's capacity for living can be defined by others is particularly haunting to a man who has been conscious of his helplessness at some other point in his life.

A few months ago, my terrified vision of helplessness was reawakened as two old friends, a husband and wife visiting the States from the Netherlands, told me what had recently happened to their oldest son. Their story had the affect of making me tremble, so intense was the rage it called forth.

From *Falling Into Life* (San Francisco: North Point, 1991): 174–95.

Let me call him Michael. We are curiously tied together, Michael and I, both of our lives radically altered by a physical handicap. We first met when I was the Fulbright lecturer at the University of Leiden during the academic year 1964–65. My wife and I and our two-year-old son were frequent visitors at Michael's parents' house. Michael was then a young man who had just turned nineteen, twelve years younger than me. We talked in a Dutch-English patois. Michael was intent not only on what the future held in store for him but on the very visible fact that, like him, I was physically crippled. Having lost the use of my legs, I walked on double long-legged braces and crutches.

Michael's own handicap was considerably more severe. He had been born in the early summer of 1945, soon after the war in Europe came to an end. His mother had been pregnant with him during the terrible final winter of that war, what people old enough to remember in western Holland still call the *Hungerwinter.* Men and women crawled in the fields and ate tulip bulbs to keep from starving. Physicians blamed the inadequate nutrition available to his mother for the overwhelming genetic weakness in Michael's arms and legs.

I had already lived for two full decades with the effect of what my virus had done to me. Diligent exercise had given me considerable strength in my arms and shoulders. I could walk mile after mile on my crutches, the fifteen pounds of leather and steel strapped to my legs no more than a metaphor for my sense of power then. Michael's mobility was extremely limited. He was dependent on his parents and his two younger brothers—both of them strong and athletic—to get around.

In August, 1968, as Russian tanks rolled into Prague, I returned to the Netherlands for a second Fulbright year. By this time I had a second son. Once again we were welcomed by Michael's family, and Michael and I renewed our conversations about life and struggle. I wasn't surprised when, a year later, soon after our return to New York, a letter from Michael announced his imminent marriage. Michael wanted me to know that my example had given him hope. He was ready to lead a "normal" life.

I am not a modest man, and I take a great deal of pride in what I have been able to make of my life despite formidable obstacles. But I never wanted to serve as anyone's model of how to live with a severe physical handicap. Looking back, however, it almost seems inevitable that I became a model for Michael. His mother had translated my first book, an account of my encounter with the polio virus, into Dutch. And when he and I talked, Michael would speak quite openly about his feelings, his thoughts, his fears and ambitions, his crippled state. Just before we left Holland in June, 1969, I learned that he had decided to study for the ministry. He had chosen to be "normal." With God's help, he now wrote, he would taste the sacrament of marriage.

A skeptic, I was more suspicious of God's help than was Michael. But in the letter I wrote back, I spoke of how splendidly he had come through, by which I meant not that he had "overcome his handicap" but that he had absorbed the pain of the cripple into his strength as a man. Michael understood what it had taken me years to learn—that a cripple validates his life by creating a sense of his selfhood out of physical pain and chaos. Of course, Michael was a Christian, and for a Christian, suffering binds one to God. But Michael also understood that it was his suffering that gave him the right to choose survival. A nonbeliever could only envy his capacity for faith. From my painfully secular position, the cripple's presence merely testified to a calculus of accident. One could accept the implications of such mathematics, since one's acceptance was beside the point. Both believers and nonbelievers were powerless to change the way things were.

Over the next ten years, I corresponded with Michael's parents. And I heard news of Michael as I heard news of their other children. Once a Christmas card from Michael himself arrived. He offered his warmest wishes on the back of a photograph showing him sitting in an oversized armchair, misshapen legs jutting out from under him, surrounded by wife and two small children. All are smiling.

Michael's father wrote to tell me that his son was minister of a small congregation in the northeastern Netherlands. Although he was, like me, a nonbeliever, with a "normal" father's pride he noted that Michael's sermons were more literate than his small-town congregation could know. He took pleasure, as I took pleasure, in the knowledge that Michael was getting on in the world.

In 1981, when I was again living in Europe, I visited Michael's parents in the small town on the Côte d'Or where they now had a summer home. Michael, I learned, had separated from his wife. But his parents believed that they might yet reconcile their differences. And Michael and his wife did reconcile. But I lost touch with his parents until this past February, when they wrote that they were coming to America for a few weeks. In April they spent three days with us in New York. And it was then that I heard the story that rekindled the primary terror of my imagination—the threat of helpless isolation imposed by someone one loves.

As I listened to Michael's parents, I felt anger, then rage. And then I felt something stronger than anger or rage, a naked, throbbing fear that came from somewhere so deep inside me that it threatened sanity. Pathologies are bred in the bone, conditioned by past expectations. In literature, Susan Sontag reminded us in *Illness as Metaphor,* illness is usually inappropriate as an image. In life, however, it can be a most appropriate definition—one that thrusts a cripple against his weakness and this strength.

Envision the scene as I envision it. Michael is now a man of forty-four, father of two grown sons, minister of the gospel. He is a respected member of the community. But his life has been defined, as it will continue to be defined, by the nutrients his mother was deprived of during the *Hungerwinter.* The war in Europe made Michael a minor irony in a world filled with irony and horror enough for all tastes. For what was Michael in the Europe of 1945? He had been conceived as Anne Frank and millions of her fellow Jews were murdered, their crime the stigma of having been born; and he sucked for the scarce nutrients that would nourish him into life as death rained ceaselessly across the skies of Europe. Heraclitus had said it thousands of years earlier: Death was everywhere, in the voices of all men. No one who survived, even survived as Michael had survived, had a right to complain.

I close my eyes and watch the scene: a woman pushing a man in a wheelchair into a small room. She takes him from the chair, forces him to the mattress on the floor. Then she takes his crutches and his wheelchair from the room, locks the door. He is to be taught a lesson by his wife-jailer. Other than the mattress on the floor and a straw-seat chair that seems to have been lifted from a Van Gogh painting and placed in the corner of the room, there is no furniture. There is no bathroom. There is no washstand.

He hears his sons, now young men of fifteen and seventeen, move through the house. His sons ignore the closed door. Beyond it lies not their father but a thing defined by their mother. Solitude is misshapen. He may talk like a man. But his sons know that a man—even a minister of the gospel—is not merely speech. A man is body, defining himself by the demands he makes upon the world. Michael demands nothing. Like Kafka's hunger artist, he finds himself more and more attracted to the aesthetics of starvation while he lies on the floor. His world has been turned inside out. His children are his guards, his wife is his jailer, his passion is now to romance his captivity.

I remain purposely calm as I listen. I envision Michael lying inside the locked room, in his own dirt, measuring time in the mind's eyes. No television set, no books, no radio, no newspaper. He can listen to the sounds of his oldest son's guitar. The sound of the guitar soothes, makes him feel part of his family again. He smiles, as if he were once more surrounded by wife and sons, posing for a picture on a Christmas card. He closes his eyes. In memory, he recites verses from the Bible. In imagination, he preaches passionate sermons to congregations hanging breathlessly on his every word.

But if he is God's voice, he can speak in imagination alone. For five days punctually at three, his wife-jailer unlocks the door and shoves a tray into the room. Focusing his eyes on the tray, he forces his face to remain expressionless. His wife grimaces her displeasure at the sight of Michael on the floor, dissatisfied with what she has created. His solitary kingdom is defined anew by the glass of water, the bread, and the cheese on the tray. He does not crawl to the tray until she has closed and relocked the door. Reduced in size, he crawls to the tray. Michael eats.

His voice survives. It survives five days of hearing itself in the mind alone. It assumes the scale imagination demands. Isaiah, Ezekiel, lamenting with Jeremiah. Never before had Michael felt comfortable with the Book of Ecclesiastes. It was always too Greek, too lacking in Christian hope. But now, in his enforced isolation, he transforms the Preacher word by word. Endurance is a form of love. And as he lies alone on the mattress in the empty room, Michael is determined to endure. If he can outlast captivity, he will, he knows, again become human.

He hears his wife and sons speaking with considerable agitation in the vestibule. He hears the front door slam. Silence descends on the house. Too weak simply to crawl, Michael twists and slithers to the door. He is not the serpent in the Garden. This is his house, not Eden. He reaches up to touch the lock and the door springs free. They have deliberately left it open. He moves to the entrance of the house, slithering to the front door. It, too, is unlocked. A neighbor spies him as he twists outside, slithering like a commando moving beneath barbed wire. Amazement on his face, the neighbor hesitantly approaches. Michael is covered with dirt. There is blood on his forehead where he scraped it against the doorjamb. He smells of feces and dried urine and sweat and stale days and nights. The neighbor reaches down, touches him, furtively, as if Michael were some jellylike blob in a low-budget horror film. Michael smiles. The neighbor will telephone the police. No, Michael insists, better if he simply helps him get into his car.

He slithers to the car. With the neighbor cradling him in a fireman's lift, he gets inside. As he suspected, the door of the car has been left open. The keys wait in the ignition. Michael feels light-headed—from hunger, from his own smell, from the unexpected gift of freedom, from the outrage and distaste so visible on his neighbor's face. Michael turns the key, touches the specially constructed hand controls, smiles his gratitude at the neighbor, who angrily slams the car door shut. Michael drives off, no longer a captive. He has been tested.

And he has been sentenced. To helplessness. But he remains a believer. "People like us," I remember him saying as he told me of his decision to enter the ministry, "have been chosen to suffer for the rest of mankind. With our lives, God demonstrates his love for the world." I remember how I resisted the temptation to make some caustic comment about God's love. Instead, I told him that I believed people chose their fates from what was available to them at the time of their choosing. Michael was adamant. God, he insisted, had chosen him. And whether I knew it or not, he had chosen me, too. If so, I remember thinking at the time, his God was capricious enough to serve as ringmaster for this century's circus. But I didn't say anything. Michael was determined to survive. His faith was the price he paid for that survival.

Michael drove to the house of a parishioner, a woman his wife insisted he was sleeping with. He saw her only for work related to church projects. Better, I thought, if they had been sleeping together. To be imprisoned for a crime committed—however ludicrous that "crime" may be—would have lent structure to Michael's ordeal. One can be grateful even for the structure.

The woman bathes him, washing away the smell of captivity. She sets the table, listens to Michael say grace. Like the neighbor, she wants to call the police. Michael refuses. She must understand. He is a minister. He is a cripple. He is a burden. To himself and to others. There will be no calls to the police. In another's house, Michael sleeps. A proper sleep in a proper bed. Without knowing it, he has read Kafka up close.

* * * * *

Thinking about that story makes me want to howl like a wounded animal, to stick my hand through glass. Thinking about that story makes me believe that only in the breaking does life make sense. I am fifty-five years old. I have created a life, built it piece by piece. And I can be thrust aside, locked away, made susceptible to the same terror as Michael. I shiver as I envision myself in Michael's place. Reeking of humiliation, imprisoned by those one loves, tested by a calculating malevolence. Michael told himself he was being tested by his God. The test is as absurd as the genetics created by the *Hungerwinter.* Accidents should not be tragic but comic—Chaplin falling through an open manhole.

I feel my sanity threatened because Michael's nightmare is also my own. Michael's fate was to become the self reduced to its scars. We are, Michael and I, creations of Susan Sontag's "more onerous citizenship." It is not a citizenship one chooses. But endemic to the life one claims from the skewered ambitions and twisted dreams of one's actual life are the choices one makes. Citizens act, think, create. In his own eyes, Michael has been singled out by his God. His problem is to prove himself worthy of having been singled out. Mine is to continue to earn a self through the everyday rigors of living with disease.

In the struggle between sickness and health, the forces of light and the forces of darkness, Michael and I are simply soldiers in the ranks. Thomas Mann pits Hans Castorp and his cousin Joachim against one another in his great novel *The Magic Mountain.* Hans is indolent in his willingness to allow disease to define his life; Joachim refuses to give in to what disease has made of him. Mann, always the master ironist, destroys Joachim because he insists on denying the defining power of disease.

What infuriates me is not the vision of Michael lying in his own filth on a bare mattress in a bare room. What infuriates me is that the genetics that defined him made him so dependent on others that his capacity to claim a self could be stolen by a bitter wife and fearful sons. To be defined as what feminists like to call an "object," a thing whose existence can be made over by others, is nightmarish. And yet, there was a time when Michael was loved, when his sons sang to him, when his wife rested her head on his childishly weak arms, seeking to unlock the self she was ultimately to lock away.

Think of Michael lying in that room. He longs for companionship, hears voices, preaches to thousands in his mind, transforms himself—like the early Christian martyrs—into a man deemed worthy of the God who has so capriciously robbed him of physical presence. Think of Michael dismissing all theories of probability, because, like Kafka, he has come to realize that whatever happened was somehow deserved. Think of Michael opening himself up to the fears of others, grafting them onto his own life.

Memory blesses terror. When I was thirteen and returned to my neighborhood from two years in an upstate hospital, my mother, I remember, walked into the apartment one September afternoon, face tear-streaked and ashen. The butcher's wife had just told her that my illness was God's judgment—on her. The butcher's wife was known throughout the neighborhood as "not right in the head," a knowledge that should have made it easy to dismiss what she said. Sitting in the sawdust-strewn butcher shop, childless, she would knit, our own Madame de Farge, mumbling incantations in Yiddish to placate a god of vengeance and to impose order on an evil, crazed universe. Her eyes would blank out the world, or else they would sparkle with the electric blue-and-green current of the mad.

Mad or sane, the butcher's wife had touched my mother's center, as Kafka touches our centers. For she had voiced precisely what my mother herself believed about disease in her own fear-ravaged heart. Illness was judgment. The slings and arrows of fortune might be outrageous; they were never undeserved. Accident, illness, war, famine, disease: punishments visited upon one by the master of the universe.

To call this superstition is useless. For the butcher's wife and my mother simply believed what far more sophisticated and rational people believe even today about disease: It is judgment rendered. Through illness, justice can be meted out. The victim of accident turns out not to be a victim by accident. It is not the meaning of illness that is beyond understanding. The meaning can easily be understood. For to dwell in Kafka's House is to discover that judgment dwells alongside one. And to be a "victim of disease" is to be tested, tried, made better, punished, reborn.

Anyone who has dealt with a long-term illness or accident soon recognizes the extent to which his or her own view of it is judgmental. In Kafka's House, a sense of mystery does not eliminate cause and effect. One loses one's body to disease, but one also loses it to memory. And it becomes increasingly difficult, as one focuses on that loss, not to read into it some greater significance than it merits. Writer and physician and theologian join hands in assigning responsibility. Disease has somehow been welcomed, accident has somehow been sought out. Psychosomatic illness may not be as fashionable an intellectual theory today as it was twenty years ago. But we continue to speak of disease-welcoming personalities and accident-embracing tendencies. A modern vocabulary makes "scientific" the fears and superstitions operating on both the butcher's mad wife and my own judgment-obsessed mother.

Did Michael, as a believer, view his treatment at the hands of his jailer-wife and guard-sons as another trial, a further test to be endured? Pain cannot be allowed to be fortuitous. Michael and his wife and sons were actors together in some metaphysical drama. In some corner of his mind, Michael achieved purgation. He had suffered, he had endured—and his suffering and endurance were meaningful. They proved him worthy.

Does Michael continue to view the body isolated from its fellow humans, assigned a place in the prison of another's making, as fit punishment for the sin of having been born with genetic defects? As he sleeps now alongside his new wife—yes, the parishioner who cleansed him—does he remember that disease, too, is a sharing, a communion of sorts? Does he recognize how it inflicts itself on others? Does he see how it spurs the imagination—Kafka's aphorisms, Poe's visions, Modigliani wandering through the night-bound streets of Europe? Incapacity can be made into a fiery judgment on the world.

How does time pass in the solitary anguish Michael experienced? Picture an insect following its antennae across wall after wall. A wall is a surface and a surface must be crawled across—up and down, right and left, circle and square, movement following movement.

When Michael first told me he had decided on the ministry, I asked him whether he had read Kafka. He hadn't. I hope he never does. Let him conceive of himself as an original. Let him think of his suffering as a reification of the self. Even the movement of an insect possesses boundaries when contained within the mind. On the blank page, Kafka stands more powerful than the father he created from memory's space. To the tubercular writer, Gregor Samsa embodies the ordinary drabness of suffering. A tedious process, illness, breeding not despair and angst but the singular determination to get through one's days and nights. Learning to live with disease is intimate, even seductive. The parts of Michael's body miraculously change themselves into animated sensors testing the world the way a blind man tests the pitch and dip of a street with his cane.

* * * * *

Illness can be a metaphor only to those determined to remain ignorant of its truth. Susan Sontag was certainly correct in that. And by the same token, illness can be therapeutic only to those determined to avoid its tedium. It is not a process by which one offers the self for assessment. But it is a state of being in which one can uncover the self, stand it naked and clear before the imagination. Has Michael learned this? He never complained, but as a believer he could never accept the sheer diceyness of what had happened to him. He accepts the responsibility of resisting the consequences of his birth, for he senses that such resistance affirms what is most human in him. But he cannot resist the temptation to make illness even more significant than it is. The truth is that the only thing he should be concerned with is not the ideology one reads into disease but the terms by which one establishes resistance to its effects. I wonder whether Michael ever learned that he cannot cure himself by endowing suffering with the theological equivalent of the Good Housekeeping Seal of Approval.

Individuals do not succumb to cancer or to heart attacks because they want to succumb. They are simply "struck down," an arbitrary striking that makes no sense and needs no justification. True, we now know that certain individuals possess a genetic susceptibility to specific diseases and conditions. But these are gamblers' odds, shaped by gamblers' recognitions. In selecting victims, disease and accident are fortuitous and illogical. Michael was born with weakened limbs because his mother was pregnant during a time of human-caused famine. Judgment was rendered here not by God but by man. Michael was the victim of the same political history that created the Holocaust and left the cities of Europe in rubble.

The mathematical probability of illness or accident can be created by any number of possible factors. For Michael, the war. For me, a prospectively innocent two weeks at summer camp. A reminder for all philosophers of chance. On the bus going to camp, we were seated according to height. I was a tall boy, taller than the two friends from the neighborhood I was going to camp with. I was made to sit next to another, taller boy. His name was Jerry, he had watery blue eyes, and by the time we arrived at the camp I had invited him to share a bunk with me and my two friends from the neighborhood. Eleven days later Jerry and I were in a small country hospital fighting to stay alive. Jerry died. I lost the use of my legs to the virus. My two friends returned to the city untouched. Was it simply a time when a capricious God or a quixotic fate had it in for taller boys? Would shorter boys have their turn next year? Did Jerry and I share an "inclination" to embrace the disease-carrying virus? Were my two neighborhood friends better prepared to resist its siren song? A simple cast of the dice is never enough: Judgment demands more magical incantations.

Think of what our age has created from such spiritual voodoo. In the name of diagnosis, the mind has been burdened with the task of saving us from illness. "Canst thou administer to a mind diseased?" cries Macbeth. In our time, he would subscribe to a journal of holistic medicine. Think healthy and you are healthy. The intensity of our interest in quackery staggers the rational mind. We peddle cures for virtually every condition know to man: cancer, acne, heart attack, impotence, stroke, hair loss, pneumonia, bad breath. We are deluged by books urging us to eat our way to health, to will our way to health, to exercise our way to health, to fuck our way to health. Physicians vie with one another for the chance to treat the soul rather than the body—or, better yet, to treat the body through treating the soul. *Amor vincit omnia!*

And we veteran denizens of Kafka's House, even we are absorbed not by the pathology of disease but by the psychology of those who "allowed" disease to enter their lives. How curious that it is Michael, not his wife, whose motives I probe. The bearer of the virus is of little interest; the victim commands our attention. In Kafka's House, one learns to view not the terrorized but terror with compassion. Just as in certain writings about the Holocaust the implicit question addressed to the Jews is, "How could you let this happen?" so Michael discovers he has been condemned to answer his wife-jailer and guard-sons as they cry out, "How could you allow us to do this?"

Ours is a century which views weakness as sin. Even those whose lives are intertwined with the lives of the weak become victims of their victimization. "Why me?" compels "Why them?" The victims of the victim become the significant bearers of his pain. His scars—the useless legs, the weak arms, the bent shoulders—are their burden. The mind of the jailer haunts the prisoner. Michael's true shame is for what he has done to those who once loved him.

It has been almost three years since Michael's sons last spoke to their father. Curiously, I can understand that. They lack the intensity of his obsession. And they lack his belief, his sense of having been selected to suffer for the rest of humanity. We do not live inside a Malamud novel. They *are* the rest of humanity. Kafka's father is the father they desire, created as need dictates. To ask them to love their father is to ask them to deny themselves. His ravaged body will forever rebuke their need for strength.

What makes their resentment understandable is that they feel trapped. Disease truly is a sharing. But its burdens and rewards are unequal. Think of Michael's two sons, men themselves now, aware from the time they were toddlers that they were physically more powerful than the man they called father. A father who is God's solitary beggar rebukes the very power they seek. What they desire is a father against whom revolt might be conventional, a father who seems powerful and overwhelming, a father like Kafka's father. What they have gotten is a father who inspires in them rage intense enough to create its own metaphysics of injustice. To assert the self, they need to pull down what is strong. A father lacking power is a father who demands not revolt but compassion. Michael's presence offends their need. His smile, his piety, his endurance all conspire to indict his sons, to deny their urgent need to test the world for themselves.

And even as I rage at her, I try to see that bare room through the eyes of Michael's jailer, his wife. Do I condemn her inability to live with her husband's bargains with God? Was locking Michael in that room her confession of failure? The idea is as soothing as it is obscene, as if Michael had to be imprisoned and humiliated, left in the dirt and smells of his affliction, so that his wife could see herself as something other than servant to his needs. Did she, I wonder, share Michael's sense that Christians are repositories of suffering? That their burden is the world's salvation? The lame, the halt, the blind: Was her anger at Michael fueled when he took the burden of being human from her heart and mind?

* * * * *

Despite Sontag's splendid effort, writers will continue to use illness as metaphor. Disease so easily springs out of control. And what better language for condemnation, for evil, for receiving one's just and unjust reward or punishment? Cancer, heart attack, AIDS, and diseases yet to be discovered—a stream of metaphors, all promising retribution against hedonism and excess. The body's unconscious revenge upon the depths of depravity available to the modern body.

And since we are creatures of paradox, we will employ the metaphors even while we continue to live in a culture that obligates man to be "healthy," a culture in which all disease can be withstood, conquered through the exertion of the individual will.

The surgeon specializing in the removal of cancerous tumors becomes a Doctor of Love specializing in the removal of moribund fears of death and dying. From a magazine cover his face stares up at me. Scalp shaved naked to the wind, eyes burning with the power and truth of his message, this is not the butcher's mad wife, finger pointing *J'accuse* at my guilt-ridden mother. Still, I cannot help wondering what the Doctor of Love would say to Michael? Or to Michael's sons? Or to Michael's ex-wife? Would he offer the power of positive thinking? New sons? New wives? New beliefs? Stabbed by reality, Michael yet hungers after salvation. He, too, searches for cause and effect. In this he is no different from the Doctor of Love.

For what did Michael want? That his faith be tested?

And the doors shall be shut in the streets,
When the sound of the grinding is low.

Well, the door was shut. But after forty-four years of living as a cripple, Michael takes the longer view. Like the Doctor of Love, he will define each stage of his life, each approaching cataclysm. The humiliated body is a mere extension of pain. Michael still believes. He still hungers after inner light. He remains an accountant of the soul, demanding spiritual compensation for a useless body.

It is a grinding obscenity, this need to authenticate suffering. Michael has become a co-conspirator in his victimization. Perhaps the "Doctor of Love" is really convinced that Michael has power over his own suffering. Perhaps he can convince Michael of the truth of what Michael already believes, that suffering itself is merely symptomatic of some breakdown in one's spiritual balance. I know better. Disease is indeed personal. And what we make of it a reflection of need. But truth is equally personal. Michael was not responsible for the barbarism that led to the *Hungerwinter* of 1944–1945 and I was not responsible for the chance encounter that allowed the virus to slip into my bloodstream in the summer of 1944. Punishment has nothing to do with the crime—unless the crime is defined as merely being human.

And perhaps it should be. To be "struck down" is a most human victimization. Given the keys to Kafka's House, one approaches prospective tenancy there prepared to confront the question of what made one's residence possible. "The romantic idea that the disease expresses the character," Sontag writes, "is invariably extended to assert that the character causes the disease—because it has not expressed itself." Even for Kafka, the voice of tuberculosis demanded that he reject disease and assert his longing for health. How he envied the self-confident and "normal," those who had neither the time nor the patience required by disease. To claim power is also to claim health.

And the man who is "successful" at creating a life out of the aftereffects of disease—as, however immodest it is to write, I have been—discovers that he must, sooner or later, fight against an inflated notion of what it is he has achieved. When a mutual friend praised Franz Rozenzweig's courage in living with pain and suffering inflicted on him by a long struggle with cancer, Freud, doomed to undergo the same long struggle, is reported to have said, "What else can he do?" Freud understood that the real question each of us must answer is no different from the question "normal" men and women face: What are the terms with which one lives with disease?

For the man or woman who has successfully "rehabilitated" the self (how awkward the vocabulary of disease, as if language were intended to keep abstract what is so intimate and personal) feels the temptation to make disease self-referential. The primacy of the self does not come from the bargains we strike with our terror: It can just as easily emerge out of what disease has wrought, out of "overcoming" disease. The man who competes in a wheelchair marathon does not view his effort as a mockery of form but as a way of turning stigma upon itself. Having "come through," having "overcome his handicap," he invests what he has done with a morality of its own. "I came, I saw, I conquered!" can so easily be transformed into "I suffered, I overcame, I endured!" It is not, finally, the life one seeks to redeem—it is the disease. For it is the disease that challenges the self to be "better" than it was.

Hans Castorp discovers that, if he is to be made conscious, he must affirm the power of disease that has snatched him from the jaws of health. In seeking shelter in Kafka's House, he deserts the humdrum and banal for the possibility of the erotic and exciting. Made physically smaller, the self suddenly looms larger. To be doomed by illness is to learn how to refuse the temptation of the ordinary and settled. Were I given to looking for signs, I would point out that as they came to the ends of their lives, Kafka and Hemingway switched roles—the one insisting on the need to "overcome" disease and accept the healthy, the other sticking a shotgun in his mouth to blow his "healthy" head away.

* * * * *

I am fifteen minutes early. I park across the street from the restaurant where my friend Ted and I are to meet for dinner. It is no more than thirty feet from where I have parked to the door. A year ago, when Ted and I last met for dinner, I walked into the restaurant on my crutches, as I had been doing for forty years. But walking has become increasingly difficult, and my mind keeps flashing on the wheelchair folded in the trunk of my car.

The question is not trivial. Ted has never seen me in a wheelchair. He has known me for thirty years as the man who has "overcome" the virus through the power of his will (*and* the crutches beneath his shoulders, *and* the braces strapped to his legs). It is how he first knew me, when we met as graduate students at Columbia. And now he has joined me in Kafka's House, each of us singular in illness. Curiously touched by shame, I reach for the crutches and carefully walk into the restaurant.

Ted arrives after I am seated at the table. He looks as he looked thirty years ago. Only he moves slowly, with trepidation, carefully placing one foot in front of the other, like a drunk trying to convince friends he has control and forcing a caution that runs against the grain of his temperament., He spots me, smiles, threads his way between tables across the nubbed industrial carpeting as if some potent unmarked danger were twisted into its fibers waiting to trip him up. "Every step I take," he said to me over the telephone, "makes me feel as if I'm about to be hit. Rheumatoid arthritis. It's a second babyhood." And then, laughing, "And no prospect of growing out of this one."

He sits down across from me, knees bending slowly, like an uncoordinated girl in the third grade preparing for her turn at jumprope. My friend Ted is afraid—and what he is afraid of, I suspect, is this sudden residence in Kafka's House, where even at dinner with an old friend, himself a resident there, he must stand alone.

Like death, disease is a personal discovery. "It's more curious than bad," he says, anticipating the question I want to ask. "I invent new ways for everything. I never thought about whether or not I was strong enough. I never had to. Now I'm always trying to outwit circumstance."

The smallest action takes on a new magnitude when one must pitch his tent in disease. It is not the halting steps of the cripple he has become that disturbs Ted. Nor even the knowledge that he will stretch memory for the Little All-American halfback he once was. Already forgotten is the party three years ago, to celebrate the ability of a man turned fifty to impose his physical presence on a birthday gathering intended to deny time's passing. No one appreciates better than my friend Ted the irony that transforms a man who loved the physical self even more than he loved Joyce's prose or John Huston's films. In Kafka's House, I remind myself, all are welcome. But the newly invited are uncomfortable, nervous, afraid to make themselves at home. One moves quickly in being forced to move slowly. Condemned now to wait for a porter to carry his bags at an airport or train station, Ted's mind hungers for its own past. At what point will it be not his luggage but himself that must be carried?

No matter how broken, my friend Ted still possesses the memory of the body he once assumed would always remain dependable, growing older into grace but not into disease. He had trusted that body more than he could possibly trust another human being. But he can accept the irony of being betrayed by that in which he had invested so much. He is a literary man, and he knew about Kafka's House long before it was decided he must live there.

As graduate students we used to meet in another restaurant. We would nurse beers after class, discussing the writers we were determined to emulate and the novels we wanted to write, arguing the world back and forth, as only the young who want to be writers can argue, circling ambition's shadow like boxers searching for an opening. Exhilarating arguments, exhausting because neither of us could bend beneath the weight of carrying the record. In such a world, health was assumed. There was no room for illness. Not when the world offered itself to be cracked apart like a walnut.

Only I was a mere eleven years beyond the confrontation with the virus that had left me without the use of my legs. I knew the dictates of disease. "Get the crutches," I say as we prepare to leave. Ted had placed my crutches behind the bar because the booth in which we sat was narrow. Ted stares at me, puzzled. "The crutches," I repeat. "You put them behind the bar."

Ted shakes his head. "I always have to remind myself you need them," he says. "I forget."

I had lived in Kafka's House for more than a decade by then. And I knew I was destined to live there for the rest of my life. That was years before I met Michael, three decades before I watched this same friend, painfully crippled himself, slip past the surety of his body into the sour comings and goings of learning to live with disease. I was still intent on "overcoming" back then, and I was as willing to accept my friend Ted's flattery as I was to make a weapon of incapacity. Perhaps that was what I had learned from the years I had already spent in Kafka's House—that while I could not will my way to health I nonetheless could create a tone for my presence out of what the virus had left. If a mind so finely tuned as Kafka's could succumb to the desire to be "normal," then perhaps I could be excused for condemning myself to project the image I was so determined to project. To tell me I had "overcome a handicap" was to affirm the self I had worked so hard to create.

Had I continued to believe I had "overcome" what would always dominate my existence, I would have been trapped in delusion. There are moments when one forgets that no one lives by choice in Kafka's House. But residence there had prepared me for the fear and bewilderment I would see in the face of my friend Ted. And residence there made unforgettable the terror of someday finding myself helpless, bound to the obligations of others as I twist and squirm in my mind. To endure is not enough. I know that, now that I have lived long enough in Kafka's House to understand that the past expects the future. Maybe what I should have said to my friend Ted, as we sat in that Greenwich Village restaurant, was that just as my terror had been Michael's nightmare, so his nightmare was already my past. For he had come to visit in Kafka's House, only to find that, like Hans Castorp on his mountain, he had earned proper residence there.

HOMAGE TO ISAAC BASHEVIS SINGER

SUSAN FROMBERG SCHAEFFER

It so happened that she began to worship Isaac Bashevis Singer. She was afflicted with a high fever that would not go down. It rose to 103 degrees in the mornings and evenings and then dropped to normal. When her fever was high, she shook all over; when it dropped, she felt healthy as a horse, but tired. The doctor said she had to go to the hospital. She said she was sure she could shake it off at home. She could take her aspirins herself. She would set her alarm to ring every four hours. Besides, one of her neighbors sat in her living room all day long, so she was not alone. She had a television and her neighbor did not and the woman was addicted to many programs. Probably, if the truth were known, Mrs. Klopstock venerated the television, which she regarded—without awareness—as the custodian of her safety.

The doctor said she could not live forever with a fever of 103 and admitted her to the hospital. That same night, her doctor came to see her. "I want to go home," she said. "Everyone's dying here." She was on a bad floor. Virtually everyone was dying. The doctor said she could go home as soon as she was finished with her tests. He told her to forget about the other patients. She was not dying. Mrs. Klopstock said she would be glad to forget about the other patients, especially since there was nothing wrong with her. She had a fever, she told the doctor, because she was upset. "You've been upset before," she said. "Being upset could cause a fever," she said. "Please," said the doctor. "No one could be that upset." "They could," she said, "if they had my daughter." "One daughter," he said, "to cause all this trouble?" "I have troubles even I don't know about," said Mrs. Klopstock. He didn't say anything.

Mrs. Klopstock remained in the hospital. In spite of herself, she grew fond of her roommate, Mrs. Smith, who was dying of brain cancer. One night, Mrs. Smith soiled herself and cried for an hour because she was afraid to call the nurse. Mrs. Klopstock

From *Jewish Currents Magazine* 40 (Nov. 1986). By permission of the publisher.

called the nurse. The nurse shouted at Mrs. Smith. She said she was worse than a baby. She said she had a 90-year-old patient who could do more for herself than Mrs. Smith could. Mrs. Smith cried for hours. She would not eat her snack; she was afraid of soiling herself again. "The patients are all dying," said Mrs. Klopstock to her doctor, "and the nurses are killing them." "Don't exaggerate," he said. She demanded to know why they were holding her there. The doctor said she was in a hospital, not a prison, and she had a fever of unknown origin. Mrs. Klopstock was worried about her health insurance; she asked if that was a disease. "Of course it's a disease," he said. She raised her eyebrows; she was not so sure.

She persuaded Mrs. Smith that she wanted to get out of bed and sit up on a chair. The nurses were always after her because she lay quietly in bed in the hospital position, curled up like a shrimp, her back to the door. Mrs. Klopstock noticed that she, too, had taken to looking out the window curled on her side, back to the door. Mrs. Smith agreed that she would like to sit up and surprise her daughter by greeting her from the chair instead of the bed. Mrs. Klopstock ran for a nurse. The nurse said she didn't have time to sit anyone up now. Mrs. Klopstock asked the nurse her name and began to write on a pad she kept near her pillow. The nurse wanted to know what she was doing. Mrs. Klopstock said she was writing to the hospital administrator. The nurse dragged Mrs. Smith from her bed and pushed her down on a chair. It was an empty victory. Mrs. Smith's daughter did not come that night and the nurse found no time in which to help Mrs. Smith back to bed. At 10 o'clock, Mrs. Klopstock buttonholed a doctor, dragged him after her and brought him over to Mrs. Smith, who was crying from exhaustion. He put her back to bed. The next day, Mrs. Smith refused to stir. Two days later, she was taken to the hospital nursing home.

Mrs. Klopstock's next roommate was a Chinese woman who made her, at 60, feel young. She did not speak a word of English and once a month came into the hospital for chemotherapy. She was a very quiet, very clean woman and Mrs. Klopstock felt she knew her. She might have been Jewish had she not been Chinese. With the help of Mrs. Wu's family, she and Mrs. Wu established a kind of sign language. When that failed, Mrs. Wu called her daughter at her place of business and told her what she wanted. Then she handed the phone to Mrs. Klopstock and her daughter translated what her mother had said. Taking care of Mrs. Wu distracted Mrs. Klopstock, who nevertheless was uncomfortably and furiously aware that the doctors did not yet know what was wrong with her. One night, Mrs. Wu, who had been attached to an intravenous, began to flail about in her bed. Mrs. Klopstock got up and went to see what the trouble was. Mrs. Wu called her daughter, spoke to her, and then gave Mrs. Klopstock the phone. "Her arm is bleeding," said the daughter, "and the needle hurts her." Mrs. Klopstock went off to get a nurse. "Her arm is not bleeding and it does not hurt," said the nurse. "There is blood on the floor," said Mrs. Klopstock. "It's old blood," said the nurse.

"I see," said Mrs. Klopstock, "the angel of death in long white robes and he's hovering over your head." She watched in fascination as the angel floated above the nurse's head and paused at the entrance to the room just before theirs. "Besides," said the nurse, who didn't seem to have heard her, "you don't speak Chinese, do you?" Mrs. Klopstock did not answer. The vision did not cheer her. On this floor, the angel of death did not come for nurses.

* * * * *

She was not surprised when she heard the Code Nine alert; the noise on the other side of the wall was no surprise to her. It took longer than she thought. "Where is Mr. Stein?" she asked the next morning. "In Intensive Care," said the first nurse. "Gone home," said the second. So she knew. Later, she heard two young doctors talking. "I didn't think he'd go down the tubes so fast," one of them said. Mrs. Klopstock planted herself in front of them. "They told him," she said, "there was nothing wrong with him and that he was just a crybaby and that he had to stop asking them for ice all the time." The doctors looked at her, appalled. They thought she was crazy. She went back to her room and curled up, back to the door. "Your programs are coming on," said a nurse. Mrs. Klopstock ignored her.

They only tolerated her because she could walk. She pretended to be asleep.

* * * * *

At last, her doctor said, they knew what was wrong with her. Mrs. Klopstock sat up. "You have an infection of the heart valves," he said. Mrs. Klopstock clutched her chest. "You're in no danger," he said. Mrs. Klopstock looked up. Nothing was hovering in the air above them. "I want to go to another hospital," she said. "They kill people here." "You have to trust your doctor," he said. "The angel of death lives here," she said. "I hate to start in with psychiatrists," said the doctor. "Wait," she said. "Someday you'll be sick and they'll put you in here and you'll see for yourself." He looked at her oddly. Silence unrolled itself between them like the map of an unknown county. "At least," he said, "we think you have an infection of the valves of the heart. We can't find any other cause of the fever. You have a murmur. People with murmurs are particularly susceptible to these infections. Sometimes the bacteria don't show up on our tests." "Then you're not sure I have it," she said. "No," said the doctor, "but we have to treat it. It's the only way to rule it out. If you have it and we don't treat it, you'll die." "I don't have it," said Mrs. Klopstock. "It's in my head." "The only thing in your head is that silly idea," he said. "Stop telling the nurses it's all in your head. They won't come when you call them." "And if you treat me and I don't have it?" she asked. "You'll have germ-free blood," he said.

"How do they treat it," she asked, "an infection of the heart?" "Oh," he said, as if waking up, "six weeks of antibiotic therapy." "I'll go home in the morning," Mrs. Klopstock said with relief. "Oh no," he said, "you have to stay here. The medication is given intravenously." Mrs. Klopstock began to protest—it would never work, the doctors were irresponsible, the nurses were worse, they never changed an I.V. bottle until the tubes from them were filled with blood. The doctor was not listening to her. He was staring into the hall. "Well?" she demanded. "I thought I saw someone in a hospital gown," he said, "on a ladder." "That was no patient," she said. He avoided her eyes.

They had her at last. She was plugged into the I.V. She was too nauseated to walk. The doctor gave her something for the nausea and she slept for three days. Her neighbor came and brought her the alarm watch she had left behind on her dresser so that she could wake herself up every three hours and remind the nurses to replace the empty I.V. bottles with full ones. Mrs. Wu was sent home. The nurse told her she would be happy to hear that her next roommate was "only" diabetic. Then why, wondered Mrs. Klopstock, when they laid the new woman on the bed next to hers, was a white figure hovering over her? Mrs. White was losing her toes and her sight. She prayed constantly, both alone and in company. Mrs. Klopstock was disgusted by the smell of her decaying feet which seemed, in some dreadful way, to incorporate the odor of prayer. She was terrified by the way Mrs. White, who was long and thin and flat, rocked and swayed in the air like a snake. Mrs. Klopstock watched her, horrified. Finally, she realized that Mrs. White swayed in the hope of seeing something more clearly.

One day, then another, passed. Mrs. Klopstock's dread of her roommate grew. Her small head at the top of the long, thin column of her body was wrapped in a turban. Mrs. White seemed about to change into something else, something not human. Mrs. Klopstock lay on her side and stared out the window. From her bed, she could see only a square of grey sky and an occasional sea gull. She lay there, hour after hour, waiting for her doctor. "You've got to get me out of here," she said. "Or get her out. I was here first." "What's wrong with her?" asked the doctor, who had inspected Mrs. White many times already. Mrs. Klopstock said that she didn't know why, but the woman gave her the creeps. "The creeps?" the doctor echoed. "Where did you get an expression like that? The creeps?" "She does, she gives me the creeps," Mrs. Klopstock insisted, starting to cry. "I'll see what I can do," he said. Mrs. Klopstock knew he wouldn't be able to do anything.

She cried harder. Later, she got up and drew the curtains around her bed. She turned on the T.V. and adjusted the curtain so that all she could see from her bed was the screen. She felt as if she had been sent into the desert.

The nurses tried to get her to draw the curtains, but she was ferocious. If no one would remove the terrifying Mrs. White, she would remove herself into her little room of striped cloth walls. Day after day went by. She heard Mrs. White pray with her minister, a faith healer and many friends. She had always hated religion. Sealed in her tent, she bit her tongue to keep from jeering at them. They loved The Book of Job. She could not avoid listening to them. They were the most unfortunate people she had ever heard of or known: their lives were plagued with calamities she never knew existed, and yet they were continually praising God. Mrs. Klopstock decided that they were either stupid or deranged. Still, something about Mrs. White awed her. Mrs. White spent half her life in hospitals. She was in the hospital or she was home. She was equally happy in either place. She was happy. Mrs. Klopstock was outraged. How could she not know what life was doing to her? Was she too stupid to be crushed? "It's quiet in here," she heard Mrs. White's current visitor say. "Too quiet," Mrs. White said pointedly. Mrs. Klopstock sighed in her tent and wrapped herself around her pillow. She looked up at her I.V. bottle. In 15 minutes, she would have to make her way through the newest group of psalm singers, into the hall, after the nurse. It was too much for her. She fell asleep.

* * * * *

When she awoke, the room was dark. She looked up at her I.V. bottles. Miraculously, they had been replaced. It was quiet. Outside, it was foggy and the traffic lights turned the mist red. She turned from the window toward the door. Something, she could see it clearly, was floating over the curtain which separated her bed from Mrs. White's. It seemed to be looking at her. She got up, and, pulling her I.V. after her, went over to inspect Mrs. White's bed. She called to her, but Mrs. White neither answered nor moved. She pushed the button and the nurse's intercom came on. "I think Mrs. White is in a coma," she said. She heard the nurses running down the hall. "Is she in a coma?" she asked. "Sure is," said the nurse. She called the office and the office paged the doctor. Mrs. Klopstock watched in fascination while the team assembled and treated Mrs. White. A white spirit rose from Mrs. White's body, floated up toward the ceiling, then sank until it touched her lips. It was as if her breath had become visible. But the thing was creature-like, human sized. She heard Mrs. White gasp and the white, vaporous being seemed to disappear into her lungs. "She'll be all right now," said the doctor. "I am completely crazy," thought Mrs. Klopstock, "or I will be if I don't get out of here." But no one seemed able to move her from Mrs. White or Mrs. White from her.

Another week went by, then another. Three weeks had passed and then a fourth, and still Mrs. Klopstock insisted on living inside her own tent. Meanwhile, she caught a cold which settled in her ears. People came into the tent and she thought they were teasing her by moving their lips without speaking. She realized that she could not always hear, but she never knew when she was going to be deprived of her hearing. Her vision, too, was becoming blurry. The eye doctor who came to examine her said the fever had irritated the membranes and nerves of her eyes. She knew she was losing interest in life. She no longer answered the phone. There was no one to whom she could talk. More and more, she left the phone off the hook altogether. What could she tell them? That she was dying? Not of the fever, which was in her mind, but of something else, something worse.

The doctors insisted that there was nothing wrong with her. They pointed at the I.V. bottles and insisted that she was getting stronger every day. Sounds reached her from far away, as if she were underwater. She stopped watching television. She lay on her bed and thought. For the first time, she thought of herself as a collection of sensors bound together by a personality. She knew, when she closed her eyes, just where her mind was attached to her body. She could put her finger on the place. The two were joined loosely, as by a large, clumsy knot. Any fingers—fingers clumsy and sticky with youth—could undo it. She could feel the threads loosening. The sensors were malfunctioning. In dreams, she was a bird whose instincts had failed. She was flying over a dark sea and no longer knew which way to fly or how to stay in the air. She was dying. It was only a matter of time. She looked up and was not surprised to see a white shape floating above her. She had no desire to breathe it back in. She woke up in Intensive Care. "Potassium shock," said the nurse. She fell asleep.

Her doctor was standing over her. "We're sending you home next week," he said, "before something really happens to you." "Do you still think I have an infection of the heart?" she asked. "No," he said. "Why?" she asked. "Your fever didn't drop the way it should have; if you'd had that kind of infection, it would have dropped down within one or two days. Once we started, we had to finish." "See?" she said. "It's all in my head! I told you! I told you from the start!" "Let's not start on that again," he said.

* * * * *

The next day, Mrs. Klopstock, who had been returned to her room, came out of her tent. "You're looking white," said Mrs. White. "Pretty pale and awful." Mrs. Klopstock said she wasn't surprised. Mrs. White said that while Mrs. Klopstock had been away in Intensive Care, she had almost signed herself out because her husband had been taken to Kings County with a seizure. Mrs. Klopstock drew the curtains back and sat on the edge of her bed. Now that she was going home, she did not fear Mrs. White. She began to like her. Mrs. White exhorted her to get up. "The bed," she said, "takes all your strength." Mrs. Klopstock suggested that it was the fever, not the bed, which had worn her down. "It's the bed," said Mrs. White. "It sucks out all your strength. You don't start in walking now, you'll be an invalid when you get home. Go get us some ice." Mrs. Klopstock, filled with foreboding, set off for ice. "I made it back!" she said, dumping some ice into Mrs. White's water pitcher. "I told you," said Mrs. White. "A few more trips and you won't even be panting like an old hound out in the swamp."

As the day of her release approached, Mrs. Klopstock grew sicker and sicker. Her hearing flickered on and off as if she were a radio with many bad tubes. She was cold, then hot. Her eyes focused unexpectedly and equally unexpectedly blurred. One morning, sitting on a chair while the nurse made her bed, she thought she would shake herself from her seat onto the floor, she was so nervous. "I've never been so jumpy," she said to Mrs. White. "You're not used to it, that's all," said Mrs. White. "I'm ready to get in that bed with you," said Mrs. Klopstock.

"Come on in," said Mrs. White, "I'm waiting for you." When Mrs. Klopstock was released, she kissed Mrs. White goodbye and promised to call her. But she knew, in leaving, she was escaping. She had begun adjusting to Mrs. White, who was losing herself, piece by piece, and when she did so, she had turned her face from the land of the living toward the land of the dead.

When she got home, she was more dead than alive. She still had a fever, although now it was considered low-grade. She was convinced that she was going to die. Nothing anyone said changed her mind. She knew how she felt.

And so it happened that she came to worship Isaac Bashevis Singer. Her daughter had left three paperback volumes of his stories in the apartment. Her eyes had improved enough so that she could now read. She had not read a word during the eight weeks she spent in the hospital, but now she read the stories one after another. They were just the right length. She read one each time she took her temperature. Gradually, she came to believe that reading the stories lowered her temperature. At first, she was annoyed by Singer's characters. So many of them seemed crazy. But then she remembered the angels she had seen floating through the air in the hospital. His characters were no crazier than she was. Gradually, she began to think of Singer as the actual creator of actual creatures who were so much like her. He was like a God. He understood his creatures; he rarely judged them. He knew more than an ordinary human. She grew to believe that God had chosen Singer as his representative on earth. He had suffered so that he could testify. He had been rewarded for fulfilling his mission by great powers. So she began to pray to Isaac Bashevis Singer.

Now Mrs. Klopstock knew that it was forbidden to pray to a living person, but she remembered her mother appealing to the spirits of dead ancestors in times of trouble. She told herself she was doing nothing her mother had not done. She was only hurrying things up. Singer was not dead yet, but someday he would be. Why wait to pray to him? So she fell into the habit of calling upon Isaac Bashevis Singer when she felt as if it were a great effort merely to breathe in and out. "Isaac Bashevis Singer, save me!" She would cry to herself. And she began to feel better. Soon, she was better. Her daughter called to say she would be coming to see her and asked how she was. "Better," said Mrs. Klopstock. "First, I could do nothing. Now I can do next to nothing." "That's progress," said her daughter in a bored voice. "When are you coming?" she asked her daughter. Her daughter was vague. Mrs. Klopstock decided to try writing stories herself. There was no point in sitting around waiting for her daughter. She would, of course, dedicate the stories to the master. She prayed to him continually, out of habit, out of devout belief.

* * * * *

Mrs. Klopstock and her daughter were sitting in the kitchen. The walls were egg-yolk yellow. Her daughter insisted that she had not visited her mother in the hospital because hospitals frightened her. Her mother knew that, she said. With a fingertip, she traced figure eights on the table. What, Mrs. Klopstock asked herself, was she doing with this large, middle-aged, alien child? She would die without ever having tried to talk to her. "You know, Elsa," she said, "those books you left here? By Singer? I read them." "That's good," said her daughter. "And now I pray to him," said Mrs. Klopstock. "He healed me." "You're not serious, of course," said her daughter. "Oh yes I am," she said. Her daughter would not look at her. "Don't worry, I'm not crazy," said Mrs. Klopstock.

"You sound," said her daughter, "crazy as a bedbug." "He has the power to answer prayers because he writes," Mrs. Klopstock said. Her daughter stared at her. "You," she began, "you haven't started writing?" "Oh yes I have!" Mrs. Klopstock said triumphantly. "Writing gives me strength." "But you can't do that!" her daughter sputtered. "You can't give away family secrets! You can't do things like that!" "What makes you think I'm writing about the family?" her mother asked. (In fact, she was.) She watched her daughter; she could hear her thinking. "Are you going to show him the stories?" her daughter asked at last. "Who?" asked Mrs. Klopstock.

"Singer?"

"Oh, Singer. God forbid. I don't want anyone, especially him, to know what they're about." Her daughter looked at her as if to say that she shouldn't worry; the stories probably weren't about anything anyway. "They are about something all right," said her mother. Her daughter looked at her with something like fear. "Ma," she said, "don't tell anyone about this business. This worshipping Singer stuff." "Whose business is it?" Mrs. Klopstock asked rhetorically. "You know," she said, "last night I had the most curious dream. I dreamed I found a beautiful doll's head right on the kitchen table and the doll had the most beautiful brown hair you ever saw. So I showed it to my parents, and to grandma, she was there too, and they all said, but the doll doesn't have a body. And that confused me because I hadn't noticed. So I put the doll's head back down on the table and I saw there were crumbs there and they would get in the doll's hair and I was afraid rats would come and chew on her hair, and I couldn't figure out how to get the crumbs out of her hair. And they kept saying that she didn't have a body, but when I looked at the doll, I could see it even if they couldn't. What do you think it means?" "God knows," said her daughter, shuddering. "I used to make dolls," said her mother. "Not the heads but the bodies. That's how you made them in those days. You bought the heads and hands and feet and made the bodies yourself." "Let's change the subject," said her daughter. "I used to keep extra heads. In case one broke," said Mrs. Klopstock. "Mother!" exclaimed Elsa.

"I know what it means," said Mrs. Klopstock. "What does it mean?" asked Elsa. "You wouldn't understand," said her mother. "Who would," asked her daughter, "Singer?" Her daughter was upset, sarcastic. This was not the mother she knew. "It's a dream about the mind and the body," said her daughter smugly. "What about them, Miss Smartypants?" asked her mother. Elsa didn't answer. "You don't know," said her mother. "Who does?" asked her daughter.

"Singer knows," said Mrs. Klopstock.

She got up and brushed some imaginary crumbs from her skirt and went to the stove to look after their tea. "Do you dream a lot?" her daughter asked wistfully, but Mrs. Klopstock was running water in the sink and did not hear her. Her daughter pressed both her hot palms to the cool enamel table. She knew she would be afraid to reread the Singer stories now. Her mother was smiling to herself and humming. A white cloud of steam rose in the air and hovered there. For a moment, the room tilted and then it seemed to right itself.

SILENT SNOW, SECRET SNOW

CONRAD AIKEN

I

Just why it should have happened, or why it should have happened just when it did, he could not, of course, possibly have said; nor perhaps would it even have occurred to him to ask. The thing was above all secret, something to be preciously concealed from Mother and Father; and to that very fact it owed an enormous part of its deliciousness. It was like a peculiarly beautiful trinket to be carried unmentioned in one's trouser-pocket,—a rare stamp, an old coin, a few tiny gold links found trodden out of shape on the path in the park, a pebble of carnelian, a sea shell distinguishable from all others by an unusual spot or stripe,—and, as if it were any one of these, he carried around with him everywhere a warm and persistent and increasingly beautiful sense of possession. Nor was it only a sense of possession—it was also a sense of protection. It was as if, in some delightful way, his secret gave him a fortress, a wall behind which he could retreat into heavenly seclusion. This was almost the first thing he had noticed about it—apart from the oddness of the thing itself—and it was this that now again, for the fiftieth time, occurred to him, as he sat in the little schoolroom. It was the half hour for geography. Miss Buell was revolving with one finger, slowly, a huge terrestrial globe which had been placed on her desk. The green and yellow continents passed and repassed, questions were asked and answered, and now the little girl in front of him, Deirdre, who had a funny little constellation of freckles on the back of her neck, exactly like the Big Dipper, was standing up and telling Miss Buell that the equator was the line that ran round the middle.

Miss Buell's face, which was old and greyish and kindly, with grey stiff curls beside the cheeks, and eyes that swam very brightly, like little minnows, behind thick glasses, wrinkled itself into a complication of amusements.

"Ah! I see. The earth is wearing a belt, or a sash. Or someone drew a line around it!"

Written by Conrad Aiken in 1932, this story is reprinted from *A Book of Contemporary Short Stories,* edited by Dorothy Brewster (New York: Macmillan, 1937): 93–114.

"Oh no—not that—I mean—"

In the general laughter, he did not share, or only a very little. He was thinking about the Arctic and Antarctic regions, which of course, on the globe, were white. Miss Buell was now telling them about the tropics, the jungles, the steamy heat of equatorial swamps, where the birds and butterflies, and even the snakes, were like living jewels. As he listened to these things, he was already, with a pleasant sense of half-effort, putting his secret between himself and the words. Was it really an effort at all? For effort implied something voluntary, and perhaps even something one did not especially want; whereas this was distinctly pleasant, and came almost of its own accord. All he needed to do was to think of that morning, the first one, and then of all the others—

But it was all so absurdly simple! It had amounted to so little. It was nothing, just an idea—and just why it should have become so wonderful, so permanent, was a mystery—a very pleasant one, to be sure, but also, in an amusing way, foolish. However, without ceasing to listen to Miss Buell, who had now moved up to the north temperate zones, he deliberately invited his memory of the first morning. It was only a moment or two after he had waked up—or perhaps the moment itself. But was there, to be exact, an exact moment? Was one awake all at once? or was it gradual? Anyway, it was after he had stretched a lazy hand up towards the headrail, and yawned, and then relaxed again among his warm covers, all the more grateful on a December morning, that the thing had happened. Suddenly, for no reason, he had thought of the postman, he remembered the postman. Perhaps there was nothing so odd in that. After all, he heard the postman almost every morning in his life—his heavy boots could be heard clumping round the corner at the top of the little cobbled hill-street, and then, progressively nearer, progressively louder, the double knock at each door, the crossings and re-crossings of the street, till finally the clumsy steps came stumbling across to the very door, and the tremendous knock came which shook the house itself.

(Miss Buell was saying "Vast wheat-growing areas in North America and Siberia." Deirdre had for the moment placed her left hand across the back of her neck.)

But on this particular morning, the first morning, as he lay there with his eyes closed, he had for some reason *waited* for the postman. He wanted to hear him come round the corner. And that was precisely the joke—he never did. He never came. He never had come—*round the corner*—again. For when at last steps *were* heard, they had already, he was quite sure, come a little down the hill, to the first house; and even so, the steps were curiously different—they were softer, they had a new secrecy about them, they were muffled and indistinct; and while the rhythm of them was the same, it now said a new thing—it said peace, it said remoteness, it said cold, it said sleep. And he had understood the situation at once—nothing could have seemed simpler—there had been snow in the night, such as all winter he had been longing for; and it was this which had rendered the postman's first footsteps inaudible, and the later ones faint. Of course! How lovely! And even now it must be snowing—it was going to be a snowy day—the long white ragged lines were drifting and sifting across the street, across the faces of the old houses, whispering and hushing, making little triangles of white in the corners between cobblestones, seething a little when the wind blew them over the ground to a drifted corner; and so it would be all day, getting deeper and deeper and silenter and silenter.

(Miss Buell was saying "Land of perpetual snow.")

All this time, of course (while he lay in bed), he had kept his eyes closed, listening to the nearer progress of the postman, the muffled footsteps thumping and slipping on the snow-sheathed cobbles; and all the other sounds—the double knocks, a frosty far-off voice or two, a bell ringing thinly and softly as if under a sheet of ice—had the same slightly abstracted quality, as if removed by one degree from actuality—as if everything in the world had been insulated by snow. But when at last, pleased, he opened his eyes, and turned them toward the window, to see for himself this long-desired and now so clearly imagined miracle—what he saw instead was brilliant sunlight on a roof; and when, astonished, he jumped out of bed and stared down into the street, expecting to see the cobbles obliterated by the snow, he saw nothing but the bare bright cobbles themselves.

Queer, the effect this extraordinary surprise had had upon him—all the following morning he had kept with him a sense as of snow falling about him, a secret screen of new snow between himself and the world. If he had not dreamed such a thing—and how could he have dreamed it while awake?—how else could one explain it? In any case, the delusion had been so vivid as to affect his entire behavior. He could not now remember whether it was on the first or the second morning—or was it even the third?—that his mother had drawn attention to some oddness in his manner.

"But my darling—" she had said at the breakfast table—"what has come over you? You don't seem to be listening. . . ."

And how often that very thing had happened since!

(Miss Buell was now asking if anyone knew the difference between the North Pole and the Magnetic Pole. Deirdre was holding up her flickering brown hand, and he could see the four white dimples that marked the knuckles.)

Perhaps it hadn't been either the second or third morning—or even the fourth or fifth. How could he be sure. How could he be sure just when the delicious *progress* had become clear? Just when it had really *begun*? The intervals weren't very precise. . . . All he now knew was, that at some point or other—perhaps the second day, perhaps the sixth—he had noticed that the presence of the snow was a little more insistent, the sound of it clearer; and, conversely, the sound of the postman's footsteps more indistinct. Not only could he not hear the steps come round the corner, he could not even hear them at the first house. It was below the first house that he heard them; and then, a few days later, it was below the second house that he had heard them; and a few days later again, below the third. Gradually, gradually, the snow was becoming heavier, the sound of its seething louder, the cobblestones more and more muffled. When he found, each morning, on going to the window, after the ritual of listening, that the roofs and cobbles were as bare as ever, it made no difference. This was, after all, only what he had expected. It was even what pleased him, what rewarded him: the thing was his own, belonged to no one else. No one else knew about it, not even his mother and father. There, outside, were the bare cobbles; and here, inside, was the snow. Snow growing heavier each day, muffling the world, hiding the ugly, and deadening increasingly—above all—the steps of the postman.

"But my darling—" she had said at the luncheon table—"what has come over you? You don't seem to listen when people speak to you. That's the third time I've asked you to pass your plate. . . ."

How was one to explain this to Mother? or to Father? There was, of course, nothing to be done about it: nothing. All one could do was to laugh embarrassedly, pretend to be a little ashamed, apologize, and take a sudden and somewhat disingenuous interest in what was being done or said. The cat had stayed out all night. He had a curious swelling on his left cheek—perhaps somebody had kicked him, or a stone had struck him. Mrs. Kempton was or was not coming to tea. The house was going to be house cleaned, or "turned out," on Wednesday instead of Friday. A new lamp was provided for his evening work—perhaps it was eyestrain which accounted for this new and so peculiar vagueness of his—Mother was looking at him with amusement as she said this, but with something else as well. A new lamp? A new lamp. Yes Mother, No Mother, Yes Mother. School is going very well. The geometry is very easy. The history is very dull. The geography is very interesting—particularly when it takes one to the North Pole. Why the North Pole? Oh, well, it would be fun to be an explorer. Another Peary or Scott or Shackleton. And then abruptly he found his interest in the talk at an end, stared at the pudding on his plate, listened, waited, and began once more—ah how heavenly, too, the first beginnings—to hear or feel—for could he actually hear it?—the silent snow, the secret snow.

(Miss Buell was telling them about the search for the Northwest Passage, about Hendrik Hudson, the *Half Moon.*)

This had been, indeed, the only distressing feature of the new experience: the fact that it so increasingly had brought him into a kind of mute misunderstanding, or even conflict, with his father and mother. It was as if he were trying to lead a double life. On the one hand he had to be Paul Hasleman, and keep up the appearance of being that person—dress, wash, and answer intelligently when spoken to—; on the other, he had to explore this new world which had been opened to him. Nor could there be the slightest doubt—not the slightest—that the new world was the profounder and more wonderful of the two. It was irresistible. It was miraculous. Its beauty was simply beyond anything—beyond speech as beyond thought—utterly incommunicable. But how then, between the two worlds, of which he was thus constantly aware, was he to keep a balance? One must get up, one must go to breakfast, one must talk with Mother, go to school, do one's lessons—and, in all this, try not to appear too much of a fool. But if all the while one was also trying to extract the full deliciousness of another and quite separate existence, one which could not easily (if at all) be spoken of—how was one to manage? How was one to explain? Would it be safe to explain? Would it be absurd? Would it merely mean that he would get into some obscure kind of trouble?

These thoughts came and went, came and went, as softly and secretly as the snow; they were not precisely a disturbance, perhaps they were even a pleasure; he liked to have them; their presence was something almost palpable, something he could stroke with his hand, without closing his eyes, and without ceasing to see Miss Buell and the school-room and the globe and the freckles on Deirdre's neck; nevertheless he did in a sense cease to see, or to see the obvious external world, and substituted for this vision the vision of snow, the sound of snow, and the slow, almost soundless, approach of the postman. Yesterday, it had been only at the sixth house that the postman had become audible; the snow was much deeper now, it was falling more swiftly and heavily, the sound of its seething was more distinct, more soothing, more persistent. And this morning, it had been—as nearly as he could figure—just above the seventh house—perhaps only a step or two above: at most, he had heard two or three footsteps before the knock had sounded. . . . And with each such narrowing of the sphere, each nearer approach of the limit at which the postman was first audible, it was odd how sharply was increased the amount of illusion which had to be carried into the ordinary business of daily life. Each day, it was harder to get out of bed, to go to the window, to look out at the—as always—perfectly empty and snowless street. Each day it was more difficult to go through the perfunctory motions of greeting Mother and Father at breakfast, to reply to their questions, to put his books together and go to school. And at school, how extraordinarily hard to conduct with success simultaneously the public life and the life that was secret. There were times when he longed—positively ached—to tell everyone about it—to burst out with it—only to be checked almost at once by a far-off feeling as of some faint absurdity which was inherent in it—but *was* it absurd?—and more importantly by a sense of mysterious power in his very secrecy. Yes: it must be kept secret. That, more and more, became clear. At whatever cost to himself, whatever pain to others—

(Miss Buell looked straight at him, smiling, and said, "Perhaps we'll ask Paul. I'm sure Paul will come out of his day-dream long enough to be able to tell us. Won't you, Paul." He rose slowly from his chair, resting one hand on the brightly varnished desk, and deliberately stared through the snow towards the blackboard. It was an effort, but it was amusing to make it. "Yes," he said slowly, "it was what we now call the Hudson River. This he thought to be the Northwest Passage. He was disappointed." He sat down again, and as he did so Deirdre half turned in her chair and gave him a shy smile, of approval and admiration.)

At whatever pain to others.

This part of it was very puzzling, very puzzling. Mother was very nice, and so was Father. Yes, that was all true enough. He wanted to be nice to them, to tell them everything—and yet, was it really wrong of him to want to have a secret place of his own?

At bedtime, the night before, Mother had said, "If this goes on, my lad, we'll have to see a doctor, we will! We can't have our boy—" But what was it she had said? "Live in another world"? "Live so far away"? The word "far" had been it, he was sure, and then Mother had taken up a magazine again and laughed a little, but with an expression which wasn't mirthful. He had felt sorry for her. . . .

The bell rang for dismissal. The sound came to him through long curved parallels of falling snow. He saw Deirdre rise, and had himself risen almost as soon—but not quite as soon—as she.

II

On the walk homeward, which was timeless, it pleased him to see through the accompaniment, or counterpoint, of snow, the items of mere externality on his way. There were many kinds of brick in the sidewalks, and laid in many kinds of pattern. The garden walls too were various, some of wooden palings, some of plaster, some of stone. Twigs of bushes leaned over the walls: the little hard green winter-buds of lilac, on grey stems, sheathed and fat; other branches very thin and fine and black and desiccated. Dirty sparrows huddled in the bushes, as dull in colour as dead fruit left in leafless trees. A single starling creaked on a weather vane. In the gutter, beside a drain, was a scrap of torn and dirty newspaper, caught in a little delta of filth: the word ECZEMA appeared in large capitals, and below it was a letter from Mrs. Amelia D. Cravath, 2100 Pine Street, Fort Worth, Texas, to the effect that after being a sufferer for years she had been cured by Caley's Ointment. In the little delta, beside the fan-shaped and deeply runnelled continent of brown mud, were lost twigs, descended from their parent trees, dead matches, a rusty horse-chestnut burr, a small concentration of sparkling gravel on the lip of the sewer, a fragment of egg-shell, a streak of yellow sawdust which had been wet and now was dry and congealed, a brown pebble, and a broken feather. Further on was a cement sidewalk, ruled into geometrical parallelograms, with a brass inlay at one end commemorating the contractors who had laid it, and, halfway across, an irregular and random series of dog-tracks, immortalized in synthetic stone. He knew these well, and always stepped on them; to cover the little hollows with his own foot had always been a queer pleasure; today he did it once more, but perfunctorily and detachedly, all the while thinking of something else. That was a dog, a long time ago, who had made a mistake and walked on the cement while it was still wet. He had probably wagged his tail, but that hadn't been recorded. Now, Paul Hasleman, aged twelve, on his way home from school, crossed the same river, which in the meantime had frozen into rock. Homeward through the snow, the snow falling in bright sunshine. Homeward?

Then came the gateway with the two posts surmounted by egg-shaped stones which had been cunningly balanced on their ends, as if by Columbus, and mortared in the very act of balance: a source of perpetual wonder. On the brick wall just beyond, the letter H had been stenciled, presumably for some purpose. H? H.

The green hydrant, with a little green-painted chain attached to the brass screw-cap.

The elm tree, with the great grey wound in the bark, kidney-shaped, into which he always put his hand—to feel the cold but living wood. The injury, he had been sure, was due to the gnawings of a tethered horse. But now it deserved only a passing palm, a merely tolerant eye. There were more important things. Miracles. Beyond the thoughts of trees, mere elms. Beyond the thoughts of sidewalks, mere stone, mere brick, mere cement. Beyond the thoughts even of his own shoes, which trod these sidewalks obediently, bearing a burden—far above—of elaborate mystery. He watched them. They were not very well polished; he had neglected them, for a very good reason: they were one of the many parts of the increasing difficulty of the daily return to daily life, the morning struggle. To get up, having at last opened one's eyes, to go to the window, and discover no snow, to wash, to dress, to descend the curving stairs to breakfast—.

At whatever pain to others, nevertheless, one must persevere in severance, since the incommunicability of the experience demanded it. It was desirable of course to be kind to Mother and Father, especially as they seemed to be worried, but it was also desirable to be resolute. If they should decide—as appeared likely—to consult the doctor, Doctor Howells, and have Paul inspected, his heart listened to through a kind of dictaphone, his lungs, his stomach—well, that was all right. He would go through with it. He would give them answer for question, too—perhaps such answers as they hadn't expected? No. That would never do. For the secret world must, at all costs, be preserved.

The bird-house in the apple-tree was empty—it was the wrong time of year for wrens. The little round black door had lost its pleasure. The wrens were enjoying other houses, other nests, remoter trees. But this too was a notion which he only vaguely and grazingly entertained—as if, for the moment, he merely touched an edge of it; there was something further on, which was already assuming a sharper importance; something which already teased at the corners of his eyes, teasing also at the corner of his mind. It was funny to think that he so wanted this, so awaited it—and yet found himself enjoying this momentary dalliance with the bird-house, as if for a quite deliberate postponement and enhancement of the approaching pleasure. He was aware of his delay, of his smiling detached and now almost uncomprehending gaze at the little bird-house; he knew what he was going to look at next: it was his own little cobbled hill-street, his own house, the little river at the bottom of the hill, the grocer's shop with the cardboard man in the window—and now, thinking of all this, he turned his head, still smiling, and looking quickly right and left through the snow-laden sunlight.

And the mist of snow, as he had foreseen, was still on it—a ghost of snow falling in the bright sunlight, softly and steadily floating and turning and pausing, soundlessly meeting the snow that covered, as with a transparent mirage, the bare bright cobbles. He loved it—he stood still and loved it. Its beauty was paralyzing—beyond all words, all experience, all dream. No fairy-story he had ever read could be compared with it—none had ever given him this extraordinary combination of ethereal loveliness with a something else, unnameable, which was just faintly and deliciously terrifying. What was this thing? As he thought of it, he looked upward toward his own bedroom window, which was open—and it was as if he looked straight into the room and saw himself lying half awake in his bed. There he was—at this very instant he was still perhaps actually there—more truly there than standing here at the edge of the cobbled hill-street, with one hand lifted to shade his eyes against the snow-sun. Had he indeed ever left his room, in all this time? Since that very first morning? Was the whole progress still being enacted there, was it still the same morning, and himself not yet wholly awake? And even now, had the postman not yet come around the corner? . . .

This idea amused him, and automatically, as he thought of it, he turned his head and looked toward the top of the hill. There was, of course, nothing there—nothing and no one. The street was empty and quiet. And all the more because of its emptiness it occurred to him to count the houses—a thing which, oddly enough, he hadn't before thought of doing. Of course, he had known there weren't many—many, that is on his own side of the street, which were the ones that figured in the postman's progress—but nevertheless it came to him as something of a shock to find that there were precisely *six,* above his own house—his own house was the seventh.

Six!

Astonished, he looked at his own house—looked at the door, on which was the number thirteen—and then realized that the whole thing was exactly and logically and absurdly what he ought to have known. Just the same, the realization gave him abruptly, and even a little frighteningly, a sense of hurry. He was being hurried—he was being rushed. For—he knit his brows—he couldn't be mistaken—it was just above the *seventh* house, his own house, that the postman had first been audible this very morning. But in that case—in that case—did it mean that tomorrow he would hear nothing? The knock he had heard must have been the knock of their own door. Did it mean—and this was an idea which gave him a really extraordinary feeling of surprise—that he would never hear the postman again?—that tomorrow morning the postman would already have passed the house, in a snow by then so deep as to render his footsteps completely inaudible? That he would have made his approach down the snow-filled street so soundlessly, so secretly, that he, Paul Hasleman, there lying in bed, would not have waked in time, or, waking, would have heard nothing?

But how could that be? Unless even the knocker should be muffled in the snow—frozen tight, perhaps? . . . But in that case—

A vague feeling of disappointment came over him; a vague sadness, as if he felt himself deprived of something which he had long looked forward to, something much prized. After all this, all this beautiful progress, the slow delicious advance of the postman through the silent and secret snow, the knock creeping closer each day, and the footsteps nearer, the audible compass of the world thus daily narrowed, narrowed, narrowed, as the snow soothingly and beautifully encroached and deepened, after all this, was he to be defrauded of the one thing he had so wanted—to be able to count, as it were, the last two or three solemn footsteps, as they finally approached his own door? Was it all going to happen, at the end, so suddenly? or indeed, had it already happened? with no slow and subtle gradations of menace, in which he could luxuriate?

He gazed upward again, toward his own window which flashed in the sun: and this time almost with a feeling that it would be better if he *were* still in bed, in that room; for in that case this must still be the first morning, and there would be six more mornings to come—or, for that matter, seven or eight or nine—how could he be sure?—or even more.

III

After supper, the inquisition began. He stood before the doctor, under the lamp, and submitted silently to the usual thumpings and tappings.

"Now will you please say 'Ah!'?"

"Ah!"

"Now again please, if you don't mind."

"Ah."

"Say it slowly, and hold it if you can—"

"Ah-h-h-h-h-h—"

"Good."

How silly all this was. As if it had anything to do with his throat! Or his heart or lungs!

Relaxing his mouth, of which the corners, after all this absurd stretching, felt uncomfortable, he avoided the doctor's eyes, and stared towards the fireplace, past his mother's feet (in grey slippers) which projected from the green chair, and his father's feet (in brown slippers) which stood neatly side by side on the hearth rug.

"Hm. There is certainly nothing wrong there. . . ."

He felt the doctor's eyes fixed upon him, and, as if merely to be polite, returned the look, but with a feeling of justifiable evasiveness.

"Now, young man, tell me—do you feel all right?"

"Yes, sir, quite right."

"No headaches? no dizziness?"

"No, I don't think so."

"Let me see. Let's get a book, if you don't mind—yes, thank you, that will do splendidly—and now, Paul, if you'll just read it, holding it as you would normally hold it—"

He took the book and read:

"And another praise have I to tell for this the city our mother, the gift of a great god, a glory of the land most high; the might of horses, the might of young horses, the might of the sea. . . . For thou, son of Cronus, our lord Poseidon, hast throned herein this pride, since in these roads first thou didst show forth the curb that cures the rage of steeds. And the shapely oar, apt to men's hands, hath a wondrous speed on the brine, following the hundred-footed Nereids. . . . O land that art praised above all lands, now is it for thee to make those bright praises seen in deeds."

He stopped, tentatively, and lowered the heavy book.

"No—as I thought—there is certainly no superficial sign of eye-strain."

Silence thronged the room, and he was aware of the focused scrutiny of the three people who confronted him. . . .

"We could have his eyes examined—but I believe it is something else."

"What could it be?" This was his father's voice.

"It's only this curious absent-mindedness—" This was his mother's voice.

In the presence of the doctor, they both seemed irritatingly apologetic.

"I believe it is something else. Now Paul—I would like very much to ask you a question or two. You will answer them, won't you—you know I'm an old, old friend of yours, eh? That's right! . . ."

His back was thumped twice by the doctor's fat fist—then the doctor was grinning at him with false amiability, while with one finger-nail he was scratching the top button of his waistcoat. Beyond the doctor's shoulder was the fire, the fingers of flame making light prestidigitation against the sooty fireback, the soft sound of their random flutter the only sound.

"I would like to know—is there anything that worries you?"

The doctor was again smiling, his eyelids low against the little black pupils, in each of which was a tiny white bead of light. Why answer him? Why answer him at all? "At whatever pain to others"—but it was all a nuisance, this necessity for resistance, this necessity for attention: it was as if one had been stood up on a brilliantly lighted stage, under a great round blaze of spotlight; as if one were merely a trained seal, or a performing dog, or a fish, dipped out of an aquarium and held up by the tail. It would serve them right if he were merely to bark or growl. And meanwhile, to miss these last few precious hours, these hours of which every minute was more beautiful than the last, more menacing—? He still looked, as if from a great distance, at the beads of light in the doctor's eyes, at the fixed false smile, and then, beyond, once more at his mother's slippers, his father's slippers, the soft flutter of the fire. Even here, even amongst these hostile presences, and in this arranged light, he could see the snow, he could hear it—it was in the corners of the room, where the shadow was deepest, under the sofa, behind the half-opened door which led to the dining-room. It was gentler here, softer, its seethe the quietest of whispers, as if, in deference to a drawing-room, it had quite deliberately put on its "manners"; it kept itself out of sight, obliterated itself, but distinctly with an air of saying, "Ah, but just wait! Wait till we are alone together! Then I will begin to tell you something new! Something white! Something cold! Something sleepy! Something of cease, and peace, and the long bright curve of space! Tell them to go away. Banish them. Refuse to speak. Leave them, go upstairs to your room, turn out the light and get into bed—I will go with you, I will be waiting for you, I will tell you a better story than *Little Kay of the Skates,* or *The Snow Ghost*—I will surround your bed, I will close the windows, pile a deep drift against the door, so that none will ever again be able to enter. Speak to them! . . ." It seemed as if the little hissing voice came from a slow white spiral of falling flakes in the corner by the front window—but he could not be sure. He felt himself smiling, then, and said to the doctor, but without looking at him, looking beyond him still—

"Oh no, I think not—"

"But are you sure, my boy?"

His father's voice came softly and coldly then—the familiar voice of silken warning. . . .

"You needn't answer at once, Paul—remember we're trying to help you—think it over and be quite sure, won't you?"

He felt himself smiling again, at the notion of being quite sure. What a joke! As if he weren't so sure that reassurance was no longer necessary, and all this cross-examination a ridiculous farce, a grotesque parody! What could they know about it? These gross intelligences, these humdrum minds so bound to the usual, the ordinary? Impossible to tell them about it! Why, even now, even now, with the proof so abundant, so formidable, so imminent, so appallingly present here in this very room, could they believe it?—could even his mother believe it? No—it was only too plain that if anything were said about it, the merest hint given, they would be incredulous—they would laugh—they would say "absurd!"—think things about him which weren't true. . . .

"Why no, I'm not worried—why should I be?"

He looked then straight at the doctor's low-lidded eyes, looked from one of them to the other, from one bead of light to the other, and gave a little laugh.

The doctor seemed to be disconcerted by this. He drew back in his chair, resting a fat white hand on either knee. The smile faded slowly from his face.

"Well, Paul!" he said, and paused gravely, "I'm afraid you don't take this quite seriously enough. I think you perhaps don't quite realize—don't quite realize—"

He took a deep quick breath, and turned, as if helplessly, at a loss for words, to the others. But Mother and Father were both silent—no help was forthcoming.

"You must surely know, be aware, that you have not been quite yourself, of late? don't you know that? . . ."

It was amusing to watch the doctor's renewed attempt at a smile, a queer disorganized look, as of confidential embarrassment.

"I feel all right, sir," he said, and again gave the little laugh.

"And we're trying to help you." The doctor's tone sharpened.

"Yes sir, I know. But why? I'm all right. I'm just *thinking,* that's all."

His mother made a quick movement forward, resting a hand on the back of the doctor's chair.

"Thinking?" she said. "But my dear, about what?"

This was a direct challenge—and would have to be directly met. But before he met it, he looked again into the corner by the door, as if for reassurance. He smiled again at what he saw, at what he heard. The little spiral was still there, still softly whirling, like the ghost of a white kitten chasing the ghost of a white tail, and making as it did so the faintest of whispers. It was all right! If only he could remain firm, everything was going to be all right.

"Oh, about anything, about nothing—*you* know the way you do!"

"You mean—day-dreaming?"

"Oh, no—thinking!"

"But thinking about *what*?"

"Anything."

He laughed a third time—but this time, happening to glance upward towards his mother's face, he was appalled at the effect his laughter seemed to have upon her. Her mouth had opened in an expression of horror. . . . This was too bad! Unfortunate! He had known it would cause pain, of course—but he hadn't expected it to be quite so bad as this. Perhaps—perhaps if he just gave them a tiny gleaming hint—?

"About the snow," he said.

"What on earth!" This was his father's voice. The brown slippers came a step nearer on the hearth-rug.

"But my dear, what do you mean!" This was his mother's voice.

The doctor merely stared.

"Just *snow,* that's all. I like to think about it."

"Tell us about it, my boy."

"But that's all it is. There's nothing to tell. *You* know what snow is?"

This he said almost angrily, for he felt that they were trying to corner him. He turned sideways so as no longer to face the doctor, and the better to see the inch of blackness between the window-sill and the lowered curtain—the cold inch of beckoning and delicious night. At once he felt better, more assured.

"Mother—can I go to bed, now, please? I've got a headache."

"But I thought you said—"

"It's just come. It's all these questions—! Can I, mother?"

"You can go as soon as the doctor has finished."

"Don't you think this thing ought to be gone into thoroughly, and *now*?" This was Father's voice. The brown slippers again came a step nearer, the voice was the well-known "punishment" voice, resonant and cruel.

"Oh, what's the use, Norman—"

Quite suddenly, everyone was silent. And without precisely facing them, nevertheless he was aware that all three of them were watching him with an extraordinary intensity—staring hard at him—as if he had done something monstrous, or was himself some kind of monster. He could hear the soft irregular flutter of the flames; the cluck-click-cluck-click of the clock; far and faint, two sudden spurts of laughter from the kitchen, as quickly cut off as begun; a murmur of water in the pipes; and then the silence seemed to deepen, to spread out, to become worldlong and worldwide, to become timeless and shapeless, and to center inevitably and rightly, with a slow and sleepy but enormous concentration of all power, on the beginning of a new sound. What this new sound was going to be, he knew perfectly well. It might begin with a hiss, but it would end with a roar—there was no time to lose—he must escape. It mustn't happen here—

Without another word, he turned and ran up the stairs.

IV

Not a moment too soon. The darkness was coming in long white waves. A prolonged sibilance filled the night—a great seamless seethe of wild influence went abruptly across it—a cold low humming shook the windows. He shut the door and flung off his clothes in the dark. The bare black floor was like a little raft tossed in waves of snow, almost overwhelmed, washed under whitely, up again, smothered in curled billows of feather. The snow was laughing: it spoke from all sides at once: it pressed closer to him as he ran and jumped exulting into his bed.

"Listen to us!" it said. "Listen! We have come to tell you the story we told you about. You remember? Lie down. Shut your eyes, now—you will no longer see much—in this white darkness who could see, or want to see? We will take the place of everything. . . . Listen—"

A beautiful varying dance of snow began at the front of the room, came forward and then retreated, flattened out toward the floor, then rose fountain-like to the ceiling, swayed, recruited itself from a new stream of flakes which poured laughing in through the humming window, advanced again, lifted long white arms. It said peace, it said remoteness, it said cold—it said—

But then a gash of horrible light fell brutally across the room from the opening door—the snow drew back hissing—something alien had come into the room—something hostile. This thing rushed at him, clutched at him, shook him—and he was not merely horrified, he was filled with such a loathing as he had never known. What was this? This cruel disturbance? This act of anger and hate? It was as if he had to reach up a hand toward another world for any understanding of it—an effort of which he was only barely capable. But of that other world he still remembered just enough to know the exorcising words. They tore themselves from his other life suddenly—

"Mother! Mother! Go away! I hate you!"

And with that effort, everything was solved, everything became all right: the seamless hiss advanced once more, the long white wavering lines rose and fell like enormous whispering sea-waves, the whisper becoming louder, the laughter more numerous.

"Listen!" it said. "We'll tell you the last, the most beautiful and secret story—shut your eyes—it is a very small story—a story that gets smaller and smaller—it comes inward instead of opening like a flower—it is a flower becoming a seed—a little cold seed—do you hear? we are leaning closer to you—"

The hiss was now becoming a roar—the whole world was a vast moving screen of snow—but even now it said peace, it said remoteness, it said cold, it said sleep.

A SENSE OF THREAT

JANE LAZARRE

I am trying to understand one experience by what it shares with another. Patterns come to me, clusters of memories that seem to belong together, and I cannot, simply for the sake of ease or sequence, keep them apart. Old memories of the months preceding and the early years after my mother's death when I was seven years old. A panic attack I experienced when Khary was attending a semester abroad, months before the cancer cells won their battle with my immune system and hardened into a tumor. And chemotherapy, which so frightened me I could write neither the word nor the name of the doctor in my journal but had to resort to initials, or watch my barely manageable fears escalate out of control.

I will not perceive the connections among these memories until all the cancer treatments are done. But I am dreaming with vague knowledge of being ashamed, and the shame is always for needing something I cannot have, or something that is not what I thought it to be. Somehow, I am humiliated, not merely disappointed; exposed, not merely wrong. A little beggar girl I saw long ago in a poverty-stricken street in Naples is in my kitchen. She looks at me with the pathetic eyes of a hungry cat and scratches on my refrigerator door with dirty, bitten nails. A river fills with blood, and long-missing bodies float to the surface while I sit in a boat aloof, even dissociated, wondering at the strangeness of what is happening right before my eyes. A distanced critic, I watch the dramas and keep track of all the themes.

Now, I turn back the pages of my journal to the day I found the lump, a surprisingly undifferentiated hardness I wasn't even sure was a lump at first. I read my brief entry the day I went for a needle biopsy and received the diagnosis. "You are the fifth person I have diagnosed with breast cancer this morning," the radiologist said to me, and it was only noon. "It's an epidemic."

But eight months before that, when I was experiencing increasingly intense panic attacks, I had written: I feel as if an actual illness inhabits me. Something at once foreign and part of me devouring myself.

I appreciate the danger of ascribing facile metaphor to illness, especially to cancer. I can become angry at the many books and acquaintances who advise one to move to northern Maine, where a hypnotic serenity presumably neutralizes the effect of sorrow and loss, to subsist on brown rice and seaweed, or "eliminate stress" from one's life (an injunction that only increases stress in me, as I become stressed by the thought of how much stress there is in my life.) I am suspicious of alternative healing methods that overemphasize the "spiritual" core of physical illness and even counsel an avoidance of Western medical knowledge. My life has been saved by Western medicine, an early, relatively small cancerous tumor removed from my breast, followed by harsh chemical treatments that have hopefully destroyed any cancer cells that might have been left behind.

But there is a sense one gains irrevocably after a life-threatening illness, that the mind, or spirit, and body are indeed one, or at least in intimate communion. I believe in the reality of the spirit and that it can be hurt as well as healed. For me, that healing always involves various forms of storytelling—the kind you recount to a therapist in that space out of ordinary space and time out of ordinary time called a "session"; the kind you write and rewrite in various formulations, experimenting with various designs; the kind you dream. It is in the perception of design that I experience healing, and if that word has been rolled around too often by shallow minds seeking instant and painless transformation so that it has lost its original power to suggest the relief of remedy, the joy of cure, I find that I still remain attached to its old-fashioned, simple promise that what is broken can, at least sometimes, be repaired.

* * * * *

Between chemotherapy treatments are three weeks during which I try to make myself as strong as possible in body and mind, not only to prepare myself for what is a terrifying encounter each time but to build up my immune system in the face of attack. Close friends offer love and gifts, and one of the most treasured is the gift of several weeks' stay in Bellport, Long Island, at the home of my friends, Sally and Bill, who are traveling in China. Reading or sleeping in these large, quiet rooms where all day and into twilight the sun alters the pale off-white colors of the walls, reflecting rosy pink, pale green, a slightly bluish lavender; swimming in the backyard pool, which is surrounded by hedges, maple, pine, and at one end, an old grape arbor; walking the hilly roads to the bay, or biking to the tiny, quiet town, I am at the same time veiled and widely opened, thinking I am perfectly composed, like an elegantly constructed story, then suddenly overwrought, bursting into unfocused tears. I am extremely frightened of cars that, in New York City and here in these quiet streets, seem always about to crash into me, and I leap out of their way as they pass, causing drivers to look at me as if I am slightly mad. My need for love and reassurance is gigantic. I try to keep it on a short leash, afraid I will lose any hope of forbearance. Fear of death races through me like a brush fire, indistinguishable from the hot flashes that have greatly intensified since I stopped taking estrogen the day of the diagnosis, so that one sets off the other by association and it all comes back, weeks of being trapped in my body, its pain, its disease, the certainty of its inevitable disintegration. The only escape is into the details of management.

Chemotherapy changes the body in many small and obvious, as well as large and mysterious, ways, and for the first time in my life I have a skin rash due to the chemicals in sunscreen lotion or to the sun itself. I use #15 to protect myself but spend large amounts of time wondering if I should escalate to #45 or return to #8. I plan my meals of spinach, broccoli, brown rice, count off a small pile of vitamin pills each morning. Despite my undiminished craving for hamburgers, vodka on ice, cigarettes, bread and cheese, I research and create a dozen vegetable dishes and I eat them. I eat them every day and I follow them with glasses of clear, purified water. Despite my desire to sit and stare, read or think or write, I walk, and I walk fast. And despite a lifelong ambivalent love affair with death, I have never been so certain that I want to live as long as I possibly can. During the months of treatment, the clearest reason for living is to see Adam and Khary develop their lives, their children born, their ambitions fulfilled, not to have to leave them. Only much later will the desire to live include the wish to see my own life develop. Now, hope is only sought after, not yet reclaimed.

I buy new sneakers for my daily walks, thick-soled, high-tops. I list the treatment dates, crossing off numbers 1 and 2, beginning the process I will continue for the next four months and beyond, of writing everything down to keep myself from succumbing to panic. But I am frequently in a state of fear. If Douglas is more than fifteen minutes late, I begin to cry with the grief of a child abandoned, incapacitated and alone, and when he returns from a run, a trip to the store, a little late from work, I sometimes have to turn my back on him, close a door behind me, hide my shame.

I try to love my body, take care of it, look at it in the mirror despite its ordinary signs of aging and the not-so-ordinary long indentation on the side of my right breast. But often, it doesn't feel like mine. It has been cut into, entered, poisoned by strangers. These assaults, I am warned in printed releases I have to sign, may have unpredictable consequences to my heart, my liver, although I am assured that "probably" everything will be fine. But I am suddenly aware of my body parts as if they were delicate infants needing my protection, part of myself and apart from myself at the same time: my liver, my heart.

One night Douglas and I make love, the first time since the surgery, and just as I knew would happen the moment he is inside me I begin to cry. Not so much cry as keen. I sound like a woman in mourning, a low wail to the heavens as she watches a coffin descend. I hear my own voice as if from far away, as I did when I was in the hardest part of labor, giving birth to my sons. In the past months of this lonely journey, I have seen how I cherish beyond measure the old love between Douglas and me. But ordinary vocabulary does not suffice. Old implies worn, or even worn out, but I mean it in the sense of an heirloom, precious, reliable, rich with history.

People say I am strong, but he has seen the fear, knows how many nights we have slept with the light on, held me when my sobs seemed bottomless, listened quietly, at times holding his head in his hands while he looks at me sadly, to my shouts of rage at the American medical system, at rude nurses and doctors who are afraid of pain and suffering, at tumors that are over one centimeter and so require chemotherapy as a treatment that perhaps, but not definitely, might stop the spread of what, I am informed repeatedly, is a systemic disease. Otherwise, I would have told them to cut the breast off, take it, I would have said, and leave me be. When he gently lays his fingers against my wounded breast or touches the still partly numb right arm, I think of blood, of vomit, of the terror of losing my hair, which I've been assured will not happen with the particular combination of chemicals being injected into me. When he moves inside me I lay my hand on my own hair as if by pressing down I might keep it rooted there, and I am lost somewhere inside my body which is vast, foreign, yet some poor fragile thing. Then in the next moment I fill it again and know the difference between his touching and entering me and all of them touching me, entering me, actually entering the flesh of my breast and cutting away tissue for testing, for saving my life, yes, but cutting parts away, parts I have never seen myself but picture as throbbing, raw, and I am unable to say how hard it has been and how dearly I love him because my need is bottomless, it will swallow us both. And so I surround myself with layers of his silence until I am inside it and can feel the words he might have been able to say at some other time, in some other life. Nor does he cry with me, but tonight I am reconciled to this habitual absence of words and in the darkness of the room, against the comforting, damp sheets, after a while I am able to say it, it has been so hard, and to repeat it and repeat it as if this simple phrase is a baptism, or a burial song.

The next morning, Ruthie, oldest intimate of my soul, arrives with her dog, Puto. We walk the narrow streets leading toward and away from the bay, talking of our lives, pressing constantly for some deeper knowledge framed in words that will enable us to escape the demons of depression and fear we have so often faced and fled together. I consider her very brave, and often dream of her exploring remote islands I am frightened to visit because of dangers lurking in ocean storms, or in the broad deserts she and her daughter are willing to cross in order to swim in some perfect lagoon. She dreams of me and the places I have lived as havens she comes upon when she is lost. Accompanied by her dog, an exceptionally intelligent animal whose only fault is that he barks incessantly when he's excited, which he always is on long walks, we wander around roads leading to mansions surrounded by gardens, expansive lawns and high hedges that make Sally's spacious and comfortable home seem like a functional cottage. As we walk we talk of love and need, and then she says, after a characteristic silence in which I know she is pondering some thought until she finds the precise words, "You have a great need of love, to receive it and to give it," and the trapdoor snaps open. I have to stop and catch my breath. I am standing at the edge of the darkness. The way down is steep. I am flushed with hot shame. I am the beggar girl with catlike paws. "No I don't," I say to her, a child's voice, as if I've been insulted and have no sensible response. "What's wrong with it?" she says. We are stopped on the road. Puto is barking at us as if he is a sheepdog and we are his wandering sheep. "What's wrong with it?" she repeats. But all I am able to say is, "I don't know. Something is wrong with it. I know that much." I am filled with images shooting through my brain like some video rewinding, spinning its pictures backward in time.

* * * * *

It is eight months earlier, the previous fall, shortly after Khary had gone to live and study in Jamaica for a semester abroad. I begin to experience panic attacks when I don't hear from him every few days. (He cannot get a phone installed for several months, and so I have to wait for him to communicate with us from pay phones, which are not very numerous in Kingston.) He is reliable and generous about calling me far more frequently than most grown children will call their mothers. Nevertheless, about a day before he is due to call I become obsessed with disaster fantasies so vivid I sometimes have to ward them off verbally, talking back to old demons, often out loud while walking down the street.

After several weeks of this, I consult a famous therapist on the recommendation of a friend who is a therapist herself. Over the course of about four weeks, for reasons I will never fully know, this woman frightens me, hurts me, and weakens me even more than I already am. She interprets my relationships with my sons critically, casting me as an overbearing, intrusive, and deeply hostile mother, a very bad mother indeed. Being fairly sophisticated about psychotherapy, its theory and practice, I twice try to defend myself, questioning her interpretations, and twice she acknowledges that she has been too harsh, apologizes, and even wonders out loud if she, a woman who does not have biological children, is too "child-identified" herself. Then she does it again. What is astonishing to me is that I do not leave immediately but remain for a month. I will never again underestimate the power of therapists, the vulnerability of patients, even the least naive. It's a dangerous business—this putting your life in the hands of a stranger—an action not to be done carelessly, or without restraint. There are ways in which I like her, of course, and keep hoping that with Gloria gone I have found someone new to help me through recurring bouts of depression and anxiety, of which these panic attacks are the worst symptoms I've experienced in years.

After some weeks, I describe her and the things she is saying to me to Leona, who is very knowledgeable about therapy herself and who becomes furious on my behalf. As soon as she begins raging at the therapist's stupidity, callousness, and downright wrongness, insisting that my sons are not only strong but devoted to me, not only "separate" in their own lives (that most overriding proof of "good mothering") but also profoundly connected to Douglas and to me (which few seem to value much at all), I understand that she is right, that I am being broken down by this strange and in some ways likable woman who for some reason dislikes me or is unbalanced by me, and that I can never return to her. I call her and tell her just this, and when she does not bill me for the sessions, I take it as an acknowledgment that she has been wrong.

Nevertheless, her accusations take root. My capacity for belief in disaster regarding my children is thoroughly tied to my fear that I have been a "bad mother," just as my surely once more malleable and ordinary belief in my badness as a child had been hardened, as if with gravel mixed into clay, by my mother's death and the circumstances surrounding it.

* * * * *

One day when I was seven years old and my sister four, we were sent away to an aunt's home, and when we returned two or three days later, our mother was gone. Gone for good. Her clothing had been cleaned out of the closets and distributed to Goodwill, or to relatives and friends. The suede and leather purses I played with, changing black for blue as she changed her elegant outfits for each day's work; the collection of artificial roses, violets, and lilies she wore in her lapels; and the stack of flowered embroidered handkerchiefs—all were gone. My father must have snatched one from the clutches of whoever was dispensing with her physical presence with such efficient dispatch, because I found one among his things when he died, and I still have it, a pattern of pink roses on a background of white, folded among the few mementos I have of her. No doubt they believed her children would be better off not witnessing the awesome dismantling that occurs after a death, as they believed, with such mistaken certainty, that we would be better off not attending the funeral. We returned to a house empty of our mother and much of what she had personally possessed.

The household she had created around her remained, however: the expensive furniture, the pale green china, the cut-crystal inkstand that sat on a graceful silver tray. She was a successful businesswoman, my father a barely paid radical activist, and over the years, with my father in charge of housekeeping and money scarce, possessions grew shabbier. A green velvet armchair that had been her favorite place to sit fell apart and disappeared. We began to use yellow plates bought in the corner hardware store for dinners that now were informal family affairs more suited to my father's working-class background and tastes than the carefully served meals of several courses, restricted to the two of them, my mother had preferred. The crystal inkstand looked more and more anachronistic on its bookshelf, surrounded by my father's dusty half-torn books on Marx, Lenin, and Soviet fiction. When my father died, and we were grown, we pulled it out from the back of the grimy shelf and gave it to my cousin, whose house and housekeeping standards would properly show it off.

But through all those years, I remained haunted by the question—where did she go? I could not comprehend the finality of her absence, and since ours was not a religious family, there was no shared mythology to attempt an explanation. I developed the idea that if I kept a close enough vigil, thinking of her every minute, I could bring her back.

At times, it seemed I was successful. A few years later, when I was in the fifth grade and a school monitor, I watched a thin, dark-haired, elegantly dressed woman kiss her child good-bye near my post at an outside door. But then, probably made uncomfortable by my relentless staring and conspiratorial smiles, she began taking leave of her son farther down the block where I could only glimpse her outline in the sun. And so I realized it hadn't been my mother after all, come back to watch over me, although, for mysterious reasons, having to pretend she was the mother of somebody else. I returned to my more controllable fantasies of her ghostly presence in my room, behind her photograph on my wall, or within my own skin.

When my vigil failed, if I thought of other things or other loves too long, I was responsible for her remaining dead, I believed, just as my desperate need of relief from her dying by hoping for her death had hastened her end. I had killed her. I was guilty of this terrible thing. Throughout my life this belief will surface, then descend into a distant shadow again. But the distancing is never remote enough to destroy my sense of culpability, the threat of punishment lurking close behind.

There were lies that reinforced both guilt and connection, the most dangerous being the idea that I looked exactly like her, was exactly like her. For a child it was an easy piece of syntactical magic to edit out the like. I was her, except that, like many mythical heroines, I had to pay a steep price for my power. She was so beautiful that people stared when she walked into a room, so brilliant she could manage a career as a successful businesswoman while still doing courageous, clandestine political work, and she possessed an indefinable and awe-inspiring quality called *dignity* I could never fully comprehend, although it seemed to have something to do with keeping your feelings under control (mine were notoriously intense, a characterization I responded to with both pride and shame), and not becoming overpowered by your sexual desires. I developed a life-shaping ambivalence to this identification, wanting to be her and thus somehow with her again, but also wanting to be different from her in order not to be dead. It was a false mythology. I recently saw an old film of her, made only one or two years before she died, and I was reminded that I didn't resemble her any more than the average child. If my interests and talents are any sign, I am not like her in temperament or character either. She was an elegant woman, deeply concerned with appearances, whose need for personal success was evidently as great as her need for love. It was my father whose passions were tropical, humid. He sweated when he was thrilled with some piece of music, actually salivated visibly when he was reunited with an old, beloved friend. He longed for my sister and me with unashamed grief when we were growing up and trying to get away from him. He gave us, whenever we asked, and when we did not, anything and everything he had.

Another sort of lie—more specific, concrete, but equally effective for my self-blaming purposes: she died not of cancer but of a "slipped disc." This distortion was perpetrated by my father while she was still alive so that I wouldn't speak the terrible word, cancer, in her presence. But several weeks before her last hospitalization, I had called to her in the night after waking from a nightmare. I heard her call back to me, shouting my name, not a comforting, maternal response but a cry of pain of her own and then I heard a crash. She had tried to get out of bed and come to me, it turned out, but her bones were already weakened by disease and when her legs could not hold her, she had fallen onto the floor. For the next ten years I remained convinced that her fall, in response to my need, was the cause of the slipped disc that killed her. This narrative itself was a distillation, of course, a representation of deeper, more complex stories, classic tales of childish rage at the withdrawal, even into illness, of a parent, especially a mother; of the influence of gender and emerging sexuality on such a wish when the father is beloved too, magnetic and powerful; of the wicked wish that the abandoning mother who is too weakened and frail to pay attention to children and their needs would be punished and die. And then there are the particularities of history, less generic, harder to unravel when the time comes. For this was a mother whose leavings began long before the final leaving, so the daughter's longing was covered over by resentment and anger long before the final anger would become entrenched, veiling the longing that seemed to form the center, which felt at times like an absence, of her life.

Easily, comfortably, I slip into the third person. Even old passions fill me with mysterious shame. Yet I believe that I must find the courage to write the story of that short, threatening breakdown as a chapter in this grief narrative, this cancer journal, must say in words again this piece of self-knowledge I learned almost talmudically with Gloria, going over it and over it, layering it with interpretations and associations, yet forgot and forget, again and again. I believe that what I love will be destroyed. I was a bad girl and my mother died. If I am a bad mother (and what mother is not a bad mother in addition to whatever and whomever else she is; the evidence can always be found) disaster will take my children.

* * * * *

On a Wednesday afternoon, there is a call on my telephone machine from the long-distance operator in Kingston, Jamaica, but no one is home and as the call is collect, Khary is not permitted to leave a message: an ordinary event that takes on extraordinary ramifications for me as soon as it happens. He was trying to call because of some emergency but couldn't get through, I decide. It is that simple, the moment that swift. A call that, at another time, might have had no effect. A moment that, in ordinary time, would have moved into the past like other moments, instead of exploding into dark smoke that remains in the air, stuck to the walls, permeating my lungs, literally shortening my breath for days. Ordinary time fractures for me, and I become an inadequate vessel for past and present, dangerously enmeshed. The idea that something is wrong takes hold and I cannot loosen it for the next four days. The only defense I have, besides talking for hours to Leona on the telephone, is writing. I write a part of a chapter for the book I am working on—an orderly, interpretive piece of nonfiction—and I still don't know how I managed to accomplish this task except that it suggests the genuine change that has taken place in my years of work with Gloria. The self that self restrains might be fragile at times, but at least she is not entirely illusory. And I write in my journal, where no restraint is required, every hour of every day.

While I am writing, I begin to feel a slight faith that he is really okay, but the faith is as ungraspable as light. I cannot gather it, or move into it, but only glimpse it as a reality next to me, from which I am somehow excluded. I only know that if I stop writing, even for a moment, I will be swept away by terror. So over and over I write down reminders of ordinary reality, signposts of ordinary time, as, less than a year later, I will do to mark the passage of weeks through chemotherapy and radiation that feel, also, like a punishment, a permanent hell that, because it is deserved, or at least destined, will never cease. I list all the late nights waiting for my sons when they return, happy and well, all the planes I thought would crash that landed safely, all the viruses that did not become some dread disease.

By Saturday morning I have cried for so many hours, pacing from one corner of our apartment to the other and back again, that Douglas has run out of sympathy and is becoming desperate and angry. I understand that I am making him feel utterly helpless, and that he is convinced I have the ability to control this madness and am refusing to do so out of some terrible self-indulgent need to over-dramatize my life. I try to come out of the terror, and I can't. Perhaps I am resisting my own best efforts in some banal need for punishment, but it feels like the opposite at the time: I am being punished for the extremity of my needs.

On Saturday night I call the Kingston, Jamaica, police station to find out if any Americans have been reported missing or murdered that week. The officer on duty is extremely pleasant, much more so than those at the 24th precinct in my neighborhood whom I have sometimes called with similar questions. No violence has been reported, the charming voice assures me. Nevertheless, I book flights to Jamaica for the coming Monday morning, just in case Khary hasn't called by Sunday night. In these mad actions and irrational plans I grope for and even find a bit of control. Finally, I call one of his professors, a number I have been given for emergencies, and although fearing Khary's anger if everything is indeed fine, I ask this man when he has last seen my son. He is as gracious as the cop, assuring me he is a parent too and understands my concerns. (But of course I am speaking to him in a normal voice, for the duration of the discussion suspending my wild tones.) He has seen him, alive and well, the previous Thursday, and although this fact undermines my theory that something disastrous happened Wednesday night when the phone message was left, it takes only a few minutes after hanging up for my panic to rise again.

I can hear my father's voice after my mother's death, pleading: Stop that crying, crying isn't going to bring her back, when my sobs and screams made him feel, no doubt, as helpless as Douglas does now. Behind my father's I hear my husband's sighs, even his breath, I imagine, furious and desperate. I listen to Leona's voice, reminding me that many losses are packed into this panic. I try to recall Gloria, literally call her up by reading old journal entries about her, and come across entry after entry describing her efforts to get me to look into the place where loss becomes abandonment and love turns murderous in its power to destroy. From that long-ago time, I try to reenter the present so I can achieve the "clarity of self-respect" she insists I deserve. But I have reached the point of no return. There is nothing between me and my savage terrors, my most vigilant obsessions, my weakest self.

When I am at the bottom, I realize that the panic itself has turned into grief, as if the worst has already happened. When I remind myself that I am frightened but really know nothing for sure, I am a little better for a few minutes, even an hour. But then the anxiety mounts back into terror and terror into grief. The future collapses with the past into the present moment where I sit alone in a room, conjuring up the image of a face until it is nearly solid flesh, keeping a ruthless vigil in my head.

Finally, late Sunday afternoon, Khary calls. He sounds normal, and why shouldn't he? He is normal. His life is normal. He said he would call by Sunday, and on Sunday he calls, so he figures his mother is normal too, and I certainly try to appear to be, instantly casting the tone of my voice into a false but familiar rhythm, as calm and low a cadence as I can manage.

We talk only a few minutes, and then I hand the phone to Douglas and leave the house to walk. I am exhausted and frightened. Anxiety remains at a low level for weeks, like muddy waters after a murderous flood. The self I re-encountered is ghostly, familiar, and powerful. I do not want to claim her, yet I am scared she is all I have ever really had. When I am diagnosed with breast cancer the following May, that ghostly other, that scratching cat-girl, is the self I fear most of all. During the week before surgery, and the harder weeks afterward, waiting through medical consultations and sleepless nights for a final diagnosis and treatment plan, I can become nearly paralyzed by the thought: What will I do if she gets out?

* * * * *

During the summer months I am not teaching, and between chemotherapy treatments I spend as much time as I can arrange near the water. Ruthie and I climb over huge white dunes striped with wide meadows of tall grass to reach a famously beautiful Wellfleet Bay. The tide is extremely low and large sandbars spotted with watery patches of seaweed and shell are visible. Walking over this damp, flat terrain, you can hardly tell where the land ends and the water begins. Both appear to be brown, then blue, then brown again. The waves are tiny and gentle, a thin sheet of sparkling wetness over sand.

In the distance a couple emerges. They undress and walk for yards until the bay is deep enough to swim, and even out there it is so shallow that when they cease swimming and stand up, the water only reaches their thighs. I can see signs of age on their bodies, white hair, a slight roundness in their shoulders, a fleshiness in his chest, a boniness in hers. And then they embrace and kiss for some time—their aging bodies, the calm, shallow water—all of it comforts so deeply my legs feel weightless, my body fluid. I can walk for miles in my sturdy high-tops. I can fall into an easy sleep in the sand.

But at the ocean I am agitated, unsatisfied, afraid to risk the cold water even at low tide. I don't know how strict I must be about the sun, as the nurse was so casual and disinterested. "Oh well," she said over her shoulder while preparing vials and tubes, "best to avoid it altogether." But when I asked if I could sit in it for short periods, since I so love the beach, she said with equal casualness, "Oh sure, but best to wear a hat."

I am covered, forehead to ankle, with #15, a hat, an umbrella, and every tiny pain is a cause of anxiety as the days move inexorably toward Treatment Number 3. When I try to risk the water, the ocean I once adored, I am filled with fear of waves and tides. I cannot go in past my knees. Only months later, when all the treatments are finished and I reenter my ordinary life again, when my days are not marked by a number checked off on a page, will I dream that I am standing on a beautiful wooden dock, watching a brave young boy dive into dark, still water where the ocean meets the bay.

At times, as if with a poisonous fluid I cannot stop, I fill up with anger: at Ruthie for sudden small distances; at people on the beach for talking too loudly; at Douglas for remaining at the house and not loving the water as much as I do; at the ocean for being too cold, and the sun merciless. The only thing I don't feel angry at—but only theorize abstractly that surely there must be anger and it must be related to all these other angers—is the disease of cancer that has threatened my life. The week before, on television, I heard the famous breast surgeon, Susan Love, describe cancer treatments as "cut, poison, and burn." I have been cut, am in the midst of being poisoned, and have the burning yet to go, and when the cutting and poisoning and burning are done, I can be given no assurances that I shall not have to go through it all again. As long as I am "in treatment" I feel I "have" cancer, and cannot seem to fully grasp that the tumor has been cut out, the surrounding tissue and lymph nodes found to be free of disease, that the treatment, which I have seen nearly kill two close friends, is "merely preventive" and, compared to other harsher chemical combinations, "mild." Anger fills me and grows into rage all day and into the evening. I try to keep it at bay, but it gathers every small dark rivulet into itself. It swells. I should probably walk out into the hills where no one can hear me or be harmed by me and scream as loudly as I can. But I keep the screams within. I freeze, grow stiff. I snarl for breath.

At about midnight, in the back bedroom Douglas and I use, with its sheer white curtains, worn flowered wallpaper, old wooden chests painted dark maroon, my anger finally dissipates and now here at last is my fear, my plain terror of the real thing. And once again, although I have been sniping at him all day, Douglas takes pity on me and holds me until my shoulders descend, my spine curves out of its tight rigidity, my muscles loosen their grip on my neck, my fingers, my arches, the cat-girl slinks away, and I begin to fall asleep.

* * * * *

A heat wave covers the East Coast as it does almost every summer for several weeks, and it combines with my altered body chemistry to make a sickliness chronic, a constant annoyance of nausea like a slimy seaweed clinging to the surface of the sea.

Back in the city, I go to see the film, *Il Postino,* partly to take my mind off things. In this story of Pablo Neruda's friendship with a simple island postman, I am moved by the power of art to influence both politics and erotic love, by the links among all three. The politics are communist in the simplest sense, a love of ordinary people, which the film connects to a sensuous passion, to the natural world, and to poetry. I am trying as much as possible to focus on art, my own and that of others, believing, like the postman, in its mysterious erotic power to redeem.

Four doctors—two oncologists, my surgeon, and my own internist whom I trust as a friend—advised me to undergo chemotherapy, although my case, with a 2-centimeter tumor, was right on the borderline. There were estrogen receptors to measure, slow-growing and fast-growing tumors to distinguish, implications of being post-or premenopausal: conditions that have been rendered dangerously ambiguous by the prevalence of estrogen replacement therapy, a regimen of hormones I was on for over ten years. There are various chemicals in different chemotherapies to consider; some cause hair to fall out, some do not. Although the studies are not yet definitive, current practice recommends chemotherapy for everyone of a certain age, except those with the tiniest of tumors, and so I decide to submit to the business of poisoning myself in hopes of killing off dangerous, ravenous cells.

Oncologists seem to feel that in their relations with patients they have to choose between falsely optimistic cheer that amounts to denial, or ruthless verbal attack. The first oncologist I consulted looked me straight in the eye and said: "This is a systemic disease. The treatment is dangerous and difficult. You will immediately lose all your hair. Don't let anyone tell you it will be easy." She then recommended a course of chemotherapy of the harshest kind and followed up by undermining my internist, a man whom she knew well and the only medical person in whom I had complete confidence. When I sought a second opinion, at first I liked the seemingly more easygoing doctor and his "chemotherapy specialist" assistant and felt encouraged by their assurances. This doctor recommended a less toxic course of treatment. My blood count would probably remain at low normal, my hair would not fall out ("maybe get a little thinner, but you have nice, thick hair, you can afford to lose some"), and although I might get "a little sick," I would probably be fine. Perhaps such reassurances enabled me to wake up one morning and, accompanied by my sister who actually held me in her arms as the subway lurched downtown, go to the oncology unit for the first time. But as the months wore on, I came to see in this attitude a denial of reality, even a deception by the medical people, because to be reassured that one was not in imminent danger of dying seemed to mean that no talk of suffering or fear was acceptable at all.

Before each treatment, I experienced almost uncontrollable anxiety. Although there was no pain involved in the event itself, and I could sit up in a bright room with the door opened, I felt trapped and imprisoned during the entire hour I was attached to the IV, and the feeling of threatening panic continued until I was back at home.

I have often wondered since then why chemotherapy was so much more frightening to me than surgery or radiation. Perhaps it was the sight of the liquid dripping into my vein, its seeping, nauseating, unstoppable penetration; or the knowledge that this form of treatment is so full of uncertainty and potential danger; or the subtle and yet dramatic physical changes one sees and feels in the body and face—the eyes cloud, the skin seems to pale, hair texture alters even if it doesn't fall out. I know how I felt completely out of control of my own physical boundaries, and the experience of nausea opened trapdoors to deeper, more primal feelings of disgust. The source of the nausea was inside my body, and became entangled with old feelings of shame. During the months of chemotherapy, I was aware of a vague, chronic sense of humiliation. I was reminded of the dead, disintegrating bodies of my dream.

After the first treatment, I was so relieved to be back home I actually felt joyful despite the weakness and queasiness I experienced for several days. After the second I engaged in a mad rush of physical activity, trying to copy a young Israeli woman who was my "treatment partner," and whose energy and optimism were both a standard and inspiration to me.

In the hospital, waiting to be called in for the third treatment, I tried not to look closely at the ill-looking, sometimes emaciated, often hairless fellow patients. I wanted to feel stoical, self-contained, and these capacities require that I also feel distanced and different from them.

Today when I enter the small treatment room, another woman is already there, attached to her IV. She has dyed blond hair, good long legs, a body that looks about forty beneath a face that looks about sixty-five. Inserted into her chest is a tube that receives the IV through which her weekly chemotherapy drips, treating her lung cancer. With tears in her eyes and the sudden intimacy I've become used to with treatment partners, she tells me how she hates and fears these weekly treatments, how she can't sleep at night for fear. Just then, the nurse, the "chemotherapy specialist," enters, a sweet but distracted woman who once inserted the needle into my right arm, the arm that has lost its lymph nodes and is never supposed to be pricked with a needle, nor even squeezed by a blood pressure monitor. Then, obviously afraid of getting in trouble, she blamed me because I had held out the wrong arm, and indeed it was my fault as much as hers. I had been advised by doctors and books since the beginning to take charge of my own illness. I knew I was never supposed to be treated in that arm. But in my anxious state, I didn't realize it until I tried to pick up my pen to write in my journal and realized I couldn't write my way through the threatening forty-five minutes, as I often did, because my right arm was attached to a needle, a long tube, and an IV.

Now, she tells the other woman that she is bringing in a new patient who will need the same implanted tube, the same weekly chemotherapy. "But we don't want to scare her," she whispers like a conspiratorial schoolgirl, "so keep your mouth shut." The new patient, who is young and frightened and who has recently had a mastectomy, is brought into the room. My partner obeys orders, perhaps believing it is kinder to lie than to terrify, and says cheerfully, "Here, have a look. See? It's nothing really." Nurse and doctor echo the mood, smiling, patting, and chattering as if we are at a party. My somber expression and tone annoy them more and more as the weeks go by, as do my questions about physical reactions that depart from their predictions. "Well, it shouldn't happen," they will say when I describe days of weakness. "Are you back at work?"—implying that I am sitting around thinking about my illness too much, and that is why I am weak and have stomach pain. "I'm a writer," I mumble, hoping they will misunderstand or ignore me, because I certainly can't explain that I am writing about my illness, rushing home after every treatment to make copious notes. "It's not so bad, is it?" I am asked repeatedly, and I am expected to answer optimistically, cheerfully. Not to do so makes me feel like a failure, purposely complaining, a bad girl, and so, like my partner, I keep my mouth shut, having learned long ago how few people can understand the emotional intensity I live with all the time, which I try to manage but can never deny. If the expression of fear and pain to a receptive, sympathetic ear is an aspect of healing, as I believe is true, these rooms are not the place to engage in such unpleasantness. I learn to wait for visits to my therapist, or to my internist, a rare doctor who is afraid neither of pain nor of the fact that he cannot always "cure" it, yet might assuage it by listening to the narrative of another's experience with its often strangely familiar detail.

In this office, the destruction of possible cancer cells is accomplished with technical efficiency based on statistical analysis. I am given computer printouts that indicate the relative normalcy of my white blood count. I am given Tylenol to lessen the headaches caused by the anti-nausea drug. When the plastic bag of chemicals is empty and the needle removed from my hand, I am always quite dizzy, but leaning on the arm of Douglas whom, I am scolded by the doctors, I should not really need to accompany me anymore, I can return home. In terms of emotional isolation, I feel very much as I did when I was pregnant and had my first child. In both experiences, all the books, doctors, and even some of the women I tried to talk to assured me of how easy it all was, and so, because it was not only difficult but often overwhelming for me, I felt alone, weaker than they were, a failure in ways as familiar and almost as old as my life. "You'll adjust," I was told by numerous people seeking to help me when I was a child and my mother disappeared for good. I did, if adjusting means one doesn't keep on crying every day. But feelings remain large in me, needing recounting, rephrasing, revising as the years go by.

My partner raises her eyebrows at me after the new patient leaves the room, her cynical smile belied by the tears filling her eyes. "I didn't pay attention to the signs of my colon cancer," she tells me, "so it went to my lung, and now I'm paying the price." Treacherously, I count off our differences, distancing myself from her with notches of relative well-being. But when I look into her eyes I see what I don't want to see. I see that this woman knows more of what I am feeling than Douglas, or my children, or my friends. She knows because she has cancer, and so I know that I have cancer, as my mother had cancer. She, too, is suddenly real to me. I have counted on our differences for too many years to know how to get along without them, that dark definitive line I first tried with all my might to cross, then growing away from her, older and older, was glad to see gathering distance behind me. But I see her now, lying in a dark room—young, in pain, and afraid—her legs too weakened to uphold her body when she gets out of bed to respond to her child's cry. I see her room, dark and eerie, the white of her sheets glowing slightly in the night. Then I see the room in the light of day, only my father's room now, her bed, her clothing, her body all gone. I can almost remember her voice, almost hear her actual scream before I back away quickly out the door and into the hall.

In the treatment room, staring at the open doorway, I am still attached to the IV that leaks its final drops into my vein. I turn back to my partner and reach out to touch her hand.

That night, I dream I am swimming in a dark, warm lake. Although I cannot lift my right arm to swim as well as I once could, I am making progress through the thick waters, and in the slow, effortful movement, I am soothed.

Three days later, the heat wave breaks. The sky is gray. Wind whips the clean light curtains in and out of the open window in my living room. I walk out onto my small terrace feeling a cool, soft rain on my face and bare feet. Newly planted flowers blow in the wind. I breathe deeply, noting the absence of nausea. A weird agitation I always feel for the first two days after the treatment is gone. I can be still, just feeling the wind, the rain.

* * * * *

And what of Ruthie's description of me as being so desperately attached to love? My grief at losing my mother is relived with each separation from my children; the passion I once felt for her has been replaced by an attachment to them so central to my being I try to hide the extremity of my own need and pretend to a freer love, more spacious and pure. The early confluence of extraordinary and even ordinary anger with guilt and punishment will haunt me as long as I live, each time I love deeply and fear abandonment, or am not loved in return. I have understood the indisputable truth of these sentences for some time. But now I am after another distinction, to unlock in myself a confusion between intensity of feeling and extremity of fear. The second, I hope, can be analyzed and perhaps diminished by retelling and renaming past losses, breaking the tie that reforms repeatedly in me between old threats and new, opening a wide chasm filled with murky rushing waters of past, never fully evaporated sorrow. The first, I am trying to see in a new way, to be brave enough to face the notion that the power of my love and need for love is neither crazy nor bad, even when reciprocation is uneven, or return denied.

Once again, I am about ten years old, a monitor at the school door. I wanted to go down on my knees, crawl on my belly, pound the concrete with my fists and beg that woman to be my mother. But she must have seen the desperation in my eyes, perhaps she was frightened of me, or thought me pitiful, when she began leaving her child farther down the block. When I see myself staring and longing, I feel both shame and anger and I try to mute the sound of my anguish by imagining the replacements I found. I am too far away to see the details of the mother's embrace, but I begin to whisper to myself about the precise way her mouth grazes the boy's cheek, her fingers moving through his hair, down to his forehead where she smooths his eyebrows with her thumb. I keep watching, turning away from my monitoring duties, even at that distance trying to feel the love, to steal it and let it fill the emptiness inside me with images and words.

HOSPITAL

MOLLY HOLDEN

They sought me out, the ancient consolations,
  now that I lay helpless in their reach,
with well-greased shoes and oily conversation,
  hoping to net me on that painful beach;

helpless indeed I lay, in that white bed, hands outspread,
  legs useless down the length before my eyes,
and could not care a deal for anything they said,
  kind though they thought themselves and wise.

Jamaican nurses spoke of Christ, wheelchair conversions,
  souls brought to God who'd never seen the light;
quietly I nodded when I could, without aspersions,
  was grateful that they cared to help me fight.

Catholic nurses said they'd pray for me, raising
  their rosaries, promising aves every day;
a priest put up a meaningless blessing, praising
  a courage I did not have, and went away.

The Church of England would have liked discussion,
  seeing I'd admitted myself: "religion none."
I held my own a while but without passion
  and asked to be excused a dialectic run.

And all the while I lay, under the words and attempted curing,
  seeking inside not out for a human grace
that would give me a strength and a courage for enduring
  against great odds in a narrow place.

SECTION TWO

BEGINNINGS AND ENDINGS

INTRODUCTION

The beginnings and endings of human experience provide some of the most evocative writings we have, speaking across generations and challenging caregivers to pay attention to the uses of memory. In its most direct form, the brief and anonymous poem, "Let Us Have Medicos of Our Own Maturity," testifies to the self-awareness and sometimes the frustrations of the aging mind and body in an ever-changing world of practices and practitioners. In a discussion of Shakespeare's monumental study of age and the disintegration of family, *King Lear,* members of a reading group focused on the rebellious daughters; in their thirties and forties, remembering the constraints and unresolved conflicts with their own parents, the readers made Shakespeare's play a forum for their own grievances. The plea of "Let Us Have Medicos of Our Own Maturity" may be heard as a call for reading beyond the limits of any generation.

Mysteriously, across age and tradition, some of us manage to forge connections. In "Black Mountain, 1977," by Donald Antrim, a grandson remembers the moments of work with his grandfather that succeeded in making it possible to remain connected to a disheartened and almost non-existent family. Edward Albee's mordant play, *The Sandbox,* is closer to today's frenzied youth culture and fear of death that have relegated the old and the dying to the margins of American life. From Canada, Emma Donoghue's study of old women, once artists and lovers, now relegated to separate floors in an old-age home, reminds us that art and memory continue despite the best efforts of regulations.

Ideology has been at work in the practices and rituals governing the beginnings of life, as it has affected the endings. Three non-fiction recollections in this section trace the ways in which individual labors and childbirths have conformed to prevailing notions; on Native American reservations and in hospitals known for their excellence, women have relinquished even the appearance of choice without awareness of their powerlessness. The subtle workings of race and class are illuminated in Eileen Pollack's short story, "Milk," a searing account of two women's contrary experiences in adjoining beds. It is an axiom of human experience that the death of a child violates the established order of the universe. Losing a child to illness, addiction, or accident shocks the generational order, and tests families and medical professionals as well. In *Tsunami Years,* Juliet S. Kono chronicles such a loss, and examines the course of generational grief.

In Flannery O'Connor's memorable short story, "The Enduring Chill," and in the much earlier story by Nathaniel Hawthorne, "Rappaccini's Daughter," generational conflict works itself out on the bodies of children; the intricate connections between emotions and bodies become only too clear. These stories raise powerful questions, too, about the boundaries between parents and children's bodies and souls.

MILK

EILEEN POLLACK

How many nurses cared for her needs? The first dressed Bea's wound, a puckered red mouth silenced with staples. A second nurse brought her a cup of chilled juice to wash away the sour taste in her mouth. A third nurse, a man, massaged her sore back.

Then a fourth nurse came in, a small dark-haired woman with a pen in her curls. She knelt beside Bea's bed and covered her feet with paper slippers, then helped Bea to stand and shuffle to the bathroom. Bea's bladder was bursting, but everything below her waist was so numb that nothing came out. When she finally gave up, the toilet bowl was gory with blood and clots of tissue. Had a mess like this really come from her body? Even as she stood there, blood dripped to the floor. She bent to wipe it up and nearly passed out. Too embarrassed to ask the nurse to do this for her, she left the blood on the tiles. The nurse handed her a belt and a sanitary napkin as thick as a book, then helped Bea lie down.

"If you need anything at all pull that cord by your bed and ask for Patrice." The nurse tapped a pill into Bea's palm. "Do you want your baby?" she said.

She was asking, of course, if Bea wanted to see him. But the question Bea heard was: Do you want to keep the baby you've just given birth to?

She hadn't conceived him on purpose. She had slept with a man without taking precautions, like any ignorant schoolgirl. But she had decided to keep him. She had worked with abstractions for so many years that she had forgotten it was possible to sometimes catch a glimpse of the thing in itself. When she realized that a fetus was growing in the universe deep in her womb, she couldn't bear to abort it. She talked to it for months, asking it questions. She looked forward to meeting it as she would have looked forward to meeting an alien who could tell her what life on another planet was like.

But for now she was tired. She swallowed the pill, then slept like a woman who has been up for three days and has just given birth to an eleven-pound child.

"Milk" was first published in *Ploughshares* 20.1 (Spring 1994); this revised version appears by permission of the author.

* * * * *

She awoke to a gong. Cheering. Applause. A floor-length blue curtain surrounded her bed. From beyond it came the sounds of a television turned up full volume.

An orderly brought soup. The warm, salty broth tasted so delicious that Bea savored each sip. Then she turned to watch the sun set above the river; the buildings dissolved until only the lights in their windows were visible. A distant observer would have guessed that the city was nothing more substantial than a few panes of glass with light bulbs behind, as earthly astronomers had assumed for so long that the universe was made of comets and stars, of things they could see. Instead, it turned out that all but a fraction of the cosmos was dark, invisible matter—black holes, some new gas, giant cold planets.

Bea looked around, as if someone could see her thinking about invisible matter instead of about her child. She heard her roommate say: "Lie still, stop your wiggling." Bea was certain that if only she could watch another mother diaper her baby she would learn to do this herself, but the heavy blue curtain blocked her roommate from view.

In fact, Bea didn't see her roommate until late that afternoon, though the woman's TV was on the whole time—soap operas, game shows, even cartoons. Every so often the woman groaned. Then, about four, the curtain rings squealed, and Bea's roommate emerged. She was short but so broad that her johnny wouldn't close, exposing a dark swatch of buttocks and spine. She was thirty, maybe older, her hair short and shapeless. Crooked in one arm was a half-naked child; in the other hand, a diaper. She scuffed to the bathroom in her blue paper slippers without glancing at Bea. After ten or fifteen minutes, she opened the door and scuffed back beyond the curtain.

When Bea hobbled to the bathroom to use the toilet herself, she saw a mustardy smear on the lid of the trash can. Why hadn't the woman wiped up her baby's feces? Well, maybe some people just weren't clean. Then she chided herself for thinking this. Wasn't it more logical that her roommate simply hadn't noticed the dirt? Or she still was too weak to juggle a baby and a wet paper towel? Probably, she had left the smear where it was in the confidence that the janitor would wipe it away. Though the next time he came, he left the smear on the can, and the stain of Bea's blood on the tiles beside the bowl.

* * * * *

The nurse rolled a Plexiglas crib through the curtain. The baby inside was swaddled in blankets. His eyes were screwed tight but his mouth was wide open, like the mouth of a pitcher waiting for someone to fill it with milk.

"He's hungry," Patrice said. She laid the child in Bea's lap, across her incision.

This is my son, Bea repeated to herself, but the fact seemed unreal. He was heavy and round, with a triple chin and jowls; she was gaunt, with high cheekbones. (Did he look like his father? She could barely recall.)

"What's his name?" Patrice asked.

"Isaac," Bea told her, and, as she named him, he suddenly seemed real.

"Isaac," Patrice repeated. "Biblical names are so full of meaning."

Bea didn't bother to explain that she had named her son after Sir Isaac Newton.

"Time to get started," Patrice said. "Your milk won't come in until tomorrow, at least, but you both need the practice."

Bea weighed a breast in one palm: it felt like a Baggie with a spoonful of milk in the bottom. She lifted her son. He was crying from hunger but wouldn't turn his head to suck.

"Here's the trick," Patrice said. Gripping Bea's nipple, she rubbed it across the baby's cheek.

As if by arrangement, Isaac turned toward the nipple and opened his mouth. But when he clamped down his gums, the pain was so intense that Bea cried out and jerked back. He was wailing more shrilly. She let him latch on again, steeling herself not to push him away. The pain abated slowly. Still, as he sucked, she felt a vague irritation, as if a beggar kept pulling at her arm.

"That's enough," Patrice said, just as Bea started to feel more at ease. "I'll take him to the nursery. Here's a pamphlet to study." The cover showed a mother in a lacy white nightgown smiling down at an infant nuzzling her breast. "A bruiser like this will want to eat every hour," Patrice said. "He'll be an eating machine. You've got to relax!"

* * * * *

It was after eleven but Bea couldn't fall sleep. In another few days she would have to take her child home. She had never been alone with a baby. Her mother lived in Cleveland and was legally blind. Few of her friends or colleagues had children. She had read books about babies, but she sensed that a new kind of knowledge was called for.

Still, she might have been able to fall asleep if only her roommate would turn off her TV. Bea hated to ask, but maybe if she asked *politely,* pleading the strains of their common ordeal. . . .

She crossed the room, barefoot, and nudged aside the curtain.

The woman sat with her knees drawn to her chest, her baby propped against her shins. She was watching a talk show whose dapper black host Bea knew she ought to recognize. He said something about a basketball player named Larry, and the woman snorted through her nose.

"I didn't mean to disturb you. It's just, well, it's late."

The woman seemed to expect that Bea would do what she had to do—take her pulse or draw blood—and leave her alone. She stared at the screen with such a fierce gravity that no light leaked out.

"Your baby," Bea said, just to make herself known. But then, to determine what to say next, she had to look at the child. It wore a frilly pink dress. Thick auburn hair curled past its ears. Its coppery brown skin was lustrous and smooth. "She's pretty," Bea said.

"Huh. That child ain't no she." The woman seemed to say this without moving her lips. Bea needed to shut her eyes to concentrate on what her roommate was saying.

"Oh, I'm sorry. I didn't—"

"Ain't your fault. Didn't I buy all these dresses? How's anyone supposed to know a baby's a boy if he's wearing a dress?"

The thought crossed Bea's mind that only a poor uneducated woman would predict her baby's sex based on some old wives' tale. "You thought you'd have a girl?"

"'Thought' nothing. Those doctors took a picture with that sound thing, said they couldn't see no johnson, I had me a girl."

Bea felt suddenly ashamed, as she did when a colleague found a mistake in a paper she had written. The baby started to fuss. Though his mother's huge breasts swelled beneath her johnny and were ringed with wet cloth, she poked a bottle in his mouth. Bea almost believed the woman did this to spite her. "What's his name?" she asked.

"Only name he's got is fit for a girl. Can't think of no new name until I ask his father. Man don't like it, his boy gets some name he ain't said he liked."

Bea couldn't help but think that a man who cared so much about his son's name ought to have attended the baby's birth. "Did you have a Cesarean?" She asked this for reasons she didn't like to admit: if the woman said no, she might leave the next day and be replaced by a roommate who wouldn't make Bea feel so self-conscious or watch TV all the time. "Or was it natural?" she said, to mask her suspicion that the woman didn't know what "Cesarean" meant.

"'Natural,' huh. Last time I was in here I had me twin girls. Doctors cut my belly open, I went home in two days. This time I had this teensy little boy, came out on his own the minute I got here, no cutting, no drugs, I can barely stand up. Hurts me down there like a sonofabitch."

The woman pushed the buttons on her remote until she found the news. A snow storm. A plane crash. The mayor of Washington had just been arrested for buying cocaine. According to his lawyer, the mayor had been framed by government officials waging a vendetta against powerful blacks.

"Huh." The woman snorted. She turned to face Bea. "What you think? Think he's guilty?"

Did Bea? Of course. "He's innocent until they prove he isn't," she said.

Whatever the test she had been given, she failed it. The woman rolled toward the curtain, her backside toward Bea and her fleshy black forearm shielding her son. Then she seemed to fall asleep as a movie about the attack on Pearl Harbor unrolled its credits over Bea's head.

* * * * *

Someone was jiggling Bea's leg.

"I'm sorry," Patrice said, "but you'll have to get used to it." Patrice handed her Isaac. He was crying again. "I don't want to worry you, but if you can't feed him soon we'll have to give him formula. Then he won't want to suck. And if that happens, well, your milk will never come in."

His mouth worked Bea's nipple. Where was this milk supposed to come from? she wondered. Why couldn't she simply will it to be?

The baby sucked at each side for exactly eight minutes; Patrice timed him, eyes trained on the watch on her sharply cocked wrist.

"You don't have to do that," Bea said. She heard an unfamiliar edge in her voice.

The nurse stopped and stood blinking. She picked at the beads trimming her sweater. It occurred to Bea then that Patrice was as uncomfortable with people as she was. Unlike the other nurses, Patrice couldn't seem to sense what a patient might want. Bea pitied her for being so poorly suited to the job she had chosen, as she pitied the student who had been her advisee for the past seven years; he thought that *having vision* meant seeing stars clearly through a telescope.

Patrice stopped picking at her sweater. "Never mind," she said. "I can be that way sometimes. We'll try again tomorrow." She wheeled the crib toward the door. Beyond the blue curtain she said to Bea's roommate: "Wake up there. Wake up. Don't you know you could crush her? Here, let me take her back to the nursery."

"Uh-uh. You leave that baby right where he is. I don't want my baby in no nursery."

Bea wondered if her roommate really believed that the nurses would purposely try to harm her son. She was being . . . what was the word? *Paranoid,* Bea thought, then she managed to fall asleep.

* * * * *

It was just after breakfast. A girl with red hair poked her face through the curtain. "Statistics," she said. She consulted her clipboard. "Are you Beatrice Weller?"

Bea nodded.

"Maiden name?"

"Beatrice Weller."

The girl regarded Bea closely. She asked what Bea "did."

"I'm a cosmologist," Bea said. She started to explain that cosmologists were scientists who studied the universe—how it formed, how it grew. But the girl interrupted.

"You do make-up? And hair?"

Bea surprised herself by saying, "Um. Sure."

"Do you mind if I ask how much you charge for making someone over? Before, you know, and after? Could you maybe do me?"

"Oh, no," Bea said. "I couldn't. I don't have my . . . tools."

The girl seemed disappointed. "Are you sure? It's important. There's this guy I just met. You'll think I'm silly, but maybe, I don't know, you could give me some beauty tips? I get paid Wednesday." She leaned forward, head cocked, her palms pressed together.

"Well. I suppose. I'll be here until Friday." She would think of something later. Already she sensed that, once you began, it was easy to say things you didn't mean.

"Oh, thanks!" the girl said. She asked a few last questions: Bea's nationality (U.S.) and her age (thirty-six). "I'm sure you had the sense not to smoke or use drugs while you were pregnant." She made a mark on a form, promised to return for her beauty consultation, then dragged a chair behind the curtain. "Hello? Coreen Jones?"

Since the name was so common it had the effect of making Bea's roommate seem less real, not more so, as if she weren't a person but a whole class of objects: chair, atom, Jones.

Bea couldn't help but eavesdrop. Coreen mumbled her answers, which the girl asked her to repeat again and again, her voice louder each time.

"You're unemployed?"

"No, I ain't."

"You've got a job?" the girl asked. "Where?"

"At a school."

"You've got a job at a school?"

"Don't worry," Coreen mumbled. "All I do is cook there."

And so on, until the girl asked Coreen for the name of her child.

"Ain't got one."

"Excuse me?"

"I said my baby doesn't have no name."

"She doesn't have a name?"

"It's a he, not a she, and he doesn't have a name."

Tell her, Bea thought. *It isn't your fault. You're not a bad mother.* But Coreen explained nothing.

The girl asked Coreen if her child had a father.

"Think I done it myself?"

"I meant are you married."

"Man never needed no piece of paper to make him a father."

The girl asked for his name. Coreen mumbled an answer. "Can you spell that?" the girl asked.

"Always make sure I can spell a man's name before I have his baby." Coreen spelled the letters slowly: "N . . . A . . . T . . . E." This ordeal over, the girl asked Coreen for her "ethnic category."

"American," Coreen said.

"Oh, no," said the girl, "I mean, where were you born?"

"America," Coreen said.

"Well, what country do you come from?"

"Come from? Way back? Guess you could say Sierra Leone."

"That's not a country. It's a mountain. In Mexico."

"Sure it's a country. Sierra Leone."

"All right then, where is it?"

"West Africa," Coreen said.

"But that's not a country! You mean South Africa."

Bea heard Coreen grunt. "You so smart, you put down whatever country you want. You got any more questions?"

"Only one," the girl said. "Now, try to think hard. Did you use alcohol, or smoke cigarettes, or take any drugs at all—heroin, or cocaine, or even marijuana—while your child was inside you?"

A pause. Bea was startled to hear Coreen laugh.

"Girl, if I done all that awful shit to my baby, he wouldn't have turned out so perfect, now would he."

* * * * *

Bea had just spent another fruitless half-hour nursing her son when a woman's harsh voice barked over the intercom that the photographer was there to take pictures of their babies, but they had to line up by the door to Room 3 within the next fifteen minutes or forfeit their chance. She usually considered taking pictures to be vulgar and vain. But if something were to happen to Isaac, she wouldn't have a picture to remember what he looked like.

From behind the blue curtain came the sounds of her roommate preparing her child. Bea took Isaac as he was, in a hospital T-shirt stamped BETH ZION, BETH ZION, as if that were his name. The two women wheeled their babies' cribs down the hall. Every few steps Coreen clutched her belly. Her forehead was wet, her face ashen.

"Are you all right?" Bea asked. "If you want, I could take him—" She was suddenly afraid that Coreen would react with the same paranoia she had shown toward Patrice.

Coreen mumbled what sounded like "tell me I'm fine" and kept pushing the crib.

They lined up behind a dozen other mothers, half Coreen's age, their hair elegantly done up in beads and braids. Their babies, like Coreen's, were dressed in fancy outfits; one of the boys wore suspenders and a bow tie. A middle-aged woman in a pink linen suit handed out brochures. When Bea saw the cheapest price she nearly turned back. But when would Isaac be a newborn again? She wiped the spittle from his mouth. He gnawed at her finger with sharply ridged gums.

"Huh," Coreen said. "How come they never tell you what things like this cost 'til you're standing in line?"

Bea expected her roommate to wheel her baby's crib back to their room. How could she afford twenty dollars for a picture? Bad enough she was spending an extra five dollars a day for TV, an expense that Bea herself, from years of living on a stipend, had elected to save.

But Coreen stayed in line. She filled out the form, holding it against the back of the woman in front of her. She let the photographer perch her son on a pillow and snap a light in his face.

"I'm not buying it right now," she told the woman in pink. "But you better take good care of it. That boy's bound to be famous. Reporters need his picture, you just might be rich."

* * * * *

Bea hadn't wanted anyone to see her until she had gotten the hang of taking care of her son. She disconnected the phone, but in the middle of the week a boy in a Mohawk brought her a towering basket of fruit. "Congratulations on your own Little Bang!" read the card, "from the crew." Her friend Modhumita, who worked in a lab not far from the hospital, stopped by every day. Bea caught herself hoping that her roommate would see Mita's dusky brown skin and think she was black.

Coreen's phone rang often, but no one came to visit. From what Bea could tell, none of Coreen's friends could get time off from work, or they couldn't leave their children. As the TV set blared, Coreen told a friend what she hadn't told Bea.

Her "pains" had begun on the subway to work. "Know what scared is?" she said. "Scared's thinking you're gonna drop your baby right there on that nasty old floor, all those white boys looking up your nookie." Instead of getting off at the stop near the school, Coreen had taken the train to her clinic. "Time I get inside I can't hardly walk, they say I'm still closed, I got a month to go, it's only false pains. I say, 'You ain't careful, you gonna have yourself a false little baby right there in your lap,' but they don't want to hear it. I go out and call Lena and ask could she keep the twins a while longer. Then I call me an ambulance. Time it pulls up, driver says, 'How come you people always waiting 'til the last minute? You like giving birth to your babies outdoors?'"

Her friend must have asked a question.

"Nate?" Coreen said. "He's away on some haul, don't even know yet." She complained she didn't feel well; she was all hot and cold and she "hurt something awful." Then she shushed whoever was on the other end because the announcer was saying that the police had a videotape of Marion Barry smoking cocaine in that Washington hotel room, and not with his wife.

"Huh," Coreen said. "They got his black ass by the balls. Just let him try to lie now."

* * * * *

After dinner that night Patrice brought in Isaac. He worked Bea's nipples so hard that he raised a welt on his lip, but still no milk came.

"He's losing weight," Patrice told her. "You'll have to calm down. Just look at his face and think loving thoughts."

But the baby kept crying. His face was red as lava; his mouth might have been a crater into which Bea had been ordered to leap. According to Patrice, if Bea's milk didn't come in within twenty-four hours they would have to give him formula.

"Hey!" Coreen called. "I need me a doctor."

Patrice shot Bea a glance, then flung the curtain aside. "You're just engorged," she said. "That means your breasts are too full. We'll have to dry you up. Then you'll feel better."

Bea wondered why her roommate wasn't nursing her child. Didn't she know that it was healthier and cheaper to breast feed? Maybe she disliked the feel of a mouth tugging at her nipple as much as Bea did. Or she couldn't afford to stay home with the baby. Bea stared at the curtain. Why could she imagine what was going on at the other end of the universe but not beyond that drape?

* * * * *

In the middle of the night Bea heard Coreen moaning, "Help me. Lord, help me. I'm freezing."

Bea stood from her bed, wobbling, and pushed aside the curtain. Coreen lay with her head thrown back on her pillow, her johnny pulled low as if she had clawed at the neck. Her breasts were exposed, hard and full, rippling with veins; they looked like twin hemispheres carved from mahogany, the North and South Pole rising from each.

"I'm freezing. I'm dying." She was shaking so violently that the bed squeaked beneath her. Her blanket lay on the floor.

Slowly, Bea bent and gathered Coreen's blanket. She drew the cotton cloth over her roommate. Her wrist brushed Coreen's arm. Bea flinched away, scorched.

She pulled the cord for the nurse, then tugged the blanket from her own bed and spread it over Coreen, whose shaking didn't stop.

Patrice came. "What's the matter? Tell me what's wrong."

"She's freezing," Bea told her. "She said she feels like she's dying."

Patrice took Bea's arm and led her back. "She's just being melodramatic," Patrice whispered. "The state gives them formula. They can't bear to turn down something for free. I'll get her an ice pack. She'll be fine, don't you worry."

Bea glanced at the curtain. "I'll get a doctor myself."

Patrice stalked from the room. Bea pushed through the drape. She didn't know what to do, so she stood there and waited. Without the window, this side of the room was so gloomy that she almost reached up to switch on the TV.

"Don't."

Her heart jumped.

"Don't let them take him." It seemed to cost Coreen a great deal to speak. "Don't," she repeated.

"I promise," Bea said. But already Coreen had started thrashing again, and she didn't seem to hear.

The baby was sleeping face-down in his crib. When Bea lifted him, he hung limp from her hands, surprisingly light compared to her own child. She carried him the way one might carry a puppy, then sat with him on her bed. Was he breathing? He hadn't stirred. She stroked his curls, then his neck. He turned toward her belly, nestling against her thigh. He moved his lips. Her breasts tingled.

A doctor came. Bea huddled closer to the child, partly for warmth and partly to protect him, from what she didn't know. What would she do if someone tried to take him?

The doctor asked Coreen this or that question; he called her "Miss Jones" and murmured "I see" after each of her answers. Then he slowly explained that she had an infection called en-do-me-tri-tis. "It's really quite rare for a natural childbirth, but sometimes it happens." He sounded offhand, though Bea knew this was something that women used to die from. "We'll put in an IV—that's an intravenous line—and you'll feel better before long."

The baby in Bea's lap looked up but didn't cry, as if he understood that it was in his interest to lie still. His smooth copper skin reminded Bea of the telescope her father had bought her for her twelfth birthday. She had cradled it for hours, until the sun set, certain it would bring her the power to see. The child in her lap seemed to hold this same promise. Unlike her own son, he appeared to want nothing. But how could that be true? How could a baby not want anything?

A sweet-faced young woman—Korean? Japanese?—wheeled an IV pole next to Bea's bed. She must have been a medical student—she had that overly serious expression of someone who is hiding how uncertain she feels.

"Here," the student said, "let me take . . . Is that your baby?"

Bea held the boy closer, hiding his face. "You want my roommate, Coreen Jones."

"Oh," the student said. She still seemed confused but wheeled the pole through the curtain. "Hello," she said. "Don't worry, I'll be done in a minute. It won't hurt one bit."

Bea could hear her roommate mutter, "You ain't got it in."

"Just a minute . . . right there . . ."

"Missed by a mile, girl. Might as well of stuck that thing in my ear." Coreen mumbled these words; if Bea hadn't grown accustomed to hearing Coreen's voice, she wouldn't have known what she had said.

The student kept up her patter—"See, that didn't hurt"—and Coreen stopped complaining. When Bea carried the baby back to his crib his mother lay snoring, the blanket Bea had given her pulled up to her chin.

* * * * *

The statistician returned. "I got paid!" She waved a check. "We've got twenty-four hours to create a new me."

Bea was changing Isaac's diaper, holding his ankles in the air with one hand and swabbing yellow stool from his bottom with the other. She hadn't washed her hair since coming to the hospital. She wore tortoiseshell glasses she had picked out in eleventh grade. "I'm really very tired."

"Just one little beauty tip?"

Bea stared at the girl. What was the name of that stuff on her eyes? Liner? Mascara? "Maybe you could use less shadow," she said. As she taped Isaac's diaper and wiped his feces from her hands she searched for a phrase from the glamour magazines her mother used to buy. "Let the real you come through."

"The real me?" The girl seemed baffled. "Well, my friends always say I'm a typical redhead."

Bea could hear Coreen groan. "I meant your best self," she said. "Let your best self shine through."

"But how?" the girl asked.

Bea shrugged. "That's the same advice I give to all my clients."

The girl nodded gravely. "I'll try it," she said. She again waved the check. "How much do I owe you?"

Bea flapped her hand, a gesture that made her feel both generous and mean.

"Thanks!" the girl said. "I'll let you know how it goes." On her way to the hall she stopped to chat with Coreen. "How *are* you?" she asked. "I looked in an atlas, and Sierra Leone was right there in West Africa, just like you said!"

* * * * *

Coreen got a visit from a tired-sounding woman who seemed to run the clinic where Coreen had received her prenatal care.

"What's this?" the doctor said. "Who put in this IV?" She summoned Patrice. "Just look at this arm, the way it's all blown up. My patient's IV has been draining into everything but her vein—for how long? Ten, fifteen hours? Where do you think all that fluid's been going?"

The doctor couldn't stay—another of her patients was about to deliver—but she gave Patrice instructions as to what to do next.

"I didn't put this in," Patrice grumbled when the doctor had gone. "I would never do a job as sloppy as this."

"Huh," Coreen said. "If I treated hamburger meat as sloppy as you treat the folks in these beds, they would fire my ass."

* * * * *

Coreen was feeling better, but her baby still was sick. "He shits all the time," she told the pediatrician.

"Oh, all newborn babies have frequent movements," he said. He sounded like the same well-meaning young intern who had given Isaac his checkup. ("The nurse tells me that you and your baby aren't bonding. Is there anything I can do?," as shy as a boy whose mother has asked him to unhook her brassiere.)

"Ain't just frequent," Coreen told him. "And the color ain't right." The pediatrician started to say that all newborn babies had odd-colored "movements," but Coreen stopped him. "Don't you think I know what a baby's shit looks like? Didn't I raise myself twins?"

His voice tensed. "I'll look into it. But I'm sure if the nurses had seen anything amiss, I would have been notified."

Bea assumed that he was right, until she remembered that even at her sickest, Coreen had changed her baby's diapers herself.

* * * * *

Coreen's boyfriend came to visit. Bea saw nothing but his running shoes, caked with dry mud, as they moved back and forth beneath the blue curtain. She could hear when he kissed his son, then kissed Coreen.

"Go on," Coreen said. "I'm too sore for that stuff."

The boyfriend, it seemed, drove a moving van or a truck. He had been away on a trip to some city out west. How could he have known that Coreen would give birth to their child five weeks early? When no one answered at home, he called the hospital from a pay phone, but someone at the switchboard kept cutting him off. He drove without stopping until he reached Boston.

They talked about names. The man suggested Mitchell, after a younger brother who had died. But Coreen wasn't sure. "This boy ain't lucky as it is." She spoke softly but didn't mumble. "I can feel it in my bones." Bea heard something in Coreen's voice that she hadn't heard before. Or maybe she was hearing Coreen's voice as it really was.

"Never mind your bones," the boyfriend said, laughing. "All you women, nothing you like better than worrying. Hell, we got us a son. Come to Daddy, little Mitchell. First thing's gonna happen now your daddy's come back, he's gonna buy you some pants!"

* * * * *

Coreen's fever returned, no one knew why. The doctors spoke to her kindly, but they said she couldn't leave the hospital. She told them that her twins were only three years old. She might lose her job if she stayed away too long. Precisely, they said. What she needed was rest, which she wouldn't get at home.

In the middle of the night, Coreen changed her baby's diaper for the third or fourth time. Then she rang for the nurse.

"Look at these diapers! You tell me his shit's supposed to be red!"

"Oh! Oh my!" Patrice said, startled. Bea heard the nurse's shoes slap the linoleum as she ran down the hall. She returned with a doctor whose voice Bea didn't recognize. He had a rich, soothing accent—English, or Australian. He paused between phrases as if to gauge the responses of someone whose reactions might be different from his.

He was . . . concerned, he told Coreen, that her son might have . . . a serious form of diarrhea. An infection in the bowel. Not so rare, really, especially for babies like hers, who had been born premature. They were taking him to Children's Hospital, just down the street. She could see him as soon as she was feeling "more perky." In the meantime, he said, they would send word how he was.

An orderly wheeled the child out the door. Bea thought of pushing through the curtain to comfort Coreen, but what could she say? That the doctors at Children's were the best in the world? That she hadn't broken her promise not to let them take him?

* * * * *

Early the next morning Bea dressed herself, then dressed her son. Bundled in the snowsuit Bea's mother had sent, Isaac seemed thoughtful, as if contemplating this latest change in his life. She took a deep breath and pushed aside the curtain, holding the gift her colleagues had sent; she had eaten one pear, but the rest of the pyramid of fruit was intact. She waited for her roommate to say *Keep your damn apples.* But Coreen didn't remove her gaze from the woman in sequins spinning a shiny wheel on TV.

Bea set the fruit on the night stand. "I hope you feel better soon. I hope your baby is all right." She tried not to wish that her roommate would thank her. "Is there anything I can do?"

Coreen turned to face her. For some reason, Bea thought that her roommate would tell her to pray. But Coreen shook her head no and turned back to the spinning wheel on TV.

* * * * *

From the moment Bea came home she had no trouble nursing. She locked the doors and pulled down the shades. She peeled off Isaac's diaper, T-shirt, and hat and gave him a bath. Seeing him naked and whole the first time, she felt a catch in her throat, a pressure in her chest. She assumed this was love, but the word seemed too weak, as if she had grown up calling pink "red," and then, in her thirties, seen crimson or scarlet.

Isaac slept by her side. Whenever he was hungry she gave him a breast. Milk spurted in his mouth so quickly it choked him; she needed to pump out the excess, which sprayed from each nipple like water from a shower head. He would have sucked half an hour at each breast, if she had let him. How could she watch his face for so long and still not be bored? Her elation, she knew, was hormonal. But who would have thought that a chemical substance could produce this effect? If vials of oxytocin could be bought at a store, who would drink or use drugs? She hadn't suspected that of all the emotions a human being could feel, this tenderness would be the one she craved most.

* * * * *

When she felt a bit stronger, Bea telephoned the hospital and asked a nurse in obstetrics if Coreen Jones had gone home. Yes, she had, the nurse said. And her baby? Bea asked. "Just a moment," the nurse said. A few minutes later she got back on the line and said that the baby had been transferred to Children's Hospital. That was all the information she could release.

When Bea called Children's, she introduced herself as Dr. Beatrice Weller, which, technically, she was, and learned that a patient listed only as "male infant Jones" had died two days earlier. She said, "Yes," then hung up.

That afternoon, she borrowed a pouch from the family next door, strapped Isaac inside, and walked to the T. As she stood by the turnstile, struggling to get some change from her pocket, someone behind her said, "Honey, don't rush. What a mother really needs isn't a pouch, it's an extra pair of hands."

The woman who had said this was at least six feet tall, with soft, sculpted hair and perfect brown skin. She wore a yellow cashmere suit and enormous brass earrings. Bea wondered if she might be one of the anchors on the local evening news, then decided that such a celebrity wouldn't be taking the T.

The woman dropped a token in the box for Bea's fare. Bea tried to repay her. But the woman lifted one palm, pushed through the gate and, briefcase to chest, ran to catch her train.

When Bea got to the hospital she went straight to Room 3. She said that she had come to buy a picture for a friend who was ill, wrote a check for twenty dollars, and was handed a portrait in a flimsy pink folder with bears along one edge. Clipped to the front was the form each mother had filled out: MOTHER'S NAME . . . ADDRESS. . . . Coreen's writing was shaky; Bea remembered her leaning on the woman in front.

She opened the folder. Yellow pinafore. Curls. Full lips. She thought of mailing the portrait but decided to follow through with her plan. To hand a person an envelope and offer your condolences for the death of her child seemed a minimum requirement for living on earth.

She took the subway to a neighborhood she had never been to before. The three-decker houses weren't all that much different from the ones where Bea lived, but the smallest details—a pair of red sneakers dangling from a telephone wire, an unopened pack of gum lying in a gutter—seemed enlarged and mysterious. Most of the houses here were enclosed by steel fences. German shepherds and Dobermans strained at their leashes and barked as Bea passed. As he slept, Isaac stirred; with her cheek to his soft spot she could feel his brain pulse.

She finally found the right address. Three rusty mailboxes hung askew on the porch, an eagle on each: HERRERO, GREEN, JONES. Had Bea really believed that she could ring Coreen's doorbell and explain why she had come? When Coreen saw the photo of her dead son, she would scream. Maybe she would faint. Besides, Bea was holding a healthy baby in her pouch, and that, more than anything, would make Coreen hate her.

A light flickered on behind a third-story window. Bea pictured Coreen lying on her bed, stone mute with grief. Her boyfriend came in. *Don't worry, sweetheart, we'll have us another baby. It wasn't your fault.* Bea wondered where the twins were. And Lena? Coreen's mother? What about Coreen's job? Would they allow her time off? How useless the eye without the imagination to inform it, to make sense of all the darkness surrounding the light.

A child started crying in the building next door. Bea's breasts began to tingle; in his pouch Isaac stirred. She slid the folder in the mailbox. Milk flowed from her nipples, soaking her blouse. She hurried to the T station, where she zippered her parka so that only Isaac's head poked from the top.

During her last night in the hospital, Bea had lain with her hands pressed against her ears as Coreen had changed her baby's diaper again and again. By then, Bea herself had come down with a fever. Every joint ached. Her breasts had swollen grossly. They were lumpy, rock hard, as if someone had pumped them full of concrete. Another few drops of milk and they would burst.

And yet they kept filling. Every time Coreen's baby whimpered, milk surged into Bea's breasts, pushing through ducts that felt tiny and clogged, like irrigation ditches silted with clay. In another few moments, she would be forced to get up and stagger down the hall and try to stop Patrice from feeding Isaac the formula she had warned Bea that she would give him. Bea longed to feel her baby's mouth sucking at her nipples, sucking and sucking, easing her pain. In the meantime, she lay there, palms against her ears, her breasts filling with milk for another woman's child.

THREE GENERATIONS OF NATIVE AMERICAN WOMEN'S BIRTH EXPERIENCE

JOY HARJO

It was still dark when I awakened in the stuffed back room of my mother-in-law's small rented house with what felt like hard cramps. At 17 years of age I had read everything I could from the Tahlequah Public Library about pregnancy and giving birth. But nothing prepared me for what was coming. I awakened my child's father and then ironed him a shirt before we walked the four blocks to the Indian hospital because we had no car and no money for a taxi. He had been working with another Cherokee artist silk-screening signs for specials at the supermarket and making $5 a day, and had to leave me alone at the hospital because he had to go to work. We didn't awaken his mother. She had to get up soon enough to fix breakfast for her daughter and granddaughter before leaving for her job at the nursing home. I knew my life was balanced at the edge of great, precarious change and I felt alone and cheated. Where was the circle of women to acknowledge and honor this birth?

It was still dark as we walked through the cold morning, under oaks that symbolized the stubbornness and endurance of the Cherokee people who had made Tahlequah their capital in the new lands. I looked for handholds in the misty gray sky, for a voice announcing this impending miracle. I wanted to change everything; I wanted to go back to a place before childhood, before our tribe's removal to Oklahoma. What kind of life was I bringing this child into? I was a poor, mixed-blood woman heavy with a child who would suffer the struggle of poverty, the legacy of loss. For the second time in my life I felt the sharp tug of my own birth cord, still connected to my mother. I believe it never pulls away, until death, and even then it becomes a streak in the sky symbolizing that most important warrior road. In my teens I had fought my mother's weaknesses with all my might, and here I was at 17, becoming as my mother, who was in Tulsa, cooking breakfasts and preparing for the lunch shift at a factory cafeteria as I walked to the hospital to give birth. I should be with her; instead, I was far from her house, in the house of a mother-in-law who later would try to use witchcraft to destroy me.

After my son's father left me I was prepped for birth. That meant my pubic area was shaved completely and then I endured the humiliation of an enema, all at the hands of strangers. I was left alone in a room painted government green. An overwhelming antiseptic smell emphasized the sterility of the hospital, a hospital built because of the U.S. government's treaty and responsibility to provide health care to Indian people.

I intellectually understood the stages of labor, the place of transition, of birth—but it was difficult to bear the actuality of it, and to bear it alone. Yet in some ways I wasn't alone, for history surrounded me. It is with the birth of children that history is given form and voice. Birth is one of the most sacred acts we take part in and witness in our lives. But sacredness seemed to be far from my lonely labor room in the Indian hospital. I heard a woman screaming in the next room with her pain, and I wanted to comfort her. The nurse used her as a bad example to the rest of us who were struggling to keep our suffering silent.

The doctor was a military man who had signed on this watch not for the love of healing or out of awe at the miracle of birth, but to fulfill a contract for medical school payments. I was another statistic to him; he touched me as if he were moving equipment from one place to another. During my last visit I was given the option of being sterilized. He explained to me that the moment of birth was the best time to do it. I was handed the form but chose not to sign it, and am amazed now that I didn't think too much of it at the time. Later I would learn that many Indian women who weren't fluent in English signed, thinking it was a form giving consent for the doctor to deliver their babies. Others were sterilized without even the formality of signing. My light skin had probably saved me from such a fate. It wouldn't be the first time in my life.

When my son was finally born I had been deadened with a needle in my spine. He was shown to me—the incredible miracle nothing prepared me for—then taken from me in the name of medical progress. I fell asleep with the weight of chemicals and awoke yearning for the child I had suffered for, had anticipated in the months proceeding from his unexpected genesis when I was still 16 and a student at Indian school. I was not allowed to sit up or walk because of the possibility of paralysis (one of the drug's side effects), and when I finally got to hold him, the nurse stood guard as if I would hurt him. I felt enmeshed in a system in which the wisdom that had carried my people from generation to generation was ignored. In that place I felt ashamed I was an Indian woman. But I was also proud of what my body had accomplished despite the rape by the bureaucracy's machinery, and I got us out of there as soon as possible. My son would flourish on beans and fry bread, and on the dreams and stories we fed him.

My daughter was born four years later, while I was an art student at the University of New Mexico. Since my son's birth I had waitressed, cleaned hospitals, filled cars with gas (while wearing a mini-skirt), worked as a nursing assistant, and led dance classes at a health spa. I knew I didn't want to cook and waitress all my life, as my mother had done. I had watched the varicose veins grow branches on her legs, and as they grew, her zest for dancing and sports dissolved into utter tiredness. She had been born with a caul over her face, the sign of a gifted visionary.

My earliest memories are of my mother writing songs on an ancient Underwood typewriter after she had washed and waxed the kitchen floor on her hands and knees. She too had wanted something different for her life. She had left an impoverished existence at age 17, bound for the big city of Tulsa. She was shamed in a time in which to be even part Indian was to be an outcast in the great U.S. system. Half her relatives were Cherokee full-bloods from near Jay, Oklahoma, who for the most part had nothing to do with white people. The other half were musically inclined "white trash" addicted to country-western music and Holy Roller fervor. She thought she could disappear in the city; no one would know her family, where she came from. She had dreams of singing and had once been offered a job singing on the radio but turned it down because she was shy. Later one of her songs would be stolen before she could copyright it and would make someone else rich. She would quit writing songs. She and my father would divorce and she would be forced to work for money to feed and clothe four children, all born within two years of each other.

As a child growing up in Oklahoma, I liked to be told the story of my birth. I would beg for it while my mother cleaned and ironed. "You almost killed me," she would say. "We almost died." That I could kill my mother filled me with remorse and shame. And I imagined the push-pull of my life, which is a legacy I deal with even now when I am twice as old as my mother was at my birth. I loved to hear the story of my warrior fight for my breath. The way it was told, it had been my decision to live. When I got older, I realized we were both nearly casualties of the system, the same system flourishing in the Indian hospital where later my son Phil would be born.

My parents felt lucky to have insurance, to be able to have their children in the hospital. My father came from a fairly prominent Muscogee Creek family. *His* mother was a full-blood who in the early 1920's got her degree in art. She was a painter. She gave birth to him in a private hospital in Oklahoma City; at least that's what I think he told me before he died at age 53. It was something of which they were proud.

This experience was much different from my mother's own birth. She and five of her six brothers were born at home, with no medical assistance. The only time a doctor was called was when someone was dying. When she was born her mother named her Wynema, a Cherokee name my mother says means beautiful woman, and Jewell, for a can of shortening stored in the room where she was born.

I wanted something different for my life, for my son, and for my daughter, who later was born in a university hospital in Albuquerque. It was a bright summer morning when she was ready to begin her journey. I still had no car, but I had enough money saved for a taxi ride to the hospital. She was born "naturally," without drugs. I could look out of the hospital window while I was in labor at the bluest sky in the world. I had support. Her father was present in the delivery room—though after her birth he disappeared on a drinking binge. I understood his despair, but did not agree with the painful means to describe it. A few days later Rainy Dawn was presented to the sun at her father's pueblo and given a name so that she will always be recognized as part of the people, as a child of the sun.

That's not to say that my experience in the hospital reached perfection. The clang of metal against metal in the delivery room had the effect of a tuning fork reverberating fear in my pelvis. After giving birth I held my daughter, but they took her from me for "processing." I refused to lie down to be wheeled to my room after giving birth; I wanted to walk out of there to find my daughter. We reached a compromise and I rode in a wheelchair. When we reached the room I stood up and walked to the nursery and demanded my daughter. I knew she needed me. That began my war with the nursery staff, who deemed me unknowledgeable because I was Indian and poor. Once again I felt the brushfire of shame, but I'd learned to put it out much more quickly, and I demanded early release so I could take care of my baby without the judgment of strangers.

I wanted something different for Rainy, and as she grew up I worked hard to prove that I could make "something" of my life. I obtained two degrees as a single mother. I wrote poetry, screenplays, became a professor, and tried to live a life that would be a positive influence for both my children. My work in this life has to do with reclaiming the memory stolen from our peoples when we were dispossessed from our lands east of the Mississippi; it has to do with restoring us. I am proud of our history, a history so powerful that it both destroyed my father and guarded him. It's a history that claims my mother as she lives not far from the place her mother was born, names her as she cooks in the cafeteria of a small college in Oklahoma.

When my daughter told me she was pregnant, I wasn't surprised. I had known it before she did, or at least before she would admit it to me. I felt despair, as if nothing had changed or ever would. She had run away from Indian school with her boyfriend and they had been living in the streets of Gallup, a border town notorious for the suicides and deaths of Indian peoples. I brought her and her boyfriend with me because it was the only way I could bring her home. At age 16, she was fighting me just as I had so fiercely fought my mother. She was making the same mistakes. I felt as if everything I had accomplished had been in vain. Yet I felt strangely empowered, too, at this repetition of history, this continuance, by a new possibility of life and love, and I steadfastly stood by my daughter.

I had a university job, so I had insurance that covered my daughter. She saw an obstetrician in town who was reputed to be one of the best. She had the choice of a birthing room. She had the finest care. Despite this, I once again battled with a system in which physicians are taught the art of healing by dissecting cadavers. My daughter went into labor a month early. We both knew intuitively the baby was ready, but how to explain that to a system in which numbers and statistics provide the base of understanding? My daughter would have her labor interrupted; her blood pressure would rise because of the drug given to her to stop the labor. She would be given an unneeded amniocentesis and would have her labor induced—after having it artificially stopped! I was warned that if I took her out of the hospital so her labor could occur naturally my insurance would cover nothing.

My daughter's induced labor was unnatural and difficult, monitored by machines, not by touch. I was shocked. I felt as if I'd come full circle, as if I were watching my mother's labor and the struggle of my own birth. But I was there in the hospital room with her, as neither my mother had been for me, nor her mother for her. My daughter and I went through the labor and birth together.

And when Krista Rae was born she was born to her family. Her father was there for her, as were both her grandmothers and my friend who had flown in to be with us. Her paternal great-grandparents and aunts and uncles had also arrived from the Navajo Reservation to honor her. Something had changed.

Four days later, I took my granddaughter to the Saguaro forest before dawn and gave her the name I had dreamed for her just before her birth. Her name looks like clouds of mist settling around a sacred mountain as it begins to speak. A female ancestor approaches on a horse. We are all together.

LABORS OF LOVE

RUTH NADELHAFT

Forty-three years ago, at about nine in the morning, I awoke in a sopping wet bed; my waters had broken, and I was about to begin the labor that would give us our daughter, Erica. Our cat, Thomas, was sleeping on the suitcase I had packed a week earlier; the baby was a few days past the due date, and Thomas had become territorial about his spot on the red and black plaid nylon suitcase right outside our bedroom. We were excited and confused, stripping the bed, bumping into each other in our small bedroom, stopping to pet Thomas, finally picking him up and moving him to a corner of our battered couch for the duration.

Nothing in the experience of labor resembled the beautiful and controlled process our classes in Natural Childbirth and Lamaze had outlined and, I thought, promised. Our baby was a breech; her position, while I was pregnant, had been a constant pleasure. I could read with my hand resting on what became more and more evidently her head, just below my rib cage. I felt as though I had company all the time, and somehow I felt that I would begin to miss her once she was born and a separate being. Nothing about her position seemed worrisome until two weeks before my due date. That day, on what I thought would be a routine visit, one of the three obstetricians in the practice tried to turn our baby into a more favorable position. It was astonishingly painful. As I would learn later, when I read up on breech presentations, the bottom of our baby was fully engaged, and she snapped back into her sitting position after each horrific attempt. We were all sweaty and exhausted when finally the doctor gave up and the nurse left the room. I had no idea what had just happened or not happened to me, but I was deeply sore and somehow as deeply indignant for my baby. Those last two weeks, after the failed attempt to turn the baby, I began to be both frightened and uncertain about what lay ahead. Something felt discordant; in the natural childbirth class I alarmed myself by being able to pretend so well to be relaxed that the instructor praised me to the whole class as my arm flopped from her grasp. The rest of my body was one ferocious contraction as I concentrated on keeping that arm utterly limp. I began to feel like a spectator trapped in a performance.

Once labor began in earnest, it was terrible. All the breathing lessons fell away; the language of discomfort and beauty and endurance was false. I was as furious as I was frightened, torn by pain unlike anything anyone had even hinted at. In the midst of the horror, some time in the evening, a resident came by and stood for a while with his hand on my writhing, twisting belly. He pronounced my labor inefficient. I was enraged.

Usually, when I tell the story of our daughter's birth, I slide over the hours of grinding exhausting pain, the humiliation of being "inefficient," the terrible feeling of being isolated in a locked world of pain for which I had no language. Usually, I skip to the delivery room, when I was finally about to produce something and was filled with excitement again and a sense of being part of all that was happening. Our baby came out feet first, and before she had emerged fully the doctor could see that she was a girl. "What's her name," he asked as I paused in my pushing, up on my elbows, watching in the mirror, finally fully alive to my own place in this world of birth. "Erica," I gasped, for we'd had only two names: Eric for a boy, Erica for a girl, after Erica Morini, the violinist. Everyone began calling to her, as she slowly slid out: "Come on Erica, come on Erica," and with a last tremendous push she was out, and we were two separate beings. I was spent but filled with joy and triumph. I had done it without anesthesia, a primary requirement in the world of *Childbirth Without Fear,* that lying bible we had all virtually memorized in preparation for painless labor and delivery in those natural childbirth classes that were part of the initiation process of the world of graduate school in Madison, Wisconsin, in the nineteen sixties. For a long time after that explosive and radiant delivery, I was charmed by my own story of the breech birth that answered the question, would it be Erica or Eric, in such a welcoming and affectionate way. It was not until almost four years later, when I was pregnant with our second child, that I was given an opportunity to understand the dangerous nature of natural childbirth for a known breech presentation. And even then, I missed it entirely, caught up in the drama of the recollection that had become almost the whole story of Erica's birth.

Our second child, Matthew, was born in a different city, a conservative place not dominated by the theories or the politics of Madison in what had been known as Red Dane County. Giving my medical history, I gave a brief account of that delivery room with its shouts of encouragement for our daughter. "Wait a minute," the new obstetrician said, stopping me before the triumphant conclusion. "I want to get my partner in here." A few moments later I took up my narrative, happily answering their rapid questions. Yes, it was my first pregnancy, and they knew it was a breech; I told my story of the attempt to turn the baby, even at this distance feeling my teeth clench with indignation at the invasion. "And it was a vaginal delivery?" Of course it had been a vaginal delivery. And I had been wide awake and the prime mover, at last. My doctor was impassive; both were listening closely. The partner patted my shoulder and left. I continued to feel triumphant. It would be decades before I came to understand that my experience had not only been rare but dangerous, bordering on malpractice and remarkably similar to the experience my mother had had with my birth twenty-five years before.

My mother was twenty-eight when I was born. Like my daughter, I was a most eagerly awaited child, conceived as soon as my parents thought they could afford to have a baby. We were in graduate school when Erica was born, and only the unexpected bequest of a thousand dollars in stocks allowed me to give up the teaching assistantship which supported us both. My parents and their closest friends were expecting their first children almost in tandem; this was true for Jerry and me as well. I loved the parallels that I knew about, not knowing those my mother chose not to tell me until years later. My mother was huge with me; she was so large that when she visited her best friend in the hospital in late February, after Edward was born, people thought my mother was there to be admitted; I was not due for another six weeks and I was a large baby, over nine pounds. The obstetrician was from Germany, already famous when he emigrated to the United States ahead of the fascists threatening him and his family. In New York he established a practice on Park Avenue and changed his name, but he brought with him and kept his theories about birth and cleanliness. Americans, he believed, attached too much value to cleanliness and to medical remedies for the pain of natural processes. Women were strong and resilient in Europe, and they could be both in America with the right doctors encouraging them. He had great faith in himself and in his patients.

Almost everything my mother told me—or didn't tell me—about her experience in childbirth was first expressed in what she went through during my labor and delivery. The day Erica was born, a hot Thursday in late June, my mother had her usual day off from work in the jewelry store my father managed and she detested. As usual, she called in the morning. But we had already dashed for the hospital, and no one was home. All day, as I went through my labor, she kept calling, knowing where I was, remembering, no doubt, the extended and unfathomable hours of her own labor twenty-five years earlier, when she had been so naive that she'd packed a deck of cards for her and my father. As Grantly Dick Read and her famous obstetrician had no doubt preached, the early hours of labor are mild and tedious; playing cards helps to pass the time.

My mother had no idea what awaited her. She was strong and athletic, a wonderful swimmer who, somewhere, had learned to do the Australian crawl stroke. When I was a child I stood on the shore at a beach on Long Island and watched her swim straight out to sea; she was so steady and strong that I imagined she would swim away forever. My mother rarely mentioned her body. By the time I knew her, it seemed that she and her body lived parallel lives in an understood and intuitive harmony that excluded the rest of the world. My mother never cried, and the pains or demands of the body seemed not to involve her. I thought she was strong and invulnerable. I think now that she was also terrified and demoralized forever by her experience of childbirth.

My mother's labor lasted twenty-eight hours. At the end of it, a tortuous breech delivery, Dr. Solomon (he was not yet Dr. Salton) had to pull my head out with forceps. When my mother finally got to see me, she saw a baby whose head had been so dented that the nurses had improvised a turban for me. My mother was exhausted; I believe she was humiliated by her own screaming, by what she thought had been cowardice or a lack of resolve, and she was frightened by the sight of her baby who looked battered and tired in her silly hat. I don't know when my mother finally saw and touched my scalp, but even now I can easily feel the ruts and dents. When my mother first saw our baby, two days after her birth, she could not stop talking about her beautiful head. We thought our baby was beautiful, so we attached no special significance to my mother's amazement, to her tentative but repeated stroking of Erica's lovely head of soft black hair.

Erica weighed seven pounds and twelve ounces; she was compact and dimpled; I had weighed nine pounds and four ounces. The pain Erica cost was as nothing compared to the joy of having her, but I was angry enough at what I remembered of the natural childbirth people and the dismissive resident to write a letter to University Hospital detailing my points of indignation. "Pain is pain," I know I wrote. "It's not 'discomfort,' and it doesn't disappear when you breathe in and out and think happy thoughts." I typed the letter out at our electric typewriter, on the kitchen table, the same typewriter on which I would later type my dissertation, as soon as I was able to sit for any length of time. I felt as though I was held together with barbed wire, and I dreaded having to go to the bathroom. Once, a few days after I got home, after an especially painful passage, I saw a chunk of material in the toilet bowl that I knew was unmistakably a segment of what we still called "the afterbirth." I was so frightened by the sight that I never told anyone, for even then I knew that women had died from the incomplete expulsion of the placenta. Squatting in our little bathroom with its sunny yellow walls and tiny corner sink, I stared at the chunk of tissue and thought of Mary Wollstonecraft, dead of puerperal fever. I flushed it away and stared after it into the swirl of pinkish water as it disappeared. I hated feeling so vulnerable all over again, knowing that I would never tell this to anyone now that I had expelled it on my own, intact (I checked). I think what I felt was that it, the it of labor and delivery and the birth of our dearly awaited mystery baby, had been spoiled, and I was alone in charge of preserving my memories intact, despite the violations inflicted by experience. My lonely scrutiny of the chunk of afterbirth was detail that I didn't divulge to the obstetrical group in Rochester, New York, when I was pregnant with the baby that turned out to be Matthew.

Earlier, when Erica was two years old and regularly called for by neighborhood children who took her off to play outside, we had decided to have another baby. It was clear that Erica was ready to join the world, and we were ready to enlarge our own little family. My own mother and father had tried to have a second child a few years after my birth, but my mother had miscarried. This was a story I had heard in some detail, and it fascinated me. Pregnant, my mother had visited a new mother in the hospital, and had been shown the baby, disfigured by a harelip. The sight had terrified my mother; each time she told this story it was apparent that she fell back into the horror which had so consumed her that she seemed to have willed herself into the miscarriage that soon followed. I never tired of hearing this story, which somehow contributed to my sense that my mother was the most powerful person in the world. She had willed that fetus out of her womb, I was convinced. The story, like the story of my birth, was both cautionary and exemplary.

My own miscarriage was as allegorical as my mother's, exposing me and the context in which I lived as surely as my mother's miscarriage told volumes about her. Early in this pregnancy, I stopped having morning sickness, a symptom that was a predictable and reassuring part of early pregnancy for me, and I began to spot. Alan Guttmacher's *Pregnancy and Birth* was my bible; it told me that most likely I was on the way towards spontaneous abortion, a term that had replaced "miscarriage" in my vocabulary. I hadn't yet consulted the Rochester gynecologists, because I was not yet, by my calculations, three months pregnant and, in what I now call the olden days, I didn't feel safely enough pregnant to confide the news to the world until I had gotten to the magical three months. So I went to a local doctor in the small town in which we lived then, and listened to absolute mumbo jumbo about rocket stages which he offered as explanation for what was happening in my body. The second stage of the rocket, he soberly informed me, needed help in firing; I should go to bed and stay there until the next stage of the rocket propelled me into a safe orbit.

An inner sanity, a sense of knowing the meaning of my own body's signals, assured me that this talk of rocket stages was lunacy, but I was reluctant to act out of what felt too much like arrogance. So I went to bed, for two horrible days, while our two-year old child went into a frenzy of demands to get me on my feet and back into her world. The small-town doctor's pastel painting of the placid mother playing games in bed with a two-year old waiting happily for a baby was almost immediately replaced by such a terrible time of enforced immobility that I only felt sane again when I climbed out of bed, compulsively making it behind me, and threw myself back into a life which would very soon bring on the "spontaneous" abortion that had been waiting to happen.

This is another birthing story that I usually tell as joyful farce; it was not joyful, especially because I understood that I would have to do it myself in the face of the wisdom I had refused to accept. It was only a matter of days before the fetus began to expel itself from my body. I felt uneasy enough about my cramping body that I let Erica go downstairs to play with Nancy, the daughter of our neighbors. Soon, my cramps became intense, and in the bathroom a convulsive spasm expelled the bloody tissue that was the fetus I had been carrying. I knelt on the linoleum floor of our bathroom and looked closely at the mass in the water; I hoped that I had gotten out all the tissue, but the edges were so ragged that I couldn't be sure, and I was still bleeding. I flushed the toilet, stuffed toilet paper in my underpants, and went to phone Jerry to tell him what had happened. I thought I was lucid and perfectly conscious, but as I talked to him I slid to the floor, pulling the highchair with me that stood under our wall phone. Our downstairs neighbors heard the crash, found me on the floor, and called the ambulance from the nearby hospital in Dansville. Actually, it was a hearse, used by the local emergency squad to transport both live patients and dead bodies. They got me downstairs in a sort of fireman's carry and then implored me not to bleed on the gurney. It's that part of the story that I usually tell, for even in my bleary state I recognized the mordantly amusing nature of that moment. "Sorry," I said, not at all sorry, really, "but bleeding is what I'm doing right now."

In the hospital, I told my story to a doctor and a nurse standing on either side of my hospital bed. I described the mass I'd seen and, as I looked at first one and then the other, I realized that they were smirking. My attempt to be helpful and descriptive was amusing; I was back in the realm of inefficient contractions, and I felt my face flush with angry embarrassment. I awoke a while later, packed with gauze from the D and C they had done "just in case," and with an intravenous needle in my hand. I was furious, and I focused my fury on that saline drip, threatening to rip it out of my hand if they didn't remove it. Another nurse, knowing no doubt that it was no longer necessary, humored me and removed it. Shortly afterwards Jerry drove me home.

Compared to my mother's miscarriage, mine was relatively undramatic. I remember the ride in the hearse as scenic; lying on my back, half-heartedly squeezing my legs together in a languid attempt not to bleed on their gurney, I could see the curves and soft outlines of the Genesee Valley out the back window. Knowing my doomed pregnancy was over, still feeling as though I had done it right, I relaxed and enjoyed the ride. Years later I read articles and poetry about the grief of abortion without a moment of identification. The fetus was only a fetus to me; the child we had was real, and I had felt entirely justified in getting out of bed and being her mother once again, not a beached whale trying to blast off into the next rocket stage described by a small-town doctor practicing in a room of his Victorian house.

Miscarriages were nature's way of rectifying mistakes; I understood and felt only relief, if indeed I felt anything at all, that we'd been spared the consequences of a mistake by nature. My mother, who never spoke directly to me of any other way to understand what had happened, sent me a book and offered to spend two nights in a hotel with me in the city as a special treat. I accepted both gestures with delight. It didn't seem strange at the time that the book was Jessamyn West's novel, based on her own life history, about one sister's loving support of another sister's decision to end her life to escape the worst ravages of an inoperable cancer. The title of the book is *The Woman Said Yes.* I read it over and over, saddened and entranced by the love and loyalty the sisters felt for one another and for the Hispanic doctor who went with them to the end that he helped to bring about. Over the years there have been times when I've literally shaken my head at what seems like a bizarre choice of a consoling story, yet I've always felt that it was perfect. In the face of a disintegrating and intractable body, two adult women and a doctor practicing at the edge of his profession outwitted the worst with courage and delight in one another. The death was a kind of birth, and I experienced the book and the two days with my mother as healing. We saw Nureyev and Fonteyn in a mawkish ballet based on the saga of Camille, their partnership transfiguring the waning days of Fonteyn's magic and Nureyev's life before AIDS destroyed him. What did I know of the bond our miscarriages provided us? When I return to the novel, which I do at least once a year, I usually skip towards the end, gravitating inevitably towards the scenes of coffee ice cream and the precisely timed shots of morphine, the childhood memories shared in the dark as the two sisters lie in their twin beds waiting for the morphine to allow them both to sleep. My mother and I shared a room with twin beds in the Hotel Tuscany, a hotel long since swallowed up by a huge chain of hotel suites. Like the sisters, we talked back and forth from our beds, and I think I was healed from the wound I hadn't even understood life had inflicted.

My mother was scrupulously honest, but she was also indirect. Filled with sadness now, I wish I had understood more particularly the gifts she offered me in our time together after my spontaneous abortion. I don't remember an embrace, even when we parted at the end of the second day, yet I knew that I was in her protection. I have never for a second wondered what that child might have been like, but I can wonder endlessly about my mother's instinct to have given me that book, those days. We learned how to eat an artichoke in a small French restaurant during those two days, and I think of that shared heart every time I prepare artichokes for cooking. I forgot about being a mother, failing to be a mother, and I was entirely a daughter, her daughter. I am still her daughter.

For me, though not, I think, for my mother, it was bliss to be a daughter. My grandmother, my mother's mother, was an Eastern European version of "the angel in the house," a woman impossible to resist and almost impossible to please. She had been thirty when my mother was born, forty when my mother's brother was born, a woman too austerely beautiful to be associated with sex, disappointed in an early romantic love, a woman who literally scrubbed floors to provide for her children when her husband went to jail for bungling his handling of union funds. From the moments of her first endless labor, I believe my mother must have vowed to do it differently, but I imagine that the rigors of the breech birth, the baby with her head swaddled in receiving blankets, pierced my mother's resolve. Perversely, my grandmother was the essence of tenderness with me; I received the tenderness that my mother yearned for. Wished for by my parents, I understood that children were wishes granted, and it wasn't until I joined my mother on the far side of pain and loss that I understood the knowledge she had chosen to withhold from me.

When finally after ten o'clock at night, our daughter swaddled in my arms, we phoned my parents to report in triumph that Erica had been born, I was incapable of registering my mother's exhausted insistence on telling me how she had phoned every hour on the hour. Knowing how much we loved our cat, she had counted on Jerry to return to feed Thomas, and as the hours passed she imagined that she knew the worst. How she must have paced and smoked, maybe even wept with frustration and fear, remembering her struggles, my father's tears, his banishment from her side which he welcomed as he fled from that noisy battlefield. My father had early on claimed his position as the sensitive one, the child with the delicate stomach, the cultured son of a highbred German family. The brutal labor to bring forth the daughter he yearned for appalled him. All their lives together, my father depended on the strength of his wife, and she in turn hid her fears and her pains from him. After her willed miscarriage, my father wrote a light-hearted note to her, assuring her that the missed package delivery could easily be made up by future promptness.

After my miscarriage, which in my mind I always called my spontaneous abortion in some attempt to define it as a natural and benign process, we began in earnest to try and conceive another child. We went back to Madison, Wisconsin, on a fellowship, to live in faculty housing and reinvent ourselves as grownups, parents determined to become parents again, armed, as we imagined, with our previous success. The team of doctors who had delivered Erica were once again our wise men. They counseled every other day intercourse and reassured me that Nature had corrected her own error. In the heat of a Madison summer as fierce as the one in which our first child had been born, we followed their instructions. Our bodies wet with sweat, making sucking noises when we pulled ourselves apart, we methodically went to bed every other morning while Erica was in nursery school. In those days, before the routine use of pregnancy tests, we had no way of knowing that I was actually pregnant when we arrived in Madison; I didn't even think to do the counting backwards that would have allowed us to enjoy the summer—and one another–without the slavish observance of a routine that made love-making a methodical drill with little to recommend it. Delayed gratification kept us going, and when we returned to our lives in upstate New York we were duly pregnant.

It was during this pregnancy that I was given the opportunity to reflect on Erica's breech presentation and my earlier experience of "natural" childbirth. I registered the lack of enthusiasm with which my new team of doctors received my account of that earlier delivery, but I think I chalked it up to easterners' condescension towards midwesterners; after all, our families had sent us CARE packages of food the whole time we lived in Madison, and my mother had insisted that I have all my dental needs taken care of before I left for graduate school.

Our new team of obstetricians were fanatics about weight gain; the old team had taken a somewhat benign position, and Guttmacher's *Pregnancy and Birth,* rich in line drawings of the developing fetus and chary of details about what might go wrong, seemed to assume that we'd all be successful if we just ate normally and took our vitamins. Once I was safely past the three-month line, we told our families and assumed all would go well. My mother, this time, made arrangements to come to stay with us in advance of this baby's expected arrival. She seemed lighthearted, and we were glad to have her nearby. This pregnancy seemed magical to me. It was as though it cancelled out the previous sadness and alienation. I was surrounded by friends in a small town, with the promise of my mother coming to be with us at the end. I ate yogurt religiously for the first time in my life, fiercely watching my weight and imagining that when the baby was born I would be slimmer than I had ever been in my life.

Because it was snow season, and we lived thirty miles from the hospital, the doctors decided to induce labor two days before my predicted date of delivery. We were between storms, and the roads were clear. The labor wing was full, it seemed, so we spent the day shopping, even stopping to see Jerry's allergist. My mother welcomed the casual and expectant mood we carried with us that day. She was our companion as we wandered through stores, and she insisted on buying me a gloriously printed shirt with decorative buttons down the front that would allow me to nurse in style and comfort. The whole day is a charmed memory for me, as I believe it was for my mother as well. It seemed to promise some restitution to us all for the fears and the pains of the past. The hospital in Rochester was participating in a trial of a new protocol for labor and delivery: this time my pubic hair wasn't shaved, a relief to us all, for it meant I could wait for a while in peace to see if my labor might start up on its own. In a little while, it did. A friend came by and took my mother back to our small town where our daughter was being cared for, leaving Jerry and me alone to experience this second labor. Up on the labor and delivery wing, in a small cubicle with a curtain hanging askew, we heard screams and shouts, voices and equipment clattering past our hospital-green sanctuary. My body and I seemed to be in some sort of tacit agreement to do this together, peacefully. There was no sense of urgency, no pain beyond meaning, no rules to try to abide by, no agony. I don't even remember a clock. The first terrible time, I watched the inexorable hands of the clock outlining the stretched out seconds of contractions that blurred my vision and made time my enemy. This time, after a while, I felt that something had changed and sent Jerry to find a nurse to check me. Astonishingly, I was ready to deliver, and I was wheeled rapidly across the hallway and into the delivery room, waving goodbye to Jerry. We never thought to have him stay. He missed a series of wonderful moments. I was, it seemed, the first woman that day to be having a baby who was desired, the first woman not to be screaming and writhing and cursing. It was evening; everyone except me seemed to be tired and grateful for this easy delivery. There was no shouting welcome to Matthew as he slid out of me, skinny and pale, lighter and leaner than his sister had been, but there was palpable delight and even expressions of gratitude from the exhausted doctor and nurses who praised me and our beautiful baby.

One conversation that I do remember having with my mother was about our inability to remember pain, especially the pain of childbirth. She told me of a woman who was in labor with her, that first time, the time that marked her forever. The other woman wasn't having her first child, and she couldn't get over her own stupidity, letting herself in for this agony for a second excruciating time. I have never forgotten, or for that matter forgiven, the pain of my first labor, but it seemed to have been redeemed by the second one. All of us, I think, shared in that feeling of accomplishment, the pleasure of giving birth, greeting a new life that seemed to come without a terrible cost. And from the start of the day, my mother had been with me, a little bewildered at the shopping frenzy and the trek through the bowels of an old but medically distinguished hospital until our friend carried her away to a good meal and the love of her adoring granddaughter.

I began to write this memory piece on my daughter's birthday; I am working towards its conclusion as we approach the birthday of my daughter's daughter, named for her two great-grandmothers. We all imagined that my mother would want to stay alive to see this child born, but, as she had willed her miscarriage, my mother willed her own death when the terms of life without my father became unendurable. My mother's almost lifelong mastery over her own body must have been especially incomprehensible and unbearable as she labored to push me backwards out into the world outside her enormous belly. As I was bashed and mashed, she must have been torn and stretched; if even today my scalp won't tolerate snug winter caps, my mother's body must have reminded her for years, decades, of its suffering. I think now that the prospect of waiting for her granddaughter to give birth must not have been the incentive to stay alive that we assumed would keep her with us. She had many reasons to flee; her memories of breech births may have been among them.

My daughter's Valentine's Day gift to us was her announcement that we were to be grandparents. I think from the very first moments of her pregnancy she saw this child as a gift to us all. I was with her in the office when the doctor did the first sonogram that clearly showed the beating heart of the baby; none of us thought of this cluster of cells as a fetus. Everything was changed, transformed by technology and desire from a technical term to the shadow of a real baby within our sight if not yet in our world.

More and more as our daughter's pregnancy advanced, I thought of my mother; I felt myself her representative in this world. Her desire not to live, her decision to die, left me alone on the border of knowledge and pain. Erica was supremely happy about her pregnancy. From the earliest moments, thanks to pregnancy tests, she was absorbed in planning and anticipating. She abandoned her dissertation work, feeling that her somber topic created an undesirable atmosphere for the child within her. I remembered how my uncle had wept and how my parents had blurted out their anxiety that my first pregnancy would put an end to my PhD work; I accepted Erica's explanation without comment, imagining that she would integrate these parts of her life in time, as I had. It had not been easy for me to hold together graduate school and motherhood; there was no one like me in my cohort at Wisconsin. When my milk dried up early in my nursing of Erica, our wonderful pediatrician, used to dealing with graduate students as parents, reminded me that "you don't get a grade for motherhood," even though the graduate students he was used to were the fathers, not the mothers; he counseled applesauce. So I knew in my body and my mind that it was possible to hold these parts together, and I chose to respond out of my own experience rather than the fears of my mother, the despair of my uncle. In this, as in all my responses to my daughter's pregnancies, I have consulted memory but have tried to feel and see beyond it: to be a mother and a daughter at once, and now a grandmother. With binocular vision, I am trying to make the images overlap, fuse, and become one of many dimensions. The effort feels literally tangible. I am giving myself headaches, and I often walk away from my keyboard and direct my vision elsewhere. Yesterday I found myself saying aloud words from John Milton's great sonnet on his blindness, his heartbroken recollection of "that one talent which is death to hide." Daughter, mother, grandmother wrestle me to silence.

Some time in advance of her expected delivery, my daughter asked me to be with her and Scott during her labor right through the birth. She asked me to take pictures, and I agreed without hesitation. I knew her obstetrician; he had been my gynecologist for many years, and as we expected he agreed without reservation that I could be present. So much had changed, I thought, from the times my mother and I had been through. We all felt nothing but joy and excitement at the prospect before us. I had no expectations to bring to this experience once I learned that the baby, whom we called Sophie Alexander to cover all contingencies, was securely head down. A series of sonograms and amniocentesis reassured us that the baby was developing normally and had no genetic defects; Erica and Scott chose not to learn the sex in advance, a decision we were happy to support. There was so much more to fear this time around, but my daughter was resolutely cheerful, especially once she had banished her Holocaust studies from her mind.

We were a small crowd in the hospital waiting room when Erica went into labor. My brother was visiting, and our closest friends, recent grandparents themselves, were with us as well. The atmosphere was excited but casual; this new generation of daughters, we thought, somehow managed to include us while remaining in charge of their labor and delivery—or so we imagined. In New York, our friends' eldest daughter had labored valiantly and painfully, only to be grateful in the end for a caesarian which denied her the sort of triumph she had imagined. Here at home, my time in the labor room with Erica and Scott stretched out endlessly, and my reports to the group in the waiting room became sketchier and less confident. My brother lost patience and went off to explore the hospital and the neighborhood. Our friends made telephone calls to report to their own daughters and stayed on to encourage us, while I went back and forth, taking pictures of a scene that became harder to watch and even harder to accept. My daughter began to moan and weep. The contractions were visibly painful and unproductive. I remembered with horror the verdict of "inefficient" that had been so casually rendered as I suffered, and I felt my throat close with remembered tears. I began to crave relief, but the terms were clear; she had to ask for an epidural, a form of pain relief that hadn't existed in my world of childbirth. And she didn't ask, but her moaning intensified, her tears came thickly. I snapped pictures furiously, my vision blurred, my mouth clenched. No one wore masks or gowns yet, for it clearly wasn't time for anything significant to happen. Yet my child was being wrenched and torn, sucking on ice chips, her hair matted with sweat. I hated being there and being ineffectual. The labor nurse smiled at me and said, "she won't remember any of this, don't worry; they never do." Then, to my daughter, in a more tender tone, "you're having back labor, sweetie; it's the worst kind. Do you want something for it?" By that time, mid-afternoon, it was apparent that my daughter's threshold for pain had long been crossed; tearfully she begged for the epidural that had always, it seemed, been an option available for the asking. Word went out for the anesthesiologist and we all began to wait with a different sense of urgency. There was a small patch of darkness showing between my daughter's legs, but it was meaningless. Still, I took its picture for the record, for something to indicate at least the idea of progress. The anesthesiologist did not arrive. The moaning and thrashing continued. Scott and I were consumed with resentment at the delay, at the nurses' relaxed conversation, at our total ineffectualness. At one moment I saw him tensing his leg, preparing to kick a heavy metal wastebasket, and I sidled up to him to stop him, to share his anger and frustration without letting him risk being asked to leave, though every cell of my body was screaming to get us out of there.

When finally the anesthesiologist arrived, the epidural wasn't the blessing we all longed for; it seemed to relieve one side of the pain but not the other. I think we were all crying when the doctor arrived, having been summoned, at last, because finally this baby was on the verge of being born. He was getting into scrubs as he entered the room, smiling and nodding, speaking confidently to Erica, giving her instructions even as he was injecting novacaine and starting an episiotomy. He was content to have me standing right behind him, my camera over his shoulder, as he instructed Erica, finally, to push and bear down. For those moments I was fully absorbed by the drama of the birth and I had some moments of freedom from the anger and frustration and anguish of all the hours of pain. Within minutes a baby squirmed out of my daughter and into the world: a girl. I took her picture as she was born and then staggered to the door which was ajar. In the hallway, my husband was waiting, and I fell into his arms, sobbing. "It's Sophie," I wept; "it's Sophie." Our friend took the camera from me and took pictures of us. I describe myself in those pictures as the five-hundred year old woman. I felt destroyed and looked it.

By the time I went back into the room, Erica was laughing with delight; as the nurses had said so confidently, she had forgotten all the pain and misery of the long day's labor. But I was nowhere near joy and delight. I had never forgotten my own first labor, and now I had experienced it again, from what seemed no distance at all, along with my mother's labor, which was somehow part of the struggle and the pain. I was overwhelmed at the cost of birth, the ability of the nurses to be in the same room with such pain without suffering it, the methodical stitching up and measuring and weighing while the baby screamed and her mother yearned for her. I was not ready to love the baby, and my day of picture-taking and presence left me empty of feeling, incapable of reflection or joy.

When I remember the birth of that child I came to love dearly, I remember in the context of my own birth, the story I came to know in fragments over the years which seemed to coalesce into one coherent narrative only after I watched my daughter's body convulse and recover. I wished that I had been able to comfort my own mother, confirm her bravery, rejoice in her delivery, as I was able eventually to do for my daughter. I longed both to comfort my mother and to be comforted by her. I knew then and know now that my mother never regretted my birth, that she withheld her story from me as though her silence could be a charm to protect me from the pain I had cost her; pain that, contrary to the serene pronouncements of the labor nurse at Sophie's birth, my mother never forgot, as I never forgot the pain of my own labor. Yet my labor came to be another version of my mother's labor, and I imagined that by bearing witness to my daughter's experience I would succeed finally in taming the wild strands of the past with the enlightened participation in the present. It hasn't concluded so neatly. Of them all, my mother's experience as I heard it and as I imagine it now is still the most salient. My sense of our labors as framed by the theories of others is more insistent now than it was when I lived through my own labors and deliveries. For now I see even our abortions as their own deliveries, experienced within our bodies but also framed by the expectations and theories of others. I want to console my mother not just for her pain but for her suffering and for her determination to protect me. As I watched my daughter, helpless, I watch my mother, and I am helpless; my understanding is hard won and worth having, but it is only by my life that I can hope to complete her work.

I'M BORN A CROW INDIAN

FRED W. VOGET

My Birth in a Tent

I was told that I began my life in a tent during our Crow Indian Fair held in October at Crow Agency in 1908. My folks were camped out in a tipi made of canvas. They moved to the fairgrounds and pitched their tipi across from the agency on October 26th, and I was born the next day. There was a hospital right across the way, but in those days Crows didn't like to go to the hospital. They called the hospital "the sick peoples' lodge," and it was a strange place from which you might not come out alive. Most kids began their lives in a tent the way I did, and when they got sick, they usually were doctored at home by a medicine man.

Once I was on the way, my mother put herself under the guidance of her mother, as old people knew what to do. They had beliefs in the old days that if a woman slept with her feet facing a doorway, she would have an easy time of it. To sleep with her feet toward a wall in a tipi or a log house would make it hard for the baby to come out. Crows also didn't like a woman to stand or sit with her backside to a fire because that heat held back the afterbirth and might cause her to die.

Mother had to get herself up at sunrise and had to drink plenty of water and soup. Each time she took water she rubbed her abdomen to keep me from getting stuck, and she walked a lot to keep me down to size. They didn't have many nine- or ten-pound babies in those days. Mother also made sure not to lift anything heavy, and she didn't do any heavy work at all for about ten days before I was to arrive. As for my father, he didn't go hunting because he knew that his shot would miss the deer anyway. That's the way it is for hunters even today when a wife is in a family way. There is something mysterious that comes between the hunter and the animal so the hunter can't shoot straight.

Chapter 2 (35–47) in *They Call Me Agnes: A Crow Narrative Based on the Life of Agnes Yellowtail Deernose,* by Fred W. Voget, with Mary K. Mee. Norman: University of Oklahoma Press, 2000.

In the old days when a baby was born in a tipi, whoever was attending the pregnant woman put up two sturdy poles at the place where a wife rested her head when sleeping. She would kneel on soft skins (especially buffalo robes), rest her elbows on the pillow, and grasp the stout poles. Once the baby was born, getting the afterbirth out was the big problem. No men or boys could be present at childbirth, for they would make it even harder on the woman. So the father-to-be would go and stay with a brother or a married sister. Some older woman, who in a dream had received a special medicine to make birth easier, was asked to take charge. She always had to be paid with something valuable, maybe a horse. A mother and grandmother usually were present, and the grandmother might be the one to cut the umbilical cord, which was measured at three fingers in breadth from the navel.

After the child was born, the older women took the buffalo robe with the afterbirth to a brushy area some distance from the camp. They drained the blood off and raised the robe four times to make the child grow. Crows always do things four times in a ritual way. Any blood that happened to get on the floor of the tipi was scraped up and thrown away outside the camp, and new dirt was brought in and the area then was smoked with sage. When everything had been cleaned up inside the tipi, the woman's mother smoked it with running cedar, fir needles, and bear root, if that was the husband's medicine. Then the tipi was finally purified and was ready for the father's return.

Although I was an old-fashioned baby, I was born in a tent, not a tipi. During early reservation days they shifted the birth to a tent instead of a tipi or log house. My sister, Amy, told me that she and my cousin played in the tent the family put up for my birth. They had a bed ready for my mother, and she could have used those poles, just as in the old days. My mother's younger sister, Mary Takes The Gun, acted as a midwife, for she was like a medicine woman and knew a lot.

In the old days the Crow women washed a newborn with water, but in my time they greased the infant with olive oil and then wiped it off. That's what my mother's sister did with me. Then she wrapped me in a blanket and brought me to my mother's bed, which was in the tipi. When my father came to see me, he called on his own mother to bring me for him to see. He didn't take me in his arms, but he did want to know if I looked like him. My father couldn't ask my mother's mother to bring me to him because he could not talk to his mother-in-law, and she couldn't talk to him either.

Mother didn't nurse me until the third day, for she did not have milk until then. My family brought in a woman who was nursing. She dropped a few drops of milk into my mouth to start me sucking. In the old days Crow women used to bring a two-week-old puppy to suck a first-time mother's nipples if they were not large enough or properly formed. Sometimes even with the second child they would get a puppy to bring on a good flow of milk.

By the time my mother began nursing me, my grandmother had pierced my ears. Crows often did it right away when first wrapping the newborn, but in my case I was two days old. Some used to wait until the fourth day. My father's mother heated the end of a metal awl to keep the blood from flowing and pierced my ears in three different places. Then she took a very small piece of the heartwood of the yellow willow, greased it, and placed it in the hole. Yellow willow was best because the wood was naturally smooth. When I was a few weeks old, my mother knew it was time to remove the willow piece from the bottom hole and to insert a small blue shell brought from the Pacific Coast. Boys got off easier than girls with their ears, and usually they had only one hole, or maybe two. Crows continued piercing girls' ears on the third or fourth day until the thirties. Nowadays girls get their ears pierced when they want to, and I don't know of any boys who have their ears pierced.

I slept with my mother's mother at first, for they were afraid my mother might roll over and smother me. Whenever I cried out of hunger, Grandma would take me to my mother and then carry me back to her bed. They didn't let me sleep with my mother until I was sitting up when I was about five months old. After that, my sleeping time was divided between a grandmother and Mother, but I came to like sleeping with my father's mother the best. She used to rock me to sleep, and when I first awakened, she whispered "tch, tch, tch" in my ears and then she sang lullabies to me. She sang one song about a colt running with his mane waving, and of his large ears and twitching tail. She also sang about the parts of a rabbit that people ate: the choice tripe, kidneys, and even the little balls. And every time they put me to bed at night, my grandmother used running cedar to smoke the house to drive away any evil spirits who might be around. Some people used bear root, or eseh, as we call it. People used a different smoke according to their medicine, but cedar is one they usually use to make sure that their prayers get through.

Protecting the Newborn

Crows always were fearful that a baby or a youngster would get sick, especially with pneumonia. If that happened, they called in a medicine man who was known for his cures. He used an ash or chokecherry tube to suck out the bad stuff, and he usually received a horse and several comforters as payment. When I was about six years old, I took sick with double pneumonia, and my parents took me to an Indian doctor by the name of Gros Ventre. My mother said I was just skin and bones by then. He sucked all the bad blood out and cured me. In those days Indian doctors were great. They could do almost anything and even could put bones together. People always tried to pay them well with four things, for the cure worked better with the spirit helpers that way. And that's the way it works today, too, if you go to a medicine man for a cure. For four things today, Crows like to give a Pendleton blanket, dress goods, tobacco, and money.

People always wanted the newborn to grow and to get tall, and so they wouldn't let anyone step over it. If some boy or girl happened to step over a baby or a growing child, the grown-ups made them step back again. Even when grown up you were not supposed to step over someone. When the Crow were moving around in the old days and came to a spring where a spirit person lived, a mother would give her infant, or young child, some beads or tobacco to throw in there so that the infant would grow to manhood or womanhood. They used to do that at a warm spring near Livingston by Yellowstone Park and at Big Spring, north of Pryor. The mother spoke to the "person" in the spring by saying, "I want this boy (or girl) to grow up to be a man (or woman)."

Medicine dreams were protective of the infant and growing child. This is where our paternal relatives come in. They dream our growth, life, and success for us. Losing a first child always was bad luck for a couple. When this happened, a man and his wife often went into the nearby hills to fast together for four days, and they often mourned for three months or more. Sometimes when they fasted, the man or the woman might receive a vision-message from a spirit person with instructions to make a necklace or other thing to keep the newborn in good health. Crows tell of one man who lost two boys in succession. In his fasting he happened to walk among some prairie dog holes, and finally he sat down. He dreamed of a large prairie dog hole, and out of it came a lot of girls. Each one had a blue and white bead necklace to which two elk teeth were attached. Besides the usual braid at each side, some of the girls had another small braid on the left side, others a small braid at the back. After that, the man had five daughters. He fixed a necklace of blue and white beads for each one of them when they were ready to start walking, for the girls he saw in his dream walked out of the prairie dog hole. All five of the girls had long lives. When a man or woman had such a medicine, others came to him or her for help so that their children might grow up healthy. But the parents or grandparents had to give the person something of value for such a medicine-blessing, usually a horse. A horse was our best gift and our standard measure of wealth. A horse is still the best gift today, and brothers-in-law usually save to give such horses to each other. These are not just ordinary horses but racehorses with papers. They do that because there is a special respect relationship between brothers-in-law and between sisters-in-law, too.

To protect their newborn, the Crow people also used a name-blessing that could bring good health and prosperity to the child. They invited a man known to have powers (usually an outstanding warrior, and often a clansman of the father), to give a name-blessing at the time when the ears were pierced. This usually was done for a boy child.

After the naming the father would invite his clan brothers to a feast, and these men would tell of their dreams. Their summer dreams always looked ahead to winter when snow was on the ground, and their winter dreams always looked ahead to the time when the grass was green and it was warm. That is how they protected their children from year to year with dream-blessings. An Indian name given by a clan uncle or a well-known clan brother is still considered important to the health and the success of Crow children.

If a child, after getting a name, turned out to be sickly, a medicine man would be called to change the name. When Cuts The Bear's Ears, a medicine man, named a boy one time, he painted the boy's face yellow with two red spots on his cheeks. He then raised the boy four times, smoking him with cedar incense, and named him High Cedar. "Here is High Cedar," he said, "and you who are present will never hear someone say that he has passed away. He will live to an old age." And that's the way it turned out. Every morning for ten years the father painted the boy's face yellow with the two red spots and prayed with tobacco that the boy would grow up healthy. He stopped the painting when High Cedar didn't want to be different from other boys of his age.

They had another way of curing a child who was sick a lot. If the parents worried that the child might die, they might make him a "throwaway" child. The parents would take a sick infant to a prearranged spot and a close friend or a relative, usually a clan aunt or uncle, would take the child home. The new parents blessed the infant and gave him a new name and new clothes. This was like a rebirth, and the new parents were now considered to be the child's real father and mother. The new mother and father were always concerned about the welfare of their child even though he might not live with them. Parents told an older child that what they were doing was a blessing wish that he get a new start, grow up strong, and become well-known. A "throwaway" child might get well right away, or it might take a longer time. By custom, the new father and mother were given four gifts, usually Pendleton blankets, three or four quilts, money, and cigarettes, and sometimes a horse.

Some children had their names changed as many as three or more times. Boys were more sickly than girls, so they had their names changed more often. Names were connected to luck and to wealth, and that is another reason boys had their names changed more often.

A medicine necklace or a medicine tied to the back of the head was usual for boys, while girls had a small braid on the left side where a medicine bead or a shell might be attached. You don't see those medicine braids much any more, but quite a few children still wear medicine necklaces to protect their health.

Taking Care of a New Mother

Mother said she didn't have much time to rest after I was born. They wouldn't let her do any cooking or work for about ten days, but my two grandmothers made her get up and walk to prevent blood poisoning. They also saw to it that she drank plenty of water and soup to produce milk. My mother said she could never seem to get enough to eat. She wanted to eat all the time, not just in the morning and evening as the Crow were used to doing. My father's mother was especially fond of natural vegetables and fruits, and she would go out in the morning and bring back wild turnips, twin grass, chokecherries, and berries for making soup when she could find them. Mother never lost her appetite for meat either, and she sucked on dried meat dipped in meat soup to increase her supply of milk. In the old days the Crow had this milkweed that they soaked in warm water. When the water turned green, the nursing mother would drink it, sipping some of it off and on all day. This never failed. Sometimes the gummy substance the plant gave out would be chewed, but you had to break up many stalks to get enough gum to chew. Nowadays rice is often used along with regular or evaporated milk to make a good flow of milk. Beef soup is also a favorite, but now most kids grow up with a bottle, especially if they are adopted.

Cradles, Colic, and Weaning

I spent my early days on a cradleboard. My father's mother made my cradleboard. In the Crow way, the father's side should do this, either his mother or his sister. Father had a sister, but his mother wanted to do it.

I was laced into my cradleboard with my arms at my sides and only my face showing. My family was still using powdered dust from rotting wood and red paint powder to help keep me dry and free from chafing and itching. Pieces of cloth soaked up my soil in place of soft hide, or my mother slipped a kind of pillow made of hide and stuffed with pine needles under me. Crows were still using that kind of pillow when Joe Medicine Crow was a baby around 1914.

My mother was a great tanner of hides, and when she went back to work in about ten days she could have given me a cow's teat to suck on to keep me quiet, for the original pacifier had been a buffalo's teat. Mothers used to give young ones some of that tough gristle from the brisket to suck on and also let them suck on the chokecherry stick used to dig marrow from the bones or used in making berry puddings. Chokecherry was good because it didn't splinter like other woods. Of course, mothers used to feed their babies just about every time the infants cried, and they always left open part of the sleeve under the arm for nursing. That's the way I did it when nursing Bobby. I never heard what my family did with my umbilical cord when it fell off. In the old days Crows sewed it up in a beaded piece and tied it to the cradleboard.

Whenever they took me out of the cradleboard for rest and play, Father like to raise me up and bounce me on his knee and give me a kiss on the cheek. When I started to sit up, around the fifth month, and showed an interest in crawling, it was time to take me out of the cradleboard. When I was able to sit up I played with a stick with a string of beads attached to it, or I was given a tin cup to knock around. Waving my arms up and down jiggled the beads and kept me quiet for a while, which was what my mother and grandmother wanted. When I started to crawl, they had to watch me all the time to make sure I didn't get burned on the kitchen stove.

Colic was a common problem for babies. In the old days there always were old women who specialists in "ass ache," as colic was called. Some mothers and grandmothers were big chewers of tobacco, while the men rolled cigarettes out of Bull Durham tobacco. Colic specialists would grease the backside of the baby and slip a wad of chewed tobacco up there. If that didn't work, they'd take a big pot and fill it with cold water. Then they'd put the colicky baby in the water, usually waist high.

They'd leave him in the cold water until he stopped crying; then they wrapped the baby in a warm skin or blanket, and usually he went right to sleep. My sister, Amy, used to do that with her baby, Joe Medicine Crow, and it worked.

Colic wasn't the only remedy the old women used chewing tobacco for. If you had sore legs, they'd rub it on, and it helped take out the ache. They also put it on cuts and then wrapped them up. Not many women of my generation took up tobacco chewing, and chewing went out pretty much with the old-timers in the forties.

When I began to make more talking sounds, Grandma Stays By The Water tried to teach me a few words, like *papa, mama,* and *give me.* She was my constant nursemaid. At our house, wooden benches and Grandmother's knees helped me to stand up, and before long I took my first steps, reaching for outstretched arms. I was about a year old when I first walked. Father sent word to the clan uncle who had named me that "his child was walking." When my clan uncle came, he brought along a lariat, sang his "glad song" for my success, and then claimed the horse owed for his good-luck blessing. Mothers were proud of children who walked early, but I didn't walk early enough for my mother to brag about. The first steps were very important, because it meant that a walking baby was on his way, protected by dream-blessings of his clan uncles. It showed they had powerful medicines for their "child."

Weaning was not a happy time, and a baby always wanted to go to the mother for food. Mother and Grandmother tried to plan ahead. Sometimes when Mother was eating and holding me in her lap, she would slip a piece of fat to me. That was around the fourth month when my lower cutting teeth made their appearance. They started me out on a watery soup, and gradually I got less water, more soup, and less breast milk. When it looked like I could take straight soup and eat solid foods with my baby teeth, Mother took some black from inside a tobacco pipe and smeared it on her nipples. That bad taste started me to crying. This happened before I began to walk. Once they began the soup-and-water diet, I was always hungry, and Grandma had to pack me around on her back, walking most of the time to keep me quiet. I used to get her up some nights, and she would have to walk and walk. Then, when they broke me with that tobacco blackening, Grandma had to do her walking at her own place, for every time I saw my mother I would cry out to be breast-fed. Crow mothers don't use that tobacco black any more. My sister, Amy, and I didn't use it either, but we fed our babies milk out of a cup and spooned in soft foods. Our mother and grandmothers were always there to help out, and even today a grandma's back is the preferred carryall for babies. In my mother's time, and even during my childhood, mothers used to nurse kids that were two and three years old and running around and playing.

Dressing Up in White Clothes

In the old days Crows dressed boys of two to three years in moccasins, hip-length leggings, and a breechcloth of soft hide. Girls wore moccasins, short leggings, and a short buckskin dress gathered at the middle with a belt. After I began to walk, I wore a simple calico dress that ended just below my knees. Little boys, especially in summer, wore a little outer shirt that barely covered the crotch. There wasn't much of the old-style dress around when I was growing up because hides for tanning were hard to get, even though the men still hunted elk and deer.

Some men, when they began to wear pants, had the seat cut out so the legs were like leggings and they could wear a cloth breechcloth. My mother cut and made dresses for herself and us girls from dress goods, and this was common for women into the thirties. During the late thirties and forties, Crows worked for wages in the WPA (Works Progress Administration) and also at jobs during the war. I think that money helped girls become more style-conscious and started them to buy dresses at the store.

Church and school had a lot to do with getting us into white man's clothes. You had to look nice when you went to church and to school. We had to give up our moccasins and put on high-topped shoes. Boys entering the government boarding school in Crow Agency had their braids cut off and wore a military uniform with a jacket, trousers, black shoes, and a round black hat. The school had the girls wear gingham dresses with the same design on so they would all look alike, too.

It wasn't like that at our Baptist mission school where I went. The mission gave out dresses, pants, shoes, socks, and underclothing sent free from people in the East. We all took what fitted best, and our mothers and grandmothers altered them to fit. In those days people didn't always know what they should wear to church, and Dr. Petzoldt (Baptist minister) used to tell how one well-known Crow warrior turned up at church one Sunday dressed in shoes, long underwear, and a high hat. He always like to tell that story because it seemed so funny to him.

THE SANDBOX

EDWARD ALBEE

The Players:

THE YOUNG MAN . . . . 25.	A good-looking, well-built boy in a bathing suit.
MOMMY . . . . 55.	A well-dressed, imposing woman.
DADDY . . . . 60.	A small man; gray, thin.
GRANDMA . . . . 86.	A tiny, wizened woman with bright eyes.
THE MUSICIAN	No particular age, but young would be nice.

Note:

When, in the course of the play, mommy and daddy call each other by these names, there should be no suggestion of regionalism. These names are empty of affection and point up the pre-senility and vacuity of their characters.

The Scene:

A bare stage, with only the following: Near the footlights, far stage-right, two simple chairs set side by side, facing the audience; near the footlights, far stage-left, a chair facing stage-right with a music stand before it; farther back, and stage-center, slightly elevated and raked, a large child's sandbox with a toy pail and shovel; the background is the sky, which alters from brightest day to deepest night.

At the beginning, it is brightest day; the YOUNG MAN is alone on stage, to the rear of the sandbox, and to one side. He is doing calesthenics; he does calesthenics until quite at the end of the play. These calesthenics, employing the arms only, should suggest the beating and fluttering of wings. The YOUNG MAN is, after all, the Angel of Death.

MOMMY and DADDY enter from stage-left, MOMMY first.

MOMMY

(*Motioning to daddy*) Well, here we are; this is the beach.

DADDY (*Whining*)

I'm cold.

MOMMY

(*Dismissing him with a little laugh*) Don't be silly; it's as warm as toast. Look at that nice young man over there: *he* doesn't think it's cold. (*Waves to the* YOUNG MAN) Hello.

YOUNG MAN

(*With an endearing smile*) Hi!

MOMMY (*Looking about*)

This will do perfectly . . . don't you think so, daddy? There's sand there . . . and water beyond. What do you think, daddy?

DADDY (*Vaguely*)

Whatever you say, mommy.

MOMMY

(*With the same little laugh*) Well, of course . . . whatever I say. Then, it's settled, is it?

DADDY (*Shrugs*)

She's *your* mother, not mine.

MOMMY

I know she's my mother. What do you take me for? (*A pause*) All right, now; let's get on with it. (*She shouts into the wings, stage left*) You! Out there! You can come in now.

(*The* MUSICIAN *enters, seats himself in the chair, stage-left, places music on the music stand, is ready to play.* MOMMY *nods approvingly*)

MOMMY

Very nice; very nice. Are you ready, daddy? Let's go get grandma.

DADDY

Whatever you say, mommy.

MOMMY

(*Leading the way out, stage-left*) Of course, whatever I say. (*To the* MUSICIAN) You can begin now.

(*The* MUSICIAN *begins playing;* MOMMY *and* DADDY *exit; the* MUSICIAN, *all the while playing, nods to the* YOUNG MAN)

YOUNG MAN

(*With the same endearing smile*) Hi!

(After a moment, MOMMY *and* DADDY *re-enter, carrying* GRANDMA. *She is borne in by their hands under her armpits; she is quite rigid; her legs are drawn up; her feet do not touch the ground; the expression on her ancient face is that of puzzlement and fear)*

DADDY

Where do we put her?

MOMMY

(*The same little laugh*) Wherever I say, of course. Let me see . . . well . . . right, over there . . . in the sandbox. (*Pause*) Well, what are you waiting for, daddy? . . . The sandbox!

(Together they carry GRANDMA *over to the sandbox and more or less dump her in)*

GRANDMA

(*Righting herself to a sitting position; her voice a cross between a baby's laugh and cry*) Ahhhhhh! Graaaaa!

DADDY (*Dusting himself*)

What do we do now?

MOMMY

(*To the* MUSICIAN) You can stop now.

(*The musician stops*)

(*Back to* DADDY) What do you mean, what do we do now? We go over there and sit down, of course. (*To the* YOUNG MAN) Hello there.

YOUNG MAN

(*Again smiling*) Hi!

(MOMMY *and* DADDY *move to the chairs, stage right, and sit down. A pause*)

GRANDMA

(*Same as before*) Ahhhhhh! Ah-haaaaaa! Graaaaaa!

DADDY

Do you think . . . do you think she's . . . comfortable?

MOMMY (*Impatiently*)

How would I know?

DADDY

(*Pause*) What do we do now?

MOMMY

(*As if remembering*) We . . . wait. We . . . sit here . . . and we wait . . . that's what we do.

DADDY

(*After a pause*) Shall we talk to each other?

MOMMY

(*With that little laugh; picking something off her dress*) Well, *you* can talk, if you want to . . . if you can think of anything to *say* . . . if you can think of anything *new*.

DADDY (*Thinks*)

No . . . I suppose not.

MOMMY

(*With a triumphant laugh*) Of course not!

GRANDMA

(*Banging the toy shovel against the pail*) Haaaaaa! Ah-haaaaaa!

MOMMY

(*Out over the audience*) Be quiet, Grandma . . . just be quiet, and wait. (GRANDMA *throws a shovelful of sand at* MOMMY)

MOMMY

(*Still out over the audience*) She's throwing sand at me! You stop that, Grandma; you stop throwing sand at Mommy! (*To* DADDY) She's throwing sand at me. (DADDY *looks around at* GRANDMA, *who screams at him*)

GRANDMA

GRAAAAA!

MOMMY

Don't look at her. Just . . . sit here . . . be very still . . . and wait. (*To the* MUSICIAN) You . . . uh . . . you go ahead and do whatever it is you do.

(*The* MUSICIAN *plays*)

(MOMMY *and* DADDY *are fixed, staring out beyond the audience.* GRANDMA *looks at them, looks at the* MUSICIAN, *looks at the sandbox, throws down the shovel*)

GRANDMA

Ah-haaaaaa! Graaaaaa! (*Looks for reaction; gets none. Now . . . directly to the audience*) Honestly! What a way to treat an old woman! Drag her out of the house . . . stick her in a car . . . bring her out here from the city . . . dump her in a pile of sand . . . and leave her here to set. I'm eighty-six years old! I was married when I was seventeen. To a farmer. He died when I was thirty. (*To the* MUSICIAN) Will you stop that, please?

(*The* MUSICIAN *stops playing*)

I'm a feeble old woman . . . how do you expect anybody to hear me over that peep! peep! peep! (*To herself*) There's no respect around here. (*To the* YOUNG MAN) There's no respect around here!

YOUNG MAN

(*Same smile*) Hi!

GRANDMA

(*After a pause, a mild double-take, continues, to the audience*) My husband died when I was thirty (*indicates* MOMMY), and I had to raise that big cow over there all by my lonesome. You can imagine what that was like. Lordy! (*To the* YOUNG MAN) Where'd they get *you*?

YOUNG MAN

Oh . . . I've been around for a while.

GRANDMA

I'll bet you have! Heh, heh, heh. Will you look at you!

YOUNG MAN

(*Flexing his muscles*) Isn't that something? (*Continues his calisthenics*)

GRANDMA

Boy, oh boy; I'll say. Pretty good.

YOUNG MAN (*Sweetly*)

I'll say.

GRANDMA

Where ya from?

YOUNG MAN

Southern California

GRANDMA (*Nodding*)

Figgers; figgers. What's your name, honey?

YOUNG MAN

I don't know . . .

GRANDMA

(*To the audience*) Bright, too!

YOUNG MAN

I mean . . . I mean, they haven't given me one yet . . . the studio . . .

GRANDMA

(*Giving him the once-over*) You don't say . . . you don't say. Well . . . uh, I've got to talk some more . . . don't you go 'way.

YOUNG MAN

Oh, no.

GRANDMA

(*Turning her attention back to the audience*) Fine; fine. (*Then, once more, back to the* YOUNG MAN) You're . . . you're an actor, hunh?

YOUNG MAN (*Beaming*)

Yes. I am.

GRANDMA

(*To the audience again; shrugs*) I'm smart that way. *Anyhow,* I had to raise . . . *that* over there all by my lonesome; and what's next to her there . . . that's what she married. Rich? I tell you . . . money, money, money. They took me off the *farm* . . . which was real decent of them . . . and they moved me into the big town house with *them* . . . fixed a nice place for me under the stove . . . gave me an army blanket . . . and my own dish . . . my very own dish! So, what have I got to complain about? Nothing, of course. I'm not complaining. (*She looks up at the sky, shouts to someone off stage*) Shouldn't it be getting dark now, dear?

(The lights dim; night comes on. The MUSICIAN *begins to play; it becomes deepest night. There are spots on all the players, including the* YOUNG MAN, *who is, of course, continuing his calisthenics)*

DADDY (*Stirring*)

It's nighttime.

MOMMY

Shhhh. Be still . . . wait.

DADDY (*Whining*)

It's so hot.

MOMMY

Shhhhhh. Be still . . . wait.

GRANDMA

(*To herself*) That's better. Night. (*To the* MUSICIAN) Honey, do you play all through this part? (*The* MUSICIAN *nods*)

Well, keep it nice and soft; that's a good boy.

(*The* MUSICIAN *nods again; plays softly*)

That's nice.

(*There is an off-stage rumble*)

DADDY (*Starting*)

What was that?

MOMMY

(*Beginning to weep*) It was nothing.

DADDY

It was . . . it was . . . thunder . . . or a wave breaking . . . or something.

MOMMY

(*Whispering, through her tears*) It was an off-stage rumble . . . and you know what *that* means . . .

DADDY

I forget. . . .

MOMMY

(*Barely able to talk*) It means the time has come for poor grandma . . . and I can't bear it!

DADDY (*Vacantly*)

I . . . I suppose you've got to be brave.

GRANDMA (*Mocking*)

That's right, kid; be brave. You'll bear up; you'll get over it.

(*Another off-stage rumble . . . louder*)

MOMMY

Ohhhhhhhhhh . . . poor grandma . . . poor grandma . . .

GRANDMA (*To* MOMMY)

I'm fine! I'm all right! It hasn't happened yet!

(*A violent off-stage rumble. All the lights go out, save the spot on the* YOUNG MAN; *the* MUSICIAN *stops playing*)

MOMMY

Ohhhhhhhhhh . . . . Ohhhhhhhhhh . . . .

(*Silence*)

GRANDMA

Don't put the lights up yet . . . I'm not ready; I'm not quite ready. (*Silence*) All right, dear . . . I'm about done.

(*The lights come up again, to brightest day; the* MUSICIAN *begins to play.* GRANDMA *is discovered, still in the sandbox, lying on her side, propped up on an elbow, half covered, busily shoveling sand over herself*)

GRANDMA (*Muttering*)

I don't know how I'm supposed to do anything with this goddam toy shovel. . . .

DADDY

Mommy! It's daylight!

MOMMY (*Brightly*)

So it is! Well! Our long night is over. We must put away our tears, take off our mourning . . . and face the future. It's our duty.

GRANDMA

(*Still shoveling; mimicking*) . . . take off our mourning . . . face the future. . . . Lordy!

(MOMMY *and* DADDY *rise, stretch.* MOMMY *waves to the young man*)

YOUNG MAN

(*With that smile*) Hi!

(GRANDMA *plays dead. (!)* MOMMY *and* DADDY *go over to look at her; she is a little more than half buried in the sand; the toy shovel is in her hands, which are crossed on her breast*)

MOMMY

(*Before the sandbox; shaking her head*) Lovely! It's . . . it's hard to be sad . . . she looks . . . so happy. (*With pride and conviction*) It pays to do things well. (*To the* MUSICIAN) All right, you can stop now, if you want to. I mean, stay around for a swim, or something; it's all right with us. (*She sighs heavily*) Well, daddy . . . off we go.

DADDY

Brave mommy!

MOMMY

Brave daddy!

(*They exit, stage-left*)

GRANDMA

(*After they leave; lying quite still*) It pays to do things well. . . . Boy, oh boy! (*She tries to sit up*) . . . well, kids . . . (*but she finds she can't*) . . . I . . . I can't get up. I . . . I can't move. . . .

(*The* YOUNG MAN *stops his calisthenics, nods to the* MUSICIAN, *walks over to* GRANDMA, *kneels down by the sandbox*)

GRANDMA

I . . . can't move. . . .

YOUNG MAN

Shhhh . . . be very still . . . .

GRANDMA

I . . . I can't move . . . .

YOUNG MAN

UH . . . ma'am; I . . . I have a line here.

GRANDMA

Oh, I'm sorry, sweetie; you go right ahead.

YOUNG MAN

I am . . . uh . . .

GRANDMA

Take your time, dear.

YOUNG MAN

(*Prepares; delivers the line like a real amateur*) I am the Angel of Death. I am . . . uh . . . I am come for you.

GRANDMA

What . . . wha . . . (*Then, with resignation*) . . . ohhhh . . . ohhhh, I see. (*The* YOUNG MAN *bends over, kisses* GRANDMA *gently on the forehead*)

GRANDMA

(*Her eyes closed, her hands folded on her breast again, the shovel between her hands, a sweet smile on her face*)

Well . . . that was very nice, dear . . .

YOUNG MAN

(*Still kneeling*) Shhhhhh . . . be still. . . .

GRANDMA

What I meant was . . . you did that very well, dear. . . .

YOUNG MAN (*Blushing*)

. . . oh . . .

GRANDMA

No, I mean it. You've got that . . . you've got a quality.

YOUNG MAN

(*With his endearing smile*) Oh . . . thank you; thank you very much . . . ma'am.

GRANDMA

(*Slowly; softly—as the* YOUNG MAN *puts his hands on top of* GRANDMA'S) You're . . . you're welcome . . . dear.

(*Tableau. The musician continues to play as the curtain slowly comes down*)

CURTAIN

THE ENDURING CHILL

FLANNERY O'CONNOR

Asbury's train stopped so that he would get off exactly where his mother was standing waiting to meet him. Her thin spectacled face below him was bright with a wide smile that disappeared as she caught sight of him bracing himself behind the conductor. The smile vanished so suddenly, the shocked look that replaced it was so complete, that he realized for the first time that he must look as ill as he was. The sky was a chill gray and a startling white-gold sun, like some strange potentate from the east, was rising beyond the black woods that surrounded Timberboro. It cast a strange light over the single block of one-story brick and wooden shacks. Asbury felt that he was about to witness a majestic transformation, that the flat of roofs might at any moment turn into the mounting turrets of some exotic temple for a god he didn't know. The illusion lasted only a moment before his attention was drawn back to his mother.

She had given a little cry; she looked aghast. He was pleased that she should see death in his face at once. His mother, at the age of sixty, was going to be introduced to reality and he supposed that if the experience didn't kill her, it would assist her in the process of growing up. He stepped down and greeted her.

"You don't look very well," she said and gave him a long clinical stare.

"I don't feel like talking," he said at once. "I've had a bad trip."

Mrs. Fox observed that his left eye was bloodshot. He was puffy and pale and his hair had receded tragically for a boy of twenty-five. The thin reddish wedge of it left on top bore down in a point that seemed to lengthen his nose and give him an irritable expression that matched his tone of voice when he spoke to her. "It must have been cold up there," she said. "Why don't you take off your coat. It's not cold down here."

"You don't have to tell me what the temperature is!" he said in a high voice. "I'm old enough to know when I want to take my coat off." The train glided silently away behind him, leaving a view of the twin blocks of dilapidated stores. He gazed after the aluminum speck disappearing into the woods. It seemed to him that his last connection with a larger world was vanishing forever. Then he turned and faced his mother grimly, irked that he had allowed himself, even for an instant, to see an imaginary temple in this collapsing country junction. He had become entirely accustomed to the thought of death, but he had not become accustomed to the thought of death *here.*

He had felt the end coming on for nearly four months. Alone in his freezing flat, huddled under his two blankets and his overcoat and with three thicknesses of the New York *Times* between, he had had a chill one night, followed by a violent sweat that left the sheets soaking and removed all doubt from his mind about his true condition. Before this there had been a gradual slackening of his energy and vague inconsistent aches and headaches. He had been absent so many days from his part-time job in the bookstore that he had lost it. Since then he had been living, or just barely so, on his savings and these, diminishing day by day, had been all he had between him and home. Now there was nothing. He was here.

"Where's the car?" he muttered.

"It's over yonder," his mother said. "And your sister is asleep in the back because I don't like to come out this early by myself. There's no need to wake her up."

"No," he said, "let sleeping dogs lie," and he picked up his two bulging suitcases and started across the road with them.

They were too heavy for him and by the time he reached the car, his mother saw that he was exhausted. He had never come home with two suitcases before. Ever since he had first gone away to college, he had come back every time with nothing but the necessities for a two-week stay and with a wooden resigned expression that said he was prepared to endure the visit for exactly fourteen days. "You've brought more than usual," she observed, but he did not answer.

He opened the car door and hoisted the two bags in beside his sister's upturned face, giving first the feet—in Girl Scout shoes—and then the rest of her a revolted look of recognition. She was packed into a black suit and had a white rag around her head with metal curlers sticking out from under the edges. Her eyes were closed and her mouth open. He and she had the same features except that hers were bigger. She was eight years older than he was and was principal of the county elementary school. He shut the door softly so she wouldn't wake up and then went around and got in the front seat and closed his eyes. His mother backed the car into the road and in a few minutes he felt it swerve into the highway. Then he opened his eyes. The road stretched between two open fields of yellow bitterweed.

"Do you think Timberboro has improved?" his mother asked. This was her standard question, meant to be taken literally.

"It's still there, isn't it?" he said in an ugly voice.

"Two of the stores have new fronts," she said. Then with a sudden ferocity, she said, "You did well to come home where you can get a good doctor! I'll take you to Doctor Block this afternoon."

"I am not," he said, trying to keep his voice from shaking, "going to Doctor Block. This afternoon or ever. Don't you think if I'd wanted to go to a doctor I'd have gone up there where they have some good ones? Don't you know they have better doctors in New York?"

"He would take a personal interest in you," she said, "None of those doctors up there would take a personal interest in you."

"I don't want him to take a personal interest in me." Then after a minute, staring out across a blurred, purple-looking field, he said, "What's wrong with me is way beyond Block," and his voice trailed off into a frayed sound, almost a sob.

He could not, as his friend Goetz had recommended, prepare to see it all as illusion, either what had gone before or the few weeks that were left to him. Goetz was certain that death was nothing at all. Goetz, whose whole face had always been purple-splotched with a million indignations, had returned from six months in Japan as dirty as ever but as bland as the Buddha himself. Goetz took the news of Asbury's approaching end with a calm indifference. Quoting something or other he said, "Although the Bodhisatva leads an infinite number of creatures into nirvana, in reality there are neither any Bodhisatvas to do the leading nor any creatures to be led." However out of some feeling for his welfare, Goetz had put forth $4.50 to take him to a lecture on Vedanta. It had been a waste of his money. While Goetz had listened enthralled to the dark little man on the platform, Asbury's bored gaze had roved among the audience. It had passed over the heads of several girls in saris, passed a Japanese youth, a blue-black man with a fez, and several girls who looked like secretaries. Finally, at the end of the row, it had rested on a lean spectacled figure in black, a priest. The priest's expression was of a polite but strictly reserved interest. Asbury identified his own feelings immediately in the taciturn superior expression. When the lecture was over a few students met in Goetz's flat, the priest among them, but he was equally reserved. He listened with a marked politeness to the discussion of Asbury's approaching death, but he said little. A girl in a sari remarked that self-fulfillment was out of the question since it meant salvation and the word was meaningless.

"Salvation," quoted Goetz, "is the destruction of a simple prejudice, and no one is saved."

"And what do you say to that?" Asbury asked the priest and returned his reserved smile over the heads of the others. The borders of this smile seemed to touch on some icy clarity.

"There is," the priest said, "a real probability of the New Man, assisted, of course," he added brittlely, "by the third Person of the Trinity."

"Ridiculous!" the girl in the sari said, but the priest only brushed her with his smile, which was slightly amused now.

When he got up to leave, he silently handed Asbury a small card on which he had written his name, Ignatius Vogle, S.J., and an address. Perhaps, Asbury thought now, he should have used it, for the priest appealed to him as a man of the world, someone who would have understood the unique tragedy of his death, a death whose meaning had been far beyond the twittering group around them. And how much more beyond Block. "What's wrong with me," he repeated, "is way beyond Block."

His mother knew at once what he meant: he meant he was going to have a nervous breakdown. She did not say a word. She did not say that this was precisely what she could have told him would happen. When people think they are smart—even when they are smart—there is nothing anybody else can say to make them see things straight, and with Asbury, the trouble was that in addition to being smart, he had an artistic temperament. She did not know where he had got it from because his father, who was a lawyer and businessman and farmer and politician all rolled into one, had certainly had his feet on the ground; and she had certainly always had hers on it. She managed after he died to get the two of them through college and beyond; but she had observed that the more education they got, the less they could do. Their father had gone to a one-room schoolhouse through the eighth grade and he could do anything.

She could have told Asbury what would help him. She could have said, "If you would get out in the sunshine, or if you would work for a month in the dairy, you'd be a different person!" but she knew exactly how that suggestion would be received. He would be a nuisance in the dairy but she would let him work in there if he wanted to. She had let him work in there last year when he had come home and was writing the play. He had been writing a play about Negroes (why anybody would want to write a play about Negroes was beyond her) and he had said he wanted to work in the dairy with them and find out what their interests were. Their interests were in doing as little as they could get by with, as she could have told him if anybody could have told him anything. The Negroes had put up with him and he had learned to put the milkers on and once he had washed all the cans and she thought that once he had mixed the feed. Then a cow had kicked him and he had not gone back to the barn again. She knew that if he would get in there now, or get out and fix fences, or do any kind of work—real work, not writing—that he might avoid the nervous breakdown. "Whatever happened to that play you were writing about the Negroes?" she asked.

"I'm not writing plays," he said. "And get this through your head: I am not working in any dairy. I am not getting out in the sunshine. I'm ill. I have fevers and chills and I'm dizzy and all I want you to do is to leave me alone."

"Then if you are really ill, you should see Doctor Block."

"And I am not seeing Block," he finished and ground himself down in the seat and stared intensely in front of him.

She turned into their driveway, a red road that ran for a quarter of a mile through the two front pastures. The dry cows were on one side and the milk herd on the other. She slowed the car and then stopped altogether, her attention caught by a cow with a bad quarter. "They haven't been attending to her," she said. "Look at that bag!"

Asbury turned his head abruptly in the opposite direction, but there a small, walleyed Guernsey was watching him steadily as if she sensed some bond between them. "Good God!" he cried in an agonized voice, "can't we go on? It's six o'clock in the morning!"

"Yes, yes," his mother said and started the car quickly.

"What's that cry of deadly pain?" his sister drawled from the back seat. "Oh, it's you," she said. "Well, well, we have the artist with us again. How utterly utterly." She had a decidedly nasal voice.

He didn't answer her or turn his head. He had learned that much. Never answer her.

"Mary George!" his mother said sharply. "Asbury is sick. Leave him alone."

"What's wrong with him?" Mary George asked.

"There's the house!" his mother said as if they were all blind but her. It rose on the crest of the hill—a white two-story farmhouse with a wide porch and pleasant columns. She always approached it with a feeling of pride and she had said more than once to Asbury, "You have a home here that half those people up there would give their eyeteeth for!"

She had been once to the terrible place he lived in New York. They had gone up five flights of dark stone steps, past open garbage cans on every landing, to arrive finally at two damp rooms and a closet with a toilet in it. "You wouldn't live like this at home," she had muttered.

"No!" he'd said with an ecstatic look, "it wouldn't be possible!"

She supposed the truth was that she simply didn't understand how it felt to be sensitive or how peculiar you were when you were an artist. His sister said he was not an artist and that he had no talent and that that was the trouble with him; but Mary George was not a happy girl herself. Asbury said she posed as an intellectual but that her I.Q. couldn't be over seventy-five, that all she really was interested in was getting a man but that no sensible man would finish a first look at her. She had tried to tell him that Mary George could be very attractive when she put her mind to it and he had said that that much strain on her mind would break her down. If she were in any way attractive, he had said, she wouldn't now be principal of a county elementary school, and Mary George had said that if Asbury had had any talent, he would by now have published something. What had he ever published, she wanted to know, and for that matter, what had he ever written?

Mrs. Fox had pointed out that he was only twenty-five years old and Mary George had said that the age most people published something at was twenty-one, which made him exactly four years overdue. Mrs. Fox was not up on things like that but she suggested that he might be writing a very *long* book. Very long book, her eye, Mary George said, he would do well if he came up with so much as a poem. Mrs. Fox hoped it wasn't going to be just a poem.

She pulled the car into the side drive and a scattering of guineas exploded into the air and sailed screaming around the house. "Home again, home again jiggity jig!" she said.

"Oh God," Asbury groaned.

"The artist arrives at the gas chamber," Mary George said in her nasal voice.

He leaned on the door and got out, and forgetting his bags he moved toward the front of the house as if he were in a daze. His sister got out and stood by the car door, squinting at his bent unsteady figure. As she watched him go up the front steps, her mouth fell slack in her astonished face. "Why," she said, "there *is* something the matter with him. He looks a hundred years old."

"Didn't I tell you so?" her mother hissed. "Now you keep your mouth shut and let him alone."

He went into the house, pausing in the hall only long enough to see his pale broken face glare at him for an instant from the pier mirror. Holding onto the banister, he pulled himself up the steep stairs, across the landing and then up the shorter second flight and into his room, a large open airy room with a faded blue rug and white curtains freshly put up for his arrival. He looked at nothing, but fell face down on his own bed. It was a narrow antique bed with a high ornamental headboard on which was carved a garlanded basket overflowing with wooden fruit.

While he was still in New York, he had written a letter to his mother which filled two notebooks. He did not mean it to be read until after his death. It was such a letter as Kafka had addressed to his father. Asbury's father had died twenty years ago and Asbury considered this a great blessing. The old man, he felt sure, had been one of the courthouse gang, a rural worthy with a dirty finger in every pie and he knew he would not have been able to stomach him. He had read some of his correspondence and had been appalled by its stupidity.

He knew, of course, that his mother would not understand the letter at once. Her literal mind would require some time to discover the significance of it, but he thought she would be able to see that he forgave her for all she had done to him. For that matter, he supposed that she would realize what she had done to him only through the letter. He didn't think she was conscious of it at all. Her self-satisfaction itself was barely conscious, but because of the letter, she might experience a painful realization and this would be the only thing of value he had to leave her.

If reading it would be painful to her, writing it had sometimes been unbearable to him—for in order to face her, he had had to face himself. "I came here to escape the slave's atmosphere of home," he had written, "to find freedom, to liberate my imagination, to take it like a hawk from its cage and set it 'whirling off into the widening gyre' (Yeats) and what did I find? It was incapable of flight. It was some bird you had domesticated, sitting huffy in its pen, refusing to come out!" The next words were underscored twice. "I have no imagination. I have no talent. I can't create. I have nothing but the desire for these things. Why didn't you kill that too? Woman, why did you pinion me?"

Writing this, he had reached the pit of despair and he thought that reading it, she would at least begin to sense his tragedy and her part in it. It was not that she had ever forced her way on him. That had never been necessary. Her way had simply been the air he breathed and when at last he had found other air, he couldn't survive in it. He felt that even if she didn't understand at once, the letter would leave her with an enduring chill and perhaps in time lead her to see herself as she was.

He had destroyed everything else he had ever written—his two lifeless novels, his half-dozen stationary plays, his prosy poems, his sketchy short stories—and kept only the two notebooks that contained the letter. They were in the black suitcase that his sister, huffing and blowing, was now dragging up the second flight of stairs. His mother was carrying the smaller bag and came on ahead. He turned over as she entered the room.

"I'll open this and get out your things," she said, "and you can go right to bed and in a few minutes I'll bring your breakfast."

He sat up and said in a fretful voice, "I don't want any breakfast and I can open my own suitcase. Leave that alone."

His sister arrived in the door, her face full of curiosity, and let the black bag fall with a thud over the doorsill. Then she began to push it around the room with her foot until she was close enough to get a good look at him. "If I looked as bad as you do," she said, "I'd go to the hospital."

Her mother cut her eyes sharply at her and she left. Then Mrs. Fox closed the door and came to the bed and sat down on it beside him. "Now this time I want you to make a long visit and rest," she said.

"This visit," he said, "will be permanent."

"Wonderful!" she cried. "You can have a little studio in your room and in the mornings, you can write plays and in the afternoons you can help in the dairy!"

He turned a white wooden face to her. "Close the blinds and let me sleep," he said.

When she was gone, he lay for some time staring at the water stains on the grey walls. Descending from the top molding, long icicle shapes had been etched by leaks and, directly over his bed on the ceiling, another leak had made a fierce bird with spread wings. It had an icicle crosswise in its beak and there were smaller icicles depending from its wings and tail. It had been there since his childhood and had always irritated him and sometimes had frightened him. He had often had the illusion that it was in motion and about to descend mysteriously and set the icicle on his head. He closed his eyes and thought: I won't have to look at it for many more days. And presently he went to sleep.

* * * * *

When he woke up in the afternoon, there was a pink open-mouthed face hanging over him and from two large familiar ears on either side of it the black tubes of Block's stethoscope extended down to his exposed chest. The doctor, seeing he was awake, made a face like a Chinaman, rolled his eyes almost out of his head and cried, "Say AHHHHH!"

Block was irresistible to children. For miles around they vomited and went into fevers to have a visit from him. Mrs. Fox was standing behind him, smiling radiantly. "Here's Doctor Block!" she said as if she had captured this angel on the rooftop and brought him in for her little boy.

"Get him out of here," Asbury muttered. He looked at the asinine face from what seemed the bottom of a black hole.

The doctor peered closer, wiggling his ears. Block was bald and had a round face as senseless as a baby's. Nothing about him indicated intelligence except two cold clinical nickel-colored eyes that hung with a motionless curiosity over whatever he looked at. "You sho do look bad, Azzberry," he murmured. He took the stethoscope off and dropped it in his bag. "I don't know when I've seen anybody your age look as sorry as you do. What you been doing to yourself?"

There was a continuous thud in the back of Asbury's head as if his heart had got trapped in it and was fighting to get out. "I didn't send for you," he said.

Block put his hand on the glaring face and pulled the eyelid down and peered into it. "You must have been on the bum up there," he said. He began to press his hand in the small of Asbury's back. "I went up there once myself," he said, "and saw exactly how little they had and came straight back home. Open your mouth."

Asbury opened it automatically and the drill-like gaze swung over it and bore down. He snapped it shut and in a wheezing breathless voice he said, "If I'd wanted a doctor, I'd have stayed up there where I could have got a good one!" "Asbury!" his mother said.

"How long you been having the so' throat?" Block asked.

"She sent for you!" Asbury said. "She can answer the questions."

"Asbury!" his mother said.

Block leaned over his bag and pulled out a rubber tube. He pushed Asbury's sleeve up and tied the tube around his upper arm. Then he took out a syringe and prepared to find the vein, humming a hymn as he pressed the needle in. Asbury lay with a rigid outraged stare while the privacy of his blood was invaded by this idiot.

"Slowly Lord but sure," Block sang in a murmuring voice, "Oh slowly Lord but sure." When the syringe was full, he withdrew the needle. "Blood don't lie," he said. He poured it in a bottle and stopped it up and put the bottle in his bag. "Asbury," he started, "how long . . ."

Asbury sat up and thrust his thudding head forward and said, "I didn't send for you. I'm not answering any questions. You're not my doctor. What's wrong with me is way beyond you."

"Most things are beyond me," Block said, "I ain't found anything yet that I thoroughly understood," and he sighed and got up. His eyes seemed to glitter at Asbury as if from a great distance.

"He wouldn't act so ugly," Mrs. Fox explained, "if he weren't really sick. And *I* want you to come back every day until you get him well."

Asbury's eyes were a fierce glaring violet. "What's wrong with me is way beyond you," he repeated and lay back down and closed his eyes until Block and his mother were gone.

* * * * *

In the next few days, though he grew rapidly worse, his mind functioned with a terrible clarity. On the point of death, he found himself existing in a state of illumination that was totally out of keeping with the kind of talk he had to listen to from his mother. This was largely about cows with names like Daisy and Bessie Button and their intimate functions—their mastitis and their screw-worms and their abortions. His mother insisted that in the middle of the day he get out and sit on the porch and "enjoy the nice view" and as his resistance was too much of a struggle, he dragged himself out and sat there in a rigid slouch, his feet wrapped in an afghan and his hands gripped on the chair arms as if he were about to spring forward into the glaring china blue sky. The lawn extended for a quarter of an acre down to a barbed-wire fence that divided it from the front pasture. In the middle of the day the dry cows rested there under a line of sweetgum trees. On the other side of the road were two hills with a pond between and his mother could sit on the porch and watch the herd walk across the dam to the hill on the other side. The whole scene was rimmed by a wall of trees which, at the time of day he was forced to sit there, was a washed-out blue that reminded him sadly of the Negroes' faded overalls.

He listened irritably while his mother detailed the faults of the help. "Those two are not stupid," she said. "They know how to look out for themselves. "They need to," he muttered, but there was no use to argue with her. Last year he had been writing a play about the Negro and he had wanted to be around them for a while to see how they really felt about their condition, but the two who worked for her had lost all their initiative over the years. They didn't talk. The one called Morgan was light brown, part Indian; the other, older one, Randall, was very black and fat. When they said anything to him, it was as if they were speaking to an invisible body located to the right or left of where he actually was, and after two days working side by side with them, he felt he had not established rapport. He decided to try something bolder than talk one afternoon as he was standing near Randall, watching him adjust a milker. He had quietly taken out his cigarettes and lit one. The Negro had stopped what he was doing and watched him. He waited until Asbury had taken two draws and then he said, "She don't 'low no smoking in here."

The other one approached and stood there, grinning.

"I know it," Asbury said and after a deliberate pause, he shook the package and held it out, first to Randall, who took one, and then to Morgan, who took one. He had then lit the cigarettes for them himself and the three of them had stood there smoking. There were no sounds but the steady click of the two milking machines and the occasional slap of a cow's tail against her side. It was one of those moments of communion when the difference between black and white is absorbed into nothing.

The next day two cans of milk had been returned from the creamery because it had absorbed the odor of tobacco. He took the blame and told his mother that it was he and not the Negroes who had been smoking. "If you were doing it, they were doing it," she had said. "Don't you think I know those two?" She was incapable of thinking them innocent; but the experience had so exhilarated him that he had been determined to repeat it in some other way.

The next afternoon when he and Randall were in the milk house pouring the fresh milk into the cans, he had picked up the jelly glass the Negroes drank out of and, inspired, had poured himself a glassful of the warm milk and drained it down. Randall had stopped pouring and had remained, half-bent, over the can, watching him. "She don't 'low that," he said. "That *the* thing she don't 'low."

Asbury poured out another glassful and handed it to him.

"She don't 'low," he repeated.

"Listen," Asbury said hoarsely, "the world is changing. There's no reason I shouldn't drink after you or you after me!"

"She don't 'low noner us to drink noner this here milk," Randall said.

Asbury continued to hold the glass out to him. "You took the cigarette," he said. "Take the milk. It's not going to hurt my mother to lose two or three glasses of milk a day. We've got to think free if we want to live free!"

The other one had come up and was standing in the door.

"Don't want noner that milk," Randall said.

Asbury swung around and held the glass out to Morgan. "Here boy, have a drink of this," he said.

Morgan stared at him; then his face took on a decided look of cunning. "I ain't seen you drink none of it yourself," he said.

Asbury despised milk. The first warm glassful had turned his stomach. He drank half of what he was holding and handed the rest to the Negro, who took it and gazed down inside the glass as if it contained some great mystery; then he set it on the floor by the cooler.

"Don't you like milk?" Asbury asked.

"I likes it but I ain't drinking noner that."

"Why?"

"She don't 'low it," Morgan said.

"My God!" Asbury exploded, "she she she!" He had tried the same thing the next day and the next and the next but he could not get them to drink the milk. A few afternoons later when he was standing outside the milk house about to go in, he heard Morgan ask, "How come you let him drink that milk every day?"

"What he do is him," Randall said. "What I do is me."

"How come he talks so ugly about his ma?"

"She ain't whup him enough when he was little," Randall said.

The insufferableness of life at home had overcome him and he had returned to New York two days early. So far as he was concerned he had died there, and the questions now was how long he could stand to linger here. He could have hastened his end but suicide would not have been a victory. Death was coming to him legitimately, as a justification, as a gift from life. That was his greatest triumph. Then too, to the fine minds of the neighborhood, a suicide son would indicate a mother who had been a failure, and while this was the case, he felt that it was a public embarrassment he could spare her. What she would learn from the letter would be a private revelation. He had sealed the notebooks in a manila envelope and had written on it: "To be opened only after the death of Asbury Porter Fox." He had put the envelope in the desk drawer in his room and locked it and the key was in his pajama pocket until he could decide on a place to leave it.

When they sat on the porch in the morning, his mother felt that some of the time she should talk about the subjects that were of interest to him. The third morning she started in on his writing. "When you get well," she said, "I think it would be nice if you wrote a book about down here. We need another good book like *Gone With the Wind.*"

He could feel the muscles in his stomach begin to tighten.

"Put the war in it," she advised. "That always makes a long book."

He put his head back gently as if he were afraid it would crack. After a moment he said, "I am not going to write any book."

"Well," she said, "if you don't feel like writing a book, you could just write poems. They're nice." She realized that what he needed was someone intellectual to talk to, but Mary George was the only intellectual she knew and he would not talk to her. She had thought of Mr. Bush, the retired Methodist minister, but she had not brought this up. Now she decided to hazard it. "I think I'll ask Dr. Bush to come to see you," she said, raising Mr. Bush's rank. "You'd enjoy him. He collects rare coins."

She was not prepared for the reaction she got. He began to shake all over and give loud spasmodic laughs. He seemed about to choke. After a minute he subsided into a cough. "If you think I need spiritual aid to die," he said, "you're quite mistaken. And certainly not from that ass Bush. My God!"

"I didn't mean that at all," she said. "He has coins dating from the time of Cleopatra."

"Well if you ask him here, I'll tell him to go to Hell," he said. "Bush! That beats all!"

"I'm glad something amuses you, " she said acidly.

For a time they sat there in silence. Then his mother looked up. He was sitting forward again and smiling at her. His face was brightening more and more as if he had just had an idea that was brilliant. She stared at him. "I'll tell you who I want to come," he said. For the first time since he had come home, his expression was pleasant; though there was also, she thought, a kind of crafty look about him.

"Who do you want to come?" she asked suspiciously.

"I want a priest," he announced.

"A priest?" his mother said in an uncomprehending voice.

"Preferably a Jesuit," he said, brightening more and more. "Yes, by all means a Jesuit. They have them in the city. You can call up and get me one."

"What's the matter with you?" his mother said.

"Most of them are very well-educated," he said, "but Jesuits are foolproof. A Jesuit would be able to discuss something besides the weather." Already, remembering Ignatius Vogle, S.J., he could picture the priest. This one would be a trifle more worldly perhaps, a trifle more cynical. Protected by their ancient institution, priests could afford to be cynical, to play both ends against the middle. He would talk to a man of culture before he died—even in this desert! Furthermore nothing would irritate his mother so much. He could not understand why he had not thought of this sooner.

"You're not a member of that church," Mrs. Fox said shortly. "It's twenty miles away. They wouldn't send one." She hoped that this would end the matter.

He sat back absorbed in the idea, determined to force her to make the call since she always did what he wanted if he kept at her. "I'm dying," he said, "and I haven't asked you to do but one thing and you refuse me that."

"You are NOT dying."

"When you realize it," he said, "it'll be too late."

There was another unpleasant silence. Presently his mother said, "Nowadays doctors don't *let* young people die. They give them some of these new medicines." She began shaking her foot with a nerve-rattling assurance. "People just don't die like they used to," she said.

"Mother," he said, "you ought to be prepared. I think even Block knows and hasn't told you yet." Block, after the first visit, had come in grimly every time, without his jokes and funny faces, and had taken his blood in silence, his nickel-colored eyes unfriendly. He was, by definition, the enemy of death and he looked now as if he knew he was battling the real thing. He had said he wouldn't prescribe until he knew what was wrong and Asbury had laughed in his face. "Mother," he said, "I AM going to die," and he tried to make each word like a hammer blow on top of her head.

She paled slightly but she did not blink. "Do you think for one minute," she said angrily, "that I intend to sit here and let you die?" Her eyes were as hard as two old mountain ranges seen in the distance. He felt the first distinct stroke of doubt.

"Do you?" she asked fiercely.

"I don't think you have anything to do with it," he said in a shaken voice.

"Humph," she said and got up and left the porch as if she could not stand to be around such stupidity an instant longer.

Forgetting the Jesuit, he went rapidly over his symptoms: his fever had increased, interspersed by chills; he barely had the energy to drag himself out on the porch; food was abhorrent to him; and Block had not been able to give her the least satisfaction. Even as he sat there, he felt the beginning of a new chill, as if death were already playfully rattling his bones. He pulled the afghan off his feet and put it around his shoulders and made his way unsteadily up the stairs to bed.

* * * * *

He continued to grow worse. In the next few days he became so much weaker and badgered her so constantly about the Jesuit that finally in desperation she decided to humor his foolishness. She made the call, explaining in a chilly voice that her son was ill, perhaps a little out of his head, and wished to speak to a priest. While she made the call, Asbury hung over the banisters, barefooted, with the afghan around him, and listened. When she hung up he called down to know when the priest was coming.

"Tomorrow sometime," his mother said irritably.

He could tell by the fact that she made the call that her assurance was beginning to shatter. Whenever she let Block in or out, there was much whispering in the downstairs hall. That evening, he heard her and Mary George talking in low voices in the parlor. He thought he heard his name and he got up and tiptoed into the hall and down the first three steps until he could hear the voices distinctly.

"I had to call that priest," his mother was saying. "I'm afraid this is serious. I thought it was just a nervous breakdown but now I think it's something real. Doctor Block thinks it's something too and whatever it is is worse because he's so rundown."

"Grow up, Mamma," Mary George said, "I've told you and I tell you again: what's wrong with him is purely psychosomatic." There was nothing she was not an expert on.

"No," his mother said, "it's a real disease. The doctor says so." He thought he detected a crack in her voice.

"Block is an idiot," Mary George said. "You've got to face the facts: Asbury can't write so he gets sick. He's going to be an invalid instead of an artist. Do you know what he needs?"

"No," his mother said.

"Two or three shock treatments," Mary George said. "Get that artist business out of his head once and for all."

His mother gave a little cry and he grasped the banister.

"Mark my words," his sister continued, "all he's going to be around here for the next fifty years is a decoration."

He went back to bed. In a sense she was right. He had failed his god, Art, but he had been a faithful servant and Art was sending him Death. He had seen this from the first with a kind of mystical clarity. He went to sleep thinking of the peaceful spot in the family burying ground where he would soon lie, and after awhile he saw that his body was being borne slowly toward it while his mother and Mary George watched without interest from their chairs on the porch. As the bier was carried across the dam, they could look up and see the procession reflected upside down in the pond. A lean dark figure in a Roman collar followed it. He had a mysterious saturnine face in which there was a subtle blend of asceticism and corruption. Asbury was laid in a shallow grave on the hillside and the indistinct mourners, after standing in silence for a while, spread out over the darkening green. The Jesuit retired to a spot beneath a dead tree to smoke and meditate. The moon came up and Asbury was aware of a presence bending over him and a gentle warmth on his cold face. He knew that this was Art come to wake him and he sat up and opened his eyes. Across the hill all the lights were on in his mother's house. The black pond was speckled with little nickel-colored stars. The Jesuit had disappeared. All around him the cows were spread out grazing in the moonlight and one large white one, violently spotted, was softly licking his head as if it were a block of salt. He awoke with a shudder and discovered that his bed was soaking from a night sweat and as he sat shivering in the dark, he realized that the end was not many days distant. He gazed down into the crater of death and fell back dizzy on his pillow.

The next day his mother noted something almost ethereal about his ravaged face. He looked like one of those dying children who must have Christmas early. He sat up in the bed and directed the rearrangement of several chairs and had her remove a picture of a maiden chained to a rock for he knew it would make the Jesuit smile. He had the comfortable rocker taken away and when he finished, the room with its severe wall stains had a certain cell-like quality. He felt it would be attractive to the visitor.

All morning he waited, looking irritably up at the ceiling where the bird with the icicle in its beak seemed poised and waiting too; but the priest did not arrive until late in the afternoon. As soon as his mother opened the door, a loud unintelligible voice began to boom in the downstairs hall. Asbury's heart beat wildly. In a second there was a heavy creaking on the stairs. Then almost at once, his mother, her expression constrained, came in followed by a massive old man who plowed straight across the room, picked up a chair by the side of the bed and put it under himself.

"I'm Father Finn—from Purrgatory," he said in a hearty voice. He had a large red face, a stiff brush of gray hair and was blind in one eye, but the good eye, blue and clear, was focused sharply on Asbury. There was a grease spot on his vest. "So you want to talk to a priest?" he said. "Very wise. None of us knows the hour Our Blessed Lord may call us." Then he cocked his good eye up at Asbury's mother and said, "Thank you, you may leave us now."

Mrs. Fox stiffened and did not budge.

"I'd like to talk to Father Finn alone," Asbury said, feeling suddenly that here he had an ally, although he had not expected a priest like this one. His mother gave him a disgusted look and left the room. He knew she would go no further than just outside the door.

"It's so nice to have you come," Asbury said. "This place is incredibly dreary. There's no one here an intelligent person can talk to. I wonder what you think of Joyce, Father?"

The priest lifted his chair and pushed closer. "You'll have to shout," he said. "Blind in one eye and deaf in one ear."

"What do you think of Joyce?" Asbury said louder.

"Joyce? Joyce who?" asked the priest.

"James Joyce," Asbury said and laughed.

The priest brushed his huge hand in the air as if he were bothered by gnats. "I haven't met him," he said. "Now. Do you say your morning and night prayers?"

Asbury appeared confused. "Joyce was a great writer," he murmured, forgetting to shout.

"You don't, eh?" said the priest. "Well you will never learn to be good unless you pray regularly. You cannot love Jesus unless you speak to Him."

"The myth of the dying god has always fascinated me," Asbury shouted, but the priest did not appear to catch it.

"Do you have trouble with purity?" he demanded, and as Asbury paled, he went on without waiting for an answer. "We all do but you must pray to the Holy Ghost for it. Mind, heart and body. Nothing is overcome without prayer. Pray with your family. Do you pray with your family?"

"God forbid," Asbury murmured. "My mother doesn't have time to pray and my sister is an atheist," he shouted.

"A shame!" said the priest. "Then you must pray for them."

"The artist prays by creating," Asbury ventured.

"Not enough!" snapped the priest. "If you do not pray daily, you are neglecting your immortal soul. Do you know your catechism?"

"Certainly not," Asbury muttered.

"Who made you?" the priest asked in a martial tone.

"Different people believe different things about that," Asbury said.

"God made you," the priest said shortly. "Who is God?"

"God is an idea created by man," Asbury said, feeling that he was getting into stride, that two could play at this.

"God is a spirit infinitely perfect," the priest said. "You are a very ignorant boy. Why did God make you?"

"God didn't . . ."

"God made you to know Him, to love Him, to serve Him in this world and to be happy with Him in the next!" the old priest said in a battering voice. "If you don't apply yourself to the catechism how do you expect to know how to save your immortal soul?"

Asbury saw he had made a mistake, and that it was time to get rid of the old fool. "Listen," he said. "I'm not a Roman."

"A poor excuse for not saying your prayers!" the old man snorted.

Asbury slumped slightly in the bed. "I'm dying," he shouted.

"But you're not dead yet!" said the priest, "and how do you expect to meet God face to face when you've never spoken to Him? How do you expect to get what you don't ask for? God does not send the Holy Ghost to those who don't ask for Him. Ask Him to send the Holy Ghost."

"The Holy Ghost?" Asbury said.

"Are you so ignorant you've never head of the Holy Ghost?" the priest asked.

"Certainly I've heard of the Holy Ghost," Asbury said furiously, "and the Holy Ghost is the last thing I'm looking for!"

"And He may be the last thing you get," the priest said, his one fierce eye inflamed. "Do you want your soul to suffer eternal damnation? Do you want to be deprived of God for all eternity? Do you want to suffer the most terrible pain, greater than fire, the pain of loss? Do you want to suffer the pain of loss for all eternity?"

Asbury moved his arms and legs helplessly as if he were pinned to the bed by the terrible eye.

"How can the Holy Ghost fill your soul when it's full of trash?" the priest roared. "The Holy Ghost will not come until you see yourself as you are—a lazy ignorant conceited youth!" he said, pounding his fist on the little bedside table.

Mrs. Fox burst in. "Enough of this!" she cried. "How dare you talk that way to a poor sick boy? You're upsetting him. You'll have to go."

"The poor lad doesn't even know his catechism," the priest said, rising. "I should think you would have taught him to say his daily prayers. You have neglected your duty as his mother." He turned back to the bed and said affably, "I'll give you my blessing and after this you must say your daily prayers without fail," whereupon he put his hand on Asbury's head and rumbled something in Latin.

"Call me anytime," he said, "and we can have another little chat," and then he followed Mrs. Fox's rigid back out. The last thing Asbury heard him say was "He's a good lad at heart but very ignorant."

When his mother had got rid of the priest, she came rapidly up the steps again to say that she had told him so, but when she saw him, pale and drawn and ravaged, sitting up in his bed, staring in front of him with large childish shocked eyes, she did not have the heart and went rapidly out again.

The next morning he was so weak that she made up her mind he must go to the hospital. "I'm not going to any hospital," he kept repeating, turning his thudding head from side to side as if he wanted to work it loose from his body. "I'm not going to any hospital as long as I'm conscious." He was thinking bitterly that once he lost consciousness, she could drag him off to the hospital and fill him full of blood and prolong his misery for days. He was convinced that the end was approaching, that it would be today, and he was tormented now thinking of his useless life. He felt as if he were a shell that had to be filled with something but he did not know what. He began to take note of everything in the room as if for the last time—the ridiculous antique furniture, the pattern in the rug, the silly picture his mother had replaced. He even looked at the fierce bird with the icicle in its beak and felt that it was there for some purpose that he could not divine.

There was something he was searching for, something that he felt he must have, some last significant culminating experience that he must make for himself before he died—and make for himself out of his own intelligence. He had always relied on himself and had never been a sniveler after the ineffable.

Once when Mary George was thirteen and he was five, she had lured him with the promise of an unnamed present into a large tent full of people and had dragged him backwards up to the front where a man in a blue suit and red and white tie was standing. "Here," she said in a loud voice. "I'm already saved but you can save him. He's a real stinker and too big for his britches." He had broken her grip and shot out of there like a small cur and later when he had asked for his present, she had said, "You would have got Salvation if you had waited for it, but since you acted the way you did, you get nothing!"

As the day wore on, he grew more and more frantic for fear he would die without making some last meaningful experience for himself. His mother sat anxiously by the side of the bed. She had called Block twice and could not get him. He thought even now she had not realized he was going to die, much less that the end was only hours off.

The light in the room was beginning to have an odd quality, almost as if it were taking on a presence. In a darkened form it entered and seemed to wait. Outside it appeared to move no farther than the edge of the faded treeline, which he could see a few inches over the sill of his window. Suddenly he thought of that experience of communion that he had had in the dairy with the Negroes when they had smoked together, and at once he began to tremble with excitement. They would smoke together one last time.

After a moment, turning his head on the pillow, he said, "Mother, I want to tell the Negroes good-bye."

His mother paled. For an instant her face seemed about to fly apart. Then the line of her mouth hardened; her brows drew together. "Good-bye?" she said in a flat voice. "Where are you going?"

For a few seconds he only looked at her. Then he said, "I think you know. Get them. I don't have long."

"This is absurd," she muttered but she got up and hurried out. He heard her try to reach Block again before she went outside. He thought her clinging to Block at a time like this was touching and pathetic. He waited, preparing himself for the encounter as a religious man might prepare himself for the last sacrament. Presently he heard their steps on the stair.

"Here's Randall and Morgan," his mother said, ushering them in. "They've come to tell you hello."

The two of them came in grinning and shuffled to the side of the bed. They stood there, Randall in front and Morgan behind. "You sho do look well," Randall said. "You looks very well."

"You look well," the other one said. "Yessuh, you looks fine."

"I ain't ever seen you lookin so well before," Randall said.

"Yes, doesn't he look well?" his mother said. "I think he looks just fine."

"Yessuh," Randall said, "I speck you ain't even sick."

"Mother," Asbury said in a forced voice. "I'd like to talk to them alone."

His mother stiffened; then she marched out. She walked across the hall and into the room on the other side and sat down. Through the open doors he could see her begin to rock in little short jerks. The two Negroes looked as if their last protection had dropped away.

Asbury's head was so heavy he could not think what he had been going to do. "I'm dying," he said.

Both their grins became gelid. "You looks fine," Randall said.

"I'm going to die," Asbury repeated. Then with some relief he remembered that they were going to smoke together. He reached for the package on the table and held it out to Randall, forgetting to shake out the cigarettes.

The Negro took the package and put it in his pocket. "I thank you," he said. "I certainly do prechat it."

Asbury stared as if he had forgotten again. After a second he became aware that the other Negro's face had turned infinitely sad; then he realized that it was not sad but sullen. He fumbled in the drawer of the table and pulled out an unopened package and thrust it at Morgan.

"I thanks you, Mister Asbury," Morgan said, brightening. "You certly does look well."

"I'm about to die," Asbury said irritably.

"You looks fine," Randall said.

"You be up and around in a few days," Morgan predicted. Neither of them seemed to find a suitable place to rest his gaze. Asbury looked wildly across the hall where his mother had her rocker turned so that her back faced him. It was apparent she had no intention of getting rid of them for him.

"I speck you might have a little cold," Randall said after a time.

"I takes a little turpentine and sugar when I has a cold," Morgan said.

"Shut your mouth," Randall said, turning on him.

"Shut your own mouth," Morgan said. "I know what I takes."

"He don't take what you take," Randall growled.

"Mother!" Asbury called in a shaking voice.

His mother stood up. "Mister Asbury has had company long enough now," she called. "You all can come back tomorrow."

"We be going," Randall said. "You sho do look well."

"You sho does," Morgan said.

They filed out agreeing with each other how well he looked but Asbury's vision became blurred before they reached the hall. For an instant he saw his mother's form as if it were a shadow in the door and then it disappeared after them down the stairs. He heard her call Block again but he heard it without interest. His head was spinning.

He knew now there would be no significant experience before he died. There was nothing more to do but give her the key to the drawer where the letter was, and wait for the end.

He sank into a heavy sleep from which he awoke about five o'clock to see her white face, very small, at the end of a well of darkness. He took the key out of his pajama pocket and handed it to her and mumbled that there was a letter in the desk to be opened when he was gone, but she did not seem to understand. She put the key down on the bedside table and left it there and he returned to his dream in which two large boulders were circling each other inside his head.

He awoke a little after six to hear Block's car stop below in the driveway. The sound was like a summons, bringing him rapidly and with a clear head out of his sleep. He had a sudden terrible foreboding that the fate awaiting him was going to be more shattering than anything he could have reckoned on. He lay absolutely motionless, as still as an animal the instant before an earthquake.

Block and his mother talked as they came up the stairs but he did not distinguish their words. The doctor came in making faces; his mother was smiling. "Guess what you've got, Sugarpie!" she cried. Her voice broke in on him with the force of a gunshot.

"Found thet there ol'bug, did old Block," Block said, sinking down into the chair by the bed. He raised his hands over his head in the gesture of a victorious prizefighter and let them collapse in his lap as if the effort had exhausted him. Then he removed a red bandana handkerchief that he carried to be funny with and wiped his face thoroughly, having a different expression on it every time it appeared from behind the rag.

"I think you're just as smart as you can be!" Mrs. Fox said. "Asbury," she said, "you have undulant fever. It'll keep coming back, but it won't kill you!" Her smile was as bright and intense as a lightbulb without a shade. "I'm so relieved," she said.

Asbury sat up slowly, his face expressionless; then he fell back down again.

Block leaned over him and smiled. "You ain't going to die," he said with deep satisfaction.

Nothing about Asbury stirred except his eyes. They did not appear to move on the surface but somewhere in their blurred depths there was an almost imperceptible motion as if something were struggling feebly. Block's gaze seemed to reach down like a steel pin and hold whatever it was until the life was out of it. "Undulant fever ain't so bad Asbury," he murmured. "It's the same as Bang's in a cow."

The boy gave almost a moan and then was quiet.

"He must have drunk some unpasteurized milk up there," his mother said softly and then the two of them tiptoed out as if they thought he were about to go to sleep.

When the sound of their footsteps had faded on the stairs, Asbury sat up again. He turned his head, almost surreptitiously, to the side where the key he had given his mother was lying on the bedside table. His hand shot out and closed over it and returned it to his pocket. He glanced across the room into the small oval-framed dresser mirror. The eyes that stared back at him were the same that had returned his gaze every day from that mirror but it seemed to him that they were paler. They looked shocked clean as if they had been prepared for some awful vision about to come down on him. He shuddered and turned his head quickly the other way and stared out the window. A blinding red-gold sun moved serenely from under a purple cloud. Below it the treeline was black against the crimson sky. It formed a brittle wall, standing as if it were the frail defense he had set up in his mind to protect him from what was coming. The boy fell back on his pillow and stared at the ceiling. His limbs that had been racked for so many weeks by fever and chill were numb now. The old life in him was exhausted. He awaited the coming of new. It was then that he felt the beginning of a chill, a chill so peculiar, so light, that it was like a warm ripple across a deeper sea of cold. His breath came short. The fierce bird which through the years of his childhood and the days of his illness had been poised over his head, waiting mysteriously, appeared all at once to be in motion. Asbury blanched and the last film of illusion was torn as if by a whirlwind from his eyes. He saw that for the rest of his days, frail, racked, but enduring, he would live in the face of a purifying terror. A feeble cry, a last impossible protest escaped him. But the Holy Ghost, emblazoned in ice instead of fire, continued, implacable, to descend.

RAPPACCINI'S DAUGHTER

NATHANIEL HAWTHORNE

[From the Writings of Aubépine.]

We do not remember to have seen any translated specimens of the productions of M. de l'Aubépine—a fact the less to be wondered at, as his very name is unknown to many of his own countrymen as well as to the student of foreign literature. As a writer, he seems to occupy an unfortunate position between the Transcendentalists (who, under one name or another, have their share in all the current literature of the world) and the great body of pen-and-ink men who address the intellect and sympathies of the multitude. If not too refined, at all events too remote, too shadowy, and unsubstantial in his modes of development to suit the taste of the latter class, and yet too popular to satisfy the spiritual or metaphysical requisitions of the former, he must necessarily find himself without an audience, except here and there an individual or possibly an isolated clique. His writings, to do them justice, are not altogether destitute of fancy and originality; they might have won him greater reputation but for an inveterate love of allegory, which is apt to invest his plots and characters with the aspect of scenery and people in the clouds, and to steal away the human warmth out of his conceptions. His fictions are sometimes historical, sometimes of the present day, and sometimes, so far as can be discovered, have little or no reference either to time or space. In any case, he generally contents himself with a very slight embroidery of outward manners—the faintest possible counterfeit of real life—and endeavors to create an interest by some less obvious peculiarity of the subject. Occasionally a breath of Nature, a raindrop of pathos and tenderness, or a gleam of humor, will find its way into the midst of his fantastic imagery, and make us feel as if, after all, we were yet within the limits of our native earth. We will only add to this very cursory notice that M. de l'Aubépine's productions, if the reader chance to take them in precisely the proper point of view, may amuse a leisure hour as well as those of a brighter man; if otherwise, they can hardly fail to look excessively like nonsense.

From *The Complete Novels and Selected Tales of Nathaniel Hawthorne*, edited by Norman Holmes Pearson (New York: Modern Library, 1937): 43–64.

Our author is voluminous; he continues to write and publish with as much praiseworthy and indefatigable prolixity as if his efforts were crowned with the brilliant success that so justly attends those of Eugene Sue. His first appearance was by a collection of stories in a long series of volumes entitled "Contes deux fois racontées." The titles of some of his more recent works (we quote from memory) are as follows: "Le Voyage Céleste à Chemin de Fer," 3 tom., 1838; "Le nouveau Père Adam et la nouvelle Mère Eve," 2 tom., 1839; "Roderic; ou le Serpent à l'estomac," 2 tom., 1840; "le Culte du Feu," a folio volume of ponderous research into the religion and ritual of the old Persian Ghebers, published in 1841; "La Soiree du Chateau en Espagne," 1 tom., 8vo, 1842; and "L'Artiste du Beau; ou le Papillon Mécanique," 5 tom., 4to, 1843. Our somewhat wearisome perusal of this startling catalogue of volumes has left behind it a certain personal affection and sympathy, though by no means admiration, for M. de l'Aubépine; and we would fain do the little in our power towards introducing him favorably to the American public. The ensuing tale is a translation of his "Beatrice; ou la Belle Empoisonneuse," recently published in "La Revue Anti-Aristocratique." This journal, edited by the Comte de Bearhaven, has for some years past led the defense of liberal principles and popular rights with a faithfulness and ability worthy of all praise.

* * * * *

A young man, named Giovanni Guasconti, came, very long ago, from the more southern region of Italy, to pursue his studies at the University of Padua. Giovanni, who had but a scanty supply of gold ducats in his pocket, took lodgings in a high and gloomy chamber of an old edifice which looked not unworthy to have been the palace of a Paduan noble, and which, in fact, exhibited over its entrance the armorial bearings of a family long since extinct. The young stranger, who was not unstudied in the great poem of his country, recollected that one of the ancestors of this family, and perhaps an occupant of this very mansion, had been pictured by Dante as a partaker of the immortal agonies of his Inferno. These reminiscences and associations, together with the tendency to heartbreak natural to a young man for the first time out of his native sphere, caused Giovanni to sigh heavily as he looked around the desolate and ill-furnished apartment.

"Holy Virgin, signor!" cried old Dame Lisabetta, who, won by the youth's remarkable beauty of person, was kindly endeavoring to give the chamber a habitable air, "what a sigh was that to come out of a young man's heart! Do you find this old mansion gloomy? For the love of Heaven, then, put your head out of the window, and you will see as bright sunshine as you have left in Naples."

Guasconti mechanically did as the old woman advised, but could not quite agree with her that the Paduan sunshine was as cheerful as that of southern Italy. Such as it was, however, it fell upon a garden beneath the window and expended its fostering influences on a variety of plants, which seemed to have been cultivated with exceeding care.

"Does this garden belong to the house?" asked Giovanni.

"Heaven forbid, signor, unless it were fruitful of better pot herbs than any that grow there now," answered old Lisabetta. "No; that garden is cultivated by the own hands of Signor Giacomo Rappaccini, the famous doctor, who, I warrant him, has been heard of as far as Naples. It is said that he distils these plants into medicines that are as potent as a charm. Oftentimes you may see the signor doctor at work, and perchance the signora, his daughter, too, gathering the strange flowers that grow in the garden."

The old woman had now done what she could for the aspect of the chamber; and, commending the young man to the protection of the saints, took her departure.

Giovanni still found no better occupation than to look down into the garden beneath his window. From its appearance, he judged it to be one of those botanic gardens which were of earlier date in Padua than elsewhere in Italy or in the world. Or, not improbably, it might once have been the pleasure-palace of an opulent family; for there was the ruin of a marble fountain in the centre, sculptured with rare art, but so wofully shattered that it was impossible to trace the original design from the chaos of remaining fragments. The water, however, continued to gush and sparkle into the sunbeams as cheerfully as ever. A little gurgling sound ascended to the young man's window, and made him feel as if the fountain were an immortal spirit that sung its song unceasingly and without heeding the vicissitudes around it, while one century embodied it in marble and another scattered the perishable garniture on the soil. All about the pool into which the water subsided grew various plants, that seemed to require a plentiful supply of moisture for the nourishment of gigantic leaves, and in some instances, flowers gorgeously magnificent. There was one shrub in particular, set in a marble vase in the midst of the pool, that bore a profusion of purple blossoms, each of which had the lustre and richness of a gem; and the whole together made a show so resplendent that it seemed enough to illuminate the garden, even had there been no sunshine. Every portion of the soil was peopled with plants and herbs, which, if less beautiful, still bore tokens of assiduous care, as if all had their individual virtues, known to the scientific mind that fostered them. Some were placed in urns, rich with old carving, and others in common garden pots; some crept serpent-like along the ground or climbed on high, using whatever means of ascent was offered them. One plant had wreathed itself round a statue of Vertumnus, which was thus quite veiled and shrouded in a drapery of hanging foliage, so happily arranged that it might have served a sculptor for a study.

While Giovanni stood at the window he heard a rustling behind a screen of leaves, and became aware that a person was at work in the garden. His figure soon emerged into view, and showed itself to be that of no common laborer, but a tall, emaciated, sallow, and sickly-looking man, dressed in a scholar's garb of black. He was beyond the middle term of life, with gray hair, a thin, gray beard, and a face singularly marked with intellect and cultivation, but which could never, even in his more youthful days, have expressed much warmth of heart.

Nothing could exceed the intentness with which this scientific gardener examined every shrub which grew in his path: it seemed as if he was looking into their inmost nature, making observations in regard to their creative essence, and discovering why one leaf grew in this shape and another in that, and wherefore such and such flowers differed among themselves in hue and perfume. Nevertheless, in spite of this deep intelligence on his part, there was no approach to intimacy between himself and these vegetable existences. On the contrary, he avoided their actual touch or the direct inhaling of their odors with a caution that impressed Giovanni most disagreeably; for the man's demeanor was that of one walking among malignant influences, such as savage beasts, or deadly snakes, or evil spirits, which, should he allow them one moment of license, would wreak upon him some terrible fatality. It was strangely frightful to the young man's imagination to see this air of insecurity in a person cultivating a garden, that most simple and innocent of human toils, and which had been alike the joy and labor of the unfallen parents of the race. Was this garden, then, the Eden of the present world? And this man, with such a perception of harm in what his own hands caused to grow—was he the Adam?

The distrustful gardener, while plucking away the dead leaves or pruning the too luxuriant growth of the shrubs, defended his hands with a pair of thick gloves. Nor were these his only armor. When, in his walk through the garden, he came to the magnificent plant that hung its purple gems beside the marble fountain, he placed a kind of mask over his mouth and nostrils, as if all this beauty did but conceal a deadlier malice; but, finding his task still too dangerous, he drew back, removed the mask, and called loudly, but in the infirm voice of a person affected with inward disease—

"Beatrice! Beatrice!"

"Here am I, my father. What would you?" cried a rich and youthful voice from the window of the opposite house—a voice as rich as a tropical sunset, and which made Giovanni, though he knew not why, think of deep hues of purple or crimson and of perfumes heavily delectable. "Are you in the garden?"

"Yes, Beatrice," answered the gardener, "and I need your help."

Soon there emerged from under a sculptured portal the figure of a young girl, arrayed with as much richness of taste as the most splendid of the flowers, beautiful as the day, and with a bloom so deep and vivid that one shade more would have been too much. She looked redundant with life, health, and energy; all of which attributes were bound down and compressed, as it were, and girdled tensely, in the luxuriance, by her virgin zone. Yet Giovanni's fancy must have grown morbid while he looked down into the garden; for the impression which the fair stranger made upon him was as if here were another flower, the human sister of those vegetable ones, as beautiful as they, more beautiful than the richest of them, but still to be touched only with a glove, not to be approached without a mask. As Beatrice came down the garden path, it was observable that she handled and inhaled the odor of several of the plants which her father had most sedulously avoided.

"Here, Beatrice," said the latter, "see how many needful offices require to be done to our chief treasure. Yet, shattered as I am, my life might pay the penalty of approaching it so closely as circumstances demand. Henceforth, I fear, this plant must be consigned to your sole charge."

"And gladly will I undertake it," cried again the rich tones of the young lady, as she bent towards the magnificent plant and opened her arms as if to embrace it. "Yes, my sister, my splendour, it shall be Beatrice's task to nurse and serve thee; and thou shalt reward her with thy kisses and perfumed breath, which to her is as the breath of life."

Then, with all the tenderness in her manner that was so strikingly expressed in her words, she busied herself with such attentions as the plant seemed to require; and Giovanni, at his lofty window, rubbed his eyes and almost doubted whether it were a girl tending her favorite flower, or one sister performing the duties of affection to another. The scene soon terminated. Whether Dr. Rappaccini had finished his labors in the garden, or that his watchful eye had caught the stranger's face, he now took his daughter's arm and retired. Night was already closing in; oppressive exhalations seemed to proceed from the plants and steal upward past the open window; and Giovanni, closing the lattice, went to his couch and dreamed of a rich flower and beautiful girl. Flower and maiden were different, and yet the same, and fraught with some strange peril in either shape.

But there is an influence in the light of morning that tends to rectify whatever errors of fancy, or even of judgment, we may have incurred during the sun's decline, or among the shadows of the night, or the less wholesome glow of moonshine. Giovanni's first movement, on starting from sleep, was to throw open the window and gaze down into the garden which his dreams had made so fertile of mysteries. He was surprised and a little ashamed to find how real and matter-of-fact an affair it proved to be, in the first rays of the sun which gilded the dew-drops that hung upon leaf and blossom, and, while giving a brighter beauty to each rare flower, brought everything within the limits of ordinary experience. The young man rejoiced that, in the heart of the barren city, he had the privilege of overlooking this spot of lovely and luxuriant vegetation. It would serve, he said to himself, as a symbolic language to keep him in communion with Nature. Neither the sickly and thoughtworn Dr. Giacomo Rappaccini, it is true, nor his brilliant daughter, were now visible; so that Giovanni could not determine how much of the singularity which he attributed to both was due to their own qualities and how much to his wonder-working fancy; but he was inclined to take a most rational view of the whole matter.

In the course of the day he paid his respects to Signor Pietro Baglioni, professor of medicine in the university, a physician of eminent repute to whom Giovanni had brought a letter of introduction. The professor was an elderly personage, apparently of genial nature, and habits that might almost be called jovial. He kept the young man to dinner, and made himself very agreeable by the freedom and liveliness of his conversation, especially when warmed by a flask or two of Tuscan wine. Giovanni, conceiving that men of science, inhabitants of the same city, must needs be on familiar terms with one another, took an opportunity to mention the name of Dr. Rappaccini. But the professor did not respond with so much cordiality as he had anticipated.

"Ill would it become a teacher of the divine art of medicine," said Professor Pietro Baglioni, in answer to a question of Giovanni, "to withhold due and well-considered praise of a physician so eminently skilled as Rappaccini; but, on the other hand, I should answer it but scantily to my conscience were I to permit a worthy youth like yourself, Signor Giovanni, the son of an ancient friend, to imbibe erroneous ideas respecting a man who might hereafter chance to hold your life and death in his hands. The truth is, our worshipful Dr. Rappaccini has as much science as any member of the faculty—with perhaps one single exception—in Padua, or all Italy; but there are certain grave objections to his professional character."

"And what are they?" asked the young man.

"Has my friend Giovanni any disease of body or heart, that he is so inquisitive about physicians?" said the professor, with a smile. "But as for Rappaccini, it is said of him—and I, who know the man well, can answer for its truth—that he cares infinitely more for science than for mankind. His patients are interesting to him only as subjects for some new experiment. He would sacrifice human life, his own among the rest, or whatever else was dearest to him, for the sake of adding so much as a grain of mustard seed to the great heap of his accumulated knowledge."

"Methinks he is an awful man indeed," remarked Guasconti, mentally recalling the cold and purely intellectual aspect of Rappaccini. "And yet, worshipful professor, is it not a noble spirit? Are there many men capable of so spiritual a love of science?"

"God forbid," answered the professor, somewhat testily; "at least, unless they take sounder views of the healing art than those adopted by Rappaccini. It is his theory that all medicinal virtues are comprised within those substances which we term vegetable poisons. These he cultivates with his own hands, and is said even to have produced new varieties of poison, more horribly deleterious than Nature, without the assistance of this learned person, would ever have plagued the world withal. That the signor doctor does less mischief than might be expected with such dangerous substances is undeniable. Now and then, it must be owned, he has effected, or seemed to effect, a marvellous cure; but, to tell you my private mind, Signor Giovanni, he should receive little credit for such instances of success—they being probably the work of chance—but should be held strictly accountable for his failures, which may justly be considered his own work."

The youth might have taken Baglioni's opinions with many grains of allowance had he known that there was a professional warfare of long continuance between him and Dr. Rappaccini, in which the latter was generally thought to have gained the advantage. If the reader be inclined to judge for himself, we refer him to certain black-letter tracts on both sides, preserved in the medical department of the University of Padua.

"I know not, most learned professor," returned Giovanni, after musing on what had been said of Rappaccini's exclusive zeal for science—"I know not how dearly this physician may love his art; but surely there is one object more dear to him. He has a daughter."

"Aha!" cried the professor, with a laugh. "So now our friend Giovanni's secret is out. You have heard of this daughter, whom all the young men in Padua are wild about, though not half a dozen have ever had the good hap to see her face. I know little of the Signora Beatrice save that Rappaccini is said to have instructed her deeply in his science, and that, young and beautiful as fame reports her, she is already qualified to fill a professor's chair. Perchance her father destines her for mine! Other absurd rumors there be, not worth talking about or listening to. So now, Signor Giovanni, drink off your glass of lachryma."

Guasconti returned to his lodgings somewhat heated with the wine he had quaffed, and which caused his brain to swim with strange fantasies in reference to Dr. Rappaccini and the beautiful Beatrice. On his way, happening to pass by a florist's, he bought a fresh bouquet of flowers.

Ascending to his chamber, he seated himself near the window, but within the shadow thrown by the depth of the wall, so that he could look down into the garden with little risk of being discovered. All beneath his eye was a solitude. The strange plants were basking in the sunshine, and now and then nodding gently to one another, as if in acknowledgment of sympathy and kindred. In the midst, by the shattered fountain, grew the magnificent shrub, with its purple gems clustering all over it; they glowed in the air, and gleamed back again out of the depths of the pool, which thus seemed to overflow with colored radiance from the rich reflection that was steeped in it. At first, as we have said, the garden was a solitude. Soon, however—as Giovanni had half hoped, half feared, would be the case—a figure appeared beneath the antique sculptured portal, and came down between the rows of plants, inhaling their various perfumes as if she were one of those beings of old classic fable that lived upon sweet odors. On again beholding Beatrice, the young man was even startled to perceive how much her beauty exceeded his recollection of it; so brilliant, so vivid, was its character, that she glowed amid the sunlight, and, as Giovanni whispered to himself, positively illuminated the more shadowy intervals of the garden path. Her face being now more revealed than on the former occasion, he was struck by its expression of simplicity and sweetness—qualities that had not entered into his idea of her character, and which made him to ask anew what manner of mortal she might be. Nor did he fail again to observe, or imagine, an analogy between the beautiful girl and the gorgeous shrub that hung its gemlike flowers over the fountain—a resemblance which Beatrice seemed to have indulged a fantastic humor in heightening, both by the arrangement of her dress and the selection of its hues.

Approaching the shrub, she threw open her arms, as with a passionate ardor, and drew its branches into an intimate embrace—so intimate that her features were hidden it its leafy bosom and her glistening ringlets all intermingled with the flowers.

"Give me thy breath, my sister," exclaimed Beatrice; "for I am faint with common air. And give me this flower of thine, which I separate with gentlest fingers from the stem and place it close beside my heart."

With these words the beautiful daughter of Rappaccini plucked one of the richest blossoms of the shrub, and was about to fasten it in her bosom. But now, unless Giovanni's draughts of wine had bewildered his senses, a singular incident occurred. A small orange-colored reptile, of the lizard or chameleon species, chanced to be creeping along the path, just at the feet of Beatrice. It appeared to Giovanni—but at the distance from which he gazed, he could scarcely have seen anything so minute—it appeared to him however, that a drop or two of moisture from the broken stem of the flower descended upon the lizard's head. For an instant the reptile contorted itself violently, and then lay motionless in the sunshine. Beatrice observed this remarkable phenomenon, and crossed herself, sadly, but without surprise; nor did she therefore hesitate to arrange the fatal flower in her bosom. There it blushed, and almost glimmered with the dazzling effect of a precious stone, adding to her dress and aspect the one appropriate charm which nothing else in the world could have supplied. But Giovanni, out of the shadow of his window, bent forward and shrank back, and murmured and trembled.

"Am I awake? Have I my senses?" said he to himself. "What is this being? Beautiful shall I call her, or inexpressibly terrible?"

Beatrice now strayed carelessly through the garden, approaching closer beneath Giovanni's window, so that he was compelled to thrust his head quite out of its concealment in order to gratify the intense and painful curiosity which she excited. At this moment there came a beautiful insect over the garden wall; it had, perhaps, wandered through the city, and found no flowers or verdure among those antique haunts of men until the heavy perfumes of Dr. Rappaccini's shrubs had lured it from afar. Without alighting on the flowers, this winged brightness seemed to be attracted by Beatrice, and lingered in the air and fluttered about her head. Now, here it could not be but that Giovanni Guasconti's eyes deceived him. Be that as it might, he fancied that, while Beatrice was gazing at the insect with childish delight, it grew faint and fell at her feet; its bright wings shivered; it was dead—from no cause that he could discern, unless it were the atmosphere of her breath. Again Beatrice crossed herself and sighed heavily as she bent over the dead insect.

An impulsive movement of Giovanni drew her eyes to the window. There she beheld the beautiful head of the young man—rather a Grecian than an Italian head, with fair, regular features, and a glistening of gold among his ringlets—gazing down upon her like a being that hovered in mid air. Scarcely knowing what he did, Giovanni threw down the bouquet which he had hitherto held in his hand.

"Signora, there are pure and healthful flowers. Wear them for the sake of Giovanni Guasconti."

"Thanks, signor," replied Beatrice, with her rich voice, that came forth as it were like a gush of music, and with a mirthful expression half childish and half woman-like.

"I accept your gift, and would fain recompense it with this precious purple flower; but if I toss it into the air it will not reach you. So Signor Guasconti must ever content himself with my thanks."

She lifted the bouquet from the ground, and then, as if inwardly ashamed at having stepped aside from her maidenly reserve to respond to a stranger's greeting, passed swiftly homeward through the garden. But few as the moments were, it seemed to Giovanni, when she was on the point of vanishing beneath the sculptured portal, that his beautiful bouquet was already beginning to wither in her grasp. It was an idle thought; there could be no possibility of distinguishing a faded flower from a fresh one at so great a distance.

For many days after this incident the young man avoided the window that looked into Dr. Rappaccini's garden, as if something ugly and monstrous would have blasted his eyesight had he been betrayed into a glance. He felt conscious of having put himself, to a certain extent, within the influence of an unintelligible power by the communication which he had opened with Beatrice. The wisest course would have been, if his heart were in any real danger, to quit his lodgings and Padua itself at once; the next wiser, to have accustomed himself, as far as possible, to the familiar and daylight view of Beatrice—thus bringing her rigidly and systematically within the limits of ordinary experience. Least of all, while avoiding her sight, ought Giovanni to have remained so near this extraordinary being that the proximity and possibility even of intercourse should have given a kind of substance and reality to the wild vagaries which his imagination ran riot continually in producing. Guasconti had not a deep heart—or, at all events, its depths were not sounded now; but he had a quick fancy, and an ardent southern temperament, which rose every instant to a higher fever pitch. Whether or no Beatrice possessed those terrible attributes, that fatal breath, the affinity with those so beautiful and deadly flowers which were indicated by what Giovanni had witnessed, she had at least instilled a fierce and subtle poison into his system. It was not love, although her rich beauty was a madness to him; nor horror, even while he fancied her spirit to be imbued with the same baneful essence that seemed to pervade her physical frame; but a wild offspring of both love and horror that had each parent in it, and burned like one and shivered like the other. Giovanni knew not what to dread; still less did he know what to hope; yet hope and dread kept a continual warfare in his breast, alternately vanquishing one another and starting up afresh to renew the contest. Blessed are all simple emotions, be they dark or bright! It is the lurid intermixture of the two that produces the illuminating blaze of the infernal regions.

Sometimes he endeavored to assuage the fever of his spirit by a rapid walk through the streets of Padua or beyond its gates: his footsteps kept time with the throbbings of his brain, so that the walk was apt to accelerate itself to a race. One day he found himself arrested; his arm was seized by a portly personage, who had turned back on recognizing the young man and expended much breath in overtaking him.

"Signor Giovanni! Stay, my young friend!" cried he. "Have you forgotten me? That might well be the case if I were as much altered as yourself."

It was Baglioni, whom Giovanni had avoided ever since their first meeting, from a doubt that the professor's sagacity would look too deeply into his secrets. Endeavoring to recover himself, he stared forth wildly from his inner world into the outer one and spoke like a man in a dream.

"Yes; I am Giovanni Guasconti. You are Professor Pietro Baglioni. Now let me pass!"

"Not yet, not yet, Signor Giovanni Guasconti," said the professor, smiling, but at the same time scrutinizing the youth with an earnest glance. "What! did I grow up side by side with your father? and shall his son pass me like a stranger in these old streets of Padua? Stand still, Signor Giovanni; for we must have a word or two before we part."

"Speedily, then most worshipful professor, speedily," said Giovanni, with feverish impatience. "Does not your worship see that I am in haste?"

Now, while he was speaking there came a man in black along the street, stooping and moving feebly like a person in inferior health. His face was all overspread with a most sickly and sallow hue, but yet so pervaded with an expression of piercing and active intellect that an observer might easily have overlooked the merely physical attributes and have seen only this wonderful energy. As he passed, this person exchanged a cold and distant salutation with Baglioni, but fixed his eyes upon Giovanni with an intentness that seemed to bring out whatever was within him worthy of notice. Nevertheless, there was a peculiar quietness in the look, as if taking merely a speculative, not a human interest, in the young man.

"It is Dr. Rappaccini!" whispered the professor when the stranger had passed. "Has he ever seen your face before?"

"Not that I know," answered Giovanni, starting at the name.

"He *has* seen you! he must have seen you!" said Baglioni, hastily. "For some purpose or other, this man of sciences is making a study of you. I know that look of his! It is the same that coldly illuminates his face as he bends over a bird, a mouse, or a butterfly, which, in pursuance of some experiment, he has killed by the perfume of a flower; a look as deep as Nature itself, but without Nature's warmth of love. Signor Giovanni, I will stake my life upon it, you are the subject of one of Rappaccini's experiments!"

"Will you make a fool of me?" cried Giovanni, passionately. "*That,* signor professor, were an untoward experiment."

"Patience! patience!" replied the imperturbable professor. "I tell thee, my poor Giovanni, that Rappaccini has a scientific interest in thee. Thou has fallen into fearful hands! And the Signora Beatrice—what part does she act in this mystery?"

But Guasconti, finding Baglioni's pertinacity intolerable, here broke away, and was gone before the professor could again seize his arm. He looked after the young man intently and shook his head.

"This must not be," said Baglioni to himself. "The youth is the son of my old friend, and shall not come to any harm from which the arcana of medical science can preserve him. Besides, it is too insufferable an impertinence in Rappaccini, thus to snatch the lad out of my own hands, as I may say, and make use of him for his infernal experiments. This daughter of his! It shall be looked to. Perchance, most learned Rappaccini, I may foil you where you little dream of it!"

Meanwhile Giovanni had pursued a circuitous route, and at length found himself at the door of his lodgings. As he crossed the threshold he was met by old Lisabetta, who smirked and smiled, and was evidently desirous to attract his attention; vainly, however, as the ebullition of his feelings had momentarily subsided into a cold and dull vacuity. He turned his eyes full upon the withered face that was puckering itself into a smile, but seemed to behold it not. The old dame, therefore, laid her grasp upon his cloak.

"Signor! signor!" whispered she, still with a smile over the whole breadth of her visage, so that it looked not unlike a grotesque carving in wood, darkened by centuries. "Listen, signor! There is a private entrance into the garden."

"What do you say?" exclaimed Giovanni, turning quickly about, as if an inanimate thing should start into feverish life. "A private entrance into Dr. Rappaccini's garden?"

"Hush! hush! not so loud!" whispered Lisabetta, putting her hand over his mouth. "Yes; into the worshipful doctor's garden, where you may see all his fine shrubbery. Many a young man in Padua would give gold to be admitted among those flowers."

Giovanni put a piece of gold into her hand.

"Show me the way," said he.

A surmise, probably excited by his conversation with Baglioni, crossed his mind, that this interposition of old Lisabetta might perchance be connected with the intrigue, whatever were its nature, in which the professor seemed to suppose that Dr. Rappaccini was involving him. But such a suspicion, though it disturbed Giovanni, was inadequate to restrain him. The instant that he was aware of the possibility of approaching Beatrice, it seemed an absolute necessity of his existence to do so. It mattered not whether she were an angel or demon; he was irrevocably within her sphere, and must obey the law that whirled him onward, in ever-lessening circles, towards a result which he did not attempt to foreshadow; and yet, strange to say, there came across him a sudden doubt whether this intense interest on his part were not delusory; whether it were really of so deep and positive a nature as to justify him in now thrusting himself into an incalculable position; whether it were not merely the fantasy of a young man's brain, only slightly or not at all connected with his heart.

He paused, hesitated, turned half about, but again went on. His withered guide led him along several obscure passages, and finally undid a door, through which, as it was opened, there came the sight and sound of rustling leaves, with the broken sunshine glimmering among them. Giovanni stepped forth, and, forcing himself through the entanglement of a shrub that wreathed its tendrils over the hidden entrance, stood beneath his own window in the open area of Dr. Rappaccini's garden.

How often is it the case that, when impossibilities have come to pass and dreams have condensed their misty substance into tangible realities, we find ourselves calm, and even coldly self-possessed, amid circumstances which it would have been a delirium of joy or agony to anticipate! Fate delights to thwart us thus. Passion will choose his own time to rush upon the scene, and lingers sluggishly behind when an appropriate adjustment of events would seem to summon his appearance. So was it now with Giovannni. Day after day his pulses had throbbed with feverish blood at the improbable idea of an interview with Beatrice, and of standing with her, face to face, in this very garden, basking in the Oriental sunshine of her beauty, and snatching from her full gaze the mystery which he deemed the riddle of his own existence. But now there was a singular and untimely equanimity within his breast. He threw a glance around the garden to discover if Beatrice or her father were present, and, perceiving that he was alone, began a critical observation of the plants.

The aspect of one and all of them dissatisfied him; their gorgeousness seemed fierce, passionate, and even unnatural. There was hardly an individual shrub which a wanderer, straying by himself through a forest, would not have been startled to find growing wild, as if an unearthly face had glared at him out of the thicket. Several also would have shocked a delicate instinct by an appearance of artificialness, indicating that there had been such commixture, and, as it were, adultery, of various vegetable species, that the production was no longer of God's making, but the monstrous offspring of man's depraved fancy, glowing with only an evil mockery of beauty. They were probably the result of experiment, which in one or two cases had succeeded in mingling plants individually lovely into a compound possessing the questionable and ominous character that distinguished the whole growth of the garden. In fine, Giovanni recognized but two or three plants in the collection, and those of a kind that he well knew to be poisonous. While busy with these contemplations he heard the rustling of a silken garment, and, turning beheld Beatrice emerging from beneath the sculptured portal.

Giovanni had not considered with himself what should be his deportment; whether he should apologize for his intrusion into the garden, or assume that he was there with the privity at least, if not by the desire, of Dr. Rappaccini or his daughter; but Beatrice's manner placed him at his ease, though leaving him still in doubt by what agency he had gained admittance. She came lightly along the path and met him near the broken fountain. There was surprise in her face, but brightened by a simple and kind expression of pleasure.

"You are a connoisseur in flowers, signor," said Beatrice, with a smile, alluding to the bouquet which he had flung her from the window. "It is no marvel, therefore, if the sight of my father's rare collection has tempted you to take a nearer view. If he were here, he could tell you many strange and interesting facts as to the nature and habits of these shrubs; for he has spent a lifetime in such studies, and this garden is his world."

"And you yourself, lady," observed Giovanni, "if fame says true—you likewise are deeply skilled in the virtues indicated by these rich blossoms and these spicy perfumes. Would you deign to be my instructress, I should prove an apter scholar than if taught by Signor Rappaccini himself."

"Are there such idle rumors?" asked Beatrice, with the music of a pleasant laugh. "Do people say that I am skilled in my father's science of plants? What a jest is there! No; though I have grown up among these flowers, I know no more of them than their hues and perfume; and sometimes methinks I would fain rid myself of even that small knowledge. There are many flowers here, and those not the least brilliant, that shock and offend me when they meet my eye. But pray, signor, do not believe these stories about my science. Believe nothing of me save what you see with your own eyes."

"And must I believe all that I have seen with my own eyes?" asked Giovanni, pointedly, while the recollection of former scenes made him shrink. "No, signora; you demand too little of me. Bid me believe nothing save what comes from your own lips."

It would appear that Beatrice understood him. There came a deep flush to her cheek; but she looked full into Giovanni's eyes, and responded to his gaze of uneasy suspicion with a queenlike haughtiness.

"I do so bid you, signor," she replied. "Forget whatever you may have fancied in regard to me. If true to the outward senses, still it may be false in its essence; but the words of Beatrice Rappaccini's lips are true from the depths of the heart outward. Those you may believe."

A fervor glowed in her whole aspect and beamed upon Giovanni's consciousness like the light of truth itself; but while she spoke there was a fragrance in the atmosphere around her, rich and delightful, though evanescent, yet which the young man, from an indefinable reluctance, scarcely dared to draw into his lungs. It might be the odor of the flowers. Could it be Beatrice's breath which thus embalmed her words with a strange richness, as if by steeping them in her heart? A faintness passed like a shadow over Giovanni and flitted away; he seemed to gaze through the beautiful girl's eyes into her transparent soul, and felt no more doubt or fear.

The tinge of passion that had colored Beatrice's manner vanished; she became gay, and appeared to derive a pure delight from her communion with the youth not unlike what the maiden of a lonely island might have felt conversing with a voyager from the civilized world. Evidently her experience of life had been confined within the limits of that garden. She talked now about matters as simple as the daylight or summer clouds, and now asked questions in reference to the city, or Giovanni's distant home, his friends, his mother, and his sisters—questions indicating such seclusion, and such lack of familiarity with modes and forms, that Giovanni responded as if to an infant. Her spirit gushed out before him like a fresh rill that was just catching its first glimpse of the sunlight and wondering at the reflections of earth and sky which were flung into its bosom. There came thought, too, from a deep source, and fantasies of a gemlike brilliancy, as if diamonds and rubies sparkled upward among the bubbles of the fountain. Ever and anon there gleamed across the young man's mind a sense of wonder that he should be walking side by side with the being who had so wrought upon his imagination, whom he had idealized in such hues of terror, in whom he had positively witnessed such manifestations of dreadful attributes—that he should be conversing with Beatrice like a brother, and should find her so human and so maidenlike. But such reflections were only momentary; the effect of her character was too real not to make itself familiar at once.

In this free intercourse they had strayed through the garden, and now, after many turns among its avenues, were come to the shattered fountain, beside which grew the magnificent shrub, with its treasury of glowing blossoms. A fragrance was diffused from it which Giovanni recognized as identical with that which he had attributed to Beatrice's breath, but incomparably more powerful. As her eyes fell upon it, Giovanni beheld her press her hand to her bosom as if her heart were throbbing suddenly and painfully.

"For the first time in my life," murmured she, addressing the shrub, "I had forgotten thee."

"I remember, signora," said Giovanni, "that you once promised to reward me with one of these living gems for the bouquet which I had the happy boldness to fling to your feet. Permit me now to pluck it as a memorial of this interview."

He made a step towards the shrub with extended hand; but Beatrice darted forward, uttering a shriek that went through his heart like a dagger. She caught his hand and drew it back with the whole force of her slender figure. Giovanni felt her touch thrilling through his fibres.

"Touch it not!" exclaimed she, in a voice of agony. "Not for thy life! It is fatal!"

Then, hiding her face, she fled from him and vanished beneath the sculptured portal. As Giovanni followed her with his eyes, he beheld the emaciated figure and pale intelligence of Dr. Rappaccini, who had been watching the scene, he knew not how long, within the shadow of the entrance.

No sooner was Guasconti alone in his chamber than the image of Beatrice came back to his passionate musings, invested with all the witchery that had been gathering around it ever since his first glimpse of her, and now likewise imbued with a tender warmth of girlish womanhood. She was human; her nature was endowed with all gentle and feminine qualities; she was worthiest to be worshipped; she was capable, surely, on her part, of the height and heroism of love. Those tokens which he had hitherto considered as proofs of a frightful peculiarity in her physical and moral system were now either forgotten, or, by the subtle sophistry of passion transmitted into a golden crown of enchantment, rendering Beatrice the more admirable by so much as she was the more unique. Whatever had looked ugly was now beautiful; or, if incapable of such a change, it stole away and hid itself among those shapeless half ideas which throng the dim region beyond the daylight of our perfect consciousness. Thus did he spend the night, nor fell asleep until the dawn had begun to awake the slumbering flowers in Dr. Rappaccini's garden, whither Giovanni's dreams doubtless led him. Up rose the sun in his due season, and, flinging his beams upon the young man's eyelids, awoke him to a sense of pain. When thoroughly aroused, he became sensible of a burning and tingling agony in his hand—in his right hand—the very hand which Beatrice had grasped in her own when he was on the point of plucking one of the gemlike flowers. On the back of that hand there was now a purple print like that of four small fingers, and the likeness of a slender thumb upon his wrist.

Oh, how stubbornly does love—or even that cunning semblance of love which flourishes in the imagination, but strikes no depth of root into the heart—how stubbornly does it hold its faith until the moment comes when it is doomed to vanish into thin mist! Giovanni wrapped a handkerchief about his hand and wondered what evil thing had stung him, and soon forgot his pain in a reverie of Beatrice.

After the first interview, a second was in the inevitable course of what we call fate. A third; a fourth; and a meeting with Beatrice in the garden was no longer an incident in Giovanni's daily life, but the whole space in which he might be said to live: for the anticipation and memory of that ecstatic hour made up the remainder. Nor was it otherwise with the daughter of Rappaccini. She watched for the youth's appearance, and flew to his side with confidence as unreserved as if they had been playmates from early infancy—as if they were playmates still. If, by any unwonted chance, he failed to come at the appointed moment, she stood beneath the window and sent up the rich sweetness of her tones to float around him in his chamber and echo and reverberate throughout his heart: "Giovanni! Giovanni! Why tarriest thou? Come down!" And down he hastened into that Eden of poisonous flowers.

But, with all this intimate familiarity, there was still a reserve in Beatrice's demeanor, so rigidly and invariably sustained that the idea of infringing it scarcely occurred to his imagination. By all appreciable signs, they loved; they had looked love with eyes that conveyed the holy secret from the depths of one soul into the depths of the other, as if it were too sacred to be whispered by the way; they had even spoken love in those gushes of passion when their spirits darted forth in articulated breath like tongues of long-hidden flame; and yet there had been no seal of lips, no clasp of hands, nor any slightest caress such as love claims and hallows. He had never touched one of the gleaming ringlets of her hair; her garment—so marked was the physical barrier between them—had never been waved against him by a breeze. On the few occasions when Giovanni had seemed tempted to overstep the limit, Beatrice grew so sad, so stern, and withal wore such a look of desolate separation, shuddering at itself, that not a spoken word was requisite to repel him. At such times he was startled at the horrible suspicions that rose, monster-like, out of the caverns of his heart and stared him in the face; his love grew thin and faint as the morning mist, his doubts alone had substance. But, when Beatrice's face brightened again after the momentary shadow, she was transformed at once from the mysterious, questionable being whom he had watched with so much awe and horror; she was now the beautiful and unsophisticated girl whom he felt that his spirit knew with a certainty beyond all other knowledge.

A considerable time had now passed since Giovanni's last meeting with Baglioni. One morning, however, he was disagreeably surprised by a visit from the professor, whom he had scarcely thought of for whole weeks, and would willingly have forgotten still longer. Given up as he had long been to a pervading excitement, he could tolerate no companions except upon condition of their perfect sympathy with his present state of feeling. Such sympathy was not be expected from Professor Baglioni.

The visitor chatted carelessly for a few moments about the gossip of the city and the university, and then took up another topic.

"I have been reading an old classic author lately," said he, "and met with a story that strangely interested me. Possibly you may remember it. It is of an Indian prince, who sent a beautiful woman as a present to Alexander the Great. She was as lovely as the dawn and gorgeous as the sunset; but what especially distinguished her was a certain rich perfume in her breath—richer than a garden of Persian roses. Alexander, as was natural to a youthful conqueror, fell in love at first sight with this magnificent stranger; but a certain sage physician, happening to be present, discovered a terrible secret in regard to her."

"And what was that?" asked Giovanni, turning his eyes downward to avoid those of the professor.

"That this lovely woman," continued Baglioni, with emphasis, "had been nourished with poisons from her birth upward, until her whole nature was so imbued with them that she herself had become the deadliest poison in existence. Poison was her element in life. With that rich perfume of her breath she blasted the very air. Her love would have been poison—her embrace death. Is not this a marvellous tale?"

"A childish fable," answered Giovanni, nervously starting from his chair. "I marvel how your worship finds time to read such nonsense among your graver studies."

"By the by," said the professor, looking uneasily about him, "what singular fragrance is this in your apartment? Is it the perfume of your gloves? It is faint, but delicious; and yet, after all, by no means agreeable. Were I to breathe it long, methinks it would make me ill. It is like the breath of a flower; but I see no flowers in the chamber."

"Nor are there any," replied Giovanni, who had turned pale as the professor spoke; "nor, I think, is there any fragrance except in your worship's imagination. Odors, being a sort of element combined of the sensual and the spiritual, are apt to deceive us in this manner. The recollection of a perfume, the bare idea of it, may easily be mistaken for a present reality."

"Ay; but my sober imagination does not often play such tricks," said Baglioni; "and, were I to fancy any kind of odor, it would be that of some vile apothecary drug, wherewith my fingers are likely enough to be imbued. Our worshipful friend Rappaccini, as I have heard, tinctures his medicaments with odors richer than those of Araby. Doubtless, likewise, the fair and learned Signora Beatrice would minister to her patients with draughts as sweet as a maiden's breath; but woe to him that sips them!"

Giovanni's face evinced many contending emotions. The tone in which the professor alluded to the pure and lovely daughter of Rappaccini was a torture to his soul; and yet the intimation of a view of her character, opposite to his own, gave instantaneous distinctness to a thousand dim suspicions, which now grinned at him like so many demons. But he strove hard to quell them and to respond to Baglioni with a true lover's perfect faith.

"Signor professor," said he, "you were my father's friend; perchance, too, it is your purpose to act a friendly part towards his son. I would fain feel nothing towards you save respect and deference; but I pray you to observe, signor, that there is one subject on which we must not speak. You know not the Signora Beatrice. You cannot, therefore, estimate the wrong—the blasphemy, I may even say—that is offered to her character by a light or injurious word."

"Giovanni! my poor Giovanni!" answered the professor, with a calm expression of pity, "I know this wretched girl far better than yourself. You shall hear the truth in respect to the poisoner Rappaccini and his poisonous daughter; yes, poisonous as she is beautiful. Listen; for, even should you do violence to my gray hairs, it shall not silence me. That old fable of the Indian woman has become a truth by the deep and deadly science of Rappaccini and in the person of the lovely Beatrice."

Giovanni groaned and hid his face.

"Her father," continued Baglioni, "was not restrained by natural affection from offering up his child in this horrible manner as the victim of his insane zeal for science; for, let us do him justice, he is as true a man of science as ever distilled his own heart in an alembic. What, then, will be your fate? Beyond a doubt you are selected as the material of some new experiment. Perhaps the result is to be death; perhaps a fate more awful still. Rappaccini, with what he calls the interest of science before his eyes, will hesitate at nothing."

"It is a dream," muttered Giovanni to himself; "surely it is a dream."

"But," resumed the professor, "be of good cheer, son of my friend. It is not yet too late for the rescue. Possibly we may even succeed in bringing back this miserable child within the limits of ordinary nature, from which her father's madness has estranged her. Behold this little silver vase! It was wrought by the hands of the renowned Benvenuto Cellini, and is well worthy to be a love gift to the fairest dame in Italy. But its contents are invaluable. One little sip of this antidote would have rendered the most virulent poisons of the Borgias innocuous. Doubt not that it will be as efficacious against those of Rappaccini. Bestow the vase, and the precious liquid within it, on your Beatrice, and hopefully await the result."

Baglioni laid a small, exquisitely wrought silver vial on the table and withdrew, leaving what he had said to produce its effect upon the young man's mind.

"We will thwart Rappaccini yet," thought he, chuckling to himself, as he descended the stairs; "But, let us confess the truth of him, he is a wonderful man—a wonderful man indeed; a vile empiric, however, in his practice, and therefore not to be tolerated by those who respect the good old rules of the medical profession."

Throughout Giovanni's whole acquaintance with Beatrice, he had occasionally, as we have said, been haunted by dark surmises as to her character; yet so thoroughly had she made herself felt by him as a simple, natural, most affectionate, and guileless creature, that the image now held up by Professor Baglioni looked as strange and incredible as if it were not in accordance with his own original conception. True, there were ugly recollections connected with his first glimpses of the beautiful girl; he could not quite forget the bouquet that withered in her grasp, and the insect that perished amid the sunny air, by no ostensible agency save the fragrance of her breath. These incidents, however, dissolving in the pure light of her character, had no longer the efficacy of facts, but were acknowledged as mistaken fantasies, by whatever testimony of the senses they might appear to be substantiated. There is something truer and more real than what we can see with the eyes and touch with the finger. On such better evidence had Giovanni founded his confidence in Beatrice, though rather by the necessary force of her high attributes than by any deep and generous faith of his part. But now his spirit was incapable of sustaining itself at the height to which the early enthusiasm of passion had exalted it; he fell down, grovelling among earthly doubts, and defiled therewith the pure whiteness of Beatrice's image. Not that he gave her up; he did but distrust. He resolved to institute some decisive test that should satisfy him, once for all, whether there were those dreadful peculiarities in her physical nature which could not be supposed to exist without some corresponding monstrosity of soul. His eyes, gazing down afar, might have deceived him as to the lizard, the insect, and the flowers; but if he could witness, at the distance of a few paces, the sudden blight of one fresh and healthful flower in Beatrice's hand, there would be room for no further question. With this idea he hastened to the florist's and purchased a bouquet that was still gemmed with the morning dew-drops.

It was now the customary hour of his daily interview with Beatrice. Before descending into the garden, Giovanni failed not to look at his figure in the mirror—a vanity to be expected in a beautiful young man, yet, as displaying itself at that troubled and feverish moment, the token of a certain shallowness of feeling and insincerity of character. He did gaze, however, and said to himself that his features had never before possessed so rich a grace, nor his eyes such vivacity, nor his cheeks so warm a hue of superabundant life.

"At least," thought he, "her poison has not yet insinuated itself into my system. I am no flower to perish in her grasp."

With that thought he turned his eyes on the bouquet, which he had never once laid aside from his hand. A thrill of indefinable horror shot through his frame on perceiving that those dewy flowers were already beginning to droop; they wore the aspect of things that had been fresh and lovely yesterday. Giovanni grew white as marble, and stood motionless before the mirror, staring at his own reflection there as at the likeness of something frightful. He remembered Baglioni's remark about the fragrance that seemed to pervade the chamber. It must have been the poison in his breath! Then he shuddered—shuddered at himself. Recovering from his stupor, he began to watch with curious eye a spider that was busily at work hanging its web from the antique cornice of the apartment, crossing and recrossing the artful system of interwoven lines—as vigorous and active a spider as ever dangled from an old ceiling. Giovanni bent towards the insect, and emitted a deep, long breath. The spider suddenly ceased its toil; the web vibrated with a tremor originating in the body of the small artisan. Again Giovanni sent forth a breath, deeper, longer, and imbued with a venomous feeling out of his heart: he knew not whether he were wicked, or only desperate. The spider made a convulsive gripe with his limbs and hung dead across the window.

"Accursed! accursed!" muttered Giovanni, addressing himself. "Hast thou grown so poisonous that this deadly insect perishes by thy breath?"

At that moment a rich, sweet voice came floating up from the garden.

"Giovanni! Giovanni! It is past the hour! Why tarriest thou? Come down!"

"Yes," muttered Giovanni again. "She is the only being whom my breath may not slay! Would that it might!"

He rushed down, and in an instant was standing before the bright and loving eyes of Beatrice. A moment ago his wrath and despair had been so fierce that he could have desired nothing so much as to wither her by a glance; but with her actual presence there came influences which had too real an existence to be at once shaken off: recollections of the delicate and benign power of her feminine nature, which had so often enveloped him in a religious calm; recollections of many a holy and passionate out-gush of her heart, when the pure fountain had been unsealed from its depths and made visible in its transparency to his mental eye; recollections which, had Giovanni known how to estimate them, would have assured him that all this ugly mystery was but an earthly illusion, and that, whatever mist of evil might seem to have gathered over her, the real Beatrice was a heavenly angel. Incapable as he was of such high faith, still her presence had not utterly lost its magic. Giovanni's rage was quelled into an aspect of sullen insensibility. Beatrice, with a quick spiritual sense, immediately felt that there was a gulf of blackness between them which neither he nor she could pass. They walked on together, sad and silent, and came thus to the marble fountain and to its pool of water on the ground, in the midst of which grew the shrub that bore gem-like blossoms. Giovanni was affrighted at the eager enjoyment—the appetite, as it were—with which he found himself inhaling the fragrance of the flowers.

"Beatrice," asked he, abruptly, "whence came this shrub?"

"My father created it," answered she, with simplicity.

"Created it! created it!" repeated Giovanni. "What mean you, Beatrice?"

"He is a man fearfully acquainted with the secrets of Nature," replied Beatrice; "and, at the hour when I first drew breath, this plant sprang from the soil, the offspring of his science, of his intellect, while I was but his earthly child. Approach it not!" continued she, observing with terror that Giovanni was drawing nearer to the shrub. "It has qualities that you little dream of. But I, dearest Giovanni—I grew up and blossomed with the plant and was nourished with her breath. It was my sister, and I loved it with a human affection; for, alas!—hast thou not suspected it?—there was an awful doom."

Here Giovanni frowned so darkly upon her that Beatrice paused and trembled. But her faith in his tenderness reassured her, and made her blush that she had doubted for an instant.

"There was an awful doom," she continued, "the effect of my father's fatal love of science, which estranged me from all society of my kind. Until Heaven sent thee, dearest Giovanni, oh, how lonely was thy poor Beatrice!"

"Was it a hard doom?" asked Giovanni, fixing his eyes upon her.

"Only of late have I known how hard it was," answered she, tenderly. "Oh, yes; but my heart was torpid, and therefore quiet."

Giovanni's rage broke forth from his sullen gloom like a lightning flash out of a dark cloud.

"Accursed one!" cried he, with venomous scorn and anger. "And, finding thy solitude wearisome, thou has severed me likewise from all the warmth of life and enticed me into thy region of unspeakable horror!"

"Giovanni!" exclaimed Beatrice, turning her large bright eyes upon his face. The force of his words had not found its way into her mind; she was merely thunderstruck.

"Yes, poisonous thing!" repeated Giovanni, beside himself with passion. "Thou hast done it! Thou hast blasted me! Thou hast filled my veins with poison! Thou has made me as hateful, as ugly, as loathsome and deadly a creature as thyself—a world's wonder of hideous monstrosity! Now, if our breath be happily as fatal to ourselves as to all others, let us join our lips in one kiss of unutterable hatred, and so die!"

"What has befallen me?" murmured Beatrice, with a low moan out of her heart. "Holy Virgin, pity me, a poor heart-broken child!"

"Thou—dost thou pray?" cried Giovanni, still with the same fiendish scorn. "Thy very prayers, as they come from thy lips, taint the atmosphere with death. Yes, yes; let us pray! Let us to church and dip our fingers in the holy water at the portal! They that come after us will perish as by a pestilence! Let us sign crosses in the air! It will be scattering curses abroad in the likeness of holy symbols!"

"Giovanni," said Beatrice, calmly, for her grief was beyond passion, "why dost thou join thyself with me thus in those terrible words? I, it is true, am the horrible thing thou namest me. But thou—what hast thou to do, save with one other shudder at my hideous misery to go forth out of the garden and mingle with thy race, and forget there ever crawled on earth such a monster as poor Beatrice?"

"Dost thou pretend ignorance?" asked Giovanni, scowling upon her. "Behold! this power have I gained from the pure daughter of Rappaccini."

There was a swarm of summer insects flitting through the air in search of the food promised by the flower odors of the fatal garden. They circled round Giovanni's head, and were evidently attracted towards him by the same influence which had drawn them for an instant within the sphere of several of the shrubs. He sent forth a breath among them, and smiled bitterly at Beatrice as at least a score of the insects fell dead upon the ground.

"I see it! I see it!" shrieked Beatrice. "It is my father's fatal science! No, no, Giovanni; it was not I! Never! never! I dreamed only to love thee and be with thee a little time, and so to let thee pass away, leaving but thine image in mine heart; for, Giovanni, believe it, though my body be nourished with poison, my spirit is God's creature, and craves love as its daily food. But my father—he has united us in this fearful sympathy. Yes; spurn me, tread upon, kill me! Oh, what is death after such words as thine? But it was not I. Not for a world of bliss would I have done it."

Giovanni's passion had exhausted itself in its outburst from his lips. There now came across him a sense, mournful, and not without tenderness, of the intimate and peculiar relationship between Beatrice and himself. They stood, as it were, in an utter solitude, which would be made none the less solitary by the densest throng of human life. Ought not, then, the desert of humanity around them to press this insulated pair closer together? If they should be cruel to one another, who was there to be kind to them? Besides, thought Giovanni, might there not still be a hope of his returning within the limits of ordinary nature, and leading Beatrice, the redeemed Beatrice, by the hand? O weak, and selfish, and unworthy spirit, that could dream of an earthly union and earthly happiness possible, after such deep love had been so bitterly wronged as was Beatrice's love by Giovanni's blighting words! No, no; there could be no such hope. She must pass heavily, with that broken heart, across the borders of Time—she must bathe her hurts in some fount of paradise, and forget her grief in the light of immortality, and *there* be well.

But Giovanni did not know it.

"Dear Beatrice," said he, approaching her, while she shrank away as always at his approach, but now with a different impulse, "dearest Beatrice our fate is not yet so desperate. Behold! there is a medicine, potent, as a wise physician has assured me, and almost divine in its efficacy. It is composed of ingredients the most opposite to those by which thy awful father has brought this calamity upon thee and me. It is distilled of blessed herbs. Shall we not quaff it together, and thus be purified from evil?"

"Give it me!" said Beatrice, extending her hand to receive the little silver vial which Giovanni took from his bosom. She added, with a peculiar emphasis, "I will drink; but do thou await the result."

She put Baglioni's antidote to her lips; and, at the same moment, the figure of Rappaccini emerged from the portal and came slowly towards the marble fountain. As he drew near, the pale man of science seemed to gaze with a triumphant expression at the beautiful youth and maiden, as might an artist who should spend his life in achieving a picture or a group of statuary and finally be satisfied with his success. He paused; his bent form grew erect with conscious power; he spread out his hands over them in the attitude of a father imploring a blessing upon his children; but those were the same hands that had thrown poison into the stream of their lives. Giovanni trembled. Beatrice shuddered nervously, and pressed her hand upon her heart.

"My daughter," said Rappaccini, "thou art no longer lonely in the world. Pluck one of those precious gems from thy sister shrub and bid thy bridegroom wear it in his bosom. It will not harm him now. My science and the sympathy between thee and him have so wrought within his system that he now stands apart from common men, as thou dost, daughter of my pride and triumph, from ordinary women. Pass on, then, through the world, most dear to one another and dreadful to all besides!"

"My father," said Beatrice, feebly—and still as she spoke she kept her hand upon her heart—"wherefore didst thou inflict this miserable doom upon thy child?"

"Miserable!" exclaimed Rappaccini. "What mean you, foolish girl? Dost thou deem it misery to be endowed with marvellous gifts against which no power nor strength could avail an enemy—misery, to be able to quell the mightiest with a breath—misery, to be as terrible as thou art beautiful? Wouldst thou, then, have preferred the condition of a weak woman, exposed to all evil and capable of none?"

"I would fain have been loved, not feared," murmured Beatrice, sinking down upon the ground. "But now it matters not. I am going, father, where the evil which thou hast striven to mingle with my being will pass away like a dream—like the fragrance of these poisonous flowers, which will no longer taint my breath among the flowers of Eden. Farewell, Giovanni! Thy words of hatred are like lead within my heart; but they, too, will fall away as I ascend. Oh, was there not, from the first, more poison in thy nature than in mine?"

To Beatrice—so radically had her earthly part been wrought upon by Rappaccini's skill—as poison had been life, so the powerful antidote was death; and thus the poor victim of man's ingenuity and of thwarted nature, and of the fatality that attends all such efforts of perverted wisdom, perished there, at the feet of her father and Giovanni. Just at that moment Professor Pietro Baglioni looked forth from the window, and called loudly, in a tone of triumph mixed with horror, to the thunderstricken man of science—

"Rappaccini! Rappaccini! and is *this* the upshot of your experiment!"

BLACK MOUNTAIN, 1977

DONALD ANTRIM

When my grandfather was in his seventies and I in my twenties, we created one of those friendships that are sometimes available between non-consecutive generations in broken or unhappy families. This friendship was brokered, however inadvertently, and as so many are, by a third party who functioned largely as an object of worry and distress—common cause and a bond between the new friends. The third party was my mother, my grandfather's daughter, a woman whose lifelong pursuit of death was, arguably, a response to severe mishandling by her own mother, my grandfather's wife, a women who in her later age became a nutritionist and appeared merely stern, but who during her early years of motherhood carried out an aggressive campaign against her daughter's body, even going so far as to advocate unnecessary surgeries for her only child. It is, of course, pointless to imagine the implications of a revision in past events or behaviors—to guess at how things might have been. Nevertheless, I hatch these kinds of daydreams constantly. Had my grandfather been less cowed by his wife, less meek and alcoholic—had he been able, in other words, to intercede and protect my future mother—then it is at least likely that she (his young girl) might not have grown up to become the lonely, distrustful, ragingly self-obliterative woman she became; it is unclear, in other words, whether my grandfather and I, during those years right before he began having his heart attacks, the years of his great anxiety over his daughter's well-being, the years when everyone was still alive—it is unclear whether my grandfather and I would have been given the platform on which to build, out of guilt, sorrow, need and respect, our real love for each other.

I was a teen-ager when my grandfather retired from his job as a junior-high-school principal in Sarasota, Florida. He and my grandmother sold their large Spanish-style house on Wisteria Street and moved into a tiny, unattractive condominium, which they hated. After that, they became regular visitors to the Great Smokey Mountains, around Ashville, North Carolina—just east of the part of the world they had both

"Black Mountain, 1977" originally appeared in *The New Yorker* (25 Dec. 2000–1 Jan. 2001): 89–93.

originally come from—and in 1977, the summer I graduated from boarding school, they retired from their retirement and bought a truly derelict bungalow in Black Mountain, intending to restore it and, eventually, move in. Would I like to join them, to spend my summer before college working on the old house? My mother's alcoholism was by then reaching its advanced stages—in a few years she would be forced to attempt sobriety or die—and my parents' fighting, not only with each other but with me, had escalated to nearly heroic levels. Yes, I would be happy to come to North Carolina and work on the house.

And yet, once in Black Mountain, I had a tendency to abandon my grandparents to their painstaking and methodical, stooped over, Presbyterian labors; every day I fled the house and drove aimlessly over mountain roads that passed by indigent farms and strange, unpainted churches. I had no concept of work. What was wrong with me? When would my life begin? Looking back on that time, I have an impression of myself performing a kind of fitful, mild-mannered revolt against—what? Anhedonia? Boredom? My family? Or perhaps it was a revolt against Southern Protestantism in general, which I associated with prohibitions and taboos in a variety of forms, perversely expressed in the self-destructive or work-obsessed temperaments of, it seemed to me then, everyone I knew. But protests against the denial of pleasure bring no pleasure. In the spirit of someone with nowhere else to go, I turned the car around and returned to the house in Black Mountain, picked up steel wool or a rag, and found something to scrub.

The day came when we got around to windows. These were painted shut and badly warped. There was, for my grandfather, no question of replacing them; they would be removed, their panes razored clean, and the frames stripped with fine-grade sandpaper, or, if too profoundly rotten, disassembled and rebuilt. This was heartbreakingly deliberate work. The casements were filled with dust, dirt, and dead animals' tiny skeletons. Here, as well, were the windows' rusted pulley wheels and ancient counterweights, canvas sacks stuffed with lead shot and tied off, their ropes broken. I remember my grandfather's old-man hands worrying the wood, delicately touching, like a blind man reading, the surfaces of things; it was slow work that he seemed determined to make slower, as if work of any sort were equivalent to an act of obstinacy. My grandmother's style, by contrast, was all harshness and haste—she attacked her chores. And I remained lazy and sarcastic; the screen door was always slamming behind me. Nonetheless, I was attracted by my grandfather's tremendous patience for what people in romantic moments like to call honest labor. It wasn't that I suddenly understood the value of a job well done. Far from it. It was that for a moment—a romantic moment of my own, destined to resonate and grow in magnitude over the years –I hoped (and this may have been a fantasy that I wanted to have about the man) that my grandfather had something to pass on to me, to teach me. And I imagined (because it did not occur to me to ask him) that what he had to teach me concerned the beauty in labor that remains, at the end of the job, hidden, and that no one except the worker will see or understand or even necessarily appreciate. The windows, when they went back in, slid up or down at a touch.

Years later, when my grandfather was nearing ninety, well after he and I had been brought together by my mother's many hospitalizations, we took drives together along the roads that led over the mountains. Ours were rambling, all-day excursions, little revolts that infuriated my grandmother, who feared for his health. We'd stop on the shoulder in hollows or valleys, where my grandfather took leaks beside the car—frequent urination caused by his heart medication. Always, he drove. Bourbon was stashed in the tire well in the trunk—his guilty, exciting secret. At some point along the way, generally when we were far from home, out beyond Hendersonville, he'd ask the question we lived with every day in our family: Will your mother be all right? Will she be all right? Since by this time he had long supported not only his daughter but intermittently over the years, her son, his only grandson, the cash poor so-called writer living up North, I felt that the question might in some ways be a question not about her, or at least not about her alone, but about me. And what could I possibly tell him? That because of a way he'd once gazed at a window frame, then gradually, stubbornly, lovingly sanded smooth its torn, abused edges, I'd be all right?

LET US HAVE MEDICOS OF OUR OWN MATURITY

ANONYMOUS PATIENT

Let us have medicos of our own maturity,
for callow practitioners incline to be casual
  with a middle-aged party.

Doctors in their thirties are loath to labour
  over sick men in their sixties.
Such are near their natural end: respect nature.

To save us suffering, or them their pains,
  physicians in their fifties
Are prepared to surrender us senior citizens.

Let our medical attendants be of compatible years,
Who will think of us as in certain ways their peers,

Who know what we possibly still have to live for,
Why we are not unfailingly poised to withdraw.

Yet for the giving of enemas or injections,
  let there be youthful nurses
With steady hands, clear heads, and other attractions.

Whether physicians or patients, we all can appreciate
A pretty miss, or (it may be) her male associate.

Then permit us to be appreciative and appreciated
A little, in our final fruition, however belated.

This poem was written by an anonymous patient around 1985. It appears here from *The Faber Book of Fevers and Frets,* edited by D. J. Enright (London: Faber, 1989).

HELLO, HELLO HENRY

MAXINE KUMIN

My neighbor in the country, Henry Manley,
with a washpot warming on his woodstove,
with a heifer and two goats and yearly chickens,
has outlasted Stalin, Roosevelt and Churchill
but something's stirring in him in his dotage.

Last fall he dug a hole and moved his privy
and a year ago in April reamed his well out.
When the county sent a truck and poles and cable,
his daddy ran the linemen off with birdshot
and swore he'd die by oil lamp, and did.

Now you tell me that all yesterday in Boston
you set your city phone at mine, and had it ringing
inside a dead apartment for three hours
room after empty room, to keep yours busy.
I hear it in my head, that ranting summons.

That must have been about the time that Henry
walked up two miles, shy as a girl come calling,
to tell me he has a phone now, 264, ring two.
It rang one time last week—wrong number.
He'd be pleased if one day I would think to call him.

Hello, hello Henry? Is that you?

THE LAST WORDS OF HENRY MANLEY

MAXINE KUMIN

At first I thought I heard wrong. Was she sayen
Oil History Project, maybe somethen
about the year I put in ditchen, layen
roadbed up Stark Mountain in the CCC?
Liven alone, I'm shy of company
but then this girl comes prettied up in blue jeans
and has me talk into a tape machine
about my raisen. Seems it's history.

I was the raisen boy of Old Man Wasson.
Back then, the county farmed out all its orphans
to any who would have them for their keep.
My ma and pa both died in World War One.
It was the influenza took them, took down
half the town. I cried myself to sleep
one whole year, I missed my ma so terrible.
I weren't but six and scrawny. Weren't able
to do much more than clean the chicken coop

and toss hay to the goats. I weren't much good
but Old Man Wasson never used me wrong.
Because he lived alone, there were some said
he weren't right upstairs, and then they'd nod.

He fed me up on eggs and goat's milk, taught
me thirty different birds to know by song
and every plant that came. First one's coltsfoot.
Lamb's quarters is good to eat. So's cattail shoots.
Cobwebs is for cuts. Jewelweed's for the sting
of nettles. Asters bloom last. Most everythen

we ate we grew. And bartered for the rest
hayen in summer, all fall choppen wood.
Whilst I was small I stacked as best I could:
hickory, oak, maple, ash. (White birch
is only fit for tourists from the city.)
I saved my dimes for the country fair. Went dressed
up clean in Sunday clothes as if for church,
a place we never went nor never prayed.
We was a scandal to the Ladies Aid.

If there's one thing I still can't stand it's pity.
We had a handpump in the yard, a privy
a cookstove in the kitchen, a potbelly
in the front room, lamps enough to read by.
Kerosene burns yellow. I miss it still.
Not steady like a bulb, it's flickery
like somethen alive: a bird, a swallowtail.
You won't think that about 'lectricity.
And we had flowers too, old-timey ones

you hardly see these days, like hollyhocks
and red tobacco plants the hummenbirds
come to. Old Man Wasson had me listen
how those ruby throats would speak—chrk chrk—
to every bloom before they'd poke their beaks
inside. There's lots to say that don't need words.
I guess I was *his* father at the end.
He wouldn't have a doctor on the place.
I got in bed and held him tell he went.

Winter of '44, private first class
in uniform like in the CCC
homesick and seasick I shipped across.
What made me famous was goen to the camps
where they'd outright starved most the men to death
and gassed the rest. Those piles of shoes and teeth?

They still come up. I dream them up in clumps.
Back home, the papers got aholt of me.
Local boy a hero in Germany.

Right here the tape clicks off. She says she's *thrilled.*
I want to say I've hardly started in
but she's packed up and standen on the doorsill
and I'm the boy whose time ran out for courten.

WHAT REMAINS

EMMA DONOGHUE

She hasn't asked for me in two months. I check with her nurses, though it's a little humiliating. "Has Miss Loring by any chance asked for me?" I say. Lightly, as if it doesn't matter either way.

That's what they call her: Miss Loring, or sometimes Frances. She's not Queenie to anyone but me.

I wheeled myself in to her room today. She was lying there like a whale ready for the axe. "Queenie," I said, "it's me. It's Florence." Which sounded absurd, as I've never had to tell her who I am before, she always knew. What a pass we've come to, if I need to introduce myself! Like that line in the Bible. *The people who walk in darkness.* Brains rot like fruit in the end. I don't pity her for going senile. It's worse being a witness.

I try to keep a grip on the numbers myself. The nurses start to worry if you get the numbers wrong. It's 1967 and I'm eighty-five years old. I should by rights be dead. Queenie's not even eighty. I ought to have gone first. It shouldn't be like this.

I always thought it would be all right so long as we ended up in the same place. She collapsed just before our final exhibition, and I fell sick a week later, and when we were both moved to this Home just north of Toronto, I thought, Well, at least we'll be together. No need to fuss with cooking or shovel our own snow anymore; we'll get to talk all day if we want.

But there's more than one kind of distance that can come between people. This is our third year here. Her door says Miss F. Loring, mine says Miss F. Wyle, and they might as well be a thousand miles apart, instead of a fifty-foot corridor. Since Queenie's last attack, her eyes barely move when I wheel into her room, and she doesn't seem to recognize my name.

What's important, I suppose, is for me to keep remembering. What matters is to hold on to what's left.

Each one must go alone down the dark valley.

I wrote that poem a long time ago, before I knew what I was talking about. My father used to say Man was the only creature capable of sleeping on his back, so that was how we should sleep. To mark the difference, you see; to show that we were a Higher Form. I did try; I started every night flat on my back but it hurt my bones and I couldn't breathe. My father would come to wake me in the morning and find me curled up on my side and shake me awake. "Florence," he'd roar, "you look like an animal!"

When I was six I found a rooster with a broken leg. I fixed him just fine, mostly because my father said I'd never manage it. It was animals that turned me towards art. I saw a bird, and then a picture of a bird, and it all came together. If I couldn't be a bird then at least I could make one. Once a cat of ours died, and I asked if God had taken her to heaven, and my father said there was no room for animals in heaven. That's the day I stopped believing in God. Rosa Bonheur the French sculptor believed in metempsychosis, which means that human souls migrate into animal forms. She lived with her friend and a whole ark of animals and painted them. I suppose it seemed to her that we're all just creatures in the end.

Mind you, I'd shoot a dog if it got as crazy as Queenie.

* * * * *

Sixty years this month since we met in that Clay Modelling class in Chicago. She was big and I was small. She was beautiful and I was not. Her family adored her and mine didn't care for me. She grew up in Geneva, Switzerland; I came from Waverly, Illinois. She thought she liked men and I thought I hated them. She had faith in politics and I wrote poems about trees. She worked in spurts; I did a little every day. All we had in common was a taste for clay.

Today her hands lie on the sheet like withered bananas. I remember a time when they were swift and sure and tireless. Like the Skeena River in full flood, that time I went to the Indian village to model the old totem poles. When was that? Back in the twenties sometime? Damn it. Gone.

That's us these days, a couple of old totem poles. Tilting at mad angles, silvery as ash, fading into the forest.

At the Art Institute in Chicago, the Master used to pinch all us girls on the bottom. He called it the *droit de maître.* Queenie didn't much mind. I slapped his hand away and called him a damn fool. Later he spread a rumour we were a couple of Sapphists.

There was another thing Queenie used to say: You can't go through life worrying about what people think of you.

* * * * *

Some days she's got more of a grip than others. She still doesn't ask for me, but when I go in to her room she sometimes seems to know who I am.

I tell her uplifting stories.

"Remember Adelaide Johnson, Queenie?"

A flicker of the eyes.

"She was barely twenty when she fell down that elevator shaft in the Chicago Music Hall. Did it stop her?"

"Hell, no," says Queenie feebly.

I laugh out loud. "That's right. She won $15,000 in damages and went off to study art in Europe!"

But Queenie's face is blank, like a block of marble that's never been touched by the chisel.

I will not feed my soul with sorrow, that was her favourite line in all my poems.

Some dates are so clear in my head it's as if they're chiselled there. We came to Toronto in 1913. Canada was a young country; there seemed infinite room. But we only really got established after the Great War. The towns needed so many memorials, they had to stoop to hiring women! Queenie used to say that her career was built on dead boys.

Sculptors, we called ourselves from the start. The word sculptress sets my teeth on edge. Work like ours called for sensible clothes. We took to trousers, as early as the twenties, plus men's shoes and baggy jackets.

I'm not allowed to wear my old grey flannels here. I suspect they've been thrown in the trash. Well, they were a little decrepit, I admit. Instead the nurses give me housecoats to put on, pink or orange: hideous. "Blue was my colour, Queenie, do you remember?" I usually wore a touch of pale blue.

Queenie was always the more bohemian dresser. At our studio parties she'd appear in purple velvet with a gold fringe, or a green satin cape. I told her once she looked like something out of the comic strips—the Caped Crusader, or the Emerald Evil—and she wasn't too pleased. There was always a trail of ash across her front because she was too busy talking to remember the ashtray.

They keep her clean and tidy here; that's another reason she doesn't look like herself. And you can't get hold of a cigarette for love nor money.

I am lost in this forest of days. I can't remember when I wrote that. I go through a sort of checklist of names in my head, in case I'm forgetting anything. Our dogs were Samson and Delilah. (Delilah tore our neighbour's fur coat, but it served her right for wearing such a thing.) We had two motor cars, first Susie, then Osgoode. (Queenie always drove, and never got any better at it; I read the maps.) Some of our sculptures were—are, I mean—*Dream within a Dream, Women War Workers, Torso, Girl with Fish, The Goal Keeper, Negro Women, The Rites of Spring, Derelicts, Eskimo Mother and Child, The Miner, Sea and Shore, The Key.* There were others, I know there were others, but I can't recall their names just now. Some are sold, some are scattered, the rest are under dust-sheets in our cold locked-up studio in Toronto that was a derelict church until we moved in. I don't have any of them here, but I can see them more clearly than my own mother's face.

The thing about sculpture is, it's always a risk. It costs money to model it, cast it, carve it, even transport it. Clay's bad enough; bronze is terrible; marble's ruinous.

All this week Queenie's been yapping away in her head to old friends, dead or alive or who knows. Sometimes if I listen closely I can pick up hints of who it is. Yesterday I could tell it was A. Y. Jackson because she was thanking him for taking us out to dinner the day he sold his first picture. He and she seemed to be having a grand old time.

She always did like parties better than I did. We had forty-eight artists for Christmas, one year, as well as three beggars from the neighbourhood. Six turkeys got eaten down to the bone. In the evening there was chamber music, and I drank too much wine and was persuaded to show them all how to do an Illinois hog call.

"Remember Liz Prophet, Queenie?"

"Mm," she says, ambiguously.

"That awful gallery in Rhode Island, they said they had nothing against showing a black girl's sculptures so long as she promised not to come to the opening. Barbarians! Do you remember what she did, Queenie?"

Silence.

I fill in with barely a pause. "Ran away to gay Paree."

"That's right," whispers Queenie.

"That's right," I repeat. "Lived on tea and marmalade."

"Stole food from dogs."

This detail cheers me up immensely. Her memory's still in there, like the shape locked inside the marble. "That's right, my dear, Liz Prophet had to steal food from Parisian dogs. What was it you used to say to me in our bad winters? No one's got a right to call herself an artist until she's starved a little!" Her eyes have gone unfocused, milky blue.

* * * * *

She still keeps that photograph on her bedside table, the one of Charlie Mulligan, who taught her marble cutting back in the 1900s.

"Isn't he a fine fellow?" she's taken to asking the nurses, sometimes four times a day. I bet she doesn't remember his name either.

"Was he your young man, Miss Loring?" one of them said this morning, to humour her.

"That's right."

"Was he the love of your life?"

"That's right, that's right," Queen repeats in a whisper, like a child. "The love of my life."

She doesn't mean Charlie Mulligan, by the way. That wild German she nearly married back in 1914, he's the one she used to call the love of her life. Not that I know what that means. Which life is she talking about when she says stupid things like that? As far as I know, the life she had was the one she spent with me.

I will not feed my soul with sorrow,
Not while dark trees march in naked majesty
Across the sunset sky.

When I wrote that, ten years ago, we still had the farm: 150 acres of wild quince and poison ivy by the Rouge River. These days I have a room with a small window facing onto the parking lot. I haven't seen a tree in a while.

* * * * *

Queenie doesn't know anyone today. She's got butter on her double chin. A journalist once asked her, "Miss Loring, do you specialize in memorial sculpture because of a special sympathy for the dear departed?"

I had to cut in; I couldn't resist. "No," I said, "it's because she likes climbing ladders."

It was true. She's always liked to work on a grand scale. She's built on a grand scale too.

The local children used to call us the Clay Ladies. That was because we showed them how to make things out of clay, of course, but the phrase fitted us too, more and more as the decades went by. These days we look like works in progress, there's no point pretending otherwise. Queenie's a vast model for a monument—all two hundred pounds of her clay slapped onto a gigantic wire armature—and as for me, I'm some skinny leftover. Maybe I'm a Giacometti and she's a Henry Moore! Not that I'm a fan of the so-called moderns; most of them couldn't draw a human body if they tried, and as for beauty, I doubt they could even spell it. Boring holes in things!—that's not sculpture, that's vandalism.

To think she and I used to be something. A unit; a name. The Loring-Wyles.

I'm not saying it was all fun and games. We had a couple of bad years. We sometimes considered suicide, only half-joking. But we didn't think we should depart alone; we wanted to take at least a dozen enemies with us. On dark February evenings in the studio we amused ourselves by drawing up a list.

But if there's no heaven, what remains?

* * * * *

All this week Queenie's been having delusions. She sits up in bed, the sheets draped around her like snow on the Niagara Escarpment. She shakes her fists over her head and pants with effort. The nurses say if she doesn't calm down she's going to bring on another attack.

Finally today I figured out what she's doing. She thinks she's carving her lion, all over again.

"Why a lion?" I asked her, nearly thirty years ago.

She laughed. "Isn't it obvious, Florence? A snarling, defiant lion; rising from a crouch, ready for a fight."

Well, this was 1940.

It was to be a huge, stylized sort of lion, guarding the entrance to the new Queen Elizabeth Way near Toronto, to commemorate the visit of the King and Queen. I wouldn't have thought it was possible to do anything new with a lion, but Queenie's design was a wonder: the beast's face and ruff and whole muscled body were made up of great smooth arcs of stone.

It was just about the most gruelling project Queenie ever dragged us into, and that's saying something. I say we, but I was only doing a bas-relief of Their Majesties on the back of the column. Queenie's lion had to be carved on site, emerging from the column, as it were. She planned to use Indiana limestone—lovely flawless stuff—but no, word came down that for patriotic reasons it had to be Queenston limestone, which was twice as hard and pocked with holes. That was bad enough, but hiring a stone cutter was the worst. The top three men on our list were struck off by government order as "enemy aliens," even though the German had been reared in Canada and the Italians were the best in the trade. Instead, Queenie had to put up with a true-blue Englishman whose work she'd never trusted.

He couldn't take orders from a woman, that was his problem, and he wasn't the only one, let me tell you. We had to scour the country to find a cutting machine for the fellow, and he still didn't get started till August of that year. When we drove down in November to check his progress, the rough outlines of the lion had only half-emerged from the column. "That fellow hasn't even started on the hind quarters," muttered Queenie.

I thought the neck looked a little odd. Queenie asked him about it. "Oh, yes, actually, Miss Loring," said the fellow, evading her eyes, "I changed the line a little, to make it lie better."

The cheek of the man! I didn't blame her for firing him on the spot, even with all the horrors that followed.

Queenie couldn't find another qualified cutter in Canada. She consulted the union, who told her that only their members were permitted to cut stone for sculpture. She told the union to go to hell, she'd finish it herself.

Neither of us had ever used a cutting machine. The December winds howled in off the lake. I remember craning up at Queenie on the scaffold, which we'd swathed in tarpaulins as a feeble shelter. She was fifty-two that year and already a huge woman. Her hands were swollen with arthritis.

"Queenie!"

"Don't you fret, Florence," she shouted down.

"It's not worth it," I bawled. "Give it up!"

She pretended not to hear. I could tell, from the way she handled the machine, that she was in pain. The planks of the scaffold buckled under her weight. Specks of snow fell on her head.

I cursed her, but the wind ate up my words. "What if you fall?" I screeched.

She peered over the tarpaulin, her face drawn but hilarious. "I'll probably bounce!"

She didn't fall. Next day she abandoned the machine and picked up her biggest chisel and hammer. If I'd been a praying sort of woman, I'd have prayed then. As it was, I stood and shivered and watched, week after week. I remember wondering what would happen to us all if Hitler won the war.

The snow held off just long enough. The lion crawled from his block, metamorphosing like something out of Ovid. By the time Queenie dropped her tools, her hands were like claws, but the lion was magnificent.

On his pedestal, in deep-cut letters, it said something about "the Empire's darkest hour" and this work having been done "in full confidence of victory and a lasting peace." I remember it because it was on the day of the Highway's official opening, as we stood below the lion with the lake wind lashing our scarves against our numb faces, that it occurred to me that I was a Canadian. Not that I'd ever got around to filling in the forms; on paper I was—as I am still—a U.S. citizen. But sometimes things about you change without you noticing.

* * * * *

So that's how the story ended. Only, for Queenie, I see now, it's not over. It's 1967 but she can't be convinced her war work is done. She still straddles the scaffolding, high above Lake Ontario. Her hands grip huge imaginary tools.

"Just another quarter-inch," she mumbles hoarsely.

"Lie down, now," I tell her. "Nurse says it's time for your sponge bath."

"In a minute," she says, austere. Her arm moves as if to hammer the air, and she speaks to me as if I'm a stranger. "I don't think you appreciate the urgency of my work."

"Of course I do," I murmur.

Then her head turns, and her blue eyes bore into mine, and her voice rises.

"It may have escaped your attention," she roars, "But there's a war going on!"

"But Queenie," I say for the hundredth time, "your lion's finished." She gives me a weary look, as if she sees through all my wiles.

"Everyone loves him! They say he's the finest monumental sculpture in Canada." Well, that's not quite a lie; some people did say that, once.

She shakes her head. "I still need to do his ears. And his back paws and his tail."

"No, he's all done. I'll prove it," I say rashly. And then it occurs to me that I can.

* * * * *

I've struck a deal with the Home's handyman. But the Head Nurse says she'll have to speak to the authorities. "On the Queen Elizabeth Way, Miss Wyle?" she repeats, unconvinced.

"Just at the entrance."

"A lion?"

"You must have seen it," I tell her. "You couldn't miss it if you've ever driven down to Niagara."

And then it occurs to me that she thinks I'm the one who's gone gaga. Delusions of lions. "It's a stone lion," I clarify coldly. "You may not know that Miss Loring and I are sculptors. Our work is to be found in many cities and galleries across Canada."

"Yes," she says, as if placating me.

"Besides," I snap, "as far as I am aware we are voluntary residents here. If we choose to be taken on a drive by a kind young man on his afternoon off, I can't see that you have any right to object."

She butts in. "Miss Loring isn't strong—"

"My friend is well enough to sit in a motor car. It's her mind that's troubled. And what I propose to do will set her mind at rest."

I sound more sure than I am.

* * * * *

The air smells clean. The May sunshine dazzles me. I cover my eyes. A Bug, the young handyman calls it. Looks like a Henry Moore car to me; all bulges and holes. He lifts me out of my wheelchair and puts me in first, then I help to tug Queenie in through the other door. Occasionally she laughs. It takes us a quarter of an hour. I can tell the boy's surprised at my strength. My legs may be kaput but my skinny arms are still a sculptor's.

"Are you comfortable, Miss Loring?"

No answer from Queenie, who's examining one of her knees as if she's never seen it before. The boy gives me a doubtful glance.

"Yes, yes, she's fine, let's be off," I tell him. So he wheels our chairs back into the Home, then starts up the engine.

Toronto is a blur of sunlight and glass highrises. I glance idly into shop windows—bikinis, Muskoka chairs, sunflowers—not letting myself wonder if this is the last time I'll ever see the city.

We're at the Queen Elizabeth Way in less than an hour. The lake glitters like tinsel. Our driver looks over his shoulder, "Where do you want me to stop, Miss Wyle?"

"Just by the entrance."

"Oh. Only, I don't think it's legal. I mean, everyone else is going pretty fast."

"Let them," I say, autocratic. "Park on the verge."

"Couldn't I just slow down a bit as we go past this statue of yours?"

"No you could not. Pull over."

He wheels onto the shoulder and we come to a shuddering stop. "It's dangerous," he remarks. "What if the cops come by?"

"Tell them you've got two octogenarians having heart attacks in the back of your car."

That shuts him up. He turns off the engine. I roll down my window jerkily, and lean out, squinting into the sun.

"Look, Queenie, your lion!"

She keeps on staring into her lap. The boy sits with his arms folded, as if embarrassed by us. I lean over her bulk and tug at the handle till the dirty glass slides down.

"Go on," I say eagerly. "Put your head out and have a look. He's finished. He's splendid."

Finally she seems to hear me. She leans her head to one side, lolling out the window. Dust blows in her face as a chain of cars rushes by. I hang out the window on my side and stare at the stone beast, as good as new if a little darker. Nearly thirty years, and not a mark on him. He could stand there forever. There, I want to tell Queenie, that's what remains of us.

I reach over to take her hand. But she has her head down again; she seems to be examining an egg stain on her lapel. A dreadful thought occurs to me. I let go of her hand and wave my fingers in front of her face. She doesn't flinch.

"Queenie?"

She looks in my direction. Her eyes are calm and milky. She can't see a thing.

I should have guessed. I should have remembered her eyes were getting worse; I would have, if I'd half a brain left myself.

"What do you think of your lion now?" I ask her softly, just to be sure.

She says nothing for a minute, and then, "Lion?"

I don't answer her. After a minute I lean over to roll up her window. Then I tell the boy he can take us back to the Home now.

* * * * *

An enormous tiredness settles on me. I lay my head on the seat back at a peculiar angle. I shut my eyes to escape from the sunlight. *Each one must go alone down the dark valley.* I keep hold of Queenie's hand, but only because I can't think of anything else to do.

"Blue," she murmurs, half an hour later at a traffic light, and I don't know what she means: the lake? The sky? Or just what she remembers of the colour that used to go by that name?

"That's right," I say, "blue."

Florence Wyle (1881–1968) and Frances Loring ("Queenie," 1887–1968), the "Loring-Wyles," remain two of the most important sculptors in the history of Canadian art. Born in Illinois and Idaho respectively, they met at the Chicago Art Institute in 1907, and spent almost sixty years working and living together, mostly in Toronto. After spending several years in a nursing home in Newmarket, Ontario, where they both gradually became senile, they died within three weeks of each other.

For this story I have used information from Rebecca Sisler's biography The Girls *(1972), and have also drawn on some of Florence Wyles's published poems. But this fictional account of their declining years, and a trip to see the lion, is my own invention. Frances Loring's lion has been moved to parkland near its original site at the entrance to the Queen Elizabeth Way between Toronto and Niagara.*

A SUMMER TRAGEDY

ARNA BONTEMPS

Old Jeff Patton, the black share farmer, fumbled with his bow tie. His fingers trembled and the high stiff collar pinched his throat. A fellow loses his hand for such vanities after thirty or forty years of simple life. Once a year, or maybe twice if there's a wedding among his kinfolks, he may spruce up; but generally fancy clothes do nothing but adorn the wall of the big room and feed the moths. That had been Jeff Patton's experience. He had not worn his stiff-bosomed shirt more than a dozen times in all his married life. His swallowtailed coat lay on the bed beside him, freshly brushed and pressed, but it was as full of holes as the overalls in which he worked on weekdays. The moths had used it badly. Jeff twisted his mouth into a hideous toothless grimace as he contended with the obstinate bow. He stamped his good foot and decided to give up the struggle.

"Jennie," he called.

"What's that, Jeff?" His wife's shrunken voice came out of the adjoining room like an echo. It was hardly bigger than a whisper.

"I reckon you'll have to help me wid this heah bow tie, baby," he said meekly. "Dog if I can hitch it up."

Her answer was not strong enough to reach him, but presently the old woman came to the door, feeling her way with a stick. She had a wasted, dead-leaf appearance. Her body, as scrawny and gnarled as a string bean, seemed less than nothing in the ocean of frayed and faded petticoats that surrounded her. These hung an inch or two above the tops of her heavy unlaced shoes and showed little grotesque piles where the stockings had fallen down from her negligible legs.

"You oughta could do a heap mo' wid a thing like that'n me—beingst as you got yo' good sight."

"Looks like I oughta could," he admitted. "But ma fingers is gone democrat on me. I get all mixed up in the looking glass and can't tell wicha way to twist the devilish thing."

Jennie sat on the side of the bed and old Jeff Patton got down on one knee while she tied the bow knot. It was a slow and painful ordeal for each of them in this position. Jeff's bones cracked, his knee ached, and it was only after a half dozen attempts that Jennie worked a semblance of a bow into the tie.

"I got to dress maself now," the old woman whispered. "These is ma old shoes and stockings, and I ain't so much as unwrapped ma dress."

"Well, don't worry 'bout me no mo', baby," Jess said. "That 'bout finishes me. All I gotta do now is slip on that old coat 'n ves' an' I'll be fixed to leave."

Jennie disappeared again through the dim passage into the shed room. Being blind was no handicap to her in that black hole. Jeff heard the cane placed against the wall beside the door and knew that his wife was on easy ground. He put on his coat, took a battered top hat from the bedpost and hobbled to the front door. He was ready to travel. As soon as Jennie could get on her Sunday shoes and her old black silk dress, they would start.

Outside the tiny log house, the day was warm and mellow with sunshine. A host of wasps were humming with busy excitement in the trunk of a dead sycamore. Gray squirrels were searching through the grass for hickory nuts and blue jays were in the trees, hopping from branch to branch. Pine woods stretched away to the left like a black sea. Among them were scattered scores of log houses like Jeff's, houses of black share farmers. Cows and pigs wandered freely among the trees. There was no danger of loss. Each farmer knew his own stock and knew his neighbor's as well as he knew his neighbor's children.

Down the slope to the right were the cultivated acres on which the colored folks worked. They extended to the river, more than two miles away, and they were today green with the unmade cotton crop. A tiny thread of a road, which passed directly in front of Jeff's place, ran through these green fields like a pencil mark.

Jeff, standing outside the door, with his absurd hat in his left hand, surveyed the wide scene tenderly. He had been forty-five years on these acres. He loved them with the unexplained affection that others have for the countries to which they belong.

The sun was hot on his head, his collar still pinched his throat, and the Sunday clothes were intolerably hot. Jeff transferred the hat to his right hand and began fanning with it. Suddenly the whisper that was Jennie's voice came out of the shed room.

"You can bring the car round front whilst you's waitin'," it said feebly. There was a tired pause; then it added, "I'll soon be fixed to go."

"A'right, baby," Jeff answered. "I'll get it in a minute."

But he didn't move. A thought struck him that made his mouth fall open. The mention of the car brought to his mind, with new intensity, the trip he and Jennie were about to take. Fear came into his eyes; excitement took his breath. Lord, Jesus!

"Jeff . . . O Jeff," the old woman's whisper called.

He awakened with a jolt. "Hunh, baby?"

"What you doin'?"

"Nuthin'. Jes studyin'. I jes been turnin' things round 'n round in ma mind."

"You could be gettin' the car," she said.

"Oh yes, right away, baby."

He started round to the shed, limping heavily on his bad leg. There were three frizzly chickens in the yard. All his other chickens had been killed or stolen recently. But the frizzly chickens had been saved somehow. That was fortunate indeed, for these curious creatures had a way of devouring "Poison" from the yard and in that way protecting against conjure and black luck and spells. But even the frizzly chickens seemed to be now in a stupor. Jeff thought they had some ailment; he expected all three of them to die shortly.

The shed in which the old T-model Ford stood was only a grass roof held up by four corner poles. It had been built by tremulous hands at a time when the little rattletrap car had been regarded as a peculiar treasure. And, miraculously, despite wind and downpour, it still stood.

Jeff adjusted the crank and put his weight upon it. The engine came to life with a sputter and bang that rattled the old car from radiator to taillight. Jeff hopped into the seat and put his foot on the accelerator. The sputtering and banging increased. The rattling became more violent. That was good. It was good banging, good sputtering and rattling, and it meant that the aged car was still in running condition. She could be depended on for this trip.

Again Jeff's thought halted as if paralyzed. The suggestion of the trip fell into the machinery of his mind like a wrench. He felt dazed and weak. He swung the car out into the yard, made a half turn and drove around to the front door. When he took his hands off the wheel, he noticed that he was trembling violently. He cut off the motor and climbed to the ground to wait for Jennie.

A few minutes later she was at the window, her voice rattling against the pane like a broken shutter.

"I'm ready, Jeff."

He did not answer, but limped into the house and took her by the arm. He led her slowly through the big room, down the step and across the yard.

"You reckon I'd oughta lock the do'?" he asked softly.

They stopped and Jennie weighed the question. Finally she shook her head.

"Ne' mind the do'," she said. "I don't see no cause to lock up things."

"You right," Jeff agreed. "No cause to lock up."

Jeff opened the door and helped his wife into the car. A quick shudder passed over him. Jesus! Again he trembled.

"How come you shaking so?" Jennie whispered.

"I don't know," he said.

"You mus' be scairt, Jeff."

"No, baby, I ain't scairt."

He slammed the door after her and went around to crank up again. The motor started easily. Jeff wished that it had not been so responsive. He would have liked a few more minutes in which to turn things around in his head. As it was, with Jennie chiding him about being afraid, he had to keep going. He swung the car into the little pencil-mark road and started off toward the river, driving very slowly, very cautiously.

Chugging across the green countryside, the small battered Ford seemed tiny indeed. Jeff felt a familiar excitement, a thrill, as they came down the first slope to the immense levels on which the cotton was growing. He could not help reflecting that the crops were good. He knew what that meant, too; he had made forty-five of them with his own hands. It was true that he had worn out nearly a dozen mules, but that was the fault of old man Stevenson, the owner of the land. Major Stevenson had the odd notion that one mule was all a share farmer needed to work a thirty-acre plot. It was an expensive notion, the way it killed mules from overwork, but the old man held to it. Jeff thought it killed a good many share farmers as well as mules, but he had no sympathy for them. He had always been strong, and he had always been taught to have no patience with weakness in men. Women or children might be tolerated if they were puny, but a weak man was a curse. Of course, his own children—

Jeff's thought halted there. He and Jennie never mentioned their dead children any more. And naturally he did not wish to dwell upon them in his mind. Before he knew it, some remark would slip out of his mouth and that would make Jennie feel blue. Perhaps she would cry. A woman like Jennie could not easily throw off the grief that comes from losing five grown children within two years. Even Jeff was still staggered by the blow. His memory had not been much good recently. He frequently talked to himself. And, although he had kept it a secret, he knew that his courage had left him. He was terrified by the least unfamiliar sound at night. He was reluctant to venture far from home in the daytime. And that habit of trembling when he felt fearful was now far beyond his control. Sometimes he became afraid and trembled without knowing what had frightened him. The feeling would just come over him like a chill.

The car rattled slowly over the dusty road. Jennie sat erect and silent, with a little absurd hat pinned to her hair. Her useless eyes seemed very large, very white in their deep sockets. Suddenly Jeff heard her voice, and he inclined his head to catch the words.

"Is we passed Delia Moore's house yet?" she asked.

"Not yet," he said.

"You must be driven' mighty slow, Jeff."

"We might just as well take our time, baby."

There was a pause. A little puff of steam was coming out of the radiator of the car. Heat wavered above the hood. Delia Moore's house was nearly half a mile away. After a moment Jennie spoke again.

"You ain't really scairt, is you, Jeff?"

"Nah, baby, I ain't scairt."

"You know how we agreed—we gotta keep on goin'."

Jewels of perspiration appeared on Jeff's forehead. His eyes rounded, blinked, became fixed on the road.

"I don't know," he said with a shiver. "I reckon it's the only thing to do."

"Hm."

A flock of guinea fowls, pecking in the road, were scattered by the passing car. Some of them took to their wings; others hid under bushes. A blue jay, swaying on a leafy twig, was annoying a roadside squirrel. Jeff held an even speed till he came near Delia's place. Then he slowed down noticeably.

Delia's house was really no house at all, but an abandoned store building converted into a dwelling. It sat near a crossroads, beneath a single black cedar tree. There Delia, a catish old creature of Jennie's age, lived alone. She had been there more years than anybody could remember, and long ago had won the disfavor of such women as Jennie. For in her young days Delia had been gayer, yellower and saucier than seemed proper in those parts. Her ways with menfolks had been dark and suspicious. And the fact that she had had as many husbands as children did not help her reputation.

"Yonder's old Delia," Jeff said as they passed.

"What she doin'?"

"Jes sittin' in the do'," he said.

"She see us?"

"Hm," Jeff said. "Musta did."

That relieved Jennie. It strengthened her to know that her old enemy had seen her pass in her best clothes. That would give the old she-devil something to chew her gums and fret about, Jennie thought. Wouldn't she have a fit if she didn't find out? Old evil Delia!

This would be just the thing for her. It would pay her back for being so evil. It would also pay her, Jennie thought, for the way she used to grin at Jeff—long ago when her teeth were good.

The road became smooth and red, and Jeff could tell by the smell of the air that they were nearing the river. He could see the rise where the road turned and ran along parallel to the stream. The car chugged on monotonously. After a long silent spell, Jennie leaned against Jeff and spoke.

"How many bale o' cotton you think we got standin'?" she said.

Jeff wrinkled his forehead as he calculated.

"'Bout twenty-five, I reckon."

"How many you make las' year?"

"Twenty-eight," he said. "How come you ask that?"

"I's jes thinkin'," Jennie said quietly.

"It don't make a speck o' difference though," Jeff reflected. "If we get much or if we get little, we still gonna be in debt to old man Stevenson when he gets through counting up agin us. It's took us a long time to learn that."

Jennie was not listening to these words. She had fallen into a trance-like meditation. Her lips twitched. She chewed her gums and rubbed her gnarled hands nervously. Suddenly she leaned forward, buried her face in the nervous hands and burst into tears. She cried aloud in a dry cracked voice that suggested the rattle of fodder on dead stalks. She cried aloud like a child, for she had never learned to suppress a genuine sob. Her slight old frame shook heavily and seemed hardly able to sustain such violent grief.

"What's the matter, baby?" Jeff asked awkwardly. "Why you cryin' like all that?"

"I's jes thinkin'," she said.

"So you the one what's scairt now, hunh?"

"I ain't scairt, Jeff. I's jes thinkin' 'bout leavin' eve'thing like this—eve'thing we been used to. It's right sad-like."

Jeff did not answer, and presently Jennie buried her face again and cried.

The sun was almost overhead. It beat down furiously on the dusty wagon-path road, on the parched roadside grass and the tiny battered car. Jeff's hands, gripping the wheel, became wet with perspiration; his forehead sparkled. Jeff's lips parted. His mouth shaped a hideous grimace. His face suggested the face of a man being burned. But the torture passed and his expression softened again.

"You mustn't cry, baby," he said to his wife. "We gotta be strong. We can't break down."

Jennie waited a few seconds, then said, "You reckon we oughta do it, Jeff? You reckon we oughta go 'head an' do it, really?"

Jeff's voice choked; his eyes blurred. He was terrified to hear Jennie say the thing that had been in his mind all morning. She had egged him on when he had wanted more than anything in the world to wait, to reconsider, to think things over a little longer. Now she was getting cold feet. Actually there was no need of thinking the question through again. It would only end in making the same painful decision once more. Jeff knew that. There was no need of fooling around longer.

"We jes as well to do like we planned," he said. "They ain't nothin' else for us now—it's the bes' thing."

Jeff thought of the handicaps, the near impossibility, of making another crop with his leg bothering him more and more each week. Then there was always the chance that he would have another stroke, like the one that had made him lame. Another one might kill him. The least it could do would be to leave him helpless. Jeff gasped—Lord, Jesus! He could not bear to think of being helpless, like a baby, on Jennie's hands. Frail, blind Jennie.

The little pounding motor of the car worked harder and harder. The puff of steam from the cracked radiator became larger. Jeff realized that they were climbing a little rise. A moment later the road turned abruptly and he looked down upon the face of the river.

"Jeff."

"Hunh?"

"Is that the water I hear?"

"Hm. Tha's it."

"Well, which way you goin' now?"

"Down this a way," he said. "The road runs 'longside o' the water a lil piece."

She waited a while calmly. Then she said, "Drive faster."

"A'right, baby," Jeff said.

The water roared in the bed of the river. It was fifty or sixty feet below the level of the road. Between the road and the water there was a long smooth slope, sharply inclined. The slope was dry, the clay hardened by prolonged summer heat. The water below, roaring in a narrow channel, was noisy and wild.

"Jeff."

"Hunh?"

"How far you goin'?"

"Jes a lil piece down the road."

"You ain't scairt, is you, Jeff?"

"Nah, baby," he said trembling. "I ain't scairt."

"Remember how we planned it, Jeff. We gotta do it like we said. Brave-like."

"Hm."

Jeff's brain darkened. Things suddenly seemed unreal, like figures in a dream. Thoughts swam in his mind foolishly, hysterically, like little blind fish in a pool within a dense cave. They rushed, crossed one another, jostled, collided, retreated and rushed again. Jeff soon became dizzy. He shuddered violently and turned to his wife.

"Jennie, I can't do it. I can't." His voice broke pitifully.

She did not appear to be listening. All the grief had gone from her face. She sat erect, her unseeing eyes wide open, strained and frightful. Her glossy black skin had become dull. She seemed as thin, as sharp and bony, as a starved bird. Now having suffered and endured the sadness of tearing herself away from beloved things, she showed no anguish. She was absorbed with her own thoughts, and she didn't even hear Jeff's voice shouting in her ear.

Jeff said nothing more. For an instant there was a light in his cavernous brain. The great chamber was, for less than a second, peopled by characters he knew and loved. They were simple, healthy creatures, and they behaved in a manner that he could understand. They had quality. But since he had already taken leave of them long ago, the remembrance did not break his heart again. Young Jeff Patton was among them, the Jeff Patton of fifty years ago who went down to New Orleans with a crowd of country boys to the Mardi Gras doings. The gay young crowd, boys with candy-striped shirts and rouged-brown girls in noisy silks, was like a picture in his head. Yet it did not make him sad. On that very trip Slim Burns had killed Joe Beasley—the crowd had been broken up. Since then Jeff Patton's world had been the Greenbriar Plantation. If there had been other Mardi Gras carnivals, he had not heard of them.

Since then there had been no time; the years had fallen on him like waves. Now he was old, worn out. Another paralytic stroke (like the one he had already suffered) would put him on his back for keeps. In that condition, with a frail blind woman to look after him, he would be worse off than if he were dead.

Suddenly Jeff's hands became steady. He actually felt brave. He slowed down the motor of the car and carefully pulled off the road. Below, the water of the stream boomed, a soft thunder in the deep channel. Jeff ran the car onto the clay slope, pointed it directly toward the stream and put his foot heavily on the accelerator. The little car leaped furiously down the steep incline toward the water. The movement was nearly as swift and direct as a fall. The two old black folks, sitting quietly side by side, showed no excitement. In another instant the car hit the water and dropped immediately out of sight.

A little later it lodged in the mud of a shallow place. One wheel of the crushed and upturned little Ford became visible above the rushing water.

ELEGY

DYLAN THOMAS

Too proud to die; broken and blind he died
The darkest way, and did not turn away,
A cold kind man brave in his narrow pride

On that darkest day. Oh, forever may
He lie lightly, at last, on the last, crossed
Hill, under the grass, in love, and there grow

Young among the long flocks, and never lie lost
Or still all the numberless days of his death, though
Above all he longed for his mother's breast

Which was rest and dust, and in the kind ground
The darkest justice of death, blind and unblessed.
Let him find no rest but be fathered and found,

I prayed in the crouching room, by his blind bed,
In the muted house, one minute before
Noon, and night, and light. The rivers of the dead

Veined his poor hand I held, and I saw
Through his unseeing eyes to the roots of the sea.
(An old tormented man three-quarters blind,

I am not too proud to cry that He and he
Will never never go out of my mind.
All his bones crying, and poor in all but pain,

Being innocent, he dreaded that he died
Hating his God, but what he was was plain:
An old kind man brave in his burning pride.

The sticks of the house were his; his books he owned.
Even as a baby he had never cried;
Nor did he now, save to his secret wound.

Out of his eyes I saw the last light glide.
Here among the light of the lording sky
An old blind man is with me where I go

Walking in the meadows of his son's eye
On whom a world of ills came down like snow.
He cried as he died, fearing at last the spheres'

Last sound, the world going out without a breath:
Too proud to cry, too frail to check the tears,
And caught between two nights, blindness and death.

O deepest wound of all that he should die
On that darkest day. Oh, he could hide
The tears out of his eyes, too proud to cry.

Until I die he will not leave my side.)

DO NOT GO GENTLE INTO THAT GOOD NIGHT

DYLAN THOMAS

Do not go gentle into that good night,
Old age should burn and rave at close of day;
Rage, rage against the dying of the light.

Though wise men at their end know dark is right,
Because their words had forked no lightning they
Do not go gentle into that good night.

Good men, the last wave by, crying how bright
Their frail deeds might have danced in a green bay,
Rage, rage against the dying of the light.

Wild men who caught and sang the sun in flight,
And learn, too late, they grieved it on its way,
Do not go gentle into that good night.

Grave men, near death, who see with blinding sight
Blind eyes could blaze like meteors and be gay,
Rage, rage against the dying of the light.

And you, my father, there on the sad height,
Curse, bless, me now with your fierce tears, I pray.
Do not go gentle into that good night.
Rage, rage against the dying of the light.

AND DEATH SHALL HAVE NO DOMINION

DYLAN THOMAS

And death shall have no dominion.
Dead men naked they shall be one
With the man in the wind and the west moon;
When their bones are picked clean and the clean bones gone,
They shall have stars at elbow and foot;
Though they go mad they shall be sane,
Though they sink through the sea they shall rise again;
Though lovers be lost love shall not;
And death shall have no dominion.

And death shall have no dominion.
Under the windings of the sea
They lying long shall not die windily;
Twisting on racks when sinews give way,
Strapped to a wheel, yet they shall not break;
Faith in their hands shall snap in two,
And the unicorn evils run them through;
Split all ends up they shan't crack;
And death shall have no dominion.

And death shall have no dominion.
No more may gulls cry at their ears
Or waves break loud on the seashores;
Where blew a flower may a flower no more
Lift its head to the blows of the rain;
Though they be mad and dead as nails,
Heads of the characters hammer through daisies;
Break in the sun till the sun breaks down,
And death shall have no dominion.

A REFUSAL TO MOURN THE DEATH, BY FIRE, OF A CHILD IN LONDON

DYLAN THOMAS

Never until the mankind making
Bird beast and flower
Fathering and all humbling darkness
Tells with silence the last light breaking
And the still hour
Is come of the sea tumbling in harness

And I must enter again the round
Zion of the water bead
And the synagogue of the ear of corn
Shall I let pray the shadow of a sound
Or sow my salt seed
In the least valley of sackcloth to mourn

The majesty and burning of the child's death.
I shall not murder
The mankind of her going with a grave truth
Nor blaspheme down the stations of the breath
With any further
Elegy of innocence and youth.

Deep with the first dead lies London's daughter,
Robed in the long friends,
The grains beyond age, the dark veins of her mother,
Secret by the unmourning water
Of the riding Thames.
After the first death, there is no other.

THE SMILE WAS

DANNIE ABSE

one thing I waited for always
after the shouting
after the palaver
the perineum stretched to pain
the parched voice of the midwife
            Push!Push!
and I can't and the rank
sweet smell of the gas
and
            I can't
as she whiffed cotton wool
inside her head
as the hollow stones of gas
dragged
   her
      down
from the lights above
to the river-bed, to the real stones.
            Push! Push!
as she floated up again
muscles tensed, to the electric
till the little head was crowned;
and I shall wait again
for the affirmation.

For it is such:
that effulgent, tender, satisfied
smile of a woman
who, for the first time,
hears the child crying the world
for the very first time.

That agreeable, radiant smile—
no man can smile it
no man can paint it
as it develops without fail,
after the gross, physical, knotted,
granular, bloody endeavour.
  Such a pure spirituality, from all that!
It occupies the face
and commands it.
          Out of relief
you say, reasonably thinking of the reasonable,
swinging lightness of any reprieve,
the joy of it, almost helium in the head.

          So wouldn't you?
And truly there's always the torture of the unknown.
There's always the dream of pregnant women,
blood of the monster in the blood of the child;
and we know of generations lost
like words faded on a stone,
of minds blank or wild with genetic mud.
          And couldn't you
smile like that?

Not like that, no, never,
not with such indefinable
dulcitude as that.
And so she smiles
with eyes as brown as a dog's
or eyes blue-mad as a doll's
it makes no odds
whore, beauty, or bitch,

it makes no odds
illimitable chaste happiness
in that smile
as new life-in-the-world
for the first time cries the world.
No man can smile like that.

2

No man can paint it.
Da Vinci sought it out
yet was far, far, hopelessly.
Leonardo, you only made
Mona Lisa look six months gone!

I remember the smile of the Indian.
I told him
          Fine, finished,
you are cured
and he sat there smiling sadly.
Any painter could paint it
the smile of a man resigned
saying
          Thank you, doctor,
you have been kind
and then, as in melodrama,
          How long
have I to live?
The Indian smiling, resigned,
all the fatalism of the East.

So one starts again, also smiling,
          All is well
you are well, you are cured.
And the Indian still smiling
his assignations with death
still shaking his head, resigned.
          Thank you
for telling me the truth, doctor.
Two months? Three months?

And beginning again
  and again
whatever I said, thumping the table,
however much I reassured him
the more he smiled the conspiratorial
smile of a damned, doomed man.

Now a woman, a lady, a whore,
a bitch, a beauty, whatever,
  the child's face crumpled
as she becomes the mother
she smiles differently, ineffably.

3

As different as
the smile of my colleague,
his eyes reveal it,
his ambiguous assignations,
good man, good surgeon,
whose smile arrives of its own accord
  from nowhere
like flies to a dead thing
when he makes the first incision.

Who draws a line of blood
across the soft, white flesh
as if something beneath,
desiring violence, had beckoned him;
who draws a ritual wound,
a calculated wound
to heal—to heal,
but still a wound—
good man, good surgeon,
his smile as luxuriant
as the smile of Peter Lorre.

So is the smile of my colleague,
the smile of a man
secretive behind the mask.

The smile of war.

But the smile, the smile
of the new mother,
what
  an extraordinary
        open thing
              it is.

4

Walking home tonight I saw
an ordinary occurrence
hardly worth remarking on:
an unhinged star, a streaking gas,
and I thought how lovely
destruction is when it is far.
Ruined it slid
on the dead dark towards fiction:
its lit world disappeared
phut, through one punched hole or another,
slipped unseen down the back of the sky
into another time.

Never,
not for one single death
can I forget we die with the dead,
and the world dies with us;
yet
in one, lonely,
small child's birth
all the tall dead rise
to break the crust of the imperative earth.

No wonder the mother smiles
a wonder like that,
a lady, a whore, a bitch, a beauty.
Eve smiled like that
when she heard Seth cry out Abel's dark,
earth dark, the first dark
eeling on the deep sea-bed,
struggling on the real stones.
Hecuba, Cleopatra, Lucretia Borgia,
Annette Vallon smiled like that.

They all, still, smile like that,
when the child first whimpers like a seagull
the ancient smile reasserts itself
instinct with a return
so outrageous and so shameless;
the smile the smile
always the same
          an uncaging
                    a freedom.

DELIVERY

TOI DERRICOTTE

i was in the delivery room. PUT YOUR
FEET UP IN THE STIRRUPS. i put them up, obedient
still humbled, though the spirit was growing larger
in me, that black woman was in my throat, her thin
song, high pitched like a lark, and all the muscles
were starting to constrict around her.
I tried to push just a little. it
didn't hurt. i tried a little more.

ROLL UP, guzzo said. he wanted to give me
a spinal. NO. I DON'T WANT A SPINAL. (same
doctor as ax handle up my butt, same as shaft
of split wood, doctor spike, driving the
head home where my soft animal cowered and prayed and
cried for his mother.)

or was the baby
part of this
whole damn
conspiracy,
in on it with
guzzo,
the two of them
wanting to shoot
the wood
up me for
nothing,

"Delivery" originally appeared in *Natural Birth: Poems*, by Toi Derricotte (Trumansburg, NY: Crossing Press, 1983). Reprinted by permission of the author.

for playing
music to him
in the dark
for singing
to my round
clasped
belly for filling
up with
pizza on a cold
night, dough
warm.

maybe
he
wanted
out,
was saying
give her
a needle
and let me/the hell/
out of here
who cares
what she
wants
put her
to sleep.

(my baby
pushing off
with his black
feet
from the dark
shore, heading
out, not
knowing
which way and trusting,
oarless and eyeless, so
hopeless
it didn't matter.)

no. not
my baby.
this
loved
thing
in/and of
myself
so i balled up
and let him
try to
stick it in.
  maybe
something was
wrong

  ROLL UP
he said
  ROLL UP
but i don't want it
  ROLL UP ROLL UP
but it doesn't hurt

we all stood,
nurses, round the white
light
hands
hanging
empty at our sides
  ROLL UP IN A BALL
all of us not
knowing
how
or if
in such a world without
false promises
we could say
anything
but, *yes,*
yes.
come take it
and be quick.

i put my belly in my hand
gave him that
thin side
of my back
the bones
intruding on the air
in little knobs
in joints
he might
crack
down my spine
his knuckles
rap
each twisted
symmetry
put me on
the rack,
each
nerve
bright
and stretched
like canvas.

he couldn't get it in!
three times, he tried
ROLL UP, he cried, ROLL UP
three times
he couldn't get it in!

dr. y (the head obstetrician)
came in

"what are you
doing, guzzo,
i thought she
wanted
natural . . .

(to me) do
you want
a shot . . . no? well,

PUT YOUR LEGS UP,
GIRL, AND
PUSH!"

and suddenly, the light
went out
the nurses
laughed
and nothing
mattered
in this 10
a.m. sun
shiny morning
we were well
the nurses and the
doctors cheering
that girl
combing hair
all in one
direction
shining
bright as water.

i
grew deep
in me
like fist and i
grew deep
in me
like death
and i
grew deep
in me
like hiding in the sea and
i was
over me
like
sun and i
was under
me

like sky and i
could look
into myself
like one
dark eye.

  i was her
and she was me
and we were
scattered around
like light
  nurses
  doctors
cheering

  such waves

my face
contorted,
never
wore
such mask, so
rigid
and so dark
  so
bright, un-
compromising
brave
no turning
back/no
no's.

i was so
beautiful. i
could look
up in the
light and
see my huge-
ness,
arc,
electric,
heavy, fleshy, living
light.

no wonder they
praised me,
a gesture
one makes
helpless and
urgent, praising
what goes on
without our praise.

when there
was nowhere
i could go, when i
was so deep
in myself
so large
i had to
let it out
they said
   drop back. i

dropped back
on the table
panting,
they moved
the head, swiveled
it correctly

   but i

      i

was
loosing
her. something
   a head
coming through
the door.
NAME PLEASE/
PLEASE /NAME /whose
head /i
don't know /some/
   disconnection

NAME PLEASE/

and i
am not ready:
the sudden visibility
his body,
his curly wet hair,
his arms
abandoned in that air,
an arching, squiggling thing,
his skin must be
so cold,
but there is nothing
i can do
to warm him,
his body clutches
in a wretched
spineless way.

they expect me
to sing
joy joy
a son is born,
child is given.
tongue
curled in my head
tears, cheeks
stringy with
damp hair.

this lump
of flesh,
lump of steamy
viscera.

who

is this
child

who

is his father

a child
never having
been seen
before,
without
credentials
credit cards without
employee
reference or
high school grades or
anything
to make him
human make
him mine but
skein of
pain to
chop off
at the navel.

while they could
they held him down and
chopped him, held him up
my little fish, my blueness
swallowed in the air
turned pink
and wailed.

no more. enough.
i lay back, speechless, looking
for something
to say to myself.

after you have
touched the brain,
that squirmy
lust of maggots,
after you have
pumped the heart,
that thief,
that comic, you
throw her in the trash.

and the little one
in a case
of glass . . .

he is not i
i am not him
he is not i

. . . the stranger . . .

blue
air
protects us from each other.

here.
here is the note he brings.
it says, "*mother.*"

but i do not even know
this man.

HOMELESS

JULIET S. KONO

My son lives on the streets.
We don't see each other much.
Like a mother who puts white lilies
on the headstone of a dead child,
I put money into his bank account,
clothes into E-Z Access storage
and pretend he's far away—
at a boarding school, or in a foreign country.
Nights, I dream fairy tales about him.
I dream he becomes a prince,
scholar or warrior who rescues me
from sorrow, the way he rescued me
when he was a child and said,
"Mommy, don't cry," and brought tea
into the room of his father's acrimony—
brave, standing tall in the forest
fire of his father's scorn. I wake
to the empty sound of wind in the trees.
He says he want to live with me.
I say I can't live with him—
but those words crash like branches in a rain storm.
Nothing can hold him in,
the walls of a house too thin.

Back home, I had seen
the "study-hard-so-you-don't-become-like-them"
street bums on Mamo Street,
and he's like *them.*
These days, in order to catch a glimpse of him,
I circle the city. One day,
I see him on his bike.
People give him a wide berth,
the same way birds avoid power lines,
oncoming cars or trees.
I park on a side street.
Wild-eyed, he flies the block
as if in a holding pattern.
Not of my body, not of my hopes,
he homes in on what can't be given or taken away.

SON, AFTER THE ATTEMPT

JULIET S. KONO

The sun dusts the nape of my neck, hotly.
Behind us, the deep-pleated Koʻolau rise.
I perspire. But you're cold in heavy
robes, sandals slapping as you pace. Our eyes
meet where I sit on a bench. You turn, size
me up, then point like some wild prophet and ask:
"Grandma Lee has Alzheimer's. When she dies,
will she be as she was, before the mask?
The paraplegic, will he be able
to walk, to pick flowers again? You do
know what it means to be alive—*stable.*
When we die, we die perfect, don't we?"
You take silence as assent. "Mom, so tell me
why do you and your miserable gods stop me?"

THE FIRST TIME

JULIET S. KONO

The hospital calls again.
You are brought in by ambulance
after you are discovered,
flopping like a fish on the sidewalk.

Every time is the first time.
I will never get used to it—
the late night calls,
the anxieties rising like tide,
the voices sounding far and fluid,
the nurses telling me
you are alive
but under observation.

But the worst time
was the first time—
the time when you took a fistful of sleeping pills,
and the nurse gave you some Ipecac
and fastened your slippery life
over the toilet bowl,
while I patted your back
in life's violent return.

Remember how the light and faces
wavered around us
detached as the moon
as if we were looking at things
from under water? To keep you awake,
I put my arms across your shoulders
like a receiving blanket
for the long walk ahead of us.
We dropped our heads, then,
to resist death,
slow-circling the room.

ROYALLY PISSED

JULIET S. KONO

"*Talk* to him. He's still here.
I know these things," pronounces the nurse
in a dispensation of her experience,
years of watching the dying die.
"The soul hangs around for awhile."
But what can I say to you—
that I'm royally pissed,
that I'm madder than hell at you
God damn kid
how dare you do the right things at the end
and that it all came too late?
I want to slap you back to life,
scream and beat the drum
of your chest with my fists,
howl in the strange, hollow
animal cry of the crazed dog
that bays at the moon
behind the old mountain house,
then cuts loose across the fields
and stream, fanning water high in its wake,
the droplets caught in the moonlight
and flung into a hive of stars.
Forgive my crown of anger.
Deliver me from this fucking pain.

NEST

JULIET S. KONO

I tighten the scarf around my neck,
grip my black coat
to resist the night's crazy wind,
the agonized air,
the whip of the branches.
Piling pillows and blankets around me,
I build a nest on a rollaway
next to your bed.
Feeding tubes and IV lines offer a covering.
Carrying its supply of air,
its smoke rings of oxygen,
your ventilator chugs,
uphill, like a train
into the broken wings of your lungs,
and departs
with your memory of what it is to be alive.
Live. Live.

I agree. Pull the plug.
What does this have to do with the heart?
Now, it's just a matter of time—
a weed in a sidewalk crack,
a gold guitar.
Tonight, hovering over you,
I'm a new mother.

I listen to you breathe—
the same way I listened
when you were a child,
and I couldn't sleep
in the fear of such a miracle.
My ears to your life.
I watch for the slightest change,
each breath's soft and shallow retreat.
And your life goes scattering.
Son who leaned too far out the window,
kicked shoes on the porch,
you who wanted more than just a breath of fresh air.
You thought you could fly.

THE STRUGGLE

JULIET S. KONO

In this rotation,
the bones of night,
Melissa, angel of mercy, works the graveyard shift.
Drifts in her whites like wind-caught sails.
Which one will go next?
Everyone on this floor is critical,
the dying beyond sleep, agony, or self-pity.
In her rounds she administers
to the anguish of the living.
She gives lozenges of comfort,
cotton pats of sympathy.
I can hear her.
"Are you comfortable?"
"May I get you something?"
"More coffee or tea?"
Next door, she sings with members
of the Samoan family
who come and go
with their ukuleles and guitars,
songs for a dying father
who sleeps on a strip of tapa
shaped like a canoe
that will spirit him away.
She comes at last to your room.

Burdened by composure and kindness,
she drops herself on my cot
and grieves for a son who is like you,
stretched out
taut as strings on a guitar,
light shiny on your forehead,
a moon cleft of fluorescence.
She tells me that children like ours
are orphans of life,
and maybe, things would be different
if we could only take them back,
again, into ourselves.
"To start all over," she says.
I nod. It is the dream
of mothers whose children
have died like this, before their time,
a wish that plays itself over and over
like a broken record,
spinning the drama of those left behind.

THE PERMISSION

JULIET S. KONO

My son is lying like a bridge
spanning himself from this life
into another.
We will take down the scaffolding
that breathes for him,
each breath a step closer
to where he will arrive.
Hands raised, the nurse snaps the latex gloves
over her hands and unplugs the ventilator.
His mouth falls open
and she takes the tubes and pulls
them out of his throat,
feeding tube from his nose,
IV from his arm.
She leaves the oxygen in for comfort,
the last suspension to his life.
His head rolls back on the pillow.
Slack from pain and tension, his eyes open
and tears roll down his face.
I hold his hand and wipe his forehead,
the things I couldn't do to love him.
You're almost there.
He breathes on his own.
It's pure reflex now.

His breathing will slow down
they tell me, then fade.
He goes on through the night,
into the next day.
It will be nice where you go.
I give him this permission of love—
to cross the bridge.
I tell him to enter Kaiwiki house.
He doesn't have to take his shoes off
or shake out his pockets,
filled with the summer he played in.

IN A RUSH

JULIET S. KONO

The day I wait for my son to die,
it's as if we are down at the harbor
watching the ships go by and the longshoremen
cart pallets of iceberg lettuce, bananas and mail across the wharf.
Our last time together, we're made whole again
as in that perfect moment,
mother and child,
child no one could have loved
or wanted, except me, his mother.
Son brought to me in a blue blanket,
face red and swollen as a wound,
the day I tied on his first booties.
We'd grown apart since then,
joined now in this pitiable end,
facing the ocean.

All day no change.
Pulse, respiration, same.
I leave to eat the meat dry as saltines,
change my sandals, wash my face.
And it is so like him
to die without me there at his bedside,
his death as impulsive as he had always been—
with no bells or clamor of the triangle—
as if he had suddenly seen a passing ship,

wasn't about to miss it,
got up and dove into the water to meet it,
going out the same way he had come,
in a rush, headlong,
pushing through water
without a clue, boarding pass, or blessing.

THE WAY

JULIET S. KONO

White candles and chrysanthemums
are an offering of continuity.
I cradle your urn to be blessed by the priest
and carry your mortuary tablet like a flame to the altar.
The seven-day service, over ashes,
inters your remains at the temple.

Mother, this is the way I come back to you.

Shoku Sho, the priest explains your Buddhist name
and places the peace you never had into your spirit.
For the sake of the living, we will hold observances:
forty-nine days, a hundred days, one year.
That your forty-ninth day, the day of compassion,
the day your spirit is released from Earth's bond
falls on my birthday is a wonderful omen.

You face the east,
the morning sun, the rise of eternity.
Each day the priest will strike the gong in a blessing
when morning breaks over Nuʻuanu,
and you will hear the song of each day's naming.
I place pictures of happier times inside the niche.
You on your bike, riding into the valley,
eating oysters at Sydney's house,
feeding the deer at Kamakura.

This is the way, mother, I come back to you.

SECTION THREE

TRAUMA AND RECOVERY

INTRODUCTION

In recent years, medical and cultural understanding about the nature of trauma has evolved; a number of recent, full-length studies, notably including Judith Herman's well-received book, *Trauma and Recovery,* illuminate the lasting effects of trauma—of all sorts of trauma, from childhood sexual abuse to trench warfare. In an age of repeated genocidal conflicts, the lasting effects of torture and ferocious conflict must be addressed in communities far from the original location of trauma. Neurologists report on lasting changes in the brains of those who have survived trauma, suggesting that the connection between mind and body is tangible, not metaphoric. Though the factual evidence is compelling, the human dimensions of these new explorations of the brain become most affecting in the hands of storytellers. For it is often in narrative that one who has experienced trauma can retrieve the fragmented self and begin to make it whole.

One of the authors whose work appears in this section, Jonathan Shay, has both a medical degree and a PhD in biochemistry; his work provides a stunning example of the healing nature of literature. In his book-length study *Achilles in Vietnam: Combat Trauma and the Undoing of Character,* from which we include chapter one, Shay brings together Homer's *Iliad* and Vietnam veterans, at once dignifying the suffering of veterans filled with rage and sorrow, and demonstrating the immediacy and relevance of our culture's oldest classic text about war. More recently, Shay has turned to Homer's *Odyssey* to help us reconstruct the narrative of the incomplete return, long after the war. The chapter of *Achilles in Vietnam* included here plunges the reader into what Shay calls "the moral world" of the soldier, providing a point of entry towards an understanding both literary and personally empathetic.

A selection such as Marisa Silver's short story, "What I Saw from Where I Stood," whose title comes from Edna St. Vincent Millay's great poem "Renascence," allows the reader to enter the process of recovery at its earliest stages. Unlike the combat veterans of Shay's studies, the scarred and scared couple in Silver's story have experienced a premature stillbirth, an event our culture is not yet able to grieve fully. For our notions of both birth and death assume the triumph of medicine over the vagaries and inadequacies of the body; the still birth has become unnatural, impossible to account for, and thus impossible to recover from.

The effects of trauma are both immediate and long lasting, and not only for the traumatized individual. As caregivers understand—both those involved professionally and those in the immediate circle of family and loved ones—trauma changes everyone. What Shay's work illuminates for the combat veteran, a short story by Pat Staten powerfully shows for the family. Her title, "The Day My Father Tried to Kill Us," is deliberately uninflected and unforgettable, as was the original trauma and its long-lasting and corrosive effect on the adult who tells the story. Because this woman narrates from memory her childhood of limited understanding but limitless pain, the reader benefits from a slow accumulation of event and understanding. Empathy arrives apparently effortlessly for the reader, but the narrative testifies to its hard-won nature, since the time of the traumatic event is long past. "Nightmares have plagued me all my life" is the opening line of the story.

All the works in this section serve also to demonstrate one of the findings of much recent research: that trauma may vary in its form but not in the significance of its consequences. So the stories range from war to domestic violence to family dissolution and reconfiguration. As healing for the survivor of trauma often includes the construction of a personal narrative, so the form of narrative helps the reader towards understanding and empathy. In poetry, the constrictions of form provide containment that is immediately evident on the page. Longer selections, such as a short story or chapter, provide more freedom for development within equally significant technical dimensions. In our time, the subject of torture has become only too relevant; the essay by Jean Améry, who was tortured during the Second World War, provides testimony that still speaks with immediacy about the long-lasting effects of such violation of body and soul. In all these works, the construction of narrative and the author's choices regarding point of view help to bring readers to new understandings of the role of trauma and recovery in everyday lives.

THE STEEL WINDPIPE

MIKHAIL BULGAKOV

So I was alone, surrounded by November gloom and whirling snow; the house was smothered in it and there was a moaning in the chimneys. I had spent all twenty-four years of my life in a huge city and thought that blizzards only howled in novels. It appeared that they howled in real life. The evenings here are unusually long, and I fell to daydreaming, staring at the reflection on the window of the lamp with its dark green shade. I dreamed of the nearest town, thirty-two miles away. I longed to leave my country clinic and go there. They had electricity, and there were four doctors whom I could consult. At all events it would be less frightening than this place. But there was no chance of running away, and at times I realized that it would be cowardly. It was for precisely this, after all, that I had been studying medicine.

"Yes, but suppose they bring me a woman in labour and there are complications? Or, say, a patient with a strangulated hernia? What shall I do then? Kindly tell me that. Forty-eight days ago I qualified "with distinction"; but distinction is one thing and hernia is another. Once I watched a professor operating on a strangulated hernia. He did it, while I sat in the amphitheatre. And I only just managed to survive. . . . "

More than once I broke out in a cold sweat down my spine at the thought of hernia. Every evening, as I drank my tea, I would sit in the same attitude: by my left hand lay all the manuals on obstetrical surgery, on top of them the small edition of Döderlein. To my right were ten different illustrated volumes on operative surgery. I groaned, smoked and drank cold tea without milk.

Once I fell asleep. I remember that night perfectly—it was 29 November, and I was woken by someone banging on the door. Five minutes later I was pulling on my trousers, my eyes glued imploringly to those sacred books on operative surgery. I could hear the creaking of sleigh-runners in the yard—my ears had become unusually sensitive. The case turned out to be, if anything, even more terrifying than a hernia or a

From *A Country Doctor's Notebook*, by Mikhail Bulgakov. Trans. Michael Glenny. London: Harvil, 1975.

transverse fetus. At eleven o'clock that night a little girl was brought to the Muryovo hospital. The nurse said tonelessly to me:

"The little girl's weak, she's dying. . . . Would you come over to the hospital, please, doctor. . . ."

I remember crossing the yard towards the hospital porch, mesmerized by the flickering light of a kerosene lamp. The lights were on in the surgery, and all my assistants were waiting for me, already dressed in their overalls: the *feldsher* Demyan Lukich, young but very capable, and two experienced midwives, Anna Nikolaevna and Pelagea Ivanovna. Only twenty-four years old, having qualified a mere two months ago, I had been placed in charge of the Muryovo hospital.

The *feldsher* solemnly flung open the door and the mother came in—or rather she seemed to fly in, slithering on her ice-covered felt boots, unmelted snow still on her shawl. In her arms she carried a bundle, from which came a steady hissing, whistling sound. The mother's face was contorted with noiseless weeping. When she had thrown off her sheepskin coat and shawl and unwrapped the bundle, I saw a little girl of about three years old. For a while the sight of her made me forget operative surgery, my loneliness, the load of useless knowledge acquired at university: it was all completely effaced by the beauty of this baby girl.

What can I liken her to? You only see children like that on chocolate boxes—hair curling naturally into big ringlets the color of ripe rye, enormous dark blue eyes, doll-like cheeks. They used to draw angels like that. But in the depths of her eyes was a strange cloudiness and I recognized it as terror—the child could not breathe. "She'll be dead in an hour," I thought with absolute certainty, feeling a sharp twinge of pity for the child.

Her throat was contracting into hollows with each breath, her veins were swollen and her face was turning from pink to a pale lilac. I immediately realized what this coloring meant. I made my first diagnosis, which was not only correct but, more important, was given at the same moment as the midwives' with all their experience: "The little girl has diphtherial croup. Her throat is already choked with membrane and soon it will be blocked completely."

"How long has she been ill?" I asked, breaking the tense silence of my assistants.

"Five days now," the mother answered, staring hard at me with dry eyes.

"Diphtheria," I said to the *feldsher* through clenched teeth, and turned to the mother:

"Why have you left it so long?"

At that moment I heard a tearful voice behind me:

"Five days, sir, five days!"

I turned round and saw that a round-faced old woman had silently come in. "I wish these old women didn't exist," I thought to myself. With an aching presentiment of trouble I said:

"Quiet, woman, you're only in the way," and repeated to the mother: "Why have you left it so long? Five days? Hmm?"

Suddenly with an automatic movement the mother handed the little girl to the grandmother and sank to her knees in front of me.

"Give her some medicine," she said and banged her forehead on the floor. "I'll kill myself if she dies."

"Get up at once," I replied, "or I won't even talk to you."

The mother stood up quickly with a rustle of her wide skirt, took the baby from the grandmother and started rocking it. The old woman turned to the doorpost and began praying, while the little girl continued to breathe with a snake-like hiss. The *feldsher* said:

"That's what they're all like. These people!" And he gave a twitch of his moustache.

"Does that mean she's going to die?" the mother asked, staring at me with what looked like black fury.

"Yes, she'll die," I said quietly and firmly.

The grandmother picked up the hem of her skirt and wiped her eyes. The mother shouted in an ugly voice:

"Give her something! Help her! Give her some medicine!"

I could see what was in store for me and remained firm.

"What medicine can I give her? Go on, you tell me. The little girl is suffocating, her throat is already blocked up. For five days you kept her ten miles away from me. Now what do you want me to do?"

"You're the one who's supposed to know," the old woman whined by my left shoulder in an affected voice which made me immediately detest her.

"Shut up!" I said to her. I turned to the *feldsher* and ordered the little girl to be taken away. The mother handed her to the midwife and the child started to struggle, evidently trying to cry, but her voice could no longer make itself heard. The mother made a protective move towards her, but we kept her away and I managed to look into the little girl's throat by the light of the pressure-lamp. I had never seen diphtheria before except for mild, forgettable cases. Her throat was full of ragged, pulsating, white substance. The little girl suddenly breathed out and spat in my face, but I was so absorbed that I did not flinch.

"Well now," I said, astonished at my own calm. "This is the situation: it's late, and the little girl is dying. Nothing will help her except one thing—an operation."

I was appalled, wondering why I had said this, but I could not help saying it. The thought flashed through my mind: "What if she agrees to it?"

"How do you mean?" the mother asked.

"I'll have to cut open her throat near the bottom of her neck and put in a silver pipe so that she can breathe, and then maybe we can save her," I explained.

The mother looked at me as if I was mad and shielded the little girl from me with her arms, while the old woman started muttering again:

"The idea! Don't you let them cut her open! What—cut her throat?"

"Go away, old woman," I said to her with hatred. "Inject the camphor!" I ordered the *feldsher.*

The mother refused to hand over the little girl when she saw the syringe, but we explained to her that there was nothing terrible about it.

"Perhaps that will cure her?"

"No, it won't cure her at all."

Then the mother burst into tears.

"Stop it," I said. I took out my watch, and added: "I'm giving you five minutes to think it over. If you don't agree in five minutes, I shall refuse to do it."

"I don't agree!" the mother said sharply.

"No, we won't agree to it," the grandmother put in.

"It's up to you," I said in a hollow voice, and thought: "Well, that's that. It makes it easier for me. I've said my piece and given them a chance. Look how dumbfounded the midwives are. They've refused and I'm saved." No sooner had I thought this than some other being spoke for me in a voice that was not mine:

"Look, have you gone mad? What do you mean by not agreeing? You're condemning the baby to death. You must consent. Have you no pity?"

"No!" the mother shouted once more. I thought to myself: "What am I doing? I shall only kill the child." But I said:

"Come on, come on—you've got to agree! You must! Look, her nails are already turning blue."

"No, no!"

"All right, take them to the ward. Let them sit there." They were led away down the half-lit passage. I could hear the weeping of the women and the hissing of the little girl. The *feldsher* returned almost at once and said:

"They've agreed!"

I felt my blood run cold, but I said in a clear voice:

"Sterilize a scalpel, scissors, hooks and a probe at once."

A minute later I was running across the yard, through a swirling, blinding snowstorm. I rushed to my room, and, counting the minutes, grabbed a book, leafed through it and found an illustration of a tracheotomy. Everything about it was clear and simple: the throat was laid open and the knife plunged into the windpipe. I started reading the text, but could take none of it in—the words seemed to jump before my eyes. I had never seen a tracheotomy performed. "Ah well, it's a bit late now," I said to myself, and looked miserably at the green lamp and the clear illustration. Feeling that I had suddenly been burdened with a most fearful and difficult task, I went back to the hospital oblivious of the snowstorm.

In the surgery a dim figure in full skirts clung to me and a voice whined:

"Oh, sir, how can you cut a little girl's throat? How can you? She's agreed to it because she's stupid. But you haven't got my permission—no you haven't. I agree to giving her medicine, but I shan't allow her throat to be cut."

"Get this woman out!" I shouted, and added vehemently: "You're the stupid one! Yes, you are. And she's the clever one. Anyway, nobody asked you! Get her out of here!"

A midwife took a firm hold of the old woman and pushed her out of the room.

"Ready!" the *feldsher* said suddenly.

We went into the small operating theatre; the shiny instruments, blinding lamplight and oilcloth seemed to belong to another world . . . for the last time I went out to the mother, and the little girl could scarcely be torn from her arms. She just said in a hoarse voice: "My husband's away in town. When he comes back and finds out what I've done he'll kill me!"

"Yes, he'll kill her," the old woman echoed, looking at me in horror.

"Don't let them into the operating theatre!" I ordered.

So we were left in the operating theatre, my assistants, myself, and Lidka, the little girl. She sat naked and pathetic on the table and wept soundlessly. They laid her on the table, strapped her down, washed her throat and painted it with iodine. I picked up a scalpel, still wondering what on earth I was doing. It was very quiet. With the scalpel I made a vertical incision down the swollen white throat. Not one drop of blood emerged. Again I drew the knife along the white strip which protruded between the slit skin. Again not a trace of blood. Slowly, trying to remember the illustrations in my textbooks, I started to part the delicate tissues with the blunt probe. At once dark blood gushed out from the lower end of the wound, flooding it instantly and pouring down her neck. The *feldsher* started to staunch it with swabs but could not stop the flow. Calling to mind everything I had seen at university, I set about clamping the edges of the wound with forceps, but this did no good either.

I went cold and my forehead broke out in a sweat. I bitterly regretted having studied medicine and having landed myself in this wilderness. In angry desperation I jabbed the forceps haphazardly into the region of the wound, snapped them shut and the flow of blood stopped immediately. We swabbed the wound with pieces of gauze; now it faced me clean and absolutely incomprehensible. There was no windpipe anywhere to be seen. This wound of mine was quite unlike any illustration. I spent the next two or three minutes aimlessly poking about in the wound, first with the scalpel and then with the probe, searching for the windpipe. After two minutes of this, I despaired of finding it. "This is the end," I thought. "Why did I ever do this? I needn't have offered to do the operation, and Lidka could have died quietly in the ward. As it is she will die with her throat slit open and I can never prove that she would have died anyway, that I couldn't have made it any worse. . . . " The midwife wiped my brow in silence. "I ought to put down my scalpel and say: I don't know what to do next." As I thought this I pictured the mother's eyes. I picked up the knife again and made a deep, undirected slash into Lidka's neck. The tissues parted and to my surprise the windpipe appeared before me.

"Hooks!" I croaked hoarsely.

The *feldsher* handed them to me. I pierced each side with a hook and handed one of them to him. Now I could see one thing only: the greyish ringlets of the windpipe. I thrust the sharp knife into it—and froze in horror. The windpipe was coming out of the incision and the *feldsher* appeared to have taken leave of his wits: he was tearing it out. Behind me the two midwives gasped. I looked up and saw what was the matter: the *feldsher* had fainted from the oppressive heat and, still holding the hook, was tearing at the windpipe. "It's fate," I thought, "everything's against me. We've certainly murdered Lidka now." And I added grimly to myself: "As soon as I get back to my room, I'll shoot myself." Then the older midwife, who was evidently very experienced, pounced on the *feldsher* and tore the hook out of his hand, saying through her clenched teeth:

"Go on, doctor. . . . "

The *feldsher* collapsed to the floor with a crash but we did not turn to look at him. I plunged the scalpel into the trachea and then inserted a silver tube. It slid in easily but Lidka remained motionless. The air did not flow into her windpipe as it should have done. I sighed deeply and stopped: I had done all I could. I felt like begging someone's forgiveness for having been so thoughtless as to study medicine. Silence reigned. I could see Lidka turning blue. I was just about to give up and weep, when the child suddenly gave a violent convulsion, expelled a fountain of disgusting clotted matter through the tube, and the air whistled into her windpipe. As she started to breathe, the little girl began to howl. That instant the *feldsher* got to his feet, pale and sweaty, looked at her throat in stupefied horror and helped me to sew it up.

Dazed, my vision blurred by a film of sweat, I saw the happy faces of the midwives and one of them said to me:

"You did the operation brilliantly, doctor."

I thought she was making fun of me and glowered at her. Then the doors were opened and a gust of fresh air blew in. Lidka was carried out wrapped in a sheet and at once the mother appeared in the doorway. Her eyes had the look of a wild beast. She asked me:

"Well?"

When I heard the sound of her voice, I felt a cold sweat run down my back as I realized what it would have been like if Lidka had died on the table. But I answered her in a very calm voice:

"Don't worry, she's alive. And she'll stay alive, I hope. Only she won't be able to talk until we take the pipe out, so don't let that upset you."

Just then the grandmother seemed to materialize from nowhere and crossed herself, bowing to the door handle, to me, and to the ceiling. This time I did not lose my temper with her, I turned away and ordered Lidka to be given a camphor injection and for the staff to take turns at watching her. Then I went across the yard to my quarters. I remember the green lamp burning in my study, Döderlein lying there and books scattered everywhere. I walked over to the couch fully dressed, lay down and was immediately lost to the world in a dreamless sleep.

A month passed, then another. I grew more experienced and some of the things I saw were rather more frightening than Lidka's throat, which passed out of my mind. Snow lay all around, and the size of my practice grew daily. Early in the new year, a woman came to my surgery holding by the hand a little girl wrapped in so many layers that she looked as round as a little barrel. The woman's eyes were shining. I took a good look and recognized them.

"Ah, Lidka! How are things?"

"Everything's fine."

The mother unwound the scarves from Lidka's neck. Though she was shy and resisted I managed to raise her chin and took a look. Her pink neck was marked with a brown vertical scar crossed by two fine stitch marks.

"All's well," I said. "You needn't come any more."

"Thank you, doctor, thank you," the mother said, and turned to Lidka: "Say thank you to the gentleman!"

But Lidka had no wish to speak to me.

I never saw her again. Gradually I forgot about her. Meanwhile my practice still grew. The day came when I had a hundred and ten patients. We began at nine in the morning and finished at eight in the evening. Reeling with fatigue, I was taking off my overall when the senior midwife said to me:

"It's the tracheotomy that has brought you all these patients. Do you know what they're saying in the villages? The story goes that when Lidka was ill a steel throat was put into her instead of her own and then sewn up. People go to her village especially to look at her. There's fame for you, doctor. Congratulations."

"So they think she's living with a steel one now, do they?" I enquired.

"That's right. But you were wonderful, doctor. You did it so coolly, it was marvelous to watch."

"Hm, well, I never allow myself to worry, you know," I said, not knowing why. I was too tired even to feel ashamed, so I just looked away. I said goodnight and went home. Snow was falling in large flakes, covering everything, the lantern was lit and my house looked silent, solitary and imposing. As I walked I had only one desire—sleep.

THIS RED OOZING

JEANNE BRYNER

I'm a nurse in emergency.
You're a hostess at Benny's Lounge,
thirty-five, divorced. After three beers,
you can never let the friend of a friend
drop you off at your apartment,
then ask him in for coffee.

Never pee with an accountant in the house,
especially one dragging his briefcase.
See how the balding sheriff shakes
his *I-told-you-so eyes*
while you tell how the man shoved
your bathroom door open,
pulled out his revolver, grinned.

We know what he said next; we hear it
nearly every week: *I'm gonna fuck you;*
you scream, I'll kill you.
We believe you cried, begged on knees,
told him your kids might be home soon.
You kneeling on the fuzzy pink rug—
he likes that—you genuflecting.

"This Red Oozing" first appeared in the *Texas Journal of Women & the Law* 3 (1994): 447–48, and was included in Jeanne Bryner's volumes *Breathless* (Kent: Kent State UP, 1995) and *Tenderly Lift Me: Nurses Honored, Celebrated and Remembered* (Kent: Kent State UP, 2004). Reprinted by permission of the *Texas Journal of Women & the Law,* 3 Tex. J. Women & L. 447–48 (1994).

The safety clicks on his forty-five.
You know guns; your father hunted—
black roundness against your right temple,
your hoop earrings clang, train whistles
in your ears and his words squeeze:
suck hard bitch.

We're sorry, but now the doctor
makes you say all of it again,
how a single lamp burns on the nightstand
and your kids smile in their school pictures.
How tight he holds the cold muzzle to your neck,
jerks your dark hair like a mane and rips
you until you bleed, your breath becomes
grunts, your face in a pillow.

Doctors in the ER speak like priests,
and they try to explain it, clean it up
when they swab, hunting for sperm, trying
to mount rage on slides—dead or alive.

This red oozing,
this trail from your buttocks to your thighs
will not fill him, and it doesn't matter
how many times you throw up green
or call on God or bruises rise
like small iris on your cheekbones,
the razor moves on.

The friend of your friend
with the pinstriped suit will probably walk.
I think you know that.
What you don't know is how he rapes you
endlessly: how he crawls out of your lipstick
tube in the morning, slithers out of the soapy
washcloth in the shower, snickers every Friday
when you dust those photos on your stand.
How his boots climb the back stairs
of your mind year after year
as he comes and comes and comes.

A JURY OF HER PEERS

SUSAN GLASPELL

When Martha Hale opened the storm-door and got a cut of the north wind, she ran back for her big woolen scarf. As she hurriedly wound that round her head her eye made a scandalized sweep of her kitchen. It was no ordinary thing that called her away—it was probably further from ordinary than anything that had ever happened in Dickson County. But what her eye took in was that her kitchen was in no shape for leaving: her bread all ready for mixing, half the flour sifted and half unsifted.

She hated to see things half done; but she had been at that when the team from town stopped to get Mr. Hale, and then the sheriff came running in to say his wife wished Mrs. Hale would come too—adding, with a grin, that he guessed she was getting scary and wanted another woman along. So she had dropped everything right where it was.

"Martha!" now came her husband's impatient voice. "Don't keep folks waiting out here in the cold."

She again opened the storm-door, and this time joined the three men and the one woman waiting for her in the big two-seated buggy.

After she had the robes tucked around her she took another look at the woman who sat beside her on the back seat. She had met Mrs. Peters the year before at the county fair, and the thing she remembered about her was that she didn't seem like a sheriff's wife. She was small and thin and didn't have a strong voice. Mrs. Gorman, sheriff's wife before Gorman went out and Peters came in, had a voice that somehow seemed to be backing up the law with every word. But if Mrs. Peters didn't look like a sheriff's wife, Peters made it up in looking like a sheriff. He was to a dot the kind of man who could get himself elected sheriff—a heavy man with a big voice, who was particularly genial with the law-abiding, as if to make it plain that he knew the difference between criminals and non-criminals. And right there it came into Mrs. Hale's

Glaspell wrote "A Jury of Her Peers" in 1917, based on her play of the previous year, *Trifles.* The version that appears here is from *Women in the Trees: U.S. Women's Short Stories about Battering and Resistance, 1839–1994,* edited by Susan Koppelman (Boston: Beacon, 1996).

mind, with a rub, that this man who was so pleasant and lively with all of them was going to the Wrights' now as sheriff.

"The country's not very pleasant this time of year," Mrs. Peters at last ventured, as if she felt they ought to be talking as well as the men.

Mrs. Hale scarcely finished her reply, for they had gone up a little hill and could see the Wright place now, and seeing it did not make her feel like talking. It looked very lonesome this cold March morning. It had always been a lonesome-looking place. It was down in a hollow, and the poplar trees around it were lonesome-looking trees. The men were looking at it and talking about what had happened. The county attorney was bending to one side of the buggy, and kept looking steadily at the place as they drew up to it.

"I'm glad you came with me," Mrs. Peters said nervously, as the two women were about to follow the men in through the kitchen door.

Even after she had her foot on the door-step, her hand on the knob, Martha Hale had a moment of feeling she could not cross that threshold. And the reason it seemed she couldn't cross it now was simply because she hadn't crossed it before. Time and time again it had been in her mind, "I ought to go over and see Minnie Foster"—she still thought of her as Minnie Foster, though for twenty years she had been Mrs. Wright. And then there was always something to do and Minnie Foster would go from her mind. But *now* she could come.

* * * * *

The men went over to the stove. The women stood close together by the door. Young Henderson, the county attorney, turned around and said, "Come up to the fire, ladies."

Mrs. Peters took a step forward, then stopped. "I'm not—cold," she said.

And so the two women stood by the door, at first not even so much as looking around the kitchen.

The men talked for a minute about what a good thing it was the sheriff had sent his deputy out that morning to make a fire for them, and then Sheriff Peters stepped back from the stove, unbuttoned his outer coat, and leaned his hands on the kitchen table in a way that seemed to mark the beginning of official business. "Now, Mr. Hale," he said in a sort of semi-official voice, "before we move things about, you tell Mr. Henderson just what it was you saw when you came here yesterday morning."

The county attorney was looking around the kitchen.

"By the way," he said, "has anything been moved?" He turned to the sheriff. "Are things just as you left them yesterday?"

Peters looked from cupboard to sink; from that to a small worn rocker a little to one side of the kitchen table.

"It's just the same."

"Somebody should have been left here yesterday," said the county attorney.

"Oh—yesterday," returned the sheriff, with a little gesture as of yesterday having been more than he could bear to think of. "When I had to send Frank to Morris Center for that man who went crazy—let me tell you, I had my hands full *yesterday.* I knew you could get back from Omaha by today, George, and as long as I went over everything here myself—"

"Well, Mr. Hale," said the county attorney, in a way of letting what was past and gone go, "tell just what happened when you came here yesterday morning."

Mrs. Hale, still leaning against the door, had that sinking feeling of the mother whose child is about to speak a piece. Lewis often wandered along and got things mixed up in a story. She hoped he would tell this straight and plain, and not say unnecessary things that would just make things harder for Minnie Foster. He didn't begin at once, and she noticed that he looked queer—as if standing in that kitchen and having to tell what he had seen there yesterday morning made him almost sick.

"Yes, Mr. Hale?" the county attorney reminded.

"Harry and I had started to town with a load of potatoes," Mrs. Hale's husband began.

Harry was Mrs. Hale's oldest boy. He wasn't with them now, for the very good reason that those potatoes never got to town yesterday and he was taking them this morning, so he hadn't been home when the sheriff stopped to say he wanted Mr. Hale to come over to the Wright place and tell the county attorney his story there, where he could point it all out. With all Mrs. Hale's other emotions came the fear now that maybe Harry wasn't dressed warm enough—they hadn't any of them realized how that north wind did bite.

"We come along this road," Hale was going on, with a motion of his hand to the road over which they had just come, "and as we got in sight of the house I says to Harry, 'I'm goin' to see if I can't get John Wright to take a telephone.' You see," he explained to Henderson, "unless I can get somebody to go in with me they won't come out this branch road except for a price I can't pay. I'd spoke to Wright about it once before; but he put me off, saying folks talked too much anyway, and all he asked was peace and quiet—guess you know about how much he talked himself. But I thought maybe if I went to the house and talked about it before his wife, and said all the women-folks liked the telephones, and that in this lonesome stretch of road it would be a good thing—well, I said to Harry that that was what I was going to say—though I said at the same time that I didn't know as what his wife wanted made much difference to John—"

Now there he was!—saying things he didn't need to say. Mrs. Hale tried to catch her husband's eye, but fortunately the county attorney interrupted with:

"Let's talk about that a little later, Mr. Hale. I do want to talk about that, but I'm anxious now to get along to just what happened when you got here."

When he began this time, it was very deliberately and carefully:

"I didn't see or hear anything. I knocked at the door. And still it was all quiet inside. I knew they must be up—it was past eight o'clock. So I knocked again, louder, and I thought I heard somebody say, 'Come in.' I wasn't sure—I'm not sure yet. But I opened the door—this door," jerking a hand toward the door by which the two women stood, "and there, in that rocker"—pointing to it—"sat Mrs. Wright."

Everyone in the kitchen looked at the rocker. It came into Mrs. Hale's mind that that rocker didn't look in the least like Minnie Foster—the Minnie Foster of twenty years before. It was a dingy red, with wooden rungs up the back, and the middle rung was gone, and the chair sagged to one side.

"How did she—look?" the county attorney was inquiring.

"Well," said Hale, "she looked—queer."

"How do you mean—queer?"

As he asked it he took out a note-book and pencil. Mrs. Hale did not like the sight of that pencil. She kept her eye fixed on her husband, as if to keep him from saying unnecessary things that would go into that note-book and make trouble.

Hale did speak guardedly, as if the pencil had affected him too.

"Well, as if she didn't know what she was going to do next. And kind of—done up."

"How did she seem to feel about your coming?"

"Why, I don't think she minded—one way or other. She didn't pay much attention. I said, 'Ho' do, Mrs. Wright? It's cold, ain't it?' And she said, 'Is it?'—and went on pleatin' at her apron.

"Well, I was surprised. She didn't ask me to come up to the stove, or to sit down, but just set there, not even lookin' at me. And so I said: 'I want to see John.'

"And then she—laughed. I guess you would call it a laugh.

"I thought of Harry and the team outside, so I said, a little sharp, 'Can I see John?' 'No,' says she—kind of dull like. 'Ain't he home?' says I. Then she looked at me. 'Yes,' says she, 'he's home.' 'Then why can't I see him?' I asked her, out of patience with her now. 'Cause he's dead,' says she, just as quiet and dull—and fell to pleatin' her apron. 'Dead?' says I, like you do when you can't take in what you've heard.

"She just nodded her head, not getting a bit excited, but rockin' back and forth.

"'Why—where is he?' says I, not knowing what to say.

"She just pointed upstairs—like this"—pointing to the room above.

"I got up, with the idea of going up there myself. By this time I—didn't know what to do. I walked from there to here; then I says: 'Why, what did he die of?'

"'He died of a rope round his neck,' says she; and just went on pleatin' at her apron."

* * * * *

Hale stopped speaking, and stood staring at the rocker, as if he were still seeing the woman who had sat there the morning before. Nobody spoke; it was as if every one were seeing the woman who had sat there the morning before.

"And what did you do then?" the county attorney at last broke the silence.

"I went out and called Harry. I thought I might—need help. I got Harry in, and we went upstairs." His voice felt almost to a whisper. "There he was—lying over the—"

"I think I'd rather have you go into that upstairs," the county attorney interrupted, "where you can point it all out. Just go on now with the rest of the story."

"Well, my first thought was to get that rope off. It looked—"

He stopped, his face twitching.

"But Harry, he went up to him, and he said, 'No, he's dead all right, and we'd better not touch anything.' So we went downstairs.

"She was still sitting that same way. 'Has anybody been notified?' I asked. 'No,' says she, unconcerned.

"'Who did this, Mrs. Wright?' said Harry. He said it businesslike, and she stopped pleatin' at her apron. 'I don't know,' she says. 'You don't *know*?' says Harry. 'Weren't you sleepin' in the bed with him?' 'Yes,' says she, 'but I was on the inside.' 'Somebody slipped a rope round his neck and strangled him, and you didn't wake up?' says Harry. 'I didn't wake up,' she said after him.

"We may have looked as if we didn't see how that could be, for after a minute she said, 'I sleep sound.'

"Harry was going to ask her more questions, but I said maybe that weren't our business: maybe we ought to let her tell her story first to the coroner or the sheriff. So Harry went fast as he could over to High Road—the Rivers' place, where there's a telephone."

"And what did she do when she knew you had gone for the coroner?" The attorney got his pencil in his hand all ready for writing.

"She moved from that chair to this one over here"—Hale pointed to a small chair in the corner—"and just sat there with her hands held together and looking down. I got a feeling that I ought to make some conversation, so I said I had come in to see if John wanted to put in a telephone; and at that she started to laugh, and then she stopped and looked at me—scared."

At the sound of a moving pencil the man who was telling the story looked up.

"I dunno—maybe it wasn't scared," he hastened; "I wouldn't like to say it was. Soon Harry got back, and then Dr. Lloyd came, and you, Mr. Peters, and so I guess that's all I know that you don't."

* * * * *

He said that last with relief, and moved a little, as if relaxing. Every one moved a little. The county attorney walked toward the stair door.

"I guess we'll go upstairs first—then out to the barn and around there."

He paused and looked around the kitchen.

"You're convinced there was nothing important here?" he asked the sheriff. "Nothing that would—point to any motive?"

The sheriff too looked all around, as if to re-convince himself.

"Nothing here but kitchen things," he said, with a little laugh for the insignificance of kitchen things.

The county attorney was looking at the cupboard—a peculiar, ungainly structure, half closet and half cupboard, the upper part of it being built in the wall, and the lower part just the old-fashioned kitchen cupboard. As if its queerness attracted him, he got a chair and opened the upper part and looked in. After a moment he drew his hand away sticky.

"Here's a nice mess," he said resentfully.

The two women had drawn nearer, and now the sheriff's wife spoke.

"Oh—her fruit," she said, looking to Mrs. Hale for sympathetic understanding. She turned back to the county attorney and explained: "She worried about that when it turned so cold last night. She said the fire would go out and her jars might burst."

Mrs. Peters' husband broke into a laugh.

"Well, can you beat the women! Held for murder, and worrying about her preserves!"

The young attorney set his lips.

"I guess before we're through with her she may have something more serious than preserves to worry about."

"Oh, well," said Mrs. Hale's husband, with good-natured superiority, "women are used to worrying over trifles."

The two women moved a little closer together. Neither of them spoke. The county attorney seemed suddenly to remember his manners—and think of his future.

"And yet," said he, with the gallantry of a young politician, "for all their worries, what would we do without the ladies?"

The women did not speak, did not unbend. He went to the sink and began washing his hands. He turned to wipe them on the roller towel—whirled it for a cleaner place.

"Dirty towels! Not much of a housekeeper, would you say, ladies?"

He kicked his foot against some dirty pans under the sink.

"There's a great deal of work to be done on a farm," said Mrs. Hale stiffly.

"To be sure. And yet"—with a little bow to her—"I know there are some Dickson County farm-houses that do not have such roller towels." He gave it a pull to expose its full length again.

"Those towels get dirty awful quick. Men's hands aren't always as clean as they might be."

"Ah, loyal to your sex, I see," he laughed. He stopped and gave her a keen look. "But you and Mrs. Wright were neighbors. I suppose you were friends, too."

Martha Hale shook her head.

"I've seen little enough of her of late years. I've not been in this house—it's more than a year."

"And why was that? You didn't like her?"

"I like her well enough." she replied with spirit. "Farmers' wives have their hands full, Mr. Henderson. And then—" She looked around the kitchen.

"Yes?" he encouraged.

"It never seemed a very cheerful place," said she, more to herself than to him.

"No," he agreed; "I don't think anyone would call it cheerful. I shouldn't say she had the home-making instinct."

"Well, I don't know as Wright had, either," she muttered.

"You mean they didn't get on very well?" he was quick to ask.

"No; I don't mean anything," she answered, with decision. As she turned a little away from him, she added: "But I don't think a place would be any the cheerfuler for John Wright's bein' in it."

"I'd like to talk to you about that a little later, Mrs. Hale," he said. "I'm anxious to get the lay of things upstairs now."

He moved toward the stair door, followed by the two men.

"I suppose anything Mrs. Peters does'll be all right?" the sheriff inquired. "She was to take in some clothes for her, you know—and a few little things. We left in such a hurry yesterday."

The county attorney looked at the two women whom they were leaving alone there among the kitchen things.

"Yes—Mrs. Peters," he said, his glance resting on the woman who was not Mrs. Peters, the big farmer woman who stood behind the sheriff's wife. "Of course Mrs. Peters is one of us," he said, in a manner of entrusting responsibility. "And keep your eye out, Mrs. Peters, for anything that might be of use. No telling: you women might come upon a clue to the motive—and that's the thing we need."

Mr. Hale rubbed his face after the fashion of a showman getting ready for a pleasantry.

"But would the women know a clue if they did come upon it?" he said; and, having delivered himself of this, he followed the others through the stair door.

* * * * *

The women stood motionless and silent, listening to the footsteps, first upon the stairs, then in the room above them.

Then, as if releasing herself from something strange, Mrs. Hale began to arrange the dirty pans under the sink, which the county attorney's disdainful push of the foot had deranged.

"I'd hate to have men comin' into my kitchen," she said testily—"snoopin' round and criticizin'."

"Of course it's no more than their duty," said the sheriff's wife, in her manner of timid acquiescence.

"Duty's all right," replied Mrs. Hale bluffly; "but I guess that deputy sheriff that come out to make the fire might have got a little of this on." She gave the roller towel a pull. "Wish I'd thought of that sooner! Seems mean to talk about her for not having things slicked up, when she has to come away in such a hurry."

She looked around the kitchen. Certainly it was not "slicked up." Her eye was held by a bucket of sugar on a low shelf. The cover was off the wooden bucket, and beside it was a paper bag—half full.

Mrs. Hale moved toward it.

"She was putting this in there," she said to herself—slowly.

She thought of the flour in her kitchen at home—half sifted, half not sifted. She had been interrupted, and had left things half done. What had interrupted Minnie Foster? Why had that work been left half done? She made a move as if to finish it—unfinished things always bothered her—and then she glanced around and saw that Mrs. Peters was watching her—and she didn't want Mrs. Peters to get that feeling she had got of work begun and then—for some reason—not finished.

"It's a shame about her fruit," she said, and walked toward the cupboard that the county attorney had opened, and got on the chair, murmuring: "I wonder if it's all gone."

It was a sorry enough looking sight, but "Here's one that's all right," she said at last. She held it toward the light. "This is cherries, too." She looked again. "I declare I believe that's the only one."

With a sigh, she got down from the chair, went to the sink, and wiped off the bottle.

"She'll feel awful bad, after all her hard work in the hot weather. I remember the afternoon I put up my cherries last summer."

She set the bottle on the table, and, with another sigh, started to sit down in the rocker. But she did not sit down. Something kept her from sitting down in that chair. She straightened—stepped back, and, half turned away, stood looking at it, seeing the woman who had sat there "pleatin' at her apron."

The thin voice of the sheriff's wife broke in upon her: "I must be getting those things from the front-room closet." She opened the door into the other room, started in, stepped back. "You coming with me, Mrs. Hale?" she asked nervously. "You—you could help me get them."

They were soon back—the stark coldness of that shut-up room was not a thing to linger in.

"My!" said Mrs. Peters, dropping the things on the table and hurrying to the stove.

Mrs. Hale stood examining the clothes the woman who was being detained in town had said she wanted.

"Wright was close!" she exclaimed, holding up a shabby black skirt that bore the marks of much making over. "I think maybe that's why she kept so much to herself. I s'pose she felt she couldn't do her part; and then, you don't enjoy things when you feel shabby. She used to wear pretty clothes and be lively—when she was Minnie Foster, one of the town girls, singing in the choir. But that—oh, that was twenty years ago."

With a carefulness in which there was something tender, she folded the shabby clothes and piled them at one corner of the table. She looked up at Mrs. Peters, and there was something in the other woman's look that irritated her.

"She don't care," she said to herself. "Much difference it makes to her whether Minnie Foster had pretty clothes when she was a girl."

Then she looked again, and she wasn't so sure; in fact, she hadn't at any time been perfectly sure about Mrs. Peters. She had that shrinking manner, and yet her eyes looked as if they could see a long way into things.

"This all you was to take in?" asked Mrs. Hale.

"No," said the sheriff's wife; "she said she wanted an apron. Funny thing to want," she ventured in her nervous little way, "for there's not much to get you dirty in jail, goodness knows. But I suppose just to make her feel more natural. If you're used to wearing an apron—. She said they were in the bottom drawer of this cupboard. Yes—here they are. And then her little shawl that always hung on the stair door."

She took the small gray shawl from behind the door leading upstairs, and stood a minute looking at it.

Suddenly Mrs. Hale took a quick step toward the other woman.

"Mrs. Peters!"

"Yes, Mrs. Hale?"

"Do you think she—did it?"

A frightened look blurred the other thing in Mrs. Peters' eyes.

"Oh, I don't know," she said, in a voice that seemed to shrink away from the subject.

"Well, I don't think she did," affirmed Mrs. Hale stoutly. "Asking for an apron, and her little shawl. Worryin' about her fruit."

"Mr. Peters says—." Footsteps were heard in the room above; she stopped, looked up, then went on in a lowered voice: "Mr. Peters says—it looks bad for her. Mr. Henderson is awful sarcastic in a speech, and he's going to make fun of her saying she didn't—wake up."

For a moment Mrs. Hale had no answer. Then, "Well, I guess John Wright didn't wake up—when they was slippin' that rope under his neck," she muttered.

"No, it's *strange,*" breathed Mrs. Peters. "They think it was such a—funny way to kill a man."

She began to laugh; at the sound of the laugh, abruptly stopped.

"That's just what Mr. Hale said," said Mrs. Hale, in a resolutely natural voice. "There was a gun in the house. He says that's what he can't understand."

"Mr. Henderson said, coming out, that what was needed for the case was a motive. Something to show anger—or sudden feeling."

"Well, I don't see any signs of anger around here," said Mrs. Hale. "I don't—"

She stopped. It was as if her mind tripped on something. Her eye was caught by a dish-towel in the middle of the kitchen table. Slowly she moved toward the table. One half of it was wiped clean, the other half messy. Her eyes made a slow, almost unwilling turn to the bucket of sugar and the half empty bag beside it. Things begun—and not finished.

After a moment she stepped back, and said, in that manner of releasing herself:

"Wonder how they're finding things upstairs? I hope she had it a little more red up up there. You know,"—she paused, and feeling gathered—"it seems kind of *sneaking*: locking her up in town and coming out here to get her own house to turn against her!"

"But, Mrs. Hale," said the sheriff's wife, "the law is the law."

"I s'pose 'tis," answered Mrs. Hale shortly.

She turned to the stove, saying something about that fire not being much to brag of. She worked with it a minute, and when she straightened up she said aggressively:

"The law is the law—and a bad stove is a bad stove. How'd you like to cook on this?"—pointing with the poker to the broken lining. She opened the oven door and started to express her opinion of the oven; but she was swept into her own thoughts, thinking of what it would mean, year after year, to have that stove to wrestle with. The thought of Minnie Foster trying to bake in that oven—and the thought of her never going over to see Minnie Foster—.

She was startled by hearing Mrs. Peters say: "A person gets discouraged—and loses heart."

The sheriff's wife had looked from the stove to the sink—to the pail of water which had been carried in from outside. The two women stood there silent, above them the footsteps of the men who were looking for evidence against the woman who had worked in that kitchen. That look of seeing into things, of seeing through a thing to something else, was in the eyes of the sheriff's wife now. When Mrs. Hale next spoke to her, it was gently:

"Better loosen up your things, Mrs. Peters. We'll not feel them when we go out."

Mrs. Peters went to the back of the room to hang up the fur tippet she was wearing. A moment later she exclaimed, "Why, she was piecing a quilt," and held up a large sewing basket piled high with quilt pieces.

Mrs. Hale spread some of the blocks on the table.

"It's log-cabin pattern," she said, putting several of them together. "Pretty, isn't it?"

They were so engaged with the quilt that they did not hear the footsteps on the stairs. Just as the stair door opened Mrs. Hale was saying:

"Do you suppose she was going to quilt it or just knot it?"

The sheriff threw up his hands.

"They wonder whether she was going to quilt it or just knot it!"

There was a laugh for the ways of women, a warming of hands over the stove, and then the county attorney said briskly:

"Well, let's go right out to the barn and get that cleared up."

"I don't see as there's anything so strange," Mrs. Hale said resentfully, after the outside door had closed on the three men—"our taking up our time with little things while we're waiting for them to get the evidence. I don't see as it's anything to laugh about."

"Of course they've got awful important things on their minds," said the sheriff's wife apologetically.

They returned to an inspection of the block for the quilt. Mrs. Hale was looking at the fine, even sewing, and preoccupied with thoughts of the woman who had done that sewing, when she heard the sheriff's wife say, in a queer tone:

"Why, look at this one."

She turned to take the block held out to her.

"The sewing," said Mrs. Peters, in a troubled way. "All the rest of them have been so nice and even—but—this one. Why it looks as if she didn't know what she was about!"

Their eyes met—something flashed to life, passed between them; then, as if with an effort, they seemed to pull away from each other. A moment Mrs. Hale sat there, her hands folded over that sewing which was so unlike all the rest of the sewing. Then she had pulled a knot and drawn the threads.

"Oh, what are you doing, Mrs. Hale?" asked the sheriff's wife, startled.

"Just pulling out a stitch or two that's not sewed very good," said Mrs. Hale mildly.

"I don't think we ought to touch things," Mrs. Peters said, a little helplessly.

"I'll just finish up this end," answered Mrs. Hale, still in that mild, matter-of-fact fashion.

She threaded a needle and started to replace bad sewing with good. For a little while she sewed in silence. Then, in that thin, timid voice, she heard:

"Mrs. Hale!"

"Yes, Mrs. Peters?"

"What do you suppose she was so—nervous about?"

"Oh, *I* don't know," said Mrs. Hale, as if dismissing a thing not important enough to spend much time on. "I don't know as she was—nervous. I sew awful queer sometimes when I'm just tired."

She cut a thread, and out of the corner of her eye looked up at Mrs. Peters. The small, lean face of the sheriff's wife seemed to have tightened up. Her eyes had that look of peering into something. But next moment she moved, and said in her thin, indecisive way:

"Well, I must get those clothes wrapped. They may be through sooner than we think. I wonder where I could find a piece of paper—and string."

"In that cupboard, maybe," suggested Mrs. Hale, after a glance around.

* * * * *

One piece of the crazy sewing remained unripped. Mrs. Peters' back turned, Martha Hale now scrutinized that piece, compared it with the dainty, accurate sewing of the other blocks. The difference was startling. Holding this block made her feel queer, as if the distracted thoughts of the woman who had perhaps turned to it to try to quiet herself were communicating themselves to her.

Mrs. Peters' voice roused her.

"Here's a bird-cage," she said. "Did she have a bird, Mrs. Hale?"

"Why, I don't know whether she did or not." She turned to look at the cage Mrs. Peters was holding up. "I've not been here in so long." She sighed. "There was a man round last year selling canaries cheap—but I don't know as she took one. Maybe she did. She use to sing real pretty herself."

Mrs. Peters looked around the kitchen.

"Seems kind of funny to think of a bird here." She half laughed—an attempt to put up a barrier. "But she must have had one—or why would she have a cage? I wonder what happened to it."

"I suppose maybe the cat got it," suggested Mrs. Hale, resuming her sewing.

"No, she didn't have a cat. She's got that feeling some people have about cats—being afraid of them. When they brought her to our house yesterday, my cat got in the room, and she was real upset and asked me to take it out."

"My sister Bessie was like that," laughed Mrs. Hale.

The sheriff's wife did not reply. The silence made Mrs. Hale turn round. Mrs. Peters was examining the bird-cage.

"Look at this door," she said slowly. "It's broke. One hinge has been pulled apart."

Mrs. Hale came nearer.

"Looks as if someone must have been—rough with it."

Again their eyes met—startled, questioning, apprehensive. For a moment neither spoke nor stirred. Then Mrs. Hale, turning away, said brusquely:

"If they're going to find any evidence, I wish they'd be about it. I don't like this place."

"But I'm awful glad you came with me, Mrs. Hale." Mrs. Peters put the bird-cage on the table and sat down. "It would be lonesome for me—sitting here alone."

"Yes, it would, wouldn't it?" agreed Mrs. Hale, a certain determined naturalness in her voice. She had picked up the sewing, but now it dropped in her lap, and she murmured in a different voice: "But I tell you what I *do* wish, Mrs. Peters. I wish I had come over sometimes when she was here. I wish—I had."

"But of course you were awful busy, Mrs. Hale. Your house—and your children."

"I could've come," retorted Mrs. Hale shortly. "I stayed away because it weren't cheerful—and that's why I ought to have come. I"—she looked around—"I've never liked this place. Maybe because it's down in a hollow and you don't see the road. I don't know what it is, but it's a lonesome place, and always was. I wish I had come over to see Minnie Foster sometimes. I can see now—" She did not put it into words.

"Well, you mustn't reproach yourself," counseled Mrs. Peters. "Somehow, we just don't see how it is with other folks till—something comes up."

"Not having children makes less work," mused Mrs. Hale, after a silence, "but it makes a quiet house—and Wright out to work all day—and no company when he did come in. Did you know John Wright, Mrs. Peters?"

"Not to know him. I've seen him in town. They say he was a good man."

"Yes—good," conceded John Wright's neighbor grimly. "He didn't drink, and kept his word as well as most, I guess, and paid his debts. But he was a hard man, Mrs. Peters. Just to pass the time of day with him—." She stopped, shivered a little. "Like a raw wind that gets to the bone." Her eye fell upon the cage on the table before her, and she added, almost bitterly: "I should think she would've wanted a bird!"

Suddenly she leaned forward, looking intently at the cage. "But what do you s'pose went wrong with it?"

"I don't know," returned Mrs. Peters; "unless it got sick and died."

But after she said it she reached over and swung the broken door. Both women watched it as if somehow held by it.

"You didn't know—her?" Mrs. Hale asked, a gentler note in her voice.

"Not till they brought her yesterday," said the sheriff's wife.

"She—come to think of it, she was kind of like a bird herself. Real sweet and pretty, but kind of timid and—fluttery. How—she—did—change."

That held her for a long time. Finally, as if struck with a happy thought and relieved to get back to everyday things, she exclaimed:

"Tell you what, Mrs. Peters, why don't you take the quilt in with you? It might take up her mind."

"Why, I think that's a real nice idea, Mrs. Hale," agreed the sheriff's wife, as if she too were glad to come into the atmosphere of a simple kindness. "There couldn't possibly be any objection to that, could there? Now, just what will I take? I wonder if her patches are in here—and her things."

They turned to the sewing basket.

"Here's some red," said Mrs. Hale, bringing out a roll of cloth. Underneath that was a box. "Here, maybe her scissors are in here—and her things." She held it up. "What a pretty box! I'll warrant that was something she had a long time ago—when she was a girl."

She held it in her hand a moment; then, with a little sigh, opened it.

Instantly her hand went to her nose.

"Why—!"

Mrs. Peters drew nearer—then turned away.

"There's something wrapped up in this piece of silk," faltered Mrs. Hale.

"This isn't her scissors," said Mrs. Peters, in a shrinking voice.

Her hand not steady, Mrs. Hale raised the piece of silk. "Oh, Mrs. Peters!" she cried. "It's—"

Mrs. Peters bent closer.

"It's the bird," she whispered.

"But, Mrs. Peters!" cried Mrs. Hale. "*Look* at it! Its *neck*—look at its neck! It's all—other side *to*."

She held the box away from her.

The sheriff's wife again bent closer.

"Somebody wrung its neck," said she, in a voice that was slow and deep.

And then again the eyes of the two women met—this time clung together in a look of dawning comprehension, of growing horror, Mrs. Peters looked from the dead bird to the broken door of the cage. Again their eyes met. And just then there was a sound at the outside door.

Mrs. Hale slipped the box under the quilt pieces in the basket, and sank into the chair before it. Mrs. Peters stood holding to the table. The county attorney and the sheriff came in from outside.

"Well, ladies," said the county attorney, as one turning from serious things to little pleasantries, "have you decided whether she was going to quilt it or knot it?"

"We think," began the sheriff's wife in a flurried voice, "that she was going to—knot it."

He was too preoccupied to notice the change that came in her voice on that last.

"Well, that's very interesting, I'm sure," he said tolerantly. He caught sight of the bird-cage. "Has the bird flown?"

"We think the cat got it," said Mrs. Hale in a voice curiously even.

He was walking up and down, as if thinking something out.

"Is there a cat?" he asked absently.

Mrs. Hale shot a look up at the sheriff's wife.

"Well, not *now,*" said Mrs. Peters. "They're superstitious; they leave."

She sank into her chair.

The county attorney did not heed her. "No sign at all of anyone having come in from the outside," he said to Peters, in the manner of continuing an interrupted conversation. "Their own rope. Now let's go upstairs again and go over it, piece by piece. It would have to have been someone who knew just the—"

The stair door closed behind them and their voices were lost.

The two women sat motionless, not looking at each other, but as if peering into something and at the same time holding back. When they spoke now it was as if they were afraid of what they were saying, but as if they could not help saying it.

"She liked the bird," said Martha Hale, low and slowly. "She was going to bury it in that pretty box."

"When I was a girl," said Mrs. Peters, under her breath, "my kitten—there was a boy took a hatchet, and before my eyes—before I could get there—" She covered her face an instant. "If they hadn't held me back I would have"—she caught herself, looked upstairs where footsteps were heard, and finished weakly—"hurt him."

Then they sat without speaking or moving.

"I wonder how it would seem," Mrs. Hale at last began, as if feeling her way over strange ground—"never to have had any children around?" Her eyes made a slow sweep of the kitchen, as if seeing what that kitchen had meant through all the years. "No, Wright wouldn't like the bird," she said after that—"a thing that sang. She used to sing. He killed that too." Her voice tightened.

Mrs. Peters moved uneasily.

"Of course we don't know who killed the bird."

"I knew John Wright," was Mrs. Hale's answer.

"It was an awful thing was done in this house that night, Mrs. Hale," said the sheriff's wife. "Killing a man while he slept—slipping a thing round his neck that choked the life out of him."

Mrs. Hale's hand went out to the bird cage.

"His neck. Choked the life out of him."

"We don't *know* who killed him," whispered Mrs. Peters wildly. "We don't *know.*"

Mrs. Hale had not moved. "If there had been years and years of—nothing, then a bird to sing to you, it would be awful—still—after the bird was still."

It was as if something within her not herself had spoken, and it found in Mrs. Peters something she did not know as herself.

"I know what stillness is," she said, in a queer, monotonous voice. "When we homesteaded in Dakota, and my first baby died—after he was two years old—and me with no other then—"

Mrs. Hale stirred.

"How soon do you suppose they'll be through looking for the evidence?"

"I know what stillness is," repeated Mrs. Peters, in just that same way. Then she too pulled back. "The law has got to punish crime, Mrs. Hale," she said in her tight little way.

"I wish you'd seen Minnie Foster," was the answer, "when she wore a white dress with blue ribbons, and stood up there in the choir and sang."

The picture of that girl, the fact that she had lived neighbor to that girl for twenty years, and had let her die for lack of life, was suddenly more than she could bear.

"Oh, I *wish* I'd come over here once in a while!" she cried. "That was a crime! That was a crime! Who's going to punish that?"

"We musn't take on," said Mrs. Peters, with a frightened look toward the stairs.

"I might 'a' *known* she needed help! I tell you, it's *queer,* Mrs. Peters. We live close together, and we live far apart. We all go through the same things—it's all just a different kind of the same thing! If it weren't—why do you and I *understand*? Why do we *know*—what we know this minute?"

She dashed her hand across her eyes. Then, seeing the jar of fruit on the table, she reached for it and choked out:

"If I was you I wouldn't *tell* her her fruit was gone! Tell her it *ain't*. Tell her it's all right—all of it. Here—take this in to prove it to her! She—she may never know whether it was broke or not."

She turned away.

Mrs. Peters reached out for the bottle of fruit as if she were glad to take it—as if touching a familiar thing, having something to do, could keep her from something else. She got up, looked about for something to wrap the fruit in, took a petticoat from the pile of clothes she had brought from the front room, and nervously started winding that around the bottle.

"My!" she began, in a high false voice, "it's a good thing the men couldn't hear us! Getting all stirred up over a little thing like a—dead canary." She hurried over that. "As if that could have anything to do with—with—My, wouldn't they *laugh*?"

Footsteps were heard on the stairs.

"Maybe they would," muttered Mrs. Hale—"maybe they wouldn't."

"No, Peters," said the county attorney incisively; "it's all perfectly clear, except the reason for doing it. But you know juries when it comes to women. If there was some definite thing—something to show. Something to make a story about. A thing that would connect up with this clumsy way of doing it."

In a covert way Mrs. Hale looked at Mrs. Peters. Mrs. Peters was looking at her. Quickly they looked away from each other. The outer door opened and Mr. Hale came in.

"I've got the team round now," he said. "Pretty cold out there."

"I'm going to stay here awhile by myself," the county attorney suddenly announced. "You can send Frank out for me, can't you?" he asked the sheriff. "I want to go over everything. I'm not satisfied we can't do better."

Again, for one brief moment, the two women's eyes found one another. The sheriff came up to the table.

"Did you want to see what Mrs. Peters was going to take in?"

The county attorney picked up the apron. He laughed.

"Oh, I guess they're not very dangerous things the ladies have picked out."

Mrs. Hale's hand was on the sewing basket in which the box was concealed. She felt she ought to take her hand off the basket. She did not seem able to. He picked up one of the quilt blocks which she had piled over to cover the box. Her eyes felt like fire. She had a feeling that if he took up the basket she would snatch it from him.

But he did not take it up. With another little laugh, he turned away, saying: "No; Mrs. Peters doesn't need supervising. For that matter, a sheriff's wife is married to the law. Ever think of it that way, Mrs. Peters?"

Mrs. Peters was standing beside the table. Mrs. Hale shot a look up at her; but she could not see her face. Mrs. Peters had turned away. When she spoke, her voice was muffled.

"Not—just that way," she said.

"Married to the law!" chuckled Mrs. Peters' husband. He moved toward the door into the front room, and said to the county attorney:

"I just want you to come in here a minute, George. We ought to take a look at these windows."

"Oh—windows," said the county attorney scoffingly.

"We'll be right out, Mr. Hale," said the sheriff to the farmer, who was still waiting by the door.

Hale went to look after the horses. The sheriff followed the county attorney into the other room. Again—for one final moment—the two women were alone in that kitchen.

Martha Hale sprang up, her hands tight together, looking at that other woman, with whom it rested. At first she could not see her eyes, for the sheriff's wife had not turned back since she turned away at the suggestion of being married to the law. But now Mrs. Hale made her turn back, her eyes made her turn back. Slowly, unwillingly, Mrs. Peters turned her head until her eyes met the eyes of the other woman. There was a moment when they held each other in a steady, burning look in which there was no evasion nor flinching. Then Martha Hale's eyes pointed the way to the basket in which was hidden the thing that would make certain the conviction of the other woman—that woman who was not there and yet who had been there with them all through that hour.

For a moment Mrs. Peters did not move. And then she did it. With a rush forward, she threw back the quilt pieces, got the box, tried to put it in her handbag. It was too big. Desperately she opened, started to take the bird out. But there she broke—she could not touch the bird. She stood there helpless, foolish.

There was the sound of a knob turning in the inner door. Martha Hale snatched the box from the sheriff's wife, and got it in the pocket of her big coat just as the sheriff and the county attorney came back into the kitchen.

"Well, Henry," said the county attorney facetiously, "at least we found out that she was not going to quilt it. She was going to—what is it you call it, ladies?"

Mrs. Hale's hand was against the pocket of her coat.

"We call it—knot it, Mr. Henderson."

BETRAYAL OF "WHAT'S RIGHT"

JONATHAN SHAY

Every instance of severe traumatic psychological injury is a standing challenge to the rightness of the social order.

–Judith Lewis Herman, 1990 Harvard Trauma Conference

We begin in the moral world of the soldier—what his culture understands to be right—and betrayal of that moral order by a commander. This is how Homer opens the *Iliad.* Agamémnon, Achilles' commander, wrongfully seizes the prize of honor voted to Achilles by the troops. Achilles' experience of betrayal of "what's right," and his reactions to it, are identical to those of American soldiers in Vietnam. I shall describe some of the many violations of what American soldiers understood to be right by holders of responsibility and trust.

> Now, there was a LURP [Long Range Reconnaissance Patrol] team from the First Brigade off of Highway One, that looked over the South China Sea. There was a bay there. . . . Now, they saw boats come in. And they suspected, now, uh—the word came down [that] they were unloading weapons off them. Three boats.
>
> At that time we moved. It was about ten o'clock at night. We moved down, across Highway One along the beach line, and it took us [until] about three or four o'clock in the morning to get on line while these people are unloading their boats. And we opened up on them—aaah.
>
> And the fucking firepower was unreal, the firepower that we put into them boats. It was just a constant, constant firepower. It seemed like no one ever ran out of ammo.
>
> Daylight came [long pause], and we found out we killed a lot of fisherman and kids.
>
> What got us thoroughly fucking confused is, at that time you turn to the team and you say to the team, "Don't worry about it. Everything's fucking fine." Because that's what you're getting from upstairs.

> The fucking colonel says, "Don't worry about it. We'll take care of it." Y'know, uh, "We got body count!" "We have body count!" So it starts working on your head.
>
> So you know in your heart it's wrong, but at the time, here's your superiors telling you that it was okay. So, I mean, that's okay then, right? This is part of war. Y'know? Gung-HO! Y'know? "AirBORNE! AirBORNE! Let's go!"
>
> So we packed up and we moved out.They wanted to give us a fucking Unit Citation—them fucking maggots. A lot of medals came down from it. The lieutenants got medals, and I know the colonel got his fucking medal. And they would have award ceremonies, y'know, I'd be standing like a fucking jerk and they'd be handing out fucking medals for killing civilians.

This veteran received his Combat Infantry Badge for participating in the action. The CIB was one of the most prized U.S. Army awards, supposed to be awarded for actual engagement in ground combat. He subsequently earned his CIB a thousand times over in four combat tours. Nonetheless, he still feels deeply dishonored by the circumstances of its official award for killing unarmed civilians on an intelligence error. He declares that the day it happened, Christmas Eve, should be stricken from the calendar.

We shall hear this man's voice and the voices of other combat veterans many times in these pages. I shall argue throughout this book that healing from trauma depends upon communalization of the trauma—being able safely to tell the story to someone who is listening and who can be trusted to retell it truthfully, to others in the community. So before thinking, before trying to *do* anything—we should *listen.* Categories and classifications play a large role in the institutions of mental health care for veterans, in the education of mental health professionals, and as tentative guides to perception. All too often, however, our mode of listening deteriorates into intellectual sorting, with the professional grabbing the veterans' words from the air and sticking them in mental bins. To some degree that is institutionally and educationally necessary, but listening this way *destroys* trust. At its worst our educational system produces counselors, psychiatrists, psychologists, and therapists who resemble museum-goers whose whole experience consists of mentally saying, "That's cubist! . . . That's El Greco!" and who never *see* anything they've looked at. "Just listen!" say the veterans when telling mental health professionals what they need to know to work with them, and I believe that is their wish for the general public as well. Passages of narrative here contain the particularity of individual men's experiences, bearing a different order of meaningfulness than any categories they might be put into. In the words of one veteran, these stories are "sacred stuff."

The mortal dependence of the modern soldier on the military organization for everything he needs to survive is as great as that of a small child on his or her parents. One Vietnam combat veteran said, "The U.S. Army [in Vietnam] was like a mother who sold out her kids to be raped by [their] father to protect her own interests."

No single English word takes in the whole sweep of a culture's definition of right and wrong; we use terms such as moral order, convention, normative expectations, ethics, and commonly understood social values. The ancient Greek word that Homer used, *thémis,* encompasses all these meanings.[1] A word of this scope is needed for the betrayals experienced by Vietnam combat veterans. In this book I shall use the phrase "what's right" as an equivalent of *thémis.* The specific content of the Homeric warriors' *thémis* was often quite different from that of American soldiers in Vietnam, but what has not changed in three millennia are violent rage and social withdrawal when deep assumptions of "what's right" are violated. The vulnerability of the soldier's moral world has increased in three thousand years because of the vast number and physical distance of people in a position to betray "what's right" in ways that threaten the survival of soldiers in battle. Homeric soldiers actually saw their commander in chief, perhaps daily.

An Army is a Moral Construction

Book 1 of the *Iliad* sets the tragedy in motion with Agamémnon's seizure of Achilles' woman, "a prize I [Achilles] sweated for, and soldiers gave me!" (1:189).[2] We must understand the cultural context to see that this episode is more than a personal squabble between two soldiers over a woman. The outrageousness of Agamémnon's behavior is repeatedly made clear. Achilles' mother, the goddess Thetis, makes her case to Zeus: "Now Lord Marshal Agamémnon has been highhanded with him, has commandeered and holds his prize of war [*géras,* portion of honor]. . . . " The prize of honor was voted by the troops for Achilles' valor in combat. A modern equivalent might be a commander telling a soldier, "I'll take that Congressional Medal of Honor of yours, because I don't have one." Obviously, Achilles' grievance was magnified by his attachment to the particular person of Brisêis, the captive woman who was the prize, but violation of "what's right" was central to the clash between Achilles and Agamémnon.[3]

Any army, ancient or modern, is a social construction defined by shared expectations and values. Some of these are embodied in formal regulations, defined authority, written orders, ranks, incentives, punishments, and formal task and occupational definitions. Others circulate as traditions, archetypal stories of things to be emulated or shunned, and accepted truth about what is praiseworthy and what is culpable. All together, these form a moral world that most of the participants most of the time regard as legitimate, "natural," and personally binding. The moral power of an army is so great that it can motivate men to get up out of a trench and step into enemy machine-gun fire.

When a leader destroys the legitimacy of the army's moral order by betraying "what's right," he inflicts manifold injuries on his men. The *Iliad* is a story of these immediate and devastating consequences. Vietnam has forced us to see that these consequences go beyond the war's "loss upon bitter loss . . . leaving so many dead men" (1:3ff.) to taint the lives of those who survive it.

Victory, Defeat and the Hovering Dead

In victory, the meaning of the dead has rarely been a problem to the living—soldiers have died "for" victory. Ancient and modern war are alike in defining the relationship between victory and the army's dead, *after the fact.* At the time of the deaths, victory has not yet been achieved, so the corpses' meaning hovers in the void until the lethal contest has been decided. Victory—and the cut, crushed, burned, impaled, suffocated, frozen, diseased, drowned, poisoned, or blown-up corpses—mutually anchor each other's meaning.[4] Homeric participants in warfare understood a very simple relationship between civilians and the soldiers who fought to protect them: In defeat, all male civilians were massacred and all female civilians were raped and carried away into slavery. In the modern world, the meaning of the dead to the defeated is a bitter, unhealed wound, where defeat rarely means obliteration of the people and civilization. As we recently witnessed in the Persian Gulf War, defeat may not even bring the fall of the opposing government. At the level of grand strategy in Vietnam, the United States had been defeated, and yet American soldiers had won every battle.

For the veterans, the unanchored dead continue to hover. They visit their surviving comrades at night like the ghost of Pátroklos, Achilles' friend, visits Achilles:

> . . . let me pass the gates of Death.
> . . . I wander
> about the wide gates and hall of Death.
> Give me your hand. I sorrow. (23: 88)

The returning Vietnam soldiers were not honored. Much of the public treated them with indifference or derision, further denying the unanchored dead a resting place.

SOME VETERANS' VIEW—WHAT IS DEFEAT? WHAT IS VICTORY?

During a group therapy session, I once blundered into a casual mention of "our defeat" in Vietnam. Many veterans returned from Vietnam and found themselves outcast and humiliated in American Legion[5] and Veterans of Foreign Wars posts where they had assumed that they would be welcomed, supported, and understood. Time and again they were assailed as "losers" by World War II veterans. The pain and rage at being blamed for defeat in Vietnam was beyond bearing and resulted in many brawls.

These feelings reflect not only outrage at the heartless wrong-headedness of such remarks but also a concept of victory in war that left Vietnam veterans bewildered. "We knew that we never lost a battle," say the veterans. Winning, as far as I have been able to determine, meant to them being in possession of the ground at the end of the battle. So the hit-and-run or hit-and-hide small-unit tactics of the enemy always meant that we had "won" after a given engagement. However, many men experienced a deep malaise that their concepts of victory, of strength embodied in fire superiority and often in great local numerical superiority, somehow didn't fit, were futile. The enemy initiated 90 percent of all engagements but "lost" them all. Even battles like Dak To and Ap Bia Mountain (Hamburger Hill) were American victories in the sense that Americans held the ground when the last shot was fired.

Larger images of victory seem to have been formed out of newsreel footage of World War II surrender ceremonies and beautiful women weeping for joy at their liberation; defeat was a document signed in a railway carriage and German troops marching in Paris.

As I listen to some veterans, there are times when it seems they believe that the Vietnamese *cannot* have won the war. Therefore, because we won all our battles, our victory was somehow stolen. Many veterans have a well-developed "stab in the back" theory akin to that developed by German veterans of World War I—that the war could have been handily won had the fighting forces not been betrayed by home-front politicians. My interest here is in the soldiers' experiences and not in the larger historical question of whether they were "sold out" by the politicians somehow brought under the spell of such still-hated figures as Jane Fonda.

Once or twice I have tried to explore with veterans these concepts of victory and defeat. I have abandoned these discussions because the sense of betrayal is still too great and the equation of defeat with abandonment by God and personal devaluation still too vivid.

To return to my blunder in group therapy, a veteran whose voice is often heard in this book turned black with anger and, glaring at me, said, "I won *my* war. It's *you* who fucking lost." He got up and left the room to remove himself from the opportunity to physically hurt me. Toward the end of the group session he returned and said, "What we lost in Vietnam was a lot of *good fucking* kids!"

More than a year after this experience I gingerly approached the subject with another veteran, prefacing what I was about to say (the paradox that we had "lost" the war while "winning" every battle) by saying that I knew that this was a very sensitive subject and that it made many vets very angry. When I had said it, he smiled in a not friendly way and drew his finger across his throat. "It makes you want to cut my throat?" I asked. "Uh-huh," he replied.

Dimensions of Betrayal of "What's Right"

To grasp the significance of betrayal we must consider two independent dimensions: first, what is at stake, and second, what *thémis* has been violated.

ON DANGER IN WAR

"To someone who has never experienced danger, the idea is attractive," wrote the famous nineteenth-century military theorist Carl von Clausewitz.[6] So it appeared to many young men who volunteered—only about 10 percent of the men I see were drafted—for military service during the Vietnam War. For some it was a way to "prove" themselves to themselves, sometimes to their fathers and uncles who were World War II veterans. For some it was attractive as an expression of patriotic and religious idealism, often understood to be equivalent to anti-Communism:

> You get brought up with God an' country and—y'know, something good turned out bad. . . . They told me I was fighting Communism. And I really believed in my country and I believed everyone served their country.

Another veteran:

> It was better to fight Communism there in Vietnam than in your own back yard. Catholics had the worst of it. We had to be the Legions of God. We were doing it for your faith. We were told: Communists don't like Catholics.

For some the war was a cause that expressed an heroic ideal of human worth, in the words of one veteran, "the highest stage of mankind, willing to put your life on the line for an idea." For others it was the excitement, the spectacle of war. One veteran described his motive for joining the Marines: "I was bored. Vietnam was where it was happening, and in the Marines everybody went to Vietnam."

All knew that war was dangerous, but none were prepared for the "final shock, the sight of men being killed and mutilated [which] moves our pounding hearts to awe and pity."[7] They went to war with the innocence built from films in which war, in Paul Fussell's words, was

> systematically sanitized and Norman Rockwellized, not to mention Disneyfied. . . . In these, no matter how severely wounded, Allied troops are never shown suffering what was termed, in the Vietnam War, traumatic amputation: everyone has all his limbs, his hands and feet and digits, not to mention expressions of courage and cheer.[8]

Danger of death and mutilation is the pervading medium of combat. It is a viscous liquid in which everything looks strangely refracted and moves about in odd ways, a powerful corrosive that breaks down many fixed contours of perception and utterly dissolves others. Without an accurate conception of danger we cannot comprehend war and cannot properly value the moral structure of an army. We must grasp what is at stake: lethal danger and the fear of it.

THE FAIRNESS ASSUMPTION

Adults rightly think that a sense of proportion about petty injustice is intrinsic to maturity and hear their children shrilling "It's not fair!" as evidence of their childishness. The culture shock of civilians entering the stratified and ritualized military world is well known. It is also the world of "chickenshit." As Paul Fussell put it:

> If you are an enlisted man, you'll know you've been the victim of chickenshit if your sergeant assigns you to K.P. not because it's your turn but because you disagreed with him on a question of taste a few evenings ago. Or, you might find your pass to town canceled at the last minute because, you finally remember, a few days ago you asked a question during the sergeant's lecture on map-reading that he couldn't answer.[9]

Civilian and noncombat veterans often equate complaints about military life to adolescent whining because of the unexamined assumption that its injustices are always of this low-stakes variety. The experiences that Fussell invokes here undoubtedly cause anger and indignation, but the essential element of mortal danger is lacking. However, Fussell, himself a World War II combat veteran, continues the passage without a change in tone:

> Or, if you uttered your . . . [indiscretion] while in combat instead of in camp, you might find yourself repeatedly selected to take out the more hazardous night patrols to secure information, the kind, a former junior officer recalls, 'we already knew from daytime observations, and had reported.'[10]

Because we have entered the realm of mortal danger, the experience of betrayal merits full, respectful attention. Paradoxically, the reader must respond *emotionally* to the reality of combat danger in order to make *rational* sense of the injury inflicted when those in charge violate "what's right." If the emotion of terror is completely absent from the reader's experience of this book, crucial information about the experience of combat is not getting through.

A veteran recalls,

> Walking point[11] was an extremely dangerous job. The decision on who was going to do it was so carefree, so carefree, yeah. The decision was made politically [laughs]. Most of the time politically. Certain people got the shit. Certain people didn't. Certain people on the right side of certain people.

Another veteran:

> The CO had his favorites. Two companies, Delta [this veteran's company] and Charlie, always got sent out. The other two always stayed back on the hill at ____.

This may sound like a child complaining, "It's not fair!" about taking turns carrying out the trash, unless one grasps what was at stake. During the course of this man's year with Delta Company, it suffered more than 100 percent casualties, taking replacements into account. The companies that were the CO's favorites suffered few casualties. Contrary to what the young men anticipated in training and in watching war films, once they encountered the reality of battle, they fervently wanted to avoid it and wanted risk to be fairly distributed. Many aspects of the *thémis* of American soldiers cluster around fairness. When they perceived that distribution of risk was unjust, they became filled with indignant rage, just as Achilles was filled with *ménis,* indignant rage.

Soldiers grow most doubtful about the fair distribution of risk when they see that their commanders shelter themselves from it. Writing of the Vietnam War, a respected military historian commented:

> Officers in every armed force must find ways of inducing their men to fight and risk their lives—a most unnatural activity. . . . In modern warfare, where automatic weapons, artillery, and air power impose dispersal, men can rarely be pushed into combat; they

> must be pulled by the prestige of their immediate leader and the officers above him. Combat expertise that soldiers recognize and personal qualities of authority are important, but so is an evident willingness to share in the . . . deadly risks of war. . . . The deadly risks of combat must unfailingly be shared whether it is tactically necessary to do so or not, and junior officers cannot do all the sharing.
>
> If soldiers see that their immediate leader is exposed to risk while his superiors stay away from combat, they will be loyal to the man but disaffected from the army. . . . In Vietnam, the mere fact that officers above the most junior rank were so abundant and mostly found in well-protected bases suggested a very unequal sharing of the risk. And statistics support the troops' suspicion. During the Second World War, the Army ground forces had a full colonel for every 672 enlisted men; in Vietnam (1971) there was a colonel for every 163 enlisted men. In the Second World War, 77 colonels died in combat, one for every 2,206 men thus killed; throughout the Vietnam war, from 1961 till 1972, only 8 colonels were killed in action, one for every 3,407 men.[12]

The *Iliad* reminds us that military and political leaders have not always been thousands of miles away from the war zone. Agamémnon, the highest Greek political and military authority, personally shares every soldier's risk on the battle field and is wounded in action (11:289ff.); the King of Lykia, a Trojan ally, is killed in action (15:568ff.). Only within the last few centuries has the era of "stone-age command" ended. Before the modern age the ruler and commander in chief were united in one person who was present and at risk in battle. Rear-echelon officers in Vietnam who attempted to micro-manage battles by radio from the rear were known as Base Camp Commandos; those who operated from a helicopter safely out of range of ground fire came to be called Great Leaders in the Sky. Martin van Creveld wrote:

> Under the conditions peculiar to the war in Vietnam, major units seldom had more than one of their subordinate outfits engage the enemy at any one time. . . . A hapless company commander engaged in a firefight on the ground was subjected to direct observation by the battalion commander circling above, who was in turn supervised by the brigade commander circling a thousand or so feet higher up, who in his turn was monitored by the division commander in the next highest chopper, who might even be so unlucky as to have his own performance watched by the Field Force (corps) commander.[13]

If American career officers in Vietnam did not share the risks of combat, cultural and institutional factors, rather than personal cowardice, were primarily responsible for this. The officers of World War II had a different culture, which focused on the substance of their *work* rather than on the institutional definition and status of their *jobs,* as in Vietnam. And compared to World War II, there were simply too many officers in Vietnam, leading them to become so absorbed in bureaucratic processes that the most elementary aspects of leadership dropped beyond their horizon.

Officers, the only soldiers we meet in the *Iliad,* went into danger in quest of "honor."

> What is the point of being honored so
> with precedence at table, choice of meat,
> and brimming cups, . . .
> And why have lands been granted you and me . . . ?
> So that we two
> at times like this in the . . . front line
> may face the blaze of battle and fight well. (12: 348ff.)

Honor was conferred by others for going into danger and fighting competently. Honor was embodied in its valuable tokens, such as the best portions of meat at feasts, land grants, or, in Achilles' case, the prize of Brisêis. And so could honor be removed; a man could be dis-honored by seizure of the tokens of honor. Homer makes it plain that men were willing to risk their lives for honor and that the material goods that symbolized honor were not *per se* what made them face "a thousand shapes of death." (12: 366) It is easy for us to caricature ancient warriors as simple brigands or booty hunters motivated by greed, but this is almost certainly a misunderstanding. The quest for social honor and avoidance of social shame are the prime motives of Homeric warriors. Achilles says,

> Only this bitterness eats at my heart
> when one man would deprive and shame his equal,
> taking back his prize by abuse of power.
> The girl whom the Akhaians chose for me
> I won by my own spear. A town with walls
> I stormed and sacked for her. Then Agamémnon
> stole her back, out of my hands, as though
> I were some vagabond held cheap. (16:61ff.)

The rage is the same, whether it is fairness, so valued by Americans, or honor, the highest good of Homer's officers, that has been violated. In both cases life is at stake. In both cases the moral constitution of the army, its cultural contract, has been impaired under risk of death and mutilating wounds.

THE FIDUCIARY ASSUMPTION

Compared to the modern soldier, the Homeric soldier hardly depended on others at all, and when he did it was upon comrades he knew personally and called on by name without technology to assist his own voice. He depended upon himself for his weapons and armor; his eyes and ears provided most of the tactical intelligence he required. He did not need to rely on the competence, mental clarity, and sense of responsibility of a chain of people he would never meet to assure that artillery or air strikes meant to protect him did not kill him by mistake.

Consider the following "routine" event of combat in Vietnam: A man on night watch on the perimeter of a landing zone, using a starlight scope, observes enemy soldiers moving toward the helicopter landing zone (LZ) through the darkness. He calls this into the command post (CP); his words awaken his comrades, lightly asleep beside him while not on watch. Meanwhile, the officer in the CP calls in a request for illumination shells and artillery fire to turn back or weaken the oncoming assault.

Note the dependency of every man on others: the sleeping men on the one on watch, the one on watch on night-vision equipment supplied by others, all of them upon the radio sets connecting the bunker with the CP. They depend upon the radio-telephone operator (RTO) on watch in the CP and the officer who calls in the request for fire support with the correct coordinates and correct munitions, upon the artillery watch officers issuing the correct orders for a fire mission to the nearby fire base, upon these being carried out with the correct munitions and the guns correctly laid—the wrong coordinants could bring the fire down *on* the Americans, ironically dubbed "friendly fire," the phrase invoked when the action of one's own arms results in any wounding or death.

The vast and distant military and civilian structure that provides a modern soldier with his orders, arms, ammunition, food, water, information, training, and fire support is ultimately a moral structure, a *fiduciary,*[14] a trustee holding the life and safety of that soldier. The need for an intact moral world increases with every added coil of a soldier's mortal dependency on others. The vulnerability of the soldier's moral world has vastly increased in three millennia.

The following narrative, which contrasts a respected company commander with his successor, illuminated both obvious and hidden dimensions of the fiduciary relationship:

> I told you about that captain I liked, he kept moving us, you know, always move. We'd set up, we'd sleep, if you could sleep, and then get out of there. I think that we walked a lot of unbroken paths, off trails, never set up—see, my second captain, he'd come up and say, "Well, that's a nice NDP [night defensive position]. It's already dug, little foxholes. It's beautiful, we'll just set up right there." My captain, wouldn't do that. He'd shake his head and say, "Uh-UH, we're going over there, and we're going to *cut.*" . . . Cutting, cutting, cutting. . . . My captain, I hated his goddamn guts, but I admired him, admired the living shit. I hated his goddamn guts because he was so hard. . . . He would always stay off trails, stay off used NDPs. Y'know, when he left and he was replaced, I thought I'd never get out of there. I'd never get out of there alive.

At first glance, this veteran appears simply to be contrasting a competent company commander with his incompetent replacement. The first captain understood that previously used NDPs were probably mined and booby-trapped, or that at the very least, enemy mortars and artillery had their coordinates. Existing trails, which would allow the company to move more quickly without the long labor of cutting through, were likewise mined and booby-trapped as well as invitations to ambush.

Why did the captain who replaced the admired commander not know these things? The answer to this question goes deep into the betrayals of trust of the higher officers who (1) designed a system of officer rotation that rotated officers (above second lieutenant) in and out of combat assignments every six months, (2) were responsible for training, evaluating, and assigning officers to combat command, and (3) placed institutional and career considerations above the lives of the soldiers under their responsibility.[15] By the time a company or battalion commander acquired knowledge of the enemy's habits, the terrain and weather, the strengths and weaknesses of his men and their arms, whose advice to heed among the junior officers and NCOs, and the arts of deception, he was replaced. Some canny commanders would set up in an existing NDP and then move out of it after dark to another position. Such skills are only slightly transferable from one officer to his replacement and mainly have to be acquired from experience.

However, these larger systemic failures such as too-rapid turnover, inadequate training, and incompetent selection of troop commanders misses another important point that was much more visible to soldiers. Was there no one to tell the new captain that he should not use existing trails? Of course there were NCOs and lieutenants to tell him. The old commander, whose way of moving was "cut, cut, cut," probably displeased his superiors who ordered him to move from point A to point B in two hours—a movement that could be done in that time only if he took his company along highly dangerous existing trails. Possibly he answered back, saying, "No, that can't be done."

Officers who *wanted* to stay in the field beyond six months were said to have "gone bush" or "gone native." They were suspected of not being "with the program" and of having nurtured a "personality cult" in which the troops were loyal to them as individuals rather than to the chain of command. The veteran quoted above continues,

> I had a lieutenant who I loved. I would've walked into hell with him, walked right into hell. . . . Now, when he was supposed to leave the field, he wouldn't leave, they had to bring two armed guards, no lie. They brought a special bird [helicopter] out. They said, "Now get on the bird! You're under orders." He didn't want to go.

Neither the admired captain nor the beloved lieutenant were cowards, avoiding the enemy out of fear. As far as I can determine from this veteran's account, both were effective officers with real loyalty both to their military tasks and to the men under them. They did not place the self-interest of "looking good" to their superiors above the safety of their men. They were not swayed by bureaucratically structured measures of "productivity" derived from industrial processes. The most fundamental incompetence in the Vietnam War was the misapplication of the social and mental model of an industrial process to human warfare.

A full analysis of how war can destroy the social contract binding soldiers to each other, to their commanders, and to the society that raised them as an army deserves a whole book in itself. My purpose here is to draw the reader's attention to the importance in itself of betrayal of *thémis,* to the soldier's reactions, and to the catastrophic outcomes that often flow from these reactions. I shall do this primarily by focusing on those things that the *Iliad* brings into view but which long familiarity has made invisible to us.

Let us look further at the extreme state of dependence of the modern soldier on his army for *everything* he needs to stay alive in combat: his arms, his training, food and water, communications, knowledge of the enemy, and the skills of his superiors:

> My personal weapon until just after this op. [Union I][16] was the M-14. It was heavy, but at least you could depend on it. Then we got the M-16. It was a piece of shit that never should have gone over there with all the malfunctions. . . . I started hating the fucking government. At least in Union I we had rifles we could depend on. The stocks [of the M-16] broke in hand-to-hand. I started feeling like the government really didn't want us to get back, that there needed to be fewer of us back home. This was a constant thing, they kept changing the spring, the buffer. It was like they was testing it. Our lives depended on them. We cleaned the damned things every day, but they were just no fucking good. There were times when we'd rather use their weapons than our own. I once took an AK [AK-47] from a dead NVA and used it instead of my Mattel toy [M-16].
>
> It was about a week or two into Union II. I was walking point. I seen this NVA soldier at a distance. We were approaching him and he spotted us. We spread out to look for him. I was coming around a stand of grass and heard noise. I couldn't tell who it was, us or him. I stuck my head in the bush and saw this NVA hiding there and told him to come out. He started to move back and I saw he had one of those commando weapons, y'know, with a pistol grip under his thigh, and he brought it up and I was looking straight down the bore. I pulled the trigger on my M-16 and nothing happened.

Obviously this soldier survived the failure of his arms to tell the story, but the experience of betrayal that he took from it has been far more destructive of his subsequent life than the grazing wound inflicted by the NVA. A vast number of military officers, civilian defense officials, and civilian contractors were involved in the specification, design, prototyping, testing, manufacture, field testing, and acceptance of the M-16. Yet as one retired military officer blandly put it, "Early models were plagued by stoppages that caused some units to request reissue of the older M-14."[17] The veteran quoted above experienced the deficiencies of design, manufacture, and especially field testing and acceptance of the M-16 as a gross betrayal of the duties of care and of loyalty by the officers who, by virtue of their office, held his life in trust.

Equipment failure is not new in modern warfare. I count nineteen instances of equipment failure in the *Iliad,* of which nine were fatal to the soldier in question. Each Homeric soldier, or his father, supplied his own equipment; its failure did not cast doubt on the moral structure of the army in which he served. The ancient soldier was far less dependent in every way on military institutions than his modern counterpart, whose dependency is as complete as that of a small child on his or her family.

> During one patrol in the dry season, _____'s squad ran out of water and was not resupplied. They walked for a day and a half in search of water in Vietcong-controlled territory. When men started to collapse from dehydration in the heat, an officer's plea for

emergency resupply was heeded: A helicopter flew over and "bombed" the squad cases of Tab, seriously injuring one of the men. The major whose helicopter dropped the Tab was recalled to evacuate the casualty. There was no enemy activity. ____ subsequently read in the division newspaper that the major had put himself in for and had received the Bronze Star for resupplying the troops and evacuating the wounded "under fire."

Extreme dependency on others is fundamental to modern combat. We have become so accustomed to this that it easily escapes notice.

Shortages of all sorts—food, water, ammunition, clothing, shelter from the elements, medical care—are intrinsic to prolonged combat, if for no other reason than enemy attacks on the army's logistical support services. The fortitude of soldiers under such conditions, for example during the siege of Dien Bien Phu or Khe Sanh, is legendary. However, when deprivation is perceived as the outcome of indifference or disrespect by superiors, it arouses *mênis* as an unbearable offense.

They had a fucking pet dog at the camp and they always got in fresh hamburger for the dog, but there were times we were out and starving, not even getting C-rations, because they wouldn't resupply us. The dog got sick and they had a chopper in there to fly it to Danang. I had a machete wound in my calf and had to walk for miles back to the base camp.

The shortage that the combat soldier finds most offensive, however, is shortage of competence.

The first deaths in ____'s platoon were caused by "friendly fire" from sectors of the defense perimeter; the officer had neglected to inform them that he was sending men out on the berm. . . . In two successive helicopter-borne combat insertions the company left the landing zone in parallel columns and after a few "klicks" in the jungle lost track of each other until they met in a furious fire fight. Two men were injured in the first one, five in the second. ____ never heard of any investigation or disciplinary action.

Another veteran:

There was just one stupid fucking thing after another. They decided to use tear gas on a ville [cluster of hamlets] after we had crossed a river neck deep, and of course everything soaked, the canisters [of the gas masks] were soaked and they decided to use tear gas. Of course the gas masks didn't work. They gassed us almost to death.

No one has successfully defined where the inescapable SNAFUs—a World War II expression: Situation Normal, All Fucked Up—of war end and culpable incompetence begins.

Is betrayal of "what's right" essential to combat trauma, or is betrayal simply one of many terrible things that happen in war? Aren't terror, shock, horror, and grief at the death of friends trauma enough? No one can conclusively answer these questions today. However, I shall argue what I've come to strongly believe through my work with Vietnam veterans: that moral injury is an essential part of any combat trauma that leads to lifelong psychological injury. Veterans can usually recover from horror, fear, and grief once they return to civilian life, so long as "what's right" has not also been violated.

We now turn our attention to the soldier's reactions to betrayal of "what's right." These are unchanged across three millennia. Indignant rage will occupy us for the remainder of this chapter. It opens the way for berserk rage, which I will describe in chapter 5.

Soldier's Rage—The Beginning

Rage is properly the title of Homer's poem, and his audience may have known it by that name, not *Iliad.*[18] King Agamémnon causes a ravaging plague in the Greek army by his refusal to accept ransom for the daughter of a priest of Apollo, god of disease and healing. The plague ends only after Achilles mobilizes moral pressure on Agamémnon to return the captive woman. In doing this, Achilles forces him to do what a pious and prudent man would have done of his own accord. Agamémnon, however, takes it as a personal attack by Achilles and seizes Achilles' prize of honor, the captive woman Brisêis, to replace the one he gave up to save the plague-devastated army. Achilles' rage at this wrong is immediate:

> . . . in his shaggy chest this way and that
> the passion of his heart ran: should he draw
> longsword from hip . . . kill
> [Agamémnon] in single combat...,
> or hold his rage in check...?
> . . . As he slid
> the big blade slowly from the sheath, Athêna
> . . . stepping
> up behind him, visible to no one
> except Akhilleus [Achilles], gripped his
> red-gold hair. . . .
> The grey-eyed goddess Athena said to him:
>
> "It was to check this killing rage I came
> from heaven. . . ." (1:221ff.)

Achilles submits and withdraws. His *mênis,* restrained at the brink of cutting down Agamémnon, is diverted to hacking away emotional bonds and driving away those he used to love. In Vietnam men were not able, as Achilles was, to withdraw physically from combat. They did, however, have the freedom to withdraw emotionally and mentally from everything beyond their small circle of combat-proven comrades.

Homer's starting point, then, is *mênis,* indignant wrath. I believe it is also the first and possibly the primary trauma that converted subsequent terror, horror, grief, and guilt into lifelong disability for Vietnam veterans. Indignant rage is uncomfortably familiar to all who work with combat veterans.

Homer uses the word *mênis* for Achilles only in connection with the wrong done to him by Agamémnon, and never in connection with his berserk rage at Hektor for killing his friend Pátroklos. I prefer "indignant rage" as a translation for *mênis*, because I can hear the word *dignity* hidden in the word *indignant*. It is the kind of rage arising from social betrayal that impairs a person's dignity through violation of "what's right." Apart from its use as a word for divine rage, Homer uses *mênis* only as the word for the rage that ruptures social attachments. We now turn to this choking-off of the social and moral world.

NOTES

1. Martha C. Nussbaum, *The Fragility of Goodness: Luck and Ethics in Greek Tragedy and Philosophy* (Cambridge: Cambridge University Press, 1986), 397–421. Nussbaum's excellent discussion centers on *nómos,* a word that largely supplanted *thémis* in this semantic range. The word *nómos,* which was much used by the Athenian tragic poets, such as Sophocles, is not found in Homer.

2. Most *Iliad* citations refer to Robert Fitzgerald's translation (New York: Anchor-Doubleday, 1974). They are in the form Book:Line Number(s). Fitzgerald's line numbers are, on average, 16 percent higher than line numbers in the original because of the poetic form of his translation. However, an interested reader will usually have little difficulty in finding quotations in the original. Multiplying Fitzgerald's line number by 0.86 usually yields a line number that is within one or two of the correct one in the original. However, occasional estimates are off by as much as twenty lines. I hope that classicists who read this book will forgive the blunt-edged anachronism of calling Achaeans, Danaäns, and Argives all "Greeks." I have followed Fitzgerald's spelling of proper names with the exception of "Akhilleus"; in this case I used the conventional English, Achilles, instead.

   Where I have used Robert Fagles's excellent new translation (New York: Viking Penguin, 1990), I have so indicated, and the line numberings refer in these passages to his translations.

   When *Iliad* citations indicate that the line numbering is to the Greek original, the edition I used was the two-volume Loeb edition prepared by A. T. Murray, with books 1–12 in vol. 1 and books 13–24 in vol. 2. *Odyssey* citations refer to the Fitzgerald translation (New York: Vintage, 1990).

3. Thetis to Zeus, 1:579ff; Brisêis, 9:41ff; also, she was arguably Achilles' betrothed, 19:328ff.

4. This analysis derives from Elaine Scarry, "The Structure of War" in *The Body in Pain: The Unmaking and Making of the World* (New York: Oxford University Press, 1985).

5. My esteemed colleague in the International Society for Traumatic Stress Studies, John Sommer, Jr., who is himself a Vietnam combat veteran and Executive Director of the Washington, D.C. office of the American Legion, has asked me to point out that the treatment experienced by my patients was contrary to the policy of the organization and by no means universal among the 16,000 posts of the American Legion. He describes his own

experiences as quite positive and regards the 800,000 Vietnam-era members (out of total of 3.1 million) as evidence of widespread support for them in the American legion.

6. Carl von Clausewitz, *On War,* ed. and trans. Michael Howard and Peter Paret (published posthumously in 1832; reprint, Princeton: Princeton University Press, 1984), 113. The title of this section is also von Clausewitz's.
7. Ibid.
8. Paul Fussell, *Wartime: Understanding and Behavior in the Second World War* (New York: Oxford University Press, 1989), 268 ff.
9. Ibid., 80.
10. Ibid., 81.
11. Patrols moved single file with space between men. The first man, who was said to be "walking point," was the first to meet mines and booby traps and often the first to be exposed to enemy fire. When enemy ambushers maintained their discipline, they often let "point" and "slack" (the second man) go through and attacked the middle of the file, creating greater shock, confusion, and disruption of unit cohesion than if the first or last ("sweep") man were attacked.
12. Edward Luttwak, *The Pentagon and the Art of War: The Question of Military Reform* (New York: Simon & Schuster, 1985), 34f.
13. Martin van Creveld, *Command in War* (Cambridge: Harvard University Press, 1985), 255f.
14. This word has now come to mean almost exclusively someone who holds someone else's money in trust. The original meaning of *fiducia,* under Roman law, was the holding of a free person in trust.
15. There are numerous writings on the various command pathologies pandemic in the Vietnam War. Among critiques from sources that are impossible to characterize as pacifistic or antimilitary are: Edward Luttwak, *The Pentagon and the Art of War,* particularly the first chapter, "The Anatomy of Military Failure"; Martin van Creveld, *Command in War,* particularly chapter 7, "The Helicopter and the Computer"; David H. Hackworth, *About Face* (New York: Simon & Schuster, 1989), 449f on "ticket punching" (Retired General Harold Moore excoriates the practice as well); and Lieutenant General Harold G. Moore and Joseph L. Galloway, *We Were Soldiers Once . . . and Young* (New York: Random House, 1992), 344.
16. Operation Union I, begun by the First Marine Division against NVA in Quang Nam and Quant Tin Provinces on April 21, 1967. Union II followed and ended on June 5.
17. Colonel Harry G. Summers, Jr., *Vietnam War Almanac* (New York: Facts on File, 1985), 234. Moore and Galloway quote one air cavalry trooper as going through three M-16s in the Ia Drang battle before finding a fourth that worked. Another describes the trigger mechanism falling out, another simply that the M-16 he tried to fire was "inoperable." Moore and Galloway, *We Were Soldiers Once,* 89, 97, 100.
18. Gregory Nagy, *The Best of the Achaeans: Concepts of the Hero in Archaic Greek Poetry* (Baltimore: Johns Hopkins University Press, 1979), 75 n. 1.

THE DAY MY FATHER TRIED TO KILL US

PAT STATEN

Nightmares have plagued me all my life. When I was young, ten or earlier, I began to look on them as a natural ailment I must learn to accept. Just as some people were born deaf or lame, I was born with nightmares (I wisely concluded). Actually, they were so much a part of my life, so routine, that I rarely thought about them at all or questioned why I had them. As I got older the nightmares at least decreased in frequency, though not particularly in intensity.

When I was small I would wake up in the old Kansas farmhouse I grew up in and cry out for my mother. As I got older, I felt foolish about such childish displays of weakness and would not cry out—except in my sleep when I had no conscious control over it. I would wake up—covered with sweat, panting like a scared, exhausted animal, too terrified to cry out, and finally after minutes of forcing myself to consciousness the fear would begin to lessen. Sometimes I would wake myself with my own screams, sobs, pleas. The lights would go on and my mother would be standing at the door. She wouldn't come to the bed to hold me or console me. She would simply stand by the door, her hand near the light switch.

"All right now?"

"Yes."

"Want the light on?"

"Yes."

"You turn it off later?"

"Yes."

She would look at me for a second before she turned to leave the room. I grew in time to understand that look. It was a look of worry, concern, a certain painful expression of helplessness, as though she wanted to reach out to help me but didn't

Reprinted from *Aphra* 5.2 (Spring 1974): 2–33. All attempts to trace the copyright holder were unsuccessful.

know how, as though she wanted to say something to me but didn't know where to begin—or maybe she was waiting for me to say something, to reach out to her, but I never could. I often wanted to sob my heart out on her breasts but something always made me pull back, unable to go on.

She never mentioned my nightmares the next day. No reference was ever made to the nightmares in the family. They were a sort of accepted fact. Occasionally a sister would complain if I had kept her from a good night's sleep.

And no one had any knowledge of Freud or the subconscious or dream symbolism. My family existed a couple of centuries behind the sophisticated, educated world. I even thought they existed apart from the rest of the world. They were farmers. Generation after generation had been farmers. Uneducated, untraveled, and incredibly innocent or ignorant of any larger world beyond the plains of western Kansas.

A television arrived late at the farm, as we could never afford it, and when we did finally get one it only picked up one station and that poorly. Books were unknown in the house. The local newspaper was all the reading done in the family and generally that remained unopened. My parents had no friends. My brother and two sisters did not invite their friends to the house. Relatives did not visit, though we had quite a number of them.

The plains stretched out to all sides of the farmhouse. Flat, empty, uneventful. Always that huge expanse of blue sky over the flat horizon. Only the clouds ever seemed to change—rolling in over the plains like prehistoric monsters, transforming themselves to gods and goddesses, to the friends I was too shy to make in real life, to the mountains and skyscrapers I had never seen. The clouds brought the winds that howled outside my bedroom window at night and the storms that popped and rolled and thundered across the endless miles of wheat fields and prairie.

If we hadn't been so isolated on that farm, perhaps I would have had some gauge of what we were all living with—but I didn't. I would have understood why the sister three years older than I had emotional, almost epileptic fits—a kind of hysteria that nearly choked her—why the oldest sister had married at fifteen and left home, why my brother left the farm at fourteen to live and work on a neighboring farm and never again returned home to live.

Through it all, it was my mother who held me together. She was always there—not with kisses or great displays of affection or even words because she was never a woman comfortable with words or exaggerated gestures. She was there simply, with a silent presence, solidarity, a completely inarticulate strength. Without her, I'm sure none of us would have survived those years as whole as we eventually turned out to be.

But as much as I loved her, depended on her, needed her, there was frequently a distance between us. A distance that I never quite understood. I never talked to her about my father. I never once thought I could just go to her and say, "I'm afraid of my father." And if I cried out for her at night during my nightmares, she quickly learned not to touch me, as I would pull violently away from her, and even I didn't understand that particular reaction in myself.

And so, at fifteen, when it began, I didn't tell her about it. I spoke to no one about it. At first I thought it was a dream because it came to me as an incident that had happened somewhere outside the usual realm of daily reality. It was a moment suspended outside myself and what I thought the "real" world to be. A funhouse image in which all the people became distorted and grotesque nearly beyond recognition.

And though I thought it must be a dream, it was not like my other dreams. Suddenly in the middle of the day—I could be at school or walking home or waking up in the morning—a part of a scene would flash into my head. I would feel a veil was slowly lifting over something, then falling back again. I would feel a light was passing through some darkness inside myself, and for a second it would hit on something, then pass on before I could really see it. The light would be gone. The veil would fall. I did not know what I had seen. But it nagged at me, disturbed me in ways my nightmares had never disturbed me.

* * * * *

I am fifteen and it's spring. I just got off the school bus and am walking toward the house on the mile-long dirt road. As I near the house, my eyes wander to the large red barn near the house. I've never liked the barn. In fact, I do everything I can to avoid going in it at any time. I've never asked myself why, but now as I'm looking at it, again, for a second it happens. The veil lifts. The light passes. I quickly shrug it off. Today I want nothing to do with this disturbing sensation. Today I must block myself off and I have already begun the process before I reach the house.

My father has been drinking solidly for three days. It's not unusual. It's as routine as my nightmares, and given the same peculiar acceptance. His ritual from the time I can remember is to drink three days, sleep three days. Occasionally there will be a day, if he's lucky, of being sober and not asleep during which he tries to work. I dread his sober days more than the others. His nerves are so raw, he yells at you for any minor thing. I welcome the moment I see him dig the bottle out. I can at least calculate his states of inebriation.

The first day of drinking he's relatively calm. Relaxed. He talks a lot about the "great" past and the "great" war. Always his war memories. He was an infantryman during World War II. At first the stories will be funny and full of practical jokes. Then heroism and patriotism. Even into the second day he is frequently humorous, good-natured, and tells stories that make me laugh till my sides ache. He is full of warmth and light-hearted teasing. He makes up games for us kids to play and joins us with all our childlike enthusiasm and total belief.

But gradually, usually into the third day, the horror stories begin. Shooting people against walls. Turning people into human torches. My father relives each episode as he talks about it, although often his sentences are so disconnected and incoherent it's difficult to make out any concrete incident behind his ravings.

He calls me as I step into the house. I expect it. I go to the living room where he sits surrounded by beer cans, overflowing ashtrays, half-eaten food on dirty plates. He's spilled food on his shirt. His hair is uncombed.

He tries to appear jolly. "Patty Sue, you come here!"

I sit down in the chair opposite him. "Hi, Dad."

"What'd you learn in school today? Huh?"

I shrug. No matter what I answer he will not hear. He's somewhere else. He barely knows I'm there.

"Nothing." I say.

He suddenly tries to struggle out of his stupor. "Huh?"

"Nothing."

"Nothing! Goddamn! Nothing!"

In a way it's comical. If he were in another mood I would laugh and he would laugh with me. But not now. I can't laugh. If I do, I risk my life. One swing from his powerful arm can knock me unconscious. I watch him closely. I say nothing. I must know when to move, when to escape. I must know when that blank look enters his eyes. My existence depends on knowing each precise change in his mood. In fifteen years, I've learned the art well. I have never miscalculated. I know that for a while I am safe. He is in the numb, half-asleep state. He will be at that state till at least my mother comes home.

Suddenly his eyes clear for a second. "I've killed men! Did you hear? Do you understand? I've killed men!"

I nod my head. A huge repressed fear nearly grabs me but I hold it down. My expression must show nothing.

"Blow the bastard's head off! . . . Son-of-a-bitch . . . he came out of there like a bat out of hell . . . but I blew the bastard's head off. One shot! That's all it takes! One shot!"

The words do not shock me. I don't even really hear them any more. I've been hearing such things for years. It has reached a level of total unimportance with me.

My father looks at me. "Kid. Just a kid. Never seen anything. Take my advice—you stay here on the farm—the good life—never see what I seen. . . . "

He drifts off again and for a second I think he has fallen asleep. I study him as he sits in the chair, his head nodding to one side. He is a big man. Six foot three, with powerful muscles he developed from his youth as a farmhand. Even the years of drinking have not given him the usual soft look of drunks. I saw pictures of him when he was young, and he had once been a handsome man (even now I see he has not lost his good looks). In the picture he had wavy red hair, penetrating blue eyes, sharp sensitive features. I saw a picture of him during the war. The sensitivity was still there, but changed, masked by a fierce expression. While, before, his gaze was penetrating, now it seemed similar to the look of well-trained dogs, ready for attack.

He comes awake abruptly. "You hear?"

"Yes."

A sudden direct intensity in his gaze. I am always shocked to suddenly encounter this penetrating, deadly sober, commanding look in his eyes. It happens without warning.

"You hear good! You stay where you belong! You stay on the land—they'll kill you. Those bastards kill everything! I seen girls like you—" He stops for a second, then continues. "Bunch of mad animals. Got to break 'em! Kick-the-bastards in the teeth! They won't do that to my kids! No sir, not my kids. I love my kids . . . all my kids . . . something they never touched. . . . "

His mind wanders and I see that beaten, defeated expression cross his face.

"You forgive me, Pat?"

I look at him and say what I always say when he asks this.

"Yes."

He nods gratefully and falls asleep, sitting in the chair.

But I do not forgive him. I hate him. And much deeper than my hatred, I fear him.

After I am sure he has fallen asleep, I slip out of the house. I walk the dirt road from our house to the main highway. Mom works at the Boeing Airplane Plant in Wichita and each night the plant bus leaves her off at the highway. And each night I wait for her. It is a ritual I established years earlier when she first took the job. Dad loses job after job and even when he can work he misses so many days his check is never substantial. We've lost all of the farm over the years but the barn and main house. There is nothing left to farm but a big plot for a garden. We still have a few chickens. But it's impossible to live off the land. So Mom took the job at the factory. Putting parts of machinery together all day. Standing on her feet eight hours. Then the two-hour trip back and forth to the plant on the factory bus.

I wait by our mailbox. The bus pulls up and stops. Mom steps off. I am always proud when I see her step off the bus. No other woman on the bus is as pretty as my Mom. Even the rich women in town with new clothes and makeup and fancy hairdos cannot compare with my mother.

She is small. Five foot two. (At ten I was as tall as she and by fifteen I've already leaped up to five eight.) She never wears anything but the same cheap dresses. Even if she had the money, I doubt that she would spend it on clothes. She is dark. Dad says she is part Indian but, if she is, she never mentions it. In the summer her skin tans to a golden bronze. Her red-auburn hair is cut at her shoulders, ending in a natural wave. She has soft, light blue eyes. And if her beauty can be called in any way startling it's in the summer when the clear blue of her eyes contrasts with her dark skin. But it is not a flashy beauty or even a beauty she is aware of possessing. I'm sure she never thinks of herself as beautiful—particularly at a time when the idea of good looks seems to depend on lots of makeup and chemical curls. She hasn't the time or money for any of this. There is nothing superficial or phony or imposed about her. It is a completely natural beauty and part of it lies in her soft grace, her strength, the gentleness and warmth in her eyes. And her smile.

She smiles, seeing me as she gets off the bus. This is the only time I have with her alone. At the house there are always my father and the other children and work to be taken care of. She has no time there. But this one-mile walk back to the house each evening is reserved for me alone. She asks me about school and I tell her and I ask her about work and she always says, "oh, it's the same as always."

It is an unusually warm day for this time of year. A strong southerly wind. As we start toward the house, Mom takes her shoes off. Unless it's cold, she will frequently do this. Mom seems to have an innate dislike of shoes. Sometimes she points out a butterfly or a flower or notes if there will be an early winter or a late summer that year.

She was raised on a farm. Born to a family of nine children. Pioneer stock. She spent the summers of her youth walking barefoot behind a horse and plow, farming the fields. Nature is still her real home. She understands it. She draws strength from it. She doesn't like the factory. It cuts her off from something essential in her life—her roots in the earth. This walk is her time to get back in touch with it.

This walk is also an important ritual in my life. It builds the bond between me and my mother, though we rarely talk of anything outside the trivial. Occasionally I will build myself up to some huge confession. But she constantly surprises me with her reaction. Her look is undisturbed, unreproachful, sometimes even amused. It's a look of: "I knew that years ago and now you're just getting around to telling me but I'm not surprised."

Not that she was without bad moods or a tired irritability at times. As she is tonight. She has been up almost constantly for two days. The weariness shows in the circles under her eyes, the tension in her face. We do not discuss my father, if he's drinking or not. She knows he is. We never discuss my father.

I know she needs time alone tonight so I begin to walk ahead of her. We are halfway to the house. I turn to look at her. She's standing right in the middle of the dirt road, her arms spread wide, her head thrown back. She sees me looking at her and turns her face into the last rays of afternoon light.

"Do you feel that wind?" she says. "Lord, do you feel that wonderful wind!"

Since my mother is rarely given to outbursts of any sort, I stand and feel the wind. I think it must be different for her to get so excited. Just a little warmer, an early spring wind. But aside from that, I decide it's the same old wind and keep walking. I hear her laughter behind me. I turn and look at her and realize how much she puzzles me. How much she has always puzzled me.

I don't understand her. I don't understand her joy, her strength, her endurance, her loves or her drive. I don't understand why she stays with my father. I don't understand how she can work all day, then come home to stay up most of the night with him. I don't understand her silent ability to endure day after day.

Why does she put up with this sort of life? The worry. The poverty. His drunks. The beatings. Is it her Puritan upbringing that suffering is good? An old-fashioned sense of duty? Or maybe she is so concerned with just surviving, so preoccupied with paying the bills and feeding the children that she long ago stopped thinking there was any other way to live.

I saw a picture of my mother soon after she was married. Both my parents look so young, neither twenty yet. There is a freshness and sensitivity to both of them. And in that picture my mother is happy. Genuinely happy. Outside that picture I have never seen my mother so happy. She is beautiful and young and holding the arm of a man she obviously loved. That picture is all that comes close to explaining something to me I've never understood—her relationship with my father.

We reach the house. Dad calls Mom into the living room. I go to my room and shut the door. It will begin now. The very worst period of his three-day drunk will begin now.

I look on these periods as something that must be endured, and my main method of endurance is fantasy. I withdraw into elaborate stories of beauty and love in exotic lands far from this shabby farmhouse and a broken man's ravings. But even my complete withdrawal into a world of make-believe does not work in those few hours when he hits his peak of violence and terror.

I lie awake and even if the night is freezing I throw all the covers off, sleep with my jeans and shirt on, make quick decisive plans of escape, keep the window half opened, calculate how long it will take me to get from the bed out of the window, across the roof, and finally into the open area beyond the house. And all the while, I am sure that when he comes I will be too terrified to move.

Sometimes if he gets particularly bad, Karie will help me barricade the door with a dresser. Karie is the sister three years older than me, and I share the bedroom with her. Usually she puts the radio to her ear or pulls the pillow over her head and falls asleep. I never understand how she can sleep then. I could no more fall asleep then than you can fall asleep on your way to the gallows.

It begins late at night. Two or three in the morning. First he listens to music. Then he talks about the war. The sound of his voice rising through the house—words so blurred, vicious I can rarely understand them. He begins to yell at my mother. Then he begins to beat her. Dishes crashing. Furniture overturned. The sound of her body hitting the walls or floor. She never cries or screams during these beatings. And the next morning there will be no sign the beating happened—aside from a large bruise or cut she will try to hide with makeup or clothes.

He stops beating her. I lie awake. Listening. Waiting. My ear tuned to every sound in the house. Silence. Only the wind howling outside and the creak and groan of the old boards in the house. I wonder if she's dead or alive. I think she is dead. I listen for any sound she might make. But I don't hear her. I think that tomorrow morning I will find her dead. But now I am too frightened to move, to help her even if she needed me. I am paralyzed with fear.

Silence. Listening to my father's footsteps downstairs. Waiting for him to climb the stairs. Waiting for him to come up and kill the rest of us. Waiting. But he never comes, and I never go through one of those nights without believing this time it will happen, this time he will kill us, this time I will not fall into exhausted sleep when the dawn comes.

But the dawn comes and I fall asleep. Mother's voice wakes me for school. She has a bruise on her forehead. She covers it with makeup. No one discusses it. No one acts as though it had ever happened.

But that day, perhaps because I'm so tired, the dream begins to come to me again. And today I have much more difficulty shaking it off than ever before. Today something is determined to come awake in me, despite all I do to ignore it.

That evening I'm in the kitchen helping mom do the dishes and I decide to mention it.

"Mom, I keep having this dream. . . ."

The words fade. I can't go on.

My mother is exhausted from the night before and the factory. She isn't paying much attention to what I'm saying. Her lack of attention makes it easier for me to continue.

"But I don't know if it's a dream. I mean, I sort of remember it like it was a dream—you know, you wake up and you can remember parts but not all—but every day now I remember a little more of this dream. Ain't that funny?"

My mother stops washing the dishes and glances at me.

"What's the dream about?"

"Oh, it's crazy. Don't make no sense."

"You want to tell me what you can remember?"

"Well, first a door slamming. It's hot and bright. I'm real little. I'm sitting under the big tree in the front yard, playing. And this door slams—I think it's the door to the porch—the screen door—and you come running out and you're real scared and you tell us all to run but I don't know why. . . ."

That part of the dream is gone so I stop. My mother hasn't stopped washing the dishes but I sense something about her then. She's waiting for something to happen. She's waiting for me to say something. But I don't know what.

I continue: "Then it's dark and I'm alone. That don't make no sense. It was bright and hot and suddenly it's dark and cold. Must be a dream, huh?"

My mother says nothing.

"I can't remember nothing else," I say.

"Nothing?"

"Well, a line—all of us are in a line in the barn and I'm last."

My mother stops washing the dishes.

"That's all?"

I nod yes.

She touches me on the arm, saying, "Off you go now."

"Don't you want me to finish drying these dishes?"

"I'll finish. You go on now."

I put the dish towel down, happy to get out of a task I hate. But as I go to my room, I think it's odd. It was my turn to dry the dishes and Mother has broken one of her strict rules of discipline by letting me out of it. But I'm too relieved to think much more about it.

It's a few days later in school that it really begins. I've had a slight headache all day. We're having our history lesson. My mind is wandering. I can't concentrate. A cold feeling begins to come over me and I wonder if I'm getting sick. But the cold isn't a kind of cold I've ever had before. I sit at my desk, struggling with feeling, trying to hide it. Afternoon. Sitting in a classroom with thirty other students. The teacher's at the blackboard, talking. I'm trying to listen to what she's saying but I can't.

All of reality seems to be retreating from me. It's not a literal hallucination. It's a feeling of being connected with nothing. I'm cold. The sun streaks through the window and falls across my desk. I suddenly look up at the sun, that blinding white light burns into my eyes.

I remembered then.

* * * * *

I'm little. No more than five years old. It's summer. The farm. A hot day. The hottest part of the day has arrived. A clear day. Not a cloud. The sky is an empty, pale blue. Only that huge ball of fire above us. The fields are burned brown. The color seems bleached out of everything, even the trees and earth.

I am with my brother and sisters in the front yard. My brother and oldest sister are playing with sticks, pretending they're swords. Karie is sitting on the steps of the porch with her doll. I'm sitting alone under the tree, playing with a toy car in the dirt. Mom's inside the house. My father is gone. He's been gone for a few days.

I look up through the branches of the tree, directly at the sun. Mother has often punished me for looking at the sun like this. She says I'll ruin my good eyes. But it fascinates me. And if I stare at it long enough it becomes a dark ball and throbs, like a big heart in the sky.

I finally look away and see black spots everywhere. The black spots begin to fade when I see the dust rising off the road to our house. The car enters the area in front of the house. The ground is hard and dry and when the car goes over it the scales of dried mud crack and pop under the tires like broken glass.

The car skids to an abrupt halt. My father gets out. Something's wrong with him. I think he must be drunk because I'm used to seeing him drunk. But there's something different this time. He does not greet us children or respond to our greeting. In fact, he doesn't even seem to notice we're there, though he walks within a few feet of us to get into the house. He walks like a blind man or someone who has had all his side vision eliminated.

I feel it then. A split second of childish premonition. A distinct feeling of something not being the same as usual (even the usual of his alcoholism, which at that age I accepted as the norm). But I'm not old enough to understand or react to the feeling. I go back to playing in the dirt. My older brother and sister continue their sword fight. Karie plays with her doll.

Remembering the scene then, I thought it odd that I could not remember any of the usual sounds of children playing. Only a heavy silence and the hot sun. A slow-motion film with the sound off.

How long did we continue to play in the front yard? I don't remember.

The front-porch door slams, like a pistol shot. I look up from where I'm playing with a sense of terror, like an alerted animal. My mother (then a young woman) runs down the steps of the porch. She grabs Karie's hand, knocking the doll out of her grasp, and pulls her to her feet, all in one swift uninterrupted gesture.

For a second my mother scans the yard, then realizes the children are too scattered to grab them all. She must grab the ones nearest her and hope the others will follow. She already has Karie in one hand. My brother is near her so she grabs his hand. None of us know what is happening, why suddenly the day is interrupted with this blind terror. I have not moved from under the tree. I am startled and bewildered at my mother's panic.

Then my mother screams, "Run! Run! Follow me!"

My older sister grabs my hand and pulls me to my feet and we follow my mother. For a second my mother glances frantically around, not sure of her direction, then starts around the house. With one sister and my brother held by each of her hands, they half stumble, then catching her panic, run after her. My older sister and I run too, but not nearly as fast. We don't know what we're running from. My sister seems to have some clearer understanding of it than I do. I can barely keep up with her. My mother keeps looking back at us, to make sure we're following. Of the five of us, I'm the last.

We round the corner of the house. I fall. My sister stops and without words grabs me to stand up and keep running. Then I look up from the ground where I have fallen and back. My father is walking toward me. Already a huge man, from my vantage point on the ground he seems gigantic. His trousers are wrinkled and worn and his white shirt dirty, half-open, sweat-stained. His face is pale. His expression is completely blank. He hasn't even seen me fall. He simply keeps advancing with that same powerful, unhindered, slow methodical gait. He's carrying an army rifle.

From the day I remembered it to now that image has never left my mind.

I struggle to my feet and run after my sister toward the barn.

The memory fades here. I have no idea how I end up under the barn, crawling through the small foot-and-a-half space between the floor of the barn and the earth. I'm crawling farther and farther back from the light. Chicken dung. Smell of animals. A few pieces of hay. Cold earth. I don't know where the rest of the family is. Somewhere in the barn.

Crawling. I'm as far back as I can go. I stop, lying flat on the earth. Suddenly the world is cool and dark and still. I do not think of my father. I wonder where my mother is. I am alone in the darkness. I can't think of anything.

(Years and years later, my early twenties, I was in the Haight-Ashbury, tripping on LSD, and I thought I heard a dog panting. I searched and searched for the dog but couldn't find it. The panting continued. It was as though the dog were right over my shoulder. By then I knew enough about drugs to know that if I was hallucinating there was a reason. Then I remembered that I frequently awaken from nightmares with the same heavy, terrified, short-breathed panting. I forced myself to think of the reason. With a sudden flash of insight I realized it was my own panting I had been hearing all these years, the panting of a five-year-old child trapped under a barn.)

Five years old again. Under the barn. The darkness is everywhere. I'm shaking from the cold. Trying to catch my breath. Trying not to breathe so he won't hear me. But he knows I'm here. I am hiding in this darkness waiting to die. I am five years old and the monumental, crushing realization that I will not live out another day of a short life hits me. Not an intellectual realization because all thoughts have stopped. It's in the coldness in my limbs, the blackness in front of my eyes, the stark terror that has paralyzed my whole body. There is nothing I can do. In this darkness smelling of chicken dung I will live out my last moments.

My father is going to kill me.

Another blank space. My sister would fill it in years later. I have no memory of it and can only relate it as she told it to me.

While we are hiding, my father fires the gun. I have no memory of a gun going off. My brother is hiding in the hayloft in the barn. My father fires into it three times. My brother is hit—a slight skin wound on one leg. He's crying out for my mother.

My memory begins again only when I hear my mother's voice: "It's all right now. You can come out now."

The nightmare's ended. It's over. Dear God, it's over! I begin to feel warm again. I can breathe again. I crawl out from under the barn. I see my sisters appearing from under the barn too though they went in at other places. I'm not afraid any more. Mother has said it's all right. It's finished.

So I and my sisters walk to the open doors of the barn, where my mother has called us from. She is telling us to come into the barn. I can't see my father. We enter the center area, where the trucks come in to unload grain.

And all of us are quietly, without protest, lined up against the wall, I don't remember if my father or mother lined us up. Since the line is arranged chronologically and I'm the youngest, I'm at the end of the line. First my mother. Then my brother. Then my oldest sister. Then Karie. Then myself. We are a good foot from one another. There's no physical contact between any of us. I don't even remember noticing that my brother is hurt, though he must have been.

My father is sitting on the barn stool, loading the gun. After we are all in position, he walks up to my mother and raises the gun. I think he will shoot her then, though I will not look. I refuse to look. I stare off through the open doors of the barn to the empty plains. I play with the grain under my feet. I'm not afraid now. It has gone beyond fear. It is just waiting.

But I don't hear the shot. It should have come by now. I turn and look at my mother. The gun barrel is pressing into the skin of her forehead. She stands straight, erect. She has the same stillness, firmness, I've always seen in my mother. She does not tremble or cry or plead. She is willing to die.

I look at my brother and sisters. I later thought it was odd that none of us made any attempt to run. Maybe we instinctively knew we couldn't. We knew we could not break that silence. We knew our lives depended on that moment.

That space of time my mother stood with a gun at her head.

If she had weakened for one instant, or if her glance had wavered, or if even an involuntary tremble had passed over her, I sincerely believe to this day my father would have pulled the trigger and then proceeded to kill us all one by one, then himself. I have absolutely no doubt that he would have done that. She reached him. By her very stillness, her direct, unflinching strength, she was able to reach through the blur of his insanity; she was able to pull him far enough back to see what he was doing.

I went through a period of doubting how much my mother could have loved any of us to play Russian roulette with our lives, and I felt betrayed that she had said that it was all right and we had come out to be lined up against a wall and executed. Then I thought she had risked us all to save my brother—that to stop my father from shooting at him, she had come out and said she would bring all the children out and he could kill us all. And she had done it.

It took me years to understand the decision my mother had made. She knew that by hiding, trying to run, we were doing exactly what would cause our deaths—that my father (trapped in the madness of a war memory) would simply have shot us all one by one where we were hiding. If he had gone far enough to shoot at my brother, eventually he would have killed him and all of us. My father was a crack shot. He had learned how to kill in the war. He could do it. It would not be the first time.

My mother took a terrible chance. Today I am not much younger than my mother was then and I doubt that I would have the courage to take such a chance. She staked her life and the lives of her children on her own strength and her belief that face to face he would not go through with it. And she won. She took the chance. She made the decision. And she won.

But at five years old, standing in a line waiting to die, I do not even vaguely think of any of those things. I only know this is the end of my life. A strange gratitude comes over me when I realize that, being the youngest, I will die last. He has to kill four people before he gets to me. I think I am very lucky. I have that much more time than the rest.

How long did my mother stand with that gun at her forehead? I don't know. Seconds. Minutes. I don't know.

Finally my father lowers the gun. He sits down on the stool again. The gun rests at his side. None of us move. He begins to cry. The bright sun streams through the door, silhouetting this huge man bent over in sobs, his hands over his face.

I can't remember anything else. It's ended.

But now I'm fifteen and sitting in a history class. The sun has gone behind the tree outside the the window. It's drawing patterns across my desk.

"Pat—."

I hear the voice from far away, like the end of a tunnel.

"Patricia! Three times is enough for anybody!"

I look up at the teacher. She's asked me a question. I don't know what it was. I don't know where I am.

The teacher is staring at me. "Are you sick?"

I don't reply. What's she talking about?

"You're white as a sheet."

I continue to stare at the teacher. I can't even think of her name now.

The teacher walks back to her desk. "Go see the school nurse."

I stand up. I feel like a robot. I walk out of the class and down the hall to the nurse's office. The nurse takes my temperature and my pulse. Not finding anything else wrong with me, she decides I'm having my first period and should be taken home. (Actually, my first period has come some months earlier). The nurse drives me to the farm.

I come into the house. My father is not there so I'm left alone. I go up to my room but I can't sleep. I'm not sick but I can't eat. I feel nauseous.

In a few hours, my sister comes home from school. She comes into the bedroom.

"Hey, I heard you come home early today."

"Yes."

"What's wrong? You sick or something?"

"No."

"Then why'd you get out of school early?"

"The nurse thought I was sick."

"That dumb nurse."

My sister sits down and begins to paint her nails. Makeup has lately become a whole ritual with her.

"Hey, Karie, can I ask you something?"

"Ask away."

She continues to paint her nails. When she was little she was known for her tantrums. Now, no matter what happens, she always "plays it cool," as she says. Nothing disturbs that surface placidity.

"Karie, did something happen when we were little?"

"What are you talking about?"

"I been having a dream—"

My sister's impatient. "Oh, you and your nightmares. You know you woke me up last night—scared me to death, you crying out like that."

"No, this is different. I keep having this dream that Dad lined us up in the barn to shoot us—"

My sister starts to laugh. She thinks I'm as naive as they come.

"If that's a dream, you and me been having the same bad dream, kid."

"Well, it ain't truth, is it? Got to be a dream," I say.

"Ain't no dream, you dummy."

I stare at her. She isn't fazed. To her it was an unimportant thing that happened. Nothing earthshaking.

She looks at me and stops painting her nails.

"Well, what you so big-eyed about? It happened a long time ago. No use getting excited about it now. You was just a kid."

I continue to stare at her, wordless.

"Don't look so stupid! All the rest of us remember. Why don't you?"

"I thought it was a dream. . . ."

"It's no dream. It's fact. Happened. Right out there. He flipped out. Cracked up. Had a breakdown, the doctors said. Bang—bang. Sure. Dad don't remember nothing about it, but ask Mom."

She goes back to painting her nails.

"Don't it bother you none?" I ask.

"Why should it?"

I don't say anything as she continues to paint her nails.

"Ah, I knew he wasn't going to do it," she says. "Shoot us all just like that? He wasn't going to. Just trying to scare us."

"I thought he was—"

"Nah, he wouldn't do that."

"Then why was we running?"

My sister stops painting her nails. She doesn't want to talk about it any more.

"Why you think about those things anyway? That's why you got them nightmares all the time—thinking about such bad things."

I lie down and pull the covers over my head.

"Hey, you really sick?" she asks.

"Go away. Go somewhere else."

"You're spoiled. You know that? Pretending sick. You ain't sick. Just spoiled."

My sister leaves the room.

A few hours later Mom gets home and calls me down to supper but I don't go. I say I don't feel well.

After supper, Mom comes up to the bedroom. She looks tired. She's been working all day. She hasn't had enough sleep. It shows in her face. Circles under her eyes, and she needs glasses, but she never has the time or money to get them, so she goes to

Woolworth's and picks out a pair on the counter that she thinks make her see better. She has those funny glasses on now, looking at me.

"Karie says you come home from school early—sick."

I don't want to see my mother. I don't want to talk to her. For the first time in my life, I hate her.

"I'm all right," I say.

I've started reading books heavily in the last few years and I pick one up now, hiding behind it.

"Missed you tonight," Mom says.

I did not come to meet the factory bus that night.

"I ain't coming no more," I say. "Ain't going to meet you no more."

My mother doesn't ask why. I am hiding behind my book. She sits down in the chair near the bed.

"You got yourself another book," she says.

I don't speak to her.

"Is it a good book?" she asks. Mom always talks about books like they're a foreign country. She never has the time to read one.

"No," I reply.

"Kind of funny to read a book you don't like, isn't it?"

Again I don't reply. My face is buried in the book.

Long pause. Finally my mother takes those bad glasses off. She rubs the area over her eyes.

"You remember much more about that dream you was telling me about?" she finally asks.

"No."

"I thought you might—"

"Didn't have no dream."

"Well, a few days ago you was saying—"

"Made it all up. Out of my head. Never happened. Just a dream that never happened. Like this book. Ain't real."

"Some things in books is real, ain't they?"

"No. It's all a lie."

I'm crying. I try to hide it.

"Why you crying then—if it ain't real?"

"Ain't crying!"

"Next you'll be telling me this chair's a dream and I'm a dream—fact, soon you'll be telling me the whole world's a dream that ain't real."

"It is! Ain't nothing real in this world."

My mother suddenly starts to laugh.

"You ain't got no right to laugh," I say.

"Child, you're making no sense to me at all."

"Not after what you did! You ain't got no right to laugh!" My face is hot with anger.

My mother's face becomes serious, tired. "Now what is it you think I did?"

"You know! You know damned well what you did!"

"You tell me."

"You—you betrayed me—all of us!"

"When?"

"You know when!"

"When?" My mother is demanding an answer.

"When he tried to kill us, when you called us out—called us out so he could line us up and kill us."

My mother doesn't say anything. She stands up and goes to the window. She looks out at the early evening, one hand on the old white curtains.

"Answer me!" I yell.

My mother turns and looks at me. It's hard for her to talk. She never discusses what she feels—her regrets, her hopes, her fears or her loves. She is a silent woman when it comes to emotions or explanations. She lives. She acts. She decides. She survives. She does not discuss any of these things. To her there's no point to endless verbal analysis. It consumes energy and time and solves nothing.

"Why don't you say something? Why you acting like you didn't hear?"

"I didn't think you'd ever remember," she says. "I thought you'd forgot and sometimes I thought it best you'd forgot."

I continue to scream out my rage. "We could have all died! He was going to kill us! Didn't you understand that?"

"I couldn't hide in the dark and listen to my children dying one by one."

"I trusted you!"

That hurt. I see the wound pass deep into her eyes.

"I did what I thought I had to do. If I was wrong, I'm sorry."

But how could I say she was wrong? I was alive. Alive enough to be furious at her in this moment, alive enough to be outraged over something that happened ten years earlier and that I had just remembered for some subconscious reason I would never guess. She was right. I was alive. I could not say she had been wrong. Yet I felt she had been wrong. I could not blame her for a decision that proved right. Yet I did blame her.

"Why didn't you leave him?" I ask.

"That first year after the hospital I couldn't."

I remember the year my father returned from the Veterans' Hospital. He was in bed most of the time. When we got home from school, we had to take our shoes off before we could come into the house. He couldn't stand the noise our shoes made on the floor. In the winter we'd come home and make a fire in the wood stove. He was so helpless then, he couldn't make a fire to keep himself warm during the day, but stayed curled up all day in bed like a baby. But that year passed. He drank more and more and over the years we all became accustomed to his drunks and semi-insanity.

"Why didn't you leave him later then?" I ask. "When he was well."

My mother says nothing. I see she is never going to answer this question for me.

"Why didn't you make them keep him in the Veterans' Hospital?" I ask.

"They said there wasn't anything they could do."

"He's crazy. He should be locked up."

"They gave me this piece of paper to sign. They said it was just so he would be taken care of. But I read it and it had this word—'frontal lobotomy.' I didn't know what that word meant so I asked. They said it was just an operation to make him better. I asked what kind of operation. They said it was on the brain—finally they said they would cut away part of his brain and that's all that could make him well again."

"Then he should'a had the operation," I say.

"Maybe."

"Then why didn't he?" I ask.

My mother goes to the other side of the room. She is searching for the words to explain something to me.

"There was men there had the operation. They was peaceful enough. Talked and made sense. But they seemed . . . I don't know . . . when you cut the pain out do you cut out part of the soul?"

For a second I don't hear the question. It's a thought far beyond anything I've considered in my fifteen years. But I'm more surprised because it's not the sort of question I had thought my mother capable of asking. Yet she has. With such clarity and directness I'm taken aback.

I have no answer so I say nothing.

She continues. "One doctor there was doing those operations all day long. Just slicing off part of the brain. I never met such people. They was educated, intelligent. Big words I didn't understand. But I never met such people that'd do something like that, not half knowing what they was doing. So maybe they could make him quiet, not somebody we'd have to be afraid of. But I couldn't do it. I couldn't sign that paper for them."

"They could'a give him some other treatment," I say. "They could'a done something else for him."

"They said they couldn't. Said they had too many veterans there after the war already. Said there wasn't no way to make them forget. Lots of veterans was having the operation. I had to agree or there wasn't nothing they could do, just release him again."

I think for a while. I don't know anything about a frontal lobotomy. I've never heard of it before.

But I say, "Well, maybe the operation was okay if it made them all better."

My mother is silent again. She's searching for the words to explain something I doubt she has ever verbally tried to articulate even to herself. She uses the words and images she understands.

"You know that old river down on the lower forty—the one you kids love to go swimming in in the summer—"

I'm paying little attention. I don't know what on earth this has to do with the subject.

She continues. "Well, let's pretend that river turns wild one day—always overflowing, ruining crops, maybe even drowning people—a mean, wild river sometimes. And someone comes up to you and says I can do something to that river to make it always quiet, now matter how bad the storm, never wild no matter how much rain falls. They say you sign this piece of paper and we'll change that river. But it won't reflect the blue sky no more and it won't sparkle and dance in the sunlight no more and it won't bring joy when it laughs and jumps over the rocks—"

"It ain't the same!"

My mother stops. "No, it ain't the same."

Abruptly I say, "You love him more than us, don't you?"

My mother is startled at what I've just said.

"I never compared the kind of love I had for him and the kind I got for my children."

"But you brought him home again."

"Yes." She says it without shame or guilt.

I am outraged at this admission.

"What about us?"

"I knew he wouldn't try to do that again. That was all broken."

I stare at her. Is she talking herself into lies to justify what she did?

"What about him beating you and getting drunk?"

"Has he ever beat you?" she asks.

"No."

It was the truth. He never had. I am silent for a moment, then stumble, trying to say something. "But—"

"But you're afraid."

I don't answer that. She needs no answer. Silence. In that silence I see the guilt in my mother's face.

Then she says, "He loves you children more than anything in this world."

I stare at her in total bewilderment. Love! A man who inflicted this kind of psychological torture on us for years.

I don't even try to restrain the words: "Like hell!"

"You forget the good times."

"What good times?" I ask.

I shouldn't have asked that. There had been good times—when Dad told us funny stories, when he dressed up in a sheet like a ghost and went out with all of us in the middle of the night to milk the cow and we laughed and laughed when the cow ran all over the pasture with Dad chasing it, when he danced with my mother all over the kitchen and without even any music playing, when he made up rhymes to go with our names, when he spent all the money he had on toys for us even when we were over our heads in debt, when he found out about the mean old woman five miles away who always sicked her dog on us everytime we came by and Dad went over in the middle of the night with some paint and wrote in big letters on the side of her barn THE GODS ARE GOING TO GET YOU—when he worried if one of us was sick. Yes, my father loved us. But I had two fathers. One was gentle and warm and light-hearted. The other was tormented, violent, frightening—a madman.

"Do you love him?" It was hard for me to ask that. I had to force myself.

Again, I know my mother will not answer.

My mother knows what I'm feeling when she says, "Don't you think I'd like you to have the father he was before he went to war? Don't you think I'd like you to see that big-hearted, laughing, strong man I married? The other kids knew him then—they was born before the war—but you didn't. You was born during the war and when he got back he was already crippled, in his mind and heart. If he'd come home without an arm or leg, you could understand. Anybody could understand. It wouldn't make him any less the man he was. But he comes home crippled some other way—in his soul. You children never understood the things that crippled him."

"Do you?" I ask.

My mother is silent for a few moments. "I never been to war. I don't know what it means to have to kill people, kill children like your own children. I don't know the guilt and hate and torment you got to live with all your life. He didn't make this world."

"I don't think that's no excuse for nothing."

"Maybe not. Maybe there ain't no excuses for him or me. I don't try to find the excuses no more."

"Mr. Jackson went to war and he ain't crazy like Dad," I say.

"Lord, child, don't you understand people ain't the same?"

"But if the war was so awful, why ain't he crazy?"

My mother is irritated, close to anger. "Yes, and Mr. Jackson's the one that goes out of his way on the highway to hit a stray dog and thinks it's funny when the high school boys poured gasoline all over that poor monkey in the town zoo and set it afire."

"But Mr. Jackson never tried to kill his family," I say.

My words stop her. She stands up, moving away.

"Besides," I say, "Mr. Craig went to war too and he's a good man."

"Yes, he's a good man."

She's standing on the dark side of the room. The afternoon sun has totally disappeared by now. Only the small light on near my bed. I have to listen hard to understand everything she begins to tell me.

"When your father was young, not even twenty, and he comes to my parents' farm for a job—it was hog-butchering time. They'd slit the hog's throat, put a bucket under it till most of the blood was out, then string it up till it bled to death. All the time the hog was screaming. The other men was going to teach your father how to do it. Your father tried but he couldn't. And the other men laughing and making jokes, him such a big man and he acts just like a woman, can't stand to see a hog die. But then your father picks up the knife and quick slits the hog's throat. He walks out of the barn and I follow him. He's so sick he's throwing up, shaking like a child."

She pauses, then says, "So he went to war and instead of hogs it was people."

There's a long silence before I ask, "Did he have to go?"

"No," she answers.

"Then why did he if he didn't have to?"

"Oh, they was making big speeches then and having parades. All the other men joined. He wanted to wear a uniform, be a hero. And I guess he was restless on the farm—wanted to see the world and come back covered with medals. He didn't know what war meant. I didn't either. I kissed him goodbye just like they did in the movies and I thought, just like in the movies, when it's over the bad guys will be dead and the good guys will still be good. The lights will go on and we'll all walk out of the theater and go back to our normal way of living with nothing changed."

I say nothing, waiting for her to continue.

"And the war ended and he come home. Still handsome. More handsome. Filled out. A man now. He come home with medals and bragging and drinking too much, like the other men. With suitcases of toys for you kids, new dresses for me. When he sees you for the first time, he grins like it was all Christmas. And that night in bed he's full of jokes and stories about Paris and all them places I never been. But I know something's wrong. He's too loud. He won't look right at me, not deep in the eyes the way he used to. Just keeps talking and laughing. He tells me some story and laughs—and all of a sudden he turns and slams his fist into the wall. He hits it so hard the plaster gives way—his fist has gone half through the wall. He turns and walks out and I don't see him again for a week, when he comes home drunk."

I say nothing. At that age I have little understanding of what my mother is trying so desperately to communicate, wants so badly for me to begin to understand.

"What did he do in the war?" I ask.

My mother looks at me but does not answer.

I ask again. "What did he do?"

"He killed—like everybody else."

"But our teachers say we was right in World War Two."

"Right? I don't know what that means any more."

"The Germans was bad."

"Yes."

"That was a awful thing they did to the Jews."

"Yes, that was awful."

"The Germans couldn't win."

"No."

"Then he had to go and he shouldn't be crazy for killing people we was supposed to kill, for killing bad people."

"No, he shouldn't."

A silence. My mother's face is drawn.

"Then why?" I ask.

My mother says nothing. She doesn't know the answer.

"The Nazis was trying to take over the free world. Somebody had to stop them," I say.

Suddenly my mother says, "They were going to court-martial him."

"Dad?"

I'm surprised. Dad court-martialed? Only traitors or cowards were court-martialed. But Dad had been brave. He hadn't run. He killed people.

"Your father was the biggest man in the outfit so they made him carry the flame-thrower. They was going through Germany. They took this village. Just farm people like us living in this village. They were hiding in the basement of the church. The sergeant tells your father to burn out the basement—that there's enemy hiding in there. But your father won't do it. He says they're just women and kids. Sergeant says it don't matter—they're Germans, ain't they? But still your father won't do it. The sergeant puts a gun to his head and says either he kills the Germans or gets killed—"

"Did he do it?"

"Yes."

An image flashes through my head. My father standing at the top of the stairs to a basement. Women and children huddled together at the opposite side of the basement. A sudden streak of orange-red flame across the basement. And again. Another streak. And again. But not even a vivid imagination can show me the agony and horror of people being burned to death. It is a scene I am incapable of visualizing, do not want to visualize.

Silence. Finally, I say, "But if he did what he was ordered, why did they want to court-martial him?"

"The next day he found the sergeant and beat him till the sergeant ended up in the hospital. I guess even that they was willing to let pass with some time in the brig. But then he started losing every flame-thrower they gave him, getting drunk all the time. But they didn't court-martial him cause after that he was the best man in the outfit—killed more Germans than anyone. So instead of a court-martial he got a medal."

A strange expression comes to my mother's face. It's not bitterness or even disbelief. Just a tired astonishment.

She gets up to leave. She has said what she wanted to say. She won't try to explain any more to me. She has tried to make me forgive and understand my father. But I can't. I can't even begin to understand at that age. If I do, I will begin to weaken. If I let myself love him, he will hurt me more than he has. And even if I could understand the reasons, it does not make the terror less for me. It does not diminish the fear. It does not erase that day from my memory.

Suddenly I say, "If he did that, he should have died in the war."

I am standing. My mother turns to face me. Though I'm six inches taller than she is, she slaps me hard across the face. It's the first and last time she ever hit me.

Tears well in my eyes as she walks out of the room.

I do not forget that slap for days. But finally one evening I go to meet the bus again. We have barely spoken to each other since the discussion. I say nothing as I stand by the highway and she gets out of the bus.

We begin to walk home. Not speaking. Separate. I'm ahead. Finally I drop back, walking beside her though still at a distance.

"How was school?" she asks.

"Okay."

We continue to walk separately. She looks off across the fields and says something about the irrigation the neighboring farmer is running to one of his fields. I nod without much response. I pay little attention to anything that has to do with crops and land. I'm not like my mother. I will not stay on the land. I will go to the cities. I only live for the day I can leave this country and never come back.

We are near the house. I stop in the middle of the road. I don't look at her when I say it.

"I'm sorry." The words barely get past my lips.

I do not look at her to see her reaction.

"Ragmuffin."

It's a term of affection she has not used since I was a child. We resume walking to the house. And for the next three years, until I'm eighteen and leave, I will meet her each night at the end of the road. The ritual is re-established. But we never again discuss the day my father tried to kill us.

* * * * *

I was home two years ago. My visits never last more than a couple of days at the most. My father had a heart attack a few years back so now he's a complete invalid. They draw a small social-security check and something from the Veteran's Administration but it's not enough to live on, so Mom still works at the same job at the factory. The house is looking a little better these days and they bought back an acre of land near the house so Mom has extended the garden. My father still drinks but his insanity has cooled. He doesn't have the physical strength to back it any more.

The children have all left home, scattered to all parts of the country. My two sisters are married, with large families, living in big cities. My brother joined the military as soon as he was of age and has become a career man. At the time of my visit he was in Vietnam. I finished college—the only one in the family that went to college. But I never seemed to find the place I fit in. I dropped out in the sixties. Drugs. Haight-Ashbury. Berkeley. The East Village. Protested. Saw the big cities.

Last time I noticed how my mother had aged. She is middle-aged and her beauty has long ago died in beatings and drunken nights and year after year in the factory. Her face is lined, aged, tired. She suffers from frequent headaches, though she did finally go to a doctor and get glasses. I always think it's amusing how she treats those glasses like a prize possession. Cleaning them, carefully putting them away at night.

I am sleeping upstairs in my old bedroom. I hear my mother get up a little before dawn. Her usual six o'clock. She always gets up at that hour even if she's been up half the night with Dad.

I hear her in the kitchen talking to the dog. She's recently found this funny mutt of a dog and, when she thinks there's no one around to hear her, she talks to it just as though it were a person.

"There now. There now. You silly dog. Don't know why I keep you. Just a big pest."

I am half awake in bed, listening to her. In this half-dream state, I begin to remember something.

* * * * *

Again, it's the day my father lined us up in the barn. He has dropped the gun. He's crying. He reaches in his pocket and hands Mom the keys to the car. There is no verbal exchange between them. . . . She takes the keys and, helping him stand, leads him to the car, where he sits in the passenger seat. He does everything without complaint. His entire body seems to have crumbled. He stares out the car window like a child.

Then she comes back, kneeling by my brother to look at his leg. She tells him to get in the car so she can take him to the doctor. My brother refuses to get in the car with my father. He seems more angry than anything else. The wound is hardly more than a slight skin cut. My brother makes an angry exit to the house. My sisters are sobbing. My mother embraces each of them, saying something to them. They go toward the house, still crying.

Then my mother turns to me. I'm standing in the same place I was during the line-up. I have not moved. My mother says my name, standing at the entrance to the barn. I do not respond. She walks toward me, then stands in front of me for a long while.

"Cry."

I can't. I don't look at her. I stare out across the plains. I don't want to look at her or anyone.

She grabs me by the shoulders. "Cry."

I pull away from her, without looking at her. I would cry if I could, but something in me is too far away for tears. When I look at her there's a faint rim of tears in her eyes. It's the only time in my life I've ever seen my mother cry. She takes her hands from my shoulders. I don't say anything to her. I barely know she's there. I turn and walk away from her.

I should have cried that day. I should have sobbed my heart out as my sisters did. I should have clung to her as I wanted to, but I couldn't. The tears, pain, fear, betrayal were buried so deep inside myself it was ten years before I could even remember that day happened.

* * * * *

But that's past. It's morning. I'm twenty-five. I get out of bed, still hearing my mother in the kitchen with the dog. I go downstairs. It's just sunrise. I stand at the kitchen door and look at Mom.

She's sitting on the back step with a cup of coffee. The little dog is beside her, wagging his tail. She pets his head now and then. The dawn catches my mother's profile—the years have revealed a strong, straight nose, high cheek-bones and firm mouth. Although she is partially gray now, the sun catches some strands of still-auburn hair around her face. I think my mother is beautiful then—in a way more beautiful than I had thought she was when she was a young woman.

I sit down beside her on the front step.

"Want some breakfast?" she asks.

"I'm okay."

"Leaving today?"

"Yes."

She will not ask me where I'm going. If I volunteer the information, that's one thing, but she makes absolutely no attempt to pry into my life. She doesn't ask me about drugs or how I'm living. She doesn't condemn my long hair and sandals. If I want to talk about my life, my plans or hopes, she will listen but she will not question me.

We sit and watch the sunrise together. I had forgotten how much I miss the plains, how deeply they had become a part of me. The sun has already broken over the bare, slight curve of the horizon. The plains seem endless now; yet I know that by that afternoon I will reach the towering peaks of the Rocky Mountains. Shadows begin to streak across the flat land. A slight wind comes up, moving the leaves of the trees near the house. The birds begin. It will be a beautiful, clear summer day.

We do not speak or touch. But I have never felt so close to my mother.

Then I hear my father's voice from inside the house. "I'm dying. . . . I'm dying. . . . Where are you?"

My mother stands up and goes to him.

I hear her voice. "You're always dying, old man. Guess we'll just have to bury you soon."

"That's what you want! You want to bury me! You want to kill me! It's dark—it's dark—"

"Morning's coming. . . ."

"It's dark."

"It's a beautiful morning coming."

My father says nothing. A silence comes over the house. He has fallen back to sleep. I only hear my mother's footsteps as she begins her day's work.

WHAT I SAW FROM WHERE I STOOD

MARISA SILVER

Dulcie is afraid of freeways. She doesn't like not being able to get off whenever she wants, and sometimes I catch her holding her breath between exits, as if she's driving through a graveyard. So even though the party we went to last week was miles from our apartment in Silver Lake, we drove home on the surface streets.

I was drunk, and Dulcie was driving my car. She'd taken one look at me as we left the party, then dug her fingers into my front pocket and pulled out my keys. I liked the feel of her hand rubbing against me, through my jeans; she hadn't been touching me much lately.

I cranked open the window to clear my head as we drove through Santa Monica. Nice houses. Pretty flowers. Volvos. Dulcie and I always say we'd never want to live out here in suburbia, but the truth is, we can't afford to, not on our salaries. Dulcie's a second-grade teacher in Glendale, and I'm a repairman for the telephone company.

When we reached Hollywood, things got livelier. There were skinny guitar punks patrolling the clubs on the strip with their pudgy girlfriends in midriff tops and thigh-high black skirts. A lot of big hair, big breasts, boredom. Further east, there were boys strutting the boulevard, waiting to slip into someone's silver Mercedes and make a buck. One leaned against a fire hydrant and picked at his sallow face, looking cold in a muscle T-shirt.

We hit a red light at Vermont, right next to the hospital where Dulcie lost the baby, a year ago. She'd started cramping badly one night. She was only six months pregnant. I called the emergency room, and the attendant said to come right over. By the time we got there, the doctors couldn't pick up a heartbeat. They gave Dulcie drugs to induce labor, and the baby was born. He was blue. He was no bigger than a football.

Dulcie looked up at the hospital and then back at the road. She's a small girl, and she sank behind the wheel, getting even smaller. I didn't say anything. The light turned green. She drove across Vermont and I nodded off.

I woke up when a car plowed into us from behind. My body flew toward the windshield, then ricocheted back against my seat. Dulcie gripped the wheel, staring straight ahead out the window.

"Something happened," she said.

"Yeah," I heard myself answer, although my voice sounded hollow. "We had an accident."

We got out to check the damage and met at the back of the car. "It's nothing," Dulcie said as we study the medium-sized dent on the fender. It was nothing to us, anyway; the car was too old and beat-up for us to feel protective of it.

Behind me, I heard the door of a van slide open. I hadn't thought about the people who'd hit us, hadn't even noticed if they'd bothered to stop. I started to wave them off. They didn't need to get out, apologize, dig around for the insurance information they probably didn't have. But when I turned, there were four or five men in front of me. They were standing very close. They were young. I was beginning to think that Dulcie and I should just get back into our car and drive away, when the van's engine cut out and a tall guy wearing a hooded sweatshirt called back toward it, "Yo, Darren! Turn it on, you motherfucker!"

His cursing seemed to make his friends nervous. Two of them looked at their feet. One hopped up and down like a fighter getting ready for a bout. Someone was saying, "Shit, shit, shit," over and over again. Then I heard "Do it, do it!" and a short, wide kid with a shaved head and glow-in-the-dark stripes on his sneakers pulled out a gun and pointed it at my face. It didn't look like the guns in movies. Dulcie screamed.

"Don't shoot. Please don't shoot us!" Her voice was so high it sounded painful, as if it were scraping her throat.

"Your keys!" the tall one shouted. "Give us your motherfucking keys!"

Dulcie threw the keys on the ground at their feet. "Please! I don't have any money!"

"I'll get it," I heard myself say, as if I were picking up the tab at a bar. I was calm. I felt like I was underwater. Everything seemed slow, and all I could hear was my own breathing. I reached into my back pocket and pulled out my wallet. I took out the bills and handed them over. The tall guy grabbed the money and ran back to the van, which made me feel better until I noticed that the kid with the shaved head was still pointing the gun at me.

That's when I got scared. As though someone had thrown a switch, all the sound returned, loud and close. I heard the cars roaring past on Sunset. I heard Dulcie screaming, "No! No! No!" I heard an argument erupt between two of the guys. "Get in their car! Get in their fucking car or I'll do you too!" I grabbed Dulcie's hand, and pulled her around the front of our car, crouching low, so I could feel the heat of the engine under the hood. The van revved up. I stood, bringing Dulcie up with me, and there, on the driver's side, no more than three feet from me, was the kid with the shaved head. He had the gun in one hand and Dulcie's keys in the other. I could see sweat glistening over the pimples on his face.

"Hey!" he said, looking confused. "What the fuck?"

Then it was as if I skipped a few minutes of my life, because the next thing I knew, Dulcie and I were racing down a side street toward the porch lights of some bungalows. We didn't look back to see if we were being followed. Sometimes Dulcie held my hand, sometimes we were separated by the row of parked cars. We had no idea where we were going.

* * * * *

After the police and their questions, and their heartfelt assurance that there was nothing at all they could do for us, we took a cab back to our apartment in Silver Lake. Dulcie was worried because the crackheads—that's what the police called them—had our keys, and our address was on the car registration. But the police had told us that the carjackers wouldn't come after us—that kind of thing almost never happened.

Still, Dulcie couldn't sleep, so we sat up all night while she went over what had happened—she'd seen the van on the street earlier, but hadn't it been in front of us, not behind? Why had they chosen our car, our sorry, broken-down mutt of a car? How close had we come to being shot?

"We saw them," she said. "We know what they look like."

"They weren't killers. They were thieves. There's a difference, I guess," I said.

"No," she said, twisting her straight brown hair around her finger so tightly the tip turned white. "It doesn't make sense."

"It doesn't. But it happened."

Dulcie needs things to be exact. You have to explain yourself clearly when you're around her, so she's probably a good teacher. For a minute I wondered whether she wished we had been shot, just for the sake of logic.

She'd done this after losing the baby too, going over and over what she might have done to kill it. Had she exercised too much? Not enough? Had she eaten something bad? She wanted an answer, and she needed to blame someone; if that person turned out to be her, that would still be better than having no one to blame at all. A few days after the delivery, a hospital social worker called to check on her. She reassured Dulcie that what had happened hadn't been her fault. It was a fluke thing, the woman said. She used the word "flukish."

"I should have noticed them tailing me," Dulcie said now. "How could I not notice a car that close?"

"Don't do that," I told her. "Don't think about what could have happened."

"I have to think about it," she said. "How can you not think about it? We were this close," she said, holding her fingers out like a gun and aiming at my chest.

* * * * *

I drove Dulcie's car to work the next day. When I got home that night, Dulcie had moved the mattress from our bed into the living room, where it lay in the middle of the floor, the sheets spilling over onto the carpet. She'd taken a personal day to recover from the holdup. Her eyes were red, and she looked as though she'd been crying all afternoon.

"It's the rat," she said. "He's back."

A month earlier, a rat had burrowed and nested in the wall behind our bed. Every night it scratched a weird, personal jazz into our ears. We told the landlord, and he said he would get on it right away, which meant *You'll be living with that rat forever, and if you don't like it there're ten other people in line for your apartment.* I checked around the house to make sure the rat couldn't find a way inside. I patched up a hole underneath the sink with plywood and barricaded the space between the dishwasher and the wall with old towels. After Dulcie was sure that there would be no midnight visitor eating our bananas, she was okay with the rat. We even named him—Mingus.

She wasn't okay with it anymore.

"He's getting louder. Closer. Like he's going to get in this time," she said.

"He can't get in. There's no way."

"Well, I can't sleep in that room."

"It's a small apartment, Dulcie." The living room was smaller than the bedroom, and the mattress nearly filled it.

"I can't do it, Charles. I can't."

"All right. We can sleep anywhere you want," I said.

"I want to sleep in the living room. And I want you to change the message on the answering machine," she said. "It has my voice on it. It should have a man's voice."

"You're worried about the rat hearing your voice on the machine?"

"Don't make fun of me, okay? Those guys know where we live."

Later that night, I discovered that she wanted to sleep with all the lights on.

"I want people to know we're home," she said. "People don't break in if they think you're there."

We were lying on the floor on our mattress. She felt tiny, so delicate that I would crush her if I squeezed too hard or rolled the wrong way.

"You don't mind, do you?" she said. "About the light. Is it too bright?"

She'd let me throw one of my shirts, an orange one, over the fixture hanging from the ceiling. It gave the room a muffled, glowy feel.

"No," I said. I kissed her forehead. She didn't turn to me. Since the baby, we've had a hard time getting together.

Dulcie sat up again. "Maybe it's a bad idea," she said. "Maybe a thief will see the light on at 4 a.m. and think that we're actually out of town. I mean, who leaves their light on all night when they're home?"

"No one."

"You know," she said, "I saw in a catalogue once that you could buy an inflatable man to put in a chair by your window. Or in your car. You could put him in the passenger seat if you were driving alone."

She looked at me, but I didn't know what to say. To me, driving with a plastic blow-up doll in the seat next to you seemed very peculiar.

"Lie down," I said, stroking her back beneath her T-shirt. Her skin was smooth and warm.

She lay down next to me. I turned over on my stomach and laid my hand across her chest. I liked the feel of the small rises of her breasts, the give of them.

Dulcie's milk had come in two days after the delivery. The doctor had warned her that this would happen and had prescribed Valium in advance. I came home from work and found Dulcie, stoned, staring at her engorged breasts in the bathroom mirror. I'd never seen anything like it. Her breasts were like boulders, and her veins spread out across them like waterways on a map. Dulcie squeezed one nipple, and a little pearl of yellowish milk appeared. She tasted it.

"It's sweet," she said. "What a waste."

For the next two days, she lay on the couch holding packs of frozen vegetables against each breast. Sometimes we laughed about it, and she posed for a few sexpot pictures, with packs of peas pressed against her chest like pasties. Other times she just stared at the living room wall, adjusting a pack when it slipped. I asked her if her breasts hurt, and she said yes, but not in the way you'd think.

I slid my hand off Dulcie's chest, turned back over, and stared at the T-shirt on the light fixture.

"Did you know," she said, "that when you're at a red light the person next to you probably has a gun in his glove compartment?"

"Defensive driving," I said, trying for a joke.

"Statistically speaking, it's true. Until yesterday, I never thought about how many people have guns," Dulcie said. "Guns in their cars, guns in their pocketbooks when they're going to the market, guns. . . ."

A fly was caught between the light and my T-shirt. I could see its shadow darting frantically back and forth until, suddenly, it was gone.

* * * * *

The next evening, as I was driving home from work, someone threw an egg at my car. I thought it was another holdup. I sucked in so much air that I started to choke and almost lost control. Two kids then ran by my window. One was wearing a Dracula mask and a cape. The other one had on a rubber monster head and green tights. I'd forgotten it was Halloween.

Dulcie takes holidays pretty seriously, and when I got home I expected to see a cardboard skeleton on the door, and maybe a carved pumpkin or two. Usually she greets the trick-or-treaters wearing a tall black witch hat that she keeps stashed in a closet the rest of the year. When she opens the door, she makes this funny cackling laugh, which is kind of embarrassing but also sweet. She's so waifish, there's not much about her that could scare anybody. But when I got home and climbed the outside stairs to our second-floor apartment, there was nothing on our door and the apartment was dark.

"What are you doing with all the lights off?" I asked when I got inside. She was sitting at the kitchen table, her hands folded in front of her as if she were praying.

"Shut the door," she said. "A whole pack of them just came. They must have rung the bell five times."

"They want their candy."

"We don't have any."

"Really? You didn't buy any?"

"Charles, we don't know who any of these people are," she said slowly, as if I were six years old. "I'm not going to open my door to perfect strangers."

"They're kids."

"What about the ones who come really late?" she asked. "All those teenagers. They're looking for trouble."

I sat down and reached across the table for her hands. "It's Halloween, Dulce. It's just kids having fun."

"Plenty of people aren't home on Halloween. This is just going to be one of those places where nobody's home."

The doorbell rang.

"Dulcie—"

"Sh-h-h!" She hissed at me like a cat.

"This is ridiculous." I got up.

"Please!" she called out after me.

The bell rang again. I grabbed a box of cookies and went to the door. A little kid was walking away, but he turned back when he heard the door open. He was six, eight years old. An old man I recognized from the neighborhood, maybe his grandfather, stood a few steps behind him.

The boy wore a cowboy outfit—a fringed orange vest over a T-shirt with a picture of Darth Vader on it, jeans mashed down into plastic cowboy boots, and a holster sliding down over his narrow hips. He took a gun out of the holster and waved it around in the air.

"Bang," he said, without enthusiasm.

"You got me," I answered, putting my hands to my chest and pretending to die.

"It's a fake gun," the boy said. "No real bullets."

"You mean I'm not dead?" I tried to sound amazed, and I got a smile out of the kid.

The grandfather said something impatiently in another language, Russian or maybe Armenian.

"Trick or treat," the boy said quietly. He held out a plastic grocery sack with his free hand.

I looked into the bag. There were only a few pieces of candy inside. Suddenly the whole thing made me sad. I offered my box of mint cookies.

The boy looked back at his grandfather, who shook his head. "I'm only allowed to have it if it's wrapped," the boy said to me.

I felt like a criminal. "We didn't have a chance to get to the store," I said, as the boy holstered his gun and moved off with his grandfather.

When I went back inside, Dulcie was standing in the middle of the dark living room, staring at me. Three months after the baby died, I came home from work and found her standing in that same place. Her belly underneath her T-shirt was huge, much bigger than when she'd actually been pregnant. For one crazy second, I thought that the whole thing had been a mistake and that she was still pregnant. I felt a kind of relief I had never felt before. Then she lifted her shirt and took out a watermelon from underneath it.

A group of kids yelled "Trick or treat!" below us. They giggled. Someone said "Boo!" then there was a chorus of dutiful thank you's. I heard small feet pound up the rickety wooden stairway to the second-floor apartments. I walked over to Dulcie and put my arms around her.

"We can't live like this," I said.

"I can," she said.

* * * * *

Dulcie went back to work three days after the carjacking. I dropped her off at school in my car, and she arranged for one of her teacher friends to give her a lift home. I took it as a good sign, her returning to work. She complains about the public school system, all the idiotic bureaucracy she has to deal with, but she loves the kids. She's always coming home with stories about cute things they did, or about how quickly they picked up something she didn't think they'd understand the first time. She was named Teacher of the Year last spring, and a couple of parents got together and gave her this little gold necklace. Her school's in a rough part of Glendale. The necklace was a big deal.

She was home when I got off work, sitting on the couch. She waved a piece of pink paper in the air.

"What's that?" I said.

"We're not allowed to touch the children anymore," she said.

"What are you talking about?"

She told me that a parent had accused a teacher of touching his daughter in the wrong way. Social Services came in, the works. When they finally got around to questioning the girl, she told them the teacher had just patted her on the back because she answered a question right.

"Now the district's in a panic—they don't want a lawsuit every time some kid exaggerates. So no touching the students."

"That's nuts," I said. "Those kids need to be hugged every once in a while. They probably don't get enough affection at home."

"That's a racist generalization, Charles," she said. "Most of the parents try hard. They love their kids just as much as you and I would."

Neither of us said anything. Dulcie hadn't brought up the idea of our having kids since we'd lost the baby. She had just stepped on a grenade, and I was waiting through those awful seconds before it explodes.

"This is a fucked-up town," she said finally.

I wasn't sure what had made her say this. The school thing? The carjacking? "Maybe if we turn on the TV we'll catch a freeway chase," I said.

"Or a riot."

"Or a celebrity bio."

She started laughing. "That's the real tragedy," she said. "The celebrity bio."

We laughed some more. When we stopped, neither of us knew what to say.

"I'm not racist," I said, at last.

"I know. I didn't mean that."

"I may be prejudiced against celebrities, though."

She squeezed out a smile. It was worth the stupid joke.

* * * * *

The next Saturday, Dulcie called an exterminator. She'd decided that we should pay for one out of our own pocket, because she'd read that some rats carry airborne viruses.

"People died in New Mexico," she said. "Children too."

It turns out that the exterminator you call to get rid of bugs is not the kind you call to get rid of a rat. That's a subspecialty—Rodent Removal. Our rodent remover was named Rod. Rod the Rodent Remover. I was scared of him already.

When he came to the door, he was wearing a clean, pressed uniform with his name on it. "Rod," I said. "Thanks for coming."

"It's really Ricardo, but I get more jobs as Rod. Ricardo is too hard for most people to remember. You have a problem with rats?" he said helpfully.

"Yeah. In here," I opened the door wider and led him into the apartment. "It's not really *in* the apartment, but we hear it from in here."

If Ricardo thought it was strange that the mattress was on the living room floor, he didn't say anything. Dulcie was waiting for us in the bedroom.

"It's there," Dulcie said, pointing to a gray smudge where the head of our bedframe met the wall. "He's in there."

Ricardo went over and tapped the wall with his knuckle. Dulcie held her breath. There was no sound from the rat.

"They usually leave the house during the day," Ricardo said.

"How does he get in?" Dulcie says.

Ricardo raised his finger toward the ceiling. "Spanish tile roof. Very pretty, but bad for the rat problem," he said. "They come in through the holes between the tiles."

"So there's nothing we can do?" Dulcie asked, alarmed.

"We can set a trap in the wall through the heating vent there," Ricardo said, pointing to the one vent in our entire apartment, which was, unhelpfully, in the hallway outside our bedroom.

"Then he'll die in the wall?"

"It's a bad smell for a few days, but then it goes away," Ricardo said.

I could see that none of this was making Dulcie feel any better.

"Or I can put a trap on the roof," Ricardo said.

"Do that," Dulcie said quickly.

"Okay," he said. "Now we have a plan."

He reached into his pockets and took out two yellow surgical gloves. Dulcie was horrified, the gloves confirming her suspicions about disease. But Ricardo smiled pleasantly. This was a guy who dealt with rats every day of his life, and it didn't seem to faze him.

"Why do they come inside?" Dulcie said as we followed Ricardo toward the door. "The rats. Why do they live in the walls? There's no food there."

"To keep warm," Ricardo said. "Sometimes to have their babies."

He smiled and gave us a courtly nod as I let him out. When I turned back, Dulcie was still staring at the closed door, her hand over her mouth.

"It's just a rat," I said. I touched her shoulder. She was shaking.

* * * * *

A month after the baby died, the mailman delivered a package that I had to sign for. We don't get a lot of packages, so it was an event. The box was from a company called La Tierra. The name sounded familiar, but I couldn't place it; I was about to call back into the apartment for Dulcie when I remembered. La Tierra was the name of the company that cremated the baby.

"What is it?" Dulcie said from behind me. "Who was at the door?"

I turned around. This will kill her, I thought.

"What is it?" she said again, holding out her hand.

I had no choice but to hand it to her. She looked at it. Her face crumpled. "It's so light," she said finally.

I went to put my arms around her, but she stepped back. Then she started laughing. Her laughter became the kind of giggling you can't turn off. She bit her lips and clenched her teeth, but the giggles kept coming back, as if they were tickling her insides in order to get out.

"You probably thought it was something from your mom," she said through her laughter. "Or some freebie from a computer company. Oh, my God," she said. "Can you believe this is our life?" I smiled, but it was that weird, embarrassed smile you offer when you feel left out of a joke.

We decided to take the ashes to the beach and scatter them on the water. We drove out to the Ventura County line, to a beach called El Pescador. You have to climb down a steep hillside to get to it, and there's usually no one there, especially in the off season. We parked and scrambled unsteadily down the trail. We were so busy concentrating on not falling that we didn't see the ocean until we were at its level. We both got quiet for a moment. The water was slate gray, pocked by the few white gulls that every so often swooped down to the surface and then rose up again. There were no boats in the ocean, only a couple of prehistoric oil derricks in the distance.

"I think we should do it now," Dulcie said.

We opened the box. Inside was some Styrofoam with a hole gouged out. Nestled inside that hole, like a tiny bird, was a plastic bag filled with brown dust. There could not have been more than a tablespoonful. I took the bag and handed the box to Dulcie. Then I kicked off my shoes, rolled up my jeans, and walked out into the water. When I was calf deep, I opened up the bag. I waited for something to happen, for some gust of wind to kick up and take the ashes out to sea. But the day was calm, so I finally dumped the ashes into the water at my feet. A tiny wave moved them toward the shore. I was worried that the ashes would end up in the sand, where somebody could step all over them, but then I felt the undertow dragging the water back out to sea.

"I think that's the bravest thing I've ever seen a person do," Dulcie said as I came out of the water.

As we headed back to the trail, she picked up a smooth stone and slipped it into her pocket. Halfway up the path, she took the stone out and let it drop to the ground.

* * * * *

A week after the holdup, the police called. They had found our stolen car. Once the kids run out of gas, the officer explained, they usually abandon the car rather than pay for more. He gave us the address of the car lot, somewhere in South Central.

"Go early in the morning," the officer warned. "Before they get up."

"They?" I asked.

"You a white guy?" the policeman asked.

"Yeah."

"You want to be down there before wake-up time. Trust me."

Dulcie said it was a self-fulfilling prophecy. Everybody expected things to be bad, so people made them bad. She saw it at her school. The kids who were expected to fail, well, they blew it every time out, even if they knew the work cold.

Still, we took the officer's advice and went down to the lot at seven in the morning. I admit I was nervous, driving through those streets. You like to think you're more open-minded than that, but I guess I'm not. I kept thinking about drive-by shootings and gangs and riots and all the things you read about, thinking, Those things don't happen near where I live, so I'm okay.

We found our car. It was a mess. It had been stripped of everything; even the steering wheel was gone. There was every kind of fast-food wrapper scattered on the back seat, and French fries and old hamburger buns on the floor. You get hungry when you're high. It wasn't worth the price of towing, so we signed it over to the pound and left it there.

As I drove Dulcie to work, I told her the police had asked us to come identify the suspects in a lineup.

"But they'll know it was us who identified them," she said. "They know where we live."

"They were busy getting high. I don't think they were memorizing our address."

"I don't even remember what they looked like. It was dark."

"Once you see some faces, it might come back."

"Charles, don't make me do this. Don't make me!" she cried.

"I'm not going to make you do anything. Jesus. What do you think I am?"

She didn't answer me. I dropped her off at the school. She got out and walked toward the front door, then turned to wave at me, as if it were any regular day, as if we weren't living like some rat trapped in our own wall.

I took the day off. I'd already used up my sick days, and I knew we couldn't throw away the money, but I thought I'd go crazy if I had to be nice to a customer or listen to some technician talk about his bodacious girlfriend or his kid's troubles in school.

I didn't have a plan. I picked up a paper and got some breakfast at a hipster coffee shop on Silver Lake Boulevard. There were a lot of tattooed and pierced people eating eggs and bacon; they looked as though they were ending a night, not beginning a day. I tried to concentrate on my paper, but nothing sank in. Then I got back into my car. I ended up driving along Vermont into Griffith Park, past the roads where guys stop to cruise, all the way to the Observatory. I parked in the empty lot and got out.

The Observatory was closed; it was still early. I was trying to think of something to do with myself when I saw a trail heading up into the hills. The path was well worn; on the weekends, it was usually packed with tourists and families making a cheap day of it. But that morning I had it to myself. I passed outcroppings where people could stand to look at the view. I wanted to walk. I walked for hours. I felt the sun rise up, and I saw the darkness that covered the canyons lift, as if someone were sliding a blanket off the ground.

By the time I stopped, others were on the trail—runners, or people walking their dogs, some kids who were probably playing hooky. I looked out over the canyon and thought about how I could go either way: I could stay with Dulcie and be as far away from life as a person could be, or I could leave.

I had been looking forward to the baby. I didn't mind talking to Dulcie about whether or not the kid should sleep in bed with us, or use a pacifier, or how long she would nurse him, or any of the things she could think about happily for days. I got excited about it too. But I had no idea what it meant, really. What was real to me was watching Dulcie's body grow bigger and bigger, watching that stripe appear on her belly, watching as her breasts got fuller and that part around her nipples got as wide and dark as pancakes. When the doctors took the baby out of her, they handed him to me without bothering to clean him up; I guess there was no point to it. Every inch of him was perfectly formed. For a second, I thought he would open his eyes and be a baby. It didn't look like anything was wrong with him, like there was any reason for him not to be breathing and crying and getting on with the business of being in the world. I kept saying to myself, This is my baby, this is my baby. But I had no idea what I was saying. The only thing I truly felt was that I would die if something happened to Dulcie.

A runner came toward me on the trail. His face was red, and sweat had made his T-shirt transparent. He gave me a pained smile as he ran past. He kicked a small rock with his shoe, and it flew over the side of the canyon. For some reason, I looked over the edge for the rock. What I saw from where I stood was amazing to me. I saw all kinds of strange cactus plants—tall ones like baseball bats, others like spiky fans. There were dry green eucalyptus trees and a hundred different kinds of bushes I couldn't name. I heard the rustle of animals, skunks or coyotes, maybe even deer. There was garbage on the ground and in the bushes—soda cans, fast-food drink cups, napkins with restaurant logos on them. I saw a condom hanging off a branch, like a burst balloon. For some reason, the garbage didn't bother me. For all I knew, this was one of those mountains that was made of trash, and it was nature that didn't belong. Maybe the trash, the dirt, the plants, bugs, condoms—maybe they were all just fighting for a little space.

I got home before Dulcie. I dragged the mattress back into the bedroom. I took my shirt off the light fixture in the living room and put it in the dresser. When Dulcie came back, she saw what I had done, but she didn't say anything. We ate dinner early. I watched a soccer game while she corrected some papers. Then I turned off the lights in the living room, and we went into the bedroom. She knew my mind was made up, and she climbed into bed like a soldier following orders. When I snapped off the bedside lamp, she gave a little gasp.

We lay quietly for a while, getting used to the dark. We listened for the rat, but he wasn't there.

"You think the traps worked?" she said.

"Maybe."

I reached for her. At first it was awkward, as though we were two people who had never had sex with each other. Truthfully, I was half ready for her to push me away. But she didn't, and after a while things became familiar again. When I rolled on top of her, though, I felt her tense up underneath me. She started to speak. "I should go and get—"

I put my fingers on her mouth to stop her. "It's okay," I said.

She looked up at me with her big, watery eyes. She was terrified. She started again to say something about her diaphragm. I stopped her once more.

"It's okay," I repeated.

I could feel her heart beating on my skin. I could feel my own heart beating even harder. We were scared, but we kept going.

MENDING

SALLIE BINGHAM

On Fifth Avenue in the middle fall, the apartment buildings stand like pyramids in the sunlight. They are expensive and well maintained, but for me their grandeur stems not from the big windows with the silk curtains where occasionally you can see a maid dusting with vague gestures but from the doctors' names in the ground-floor windows. Some buildings have bronze plaques for the doctors' names beside the entrance door. Whether those doctors are more magical than the ones who are proclaimed in the windows is one of the puzzles I amuse myself with as I ply my trade up and down the avenue.

My trade is not the trade which might be expected from the height of my red-heeled sandals or the swing of my patent-leather bag. I am, after all, a good girl, a fairly young girl, although I have a few lines and a tendency to wake up at five in the morning. Taxi drivers still comment on my down-home accent, and although for a while I tried to dispel that impression by buying my clothes at Bloomingdale's I have given up the effort.

My trade is doctors, and it is essential. I have a doctor for my eyes and another for my skin; I have a special man for my allergies—which are not crippling—and I also have a specialist for the inside of my head. For a while it seemed that my head was as far as he would go, with an occasional foray down my throat. Finally a choking sensation forced me to cancel my appointments. I suppose I should not expect anyone to take that at face value. He was a very handsome man; he is still, and it is still painful for me to imagine the man whose lap I longed to sit on presiding behind his profession, gazing with those curious green, unshadowed eyes at the women (why are they all women?)—the young ones, the old ones who hang their coats on his rack and sling their bags beside their feet as they sit down, with sighs, or in silence, on his couch.

From *Solo: Women on Woman Alone,* edited by Linda Hamalian and Leo Hamalian (New York: Delacorte, 1977): 101–112. By permission of the author.

My childhood was made to order to produce a high-heeled trader in doctors on Fifth Avenue, although my childhood would never have provided the money. My mother was blond and a beauty, and she had a penchant for changing men. My favorite was a truck driver from Georgia who used to let me ride with him on all-night trips down the coast. Mother didn't approve of that, but it took me off her hands. He would sing and I would doze in the big high cab, which seemed to me as hot and solid as a lump of molten lead—as hard to get out of, too, as I discovered when I tried to open the door. Oh, that truck cab was ecstasy. That was as close as I could come. My mother lost interest in him when I was six and replaced him with a white-collar worker. She thought Edwin was a step up, but for me, he never had any kind of appeal; he was the first of her men to carry a briefcase, and I learned an aversion then I have never been able to overcome to men who tie their shoes with very big bows and carry cow-smelling leather briefcases.

There were many others after Edwin, but they washed over me and I do not remember disliking them at all. They did not make much of an impression, as my mother would say; that was left to my first doctor, a personable Cincinnati gynecologist. My mother, who had settled in that town with a railroad man, made the appointment for me. She wanted me to know the facts, and she did not feel up to explaining them. Of course by then I knew everything, as well as the fact that if you turn a boy down, he will suffer from an excruciating disease. I did not really need to know that to be persuaded, since the interiors of those 1950 Chevrolets smelled just like the cab of Ronny's truck.

The gynecologist armed me with a strange rubber disk that flew across the room the first time I tried to insert it. The second time I was successful, but I was never able to find the thing again. It sailed like a moon through the uncharted darkness of my insides. I knew it was not right to have a foreign body sailing those seas, but it took me a month to summon the courage to call the gynecologist. I was so afraid he would be disappointed in me. He rescued the thing the next day as I lay down on his long table; he was disappointed, and the thing had turned bright green.

After that my mother married an Air Force man who was going to be stationed in Honolulu. I still think of her little black boots when I think of brave women leaving for parts unknown. She tripped up the steps to the airplane, an indomitable little mountain climber, with tears in her eyes. The Air Force man was in tears, too, and smiling as though their future lay shining on the tarmac. There was no room for me in that arrangement, and so I was farmed out to my mother's only prosperous relative, a hard-working doctor who lives in Greenwich and had the luck to marry my aunt.

I was nineteen, too old to be educated, too young to be employed. It made sense for me to do what I could to help Aunt Janey run her large house. There were people to do everything that needed to be done, but no one to organize them. Often the window washer arrived on the same day as the man who put up the screens, or the children needed to be picked up at friends just as Aunt Janey was going to bed with her second cousin. (He was no relative of mine: another briefcase man.) So it was vital to have someone she could rely on to make telephone calls and draw up schedules.

Since I was not being paid in money but in good food and a fine room with roses on the wallpaper, Aunt Janey felt responsible for finishing me. She had been a brilliant woman once, and she still had her books from those days. She wrote my assignment every morning while I started the telephoning. I had to do it before I could do the bills. I can't say the reading meant a great deal to me, but the swing of the sentences—*Jane Eyre,* for example—seemed to carry me out of my ordinary way. I had thought that life was quite plain and obvious, with people coupling and breaking apart like the little snot-colored dots I had seen under the microscope in fifth-grade biology. The only lesson I had learned so far was to stay out of the way of those dots. After I read about blind Rochester's cry, I began to want some of that for my own.

I had not been demanding until then. No one could have complained that I made a fuss over a quick one in the back hall—that was the furnace repairman—or took it more seriously than the roar of the crowd at a construction site. I was never a prude, and my body did not do me that kind of helpful disservice. At home, in the upper South, in the Midwest, in Florida, they talked about boobies or the swing on my back porch. Greenwich is more refined, even New York City is more refined, and the repairmen used to praise my eyes. When it came to seeing one of the men twice, I would shy away, not only because I was waiting for the voice across the miles but because I did not want to spend any time with a man who might begin by praising my eyes and then go on to feeling things himself—I did not mind that—but then would expect me to feel things as well.

In feeling, I was somewhat deficient. It had not mattered before. I could remember the smell of Ronny's cab and glory in it, but I was not able to enjoy the particular flavor of a man's body. A naked man, to me, was like a root or a tuber. I can't say I was afraid. But I never could see the gleam, the light before the dawn, the pot at the end of the rainbow when a naked man stood in front of me. It seemed to me that women were seemlier, more discreet, without that obtrusive member I was always called on to admire. I could not touch it without conscious effort, and that showed in my face. For a long time, it did not matter to me, but it mattered to those men. They wanted me to admire, they wanted me to feel something. Even the man who came to prune Aunt Janey's forsythia insisted that I had to feel. "What's wrong with you?" he complained, when we were lying under the bare branches of the big bush. I knew he was feeling that it was somehow his fault.

I have never wanted to hurt anyone. I have wanted to help, if possible. And so I decided I would stop going out with men.

The trouble was that I wanted a pair of arms. I needed a pair of arms with a pain that even now I can't bring myself to describe. That, of all things, I had carried out of my childhood. When my mother was between men and feeling the ache, she would call me into her bed and squeeze me until suddenly she would fall asleep. I was more the holder that the holdee. It did not matter. The warmth of her thin arms, the wrists hardly wider than milk-bottle necks, the bones as fine as glass splinters, would last me through the next day and the next. Chronic cold was one of my chief complaints. But after she had held me, I didn't even need to button my school coat. I would walk down whatever gray street we were living on in whatever more or less depressed small-city neighborhood in whatever indistinguishable section in the middle of this country with no scarf over my head, no gloves on my hands, and the wind that comes from the Great Plains or the Mississippi or the Rockies or some other invisible boundary lifting the ends of my mouse-colored hair like a lover. Of course the trick was that my mother didn't expect anything of me, except not to wet the bed. She didn't expect me to feel anything in particular or to praise the way she looked in her nylon slip. She gave me the warmth of her long, skinny arms, and I gave her the warmth of mine, and before I was ten years old, I was addicted.

When the new man moved in, I had to spend the night in my own bed with my fist in my mouth, not because the sounds they made frightened me—they were no more frightening than the chittering of the squirrels in the little-city parks—but because there was no more warmth for me. Mother got into the habit of buying me bunny pajamas and woolly sweaters before she installed a new cousin.

After the forsythia man and my decision to do without men, I started to get cold in that old way. Aunt Janey noticed the gooseflesh on my arms one morning when I brought up her breakfast tray. She made me sit down on the satin blanket cover. "We haven't had a talk in I don't know how long." She was the prettiest woman I'd even seen—the best, the brightest, with her jewelry box turned upside down on the pillow and her list of the day's duties, prepared by me, balled up and thrown on the floor. I could think of her only in silly ways—still that's the best I can do—because when I think of her eyes and the way her lips curled when her second cousin rang the doorbell, I know I will always be lonely for her. So I describe her to myself as a fickle woman who cheated on what my mother (who never had her luck) called, reverently, a perfectly good husband, and fed her children peanut butter out of the jar when I made the mistake of leaving a meal to her, and was happy. So happy. Outrageously happy. She had my mother's long, skinny arms—the only family resemblance—and although she very seldom held me in them, I knew she had the same heat. The difference a diamond wristwatch and a growth of fine blond hair made was not even worth thinking about.

(And he, the second cousin, did she make him groan with happiness, too? She used to come downstairs afterward in her Chinese kimono with her pearls hanging down her back, but I never saw much of him.)

We had our talk that morning. It was fall and Jacob the gardener was burning leaves. I insisted on opening the window, although Aunt Janey hated fresh air, and so I was able to flavor her words with the leaf smoke. She told me that I was unhappy, and there was no way I could deny that. So for once she took the pad and the telephone book and asked for the telephone, which had a crook on the receiver so that it could perch on your shoulder. And she began to make me appointments.

She had noticed my teeth, she said between dialings. Was there any implication about my breath? She had noticed that I squinted a good deal over the print in the telephone directory, and so she was sending me to have my eyes checked. She was also not certain that I should be as thin as I seemed to be growing, and so she was making an appointment with her own internist on upper Fifth Avenue. Unfortunately in his office I felt my old enemy, tears rising like an insurrection of moles, like a walking army of termites. When I cried on the leatherette chair, the doctor, who was as friendly as the repairman my mother had left after six months of too much loving, suggested that I ought to go and see the other kind.

That was all right, too, as far as I was concerned. I was ready to take anyone's advice. It did not seem possible to go through the rest of my life trying to get warmth from the eyes of construction workers; it did not seem possible to go on spreading my legs for men who took it personally that that part—"down there," as my mother called it—had no more feeling than the vegetable it so closely resembles: a radish, fancy cut.

The next waiting room was soft and beige, like the tissuey inside of an expensive shoe box, and I could have lain there forever, till the robins covered me with magazine leaves. Of course I had to get up and go and lay myself down when the time came—why this eternal lying?—on an even softer, browner couch in a smaller, safer room. I asked the doctor right away to let me stay forever. He held my hand for a moment, introducing himself, and my cold began to fade. Can it fade from the hands up and will the heart in the end be heated, like a tin pot on a gas burner turned high? I had always assumed that my body warmed up independently and that my heart, at the end, would always be safe and cold. He did not want anything from me—you can't count money in a desperate situation like this—except my compliance, so that he could try to help. And I believed him.

My mother would have said that there is no such thing as a disinterested man; she would have gone on to add that since he had green eyes, he must have other things in view. He did have green eyes, pale, finely lashed, and a pale, tired face. He seemed to have spent himself warming people up. By the second session, I hated the idea of any particle of him going to other people, and I ground my teeth when I passed the next patient—always a woman—in his little hall. I wanted him all to myself and it seemed to me that this was my last chance. My day was flooded with sights I had never seen in my life, views of my lean body folded up on his lap or the back of my neck as I knelt to kiss his feet. I had been cross and mean all my life and now, like a three-year-old with a lollypop, I was all syrup and sunshine. Shame had no part in it. As I went my rounds to the other doctors, letting them fill my teeth or put contact lenses in my eyes, as patiently as I have seen horses stand to be bridled and saddled, I imagined myself in my doctor's arms. Of course he did not respond. How could he respond? He wanted to help and, as he explained, holding me in his arms for a while or even for fifty minutes could not do me anything but harm. It is true that afterward I would never have let him go.

I thought I could push him. After all, other men had always wanted me. So I started to bring him little presents, bunches of chrysanthemums from Aunt Janey's garden, jars of my own grape jelly, poems on yellow paper that would have embarrassed a twelve-year old. He made me take them all away, always neutral, always kind, always ready to listen, but never won or even tempted. My wishes were making me wild and I wanted to gather myself up and wrap myself in a piece of flowered paper and hand myself to him—not for sex or compliments, but only to be held by him.

Aunt Janey caught me crying after three months of this and offered a trip to Paris as a distraction. I told her I couldn't go because I couldn't bear to break a single appointment with my doctor; she was taken aback. We had a long talk in the late-night kitchen where Uncle John had been making pancakes. She told me that analysis works but not in that way. "I can understand you wanting to go to bed with him, that's what everybody wants, but I can't understand you letting it get so out of hand."

"I don't want to go to bed with him," I said. "I couldn't feel him any more than I could feel the furnace repairman. I want him to hold me on his lap and put his arms around me."

"Yes, that's childish," she said, tapping her cigarette out.

"If I can't persuade him to do it, I'll die. I'll lie down and die." It was as clear to me as an item on the grocery list.

"You will not die," she said firmly. "You will go to Paris with me and we will shop for clothes and visit the museums and we will find you a nice free man."

"With green eyes and rays around his eyes and long hands with flat-tipped fingers?"

"That I can't promise," she said. "But he'll be free."

"I won't go if it means missing an appointment."

She started to figure how we could leave late on a Friday and come back on a Sunday, but then she saw it was no use and decided to go for a longer time with the second cousin.

So I was left alone for two weeks, except for Uncle John and the children. He was gone most of the time, coming back at night for his ginger ale and his smoked salmon and a spot of conversation before the late news. He wouldn't let me fix real coffee in the morning; I think, being old and tired, he was afraid of the obligation. (The quid pro quid, my mother called it; nothing was free in her world, especially first thing in the morning.) The two girls spent most of the day in school and when the bus brought them home, I would have our tea picnic ready and we would take it out to the field behind the house. Late autumn by now and not many flowers left to pick, so we found milkweed pods and split them into the air. The little girls sat on my lap, either one at a time or both together, and when I kissed them, their hair smelled of eraser dust. I was in pain because the hours between my appointments were the longest hours of my life, and yet I never saw anything as beautiful as that field with the willows at the far end and the two little girls in their navy skirts and white blouses running after the milkweed parachutes.

By then I had discovered that my doctor had a wife and three children, and they all loved one another and managed well. More than that he would not tell me, and I was forced to believe him. After all, the owners of pale green eyes and flat-ended fingers tend to find the wives and get the children they can enjoy, the way a girl I met in one of my many schools knew exactly—but exactly—what to say to win a smile, and what flavor of milkshake would bring out the angel in her.

As my mother used to say, "Those that know what they want, get it." But she had feeling all over her body, not just lodged here and there in little pockets.

Meanwhile my doctor was trying to take the bits and pieces I gave him and string them together to make me a father. I had never known or even asked which one of the cousins was my father, and so I gave him all the pieces I remembered from the whole bunch of them. Ronny and his truck. He had thick thighs that rubbed together when he walked and made him roll like a seafaring man. He like to hold me between the thighs and comb my hair. Edwin with his briefcase that reminded me of my doctor's (although Edwin's was more expensive) and which, he once told me, held a surprise. The surprise, it turned out, was my cough medicine. Louis the railroad man who said he would take me with him on the train except that white girls brought bad luck; it was just like in the mines. The Air Force regular who yelped with joy and hugged me the day my mother said she would go to Honolulu.

My doctor wanted to know which one was my father, and he proposed that I write my mother and ask. I wrote her because I did everything he even hinted at and I would have as soon slit my own throat. Word came back a week later; she thought I had known all along. My father had been a Kansas boy stationed at Fort Knox one summer when she was working at a diner called the Blue Boar. I remembered then that she had always kept a picture of a big-faced smiling boy on the mantelpiece, when there was one, or on the table by her bed. She said he had been killed in Korea.

My doctor did not try to do much with that scrap. Probably my father never even saw my mother's big stomach; if he had, he might have told her what to do about it, as a farm boy familiar with cows. So we had to start all over again with the scraps and pieces, trying to undo the way my memory simplified everything, trying to get behind the little pictures I wanted so desperately to keep: the shape of men's hands and the ways they had let me down.

We were still at work when Aunt Janey came back from Paris and she made me get on the scales that first evening. I told her the work we were doing was wearing me down; it was like ditch digging, or snaking out drains. She knew I was better, and she told me not to give up now with the end in sight. I wasn't sure what she meant, but I knew I had to keep on. There was some hope for me somewhere in all that. At my doctor's, the sweat would run down my face and I would have to pace the floor because there were months and even years of my life when all I could remember was the pattern a tree of heaven made when the sun shone through it on a linoleum floor. My doctor thought some of the scraps might have forced me into bed, but I only remember being tickled or chased with the hairbrush or locked in the car while they went into a road house. Nothing high or strange but only flat and cold. Something killed off my feeling, but it wasn't being raped by Ronny or Edwin or any of the others. Mother had sense enough to find men who wanted only her.

I told my doctor I believed I had been an ugly, squalling baby who kept my mother up at night, screeching for more milk. That was the only thing Mother ever said about me, and she said it more to criticize herself. She hadn't had sense enough, she explained, to realize I was hungry and to give me more bottles. Instead she slapped me once or twice. That wasn't enough to kill off much feeling, although it is true that if I were asked to draw a picture of myself, I would draw a great mouth.

By then I was almost in despair about getting what I wanted from my doctor, even a kiss or a lap sit or holding his hand. I kept having faith in him, the kind he didn't want, the kind that keeps you from eating and wakes you up at night. That faith woke the saints with visions of martyrdom and woke me with visions of lying in his arms. I kept believing that nature and its urges would triumph over the brittle standards of his profession; I kept believing that his calm attention was the marker for a hidden passion. I also believed that if he would take me, I would begin, magically, to feel. Or lacking that, light up like a torch: joy, like Aunt Janey with her pearls hanging straight down her back.

But he would not.

So for me it was a question of quitting—which of course I would not do, because at least during the sessions I saw him—or of going on with the work, keeping to the schedule, getting up in Greenwich in time to dress and catch the train. It was a question of opening my mind to the terrible thoughts that flashed through it like a barracuda through muddy water. It was a question of making connections between one thing and another that did not come from the expression in his eyes—the looks I called waiting, eager, pleased—but from some deep, muddy layer of my own, where the old dreams had died and lay partially decayed.

The result was that I lost what ability I had. The children went back to eating peanut butter out of the jar although I had gotten Aunt Janey to lay in a supply of bread. The little skirts and tops we had bought at Bloomingdale's began to stink with sweat, and I stopped washing my hair. It did not seem possible to stand under the shower and come out feeling alive and new. It did not seem worthwhile even to try.

I didn't care anymore about getting better—that was a sailing planet—but I did care about the little fix of warmth which I got from sitting next to my doctor. I cared about his words, which were for me and not for all the other women, and after a while I began to care about the things he said that hurt me and seemed at first unacceptable. There were, in the end, no answers. Yet he seemed to see me, clearly, remotely, as I had never seen myself, and he watered me with acceptance as regularly as he watered the sprouted avocado on his windowsill. Is it after all a kind of love? By January, I was back inside my own bleached mind; I knew it the day I went out and bought myself a bunch of flowers.

Aunt Janey washed my hair for me and insisted on new clothes and a trip to Antigua; when I said I would go, she hugged me and kissed me and gave me a garnet ring. Uncle John told me I was looking like a million dollars, and the little girls, who had been scared off by my smell, began to bring their paper dolls again so that I could cut out the clothes. I was still, and always would be, one of the walking wounded; I was an internalized scab, and when I looked at myself in the mirror, I understood why people call naked need the ugliest thing in the world. I broke two appointments with my doctor and went to Antigua with Aunt Janey, and one night, I danced with an advertising man. I was no queen, but I was somebody, two legs, two arms, a body, and a head with a mouthful of choice words. I wouldn't sleep with him because I knew that I wouldn't feel a thing, but the next day we played some fine tennis.

When I came back to New York, the pyramids on Fifth Avenue were no longer shining. The gutters were running with filth and melted snow, and the doctors' names in the windows and on the plaques were only names, like lawyers' and dentists'. My doctor was on the telephone when I walked in, and I looked at his free ear and knew he would never be mine. Never. Never. And that I would live.

TORTURE

JEAN AMÉRY

Whoever visits Belgium as a tourist may perhaps chance upon Fort Breendonk, which lies halfway between Brussels and Antwerp. The compound is a fortress from the First World War, and what its fate was at that time I don't know. In the Second World War, during the short eighteen days of resistance by the Belgian army in May 1940, Breendonk was the last headquarters of King Leopold. Then, under German occupation, it became a kind of small concentration camp, a "reception camp," as it was called in the cant of the Third Reich. Today it is a Belgian National Museum.

At first glance, the fortress Breendonk makes a very old, almost historic impression. As it lies there under the eternally rain-gray sky of Flanders, with its grass-covered domes and black-gray walls, it gives the feeling of a melancholy engraving from the 1870s war. One thinks of Gravelotte and Sedan and is convinced that the defeated Emperor Napoleon III, with kepi in hand, will immediately appear in one of the massive, low gates. One must step closer, in order that the fleeting picture from past times be replaced by another, which is more familiar to us. Watchtowers arise along the moat that rings the castle. Barbed-wire fences wrap around them. The copperplate of 1870 is abruptly obscured by horror photos from the world that David Rousset has call "l'Univers Concentrationnaire." The creators of the National Museum have left everything the way it was between 1940 and 1944. Yellowed wall cards: "Whoever goes beyond this point will be shot." The pathetic monument to the resistance movement that was erected in front of the fortress shows a man forced to his knees, but defiantly raising his head with its oddly Slavic lines. This monument would not at all have been necessary to make clear to the visitor *where* he is and *what* is recollected there.

One steps through the main gate and soon finds oneself in a room that in those days was mysteriously called the "business room." A picture of Heinrich Himmler on the wall, a swastika flag spread as a cloth over a long table, a few bare chairs. The

From *At the Mind's Limits: Contemplations by a Survivor of Auschwitz and Its Realities* (21–40), by Jean Améry. Trans. Sidney Rosenfeld and Stella Rosenfeld. Bloomington: Indiana University Press, 1980.

business room. Everyone went about his business, and theirs was murder. Then the damp, cellarlike corridors, dimly lit by the same thin and reddishly glowing bulbs as the ones that used to hang there. Prison cells, sealed by inch-thick wooden doors. Again and again one must pass through heavy barred gates before one finally stands in a windowless vault in which various iron implements lie about. From there no scream penetrated to the outside. There I experienced it: torture.

If one speaks about torture, one must take care not to exaggerate. What was inflicted on me in the unspeakable vault in Breendonk was by far not the worst form of torture. No red-hot needles were shoved under my fingernails, nor were any lit cigars extinguished on my bare breast. What did happen to me there I will have to tell about later; it was relatively harmless and it left no conspicuous scars on my body. And yet, twenty-two years after it occurred, on the basis of an experience that in no way probed the entire range of possibilities, I dare to assert that torture is the most horrible event a human being can retain within himself.

But very many people have preserved such things, and the horrible can make no claim to singularity. In most Western countries torture was eliminated as an institution and method at the end of the eighteenth century. And yet, today, two hundred years later, there are still men and women—no one knows how many—who can tell of the torture they underwent. As I am preparing this article, I come across a newspaper page with photos that show members of the South Vietnamese army torturing captured Vietcong rebels. The English novelist Graham Greene wrote a letter about it to the London *Daily Telegraph,* saying:

> The strange new feature about the photographs of torture now appearing in the British and American press is that they have been taken with the approval of the torturers and are published over captions that contain no hint of condemnation. They might have come out of a book on insect life. . . . Does this mean that the American authorities sanction torture as a means of interrogation? The photographs certainly are a mark of honesty, a sign that the authorities do not shut their eyes to what is going on, but I wonder if this kind of honesty without conscience is really to be preferred to the old hypocrisy.

Every one of us will ask himself Graham Green's question. The admission of torture, the boldness—but is it still that?—of coming forward with such photos is explicable only if it is assumed that a revolt of public conscience is no longer to be feared. One could think that this conscience has accustomed itself to the practice of torture. After all, torture was, and is, by no means being practiced only in Vietnam during these decades. I would not like to know what goes on in South African, Angolese, and Congolese prisons. But I do know, and the reader probably has also heard, what went on between 1956 and 1963 in the jails of French Algeria. There is a frighteningly exact and sober book on it, *La question* by Henri Alleg, a work whose circulation was prohibited, the report of an eyewitness who was also personally tortured and who gave evidence of the horror, sparingly and without making a fuss about himself. Around 1960 numerous other books and pamphlets on the subject appeared: the learned criminological treatise by the famous lawyer Alec Mellor, the protest of the publicist Pierre-Henri Simon, the ethical-philosophic investigation of a theologian named Vialatoux. Half the French nation rose up against the torture in Algeria. One cannot say often and emphatically enough that by this the French did honor to themselves. Leftist intellectuals protested. Catholic trade unionists and other Christian laymen warned against the torture, and at the risk of their safety and lives took action against it. Prelates raised their voices, although to our feeling much too gently.

But that was the great and freedom-loving France, which even in those dark days was not entirely robbed of its liberty. From other places the screams penetrated as little into the world as did once my own strange and uncanny howls from the vaults of Breendonk. In Hungary there presides a Party First Secretary, of whom it is said that under the regime of one of his predecessors torturers ripped out his fingernails.[5] And where and who are all the others about whom one learned nothing at all, and of whom one will probably never hear anything? Peoples, governments, authorities, names that are known, but which no one says aloud. Somewhere, someone is crying out under torture. Perhaps in this hour, this second.

And how do I come to speak of torture solely in connection with the Third Reich? Because I myself suffered it under the outspread wings of this very bird of prey, of course. But not only for that reason; rather, I am convinced, beyond all personal experiences, that torture was not an accidental quality of this Third Reich, but its essence. Now I hear violent objection being raised, and I know that this assertion puts me on dangerous ground. I will try to substantiate it later. First, however, I suppose I must tell what the content of my experience actually was and what happened in the cellar-damp air of the fortress of Breendonk.

In July 1943 I was arrested by the Gestapo. It was a matter of fliers. The group to which I belonged, a small German-speaking organization within the Belgian resistance movement, was spreading anti-Nazi propaganda among the members of the German occupation forces. We produced rather primitive agitation material, with which we imagined we could convince the German soldiers of the terrible madness of Hitler and his war. Today I know, or at least believe I know, that we were aiming our feeble message at deaf ears. I have much reason to assume that the soldiers in field-gray uniform who found our mimeographed papers in front of their barracks clicked their heels and passed them straight on to their superiors, who then, with the same official readiness, in turn notified the security agency. And so the latter rather quickly got onto our trail and raided us. One of the fliers that I was carrying at the time of my arrest bore the message, which was just as succinct as it was propagandistically ineffectual, "Death to the SS bandits and Gestapo hangmen!" Whoever was stopped with such material by the men in leather coats and with drawn pistols could have no illusions of any kind. I also did not allow myself any for a single moment. For, God knows, I regarded myself—wrongly, as I see today—as an old, hardened expert on the system, its men, and its methods. A reader of the *Neue Weltbühne* and the *Neues Tagebuch* in times past, well up on the KZ literature of the German emigration from 1933 on, I believed to anticipate what was in store for me. Already in the first days of the Third Reich I had heard of the cellars of the SA barracks on Berlin's General Pape Street. Soon thereafter I had read what to my knowledge was the first German KZ document, the little book *Oranienburg* by Gerhard Segers. Since that time so many reports by former Gestapo prisoners had reached my ears that I thought there could be nothing new for me in this area. What would take place would then have to be incorporated into the relevant literature, as it were. Prison, interrogation, blows, torture; in the end, most probably death. Thus it was written and thus it would happen. When, after my arrest, a Gestapo man ordered me to step away from the window—for he knew the trick, he said, with your chained hands you tear open the window and leap onto a nearby ledge—I was certainly flattered that he credited me with so much determination and dexterity, but, obeying the order, I politely gestured that it did not come into question. I gave him to understand that I had neither the physical prerequisites nor at all the intention to escape my fate in such an adventurous way. I knew what was coming and they could count on my consent to it. But does one really know? Only in part. "Rien n'arrive ni comme on l'espére, ni comme on le craint," Proust writes somewhere. Nothing really happens as we hope it will, nor as we fear it will. But not because the occurrence, as one says, perhaps "goes beyond the imagination" (it is not a quantitative question), but because it is reality and not phantasy. One can devote an entire life to comparing the imagined and the real, and still never accomplish anything by it. Many things do indeed happen approximately the way they were anticipated in the imagination: Gestapo men in leather coats, pistol pointed at their victim—that is correct, all right. But then, almost amazingly, it dawns on one that the fellows not only have leather coats and pistols, but also faces: not "Gestapo faces" with twisted noses, hypertrophied chins, pockmarks, and knife scars, as might appear in a book, but rather faces like anyone else's. Plain, ordinary faces. And the enormous perception at a later stage, one that destroys all abstractive imagination, makes clear to us how the plain, ordinary faces finally become Gestapo faces after all, and how evil overlays and exceeds banality. For there is no "banality of evil," and Hannah Arendt, who wrote about it in her Eichmann book, knew the enemy of mankind only from hearsay, saw him only through the glass cage.

When an event places the most extreme demands on us, one ought not to speak of banality. For at this point there is no longer any abstraction and never an imaginative power that could even approach its reality. That someone is carried away shackled in an auto is "self-evident" only when you read about it in the newspaper and you rationally tell yourself, just at the moment when you are packing fliers: well of course, and what more? It can and it will happen like that to me someday, too. But the auto is different, and the pressure of the shackles was not felt in advance, and the streets are strange, and although you may previously have walked by the gate of the Gestapo headquarters countless times, it has other perspectives, other ornaments, other ashlars when you cross its threshold as a prisoner. Everything is self-evident, and nothing is self-evident as soon as we are thrust into a reality whose light blinds us and burns us to the bone. What one tends to call "normal life" may coincide with anticipatory imagination and trivial statement. I buy a newspaper and am "a man who buys a newspaper." The act does not differ from the image through which I anticipated it, and I hardly differentiate myself personally from the millions who performed it before me. Because my imagination did not suffice to entirely capture such an event? No, rather because even in direct experience everyday reality is nothing but codified abstraction. Only in rare moments of life do we truly stand face to face with the event and, with it, reality.

It does not have to be something as extreme as torture. Arrest is enough and, if need be, the first blow one receives. "If you talk," the men with the plain, ordinary faces said to me, "then you will be put in the military police station. If you don't confess, then it's off to Breendonk, and you know what that means." I knew, and I didn't know. In any case, I acted roughly like the man who buys a newspaper, and spoke as planned. I would be most pleased to avoid Breendonk, with which I was quite familiar, and give the evidence desired of me. Except that I unfortunately knew nothing, or almost nothing. Accomplices?

I could name only their aliases. Hiding places? But one was led to them only at night, and the exact addresses were never entrusted to us. For these men, however, that was far too familiar twaddle, and it didn't pay them to go into it. They laughed contemptuously. And suddenly I felt—*the first blow.*

In an interrogation, blows have only scant criminological significance. They are tacitly practiced and accepted, a normal measure employed against recalcitrant prisoners who are unwilling to confess. If we are to believe the above-cited lawyer, Alec Mellor, and his book *La Torture*, then blows are applied in more or less heavy doses by almost all police authorities, including those of the Western-democratic countries, with the exception of England and Belgium. In America one speaks of the "third degree" of a police investigation, which supposedly entails something worse than a few punches. France has even found an argot word that nicely plays down a beating by the police. One speaks of the prisoner's "passage à tabac." After the Second World War a high French criminal investigator, in a book intended for his subordinates, still explained in extravagant detail that it would not be possible to forgo physical compulsion at interrogations, "within the bounds of legality."

Mostly, the public does not prove to be finicky when such occurrences in police stations are revealed now and then in the press. At best, there may be an interpellation in Parliament by some leftist-oriented deputy. But then the stories fizzle out; I have never yet heard of a police official who had beaten a prisoner and was not energetically covered by his superior officers. Simple blows, which really are entirely incommensurable with actual torture, may almost never create a far-reaching echo among the public, but for the person who suffers them they are still experiences that leave deep marks—if one wishes not to use up the high-sounding words already and clearly say: enormities. The first blow brings home to the prisoner that he is *helpless,* and thus it already contains in the bud everything that is to come. One may have known about torture and death in the cell, without such knowledge having possessed the hue of life; but upon the first blow they are anticipated as real possibilities, yes, as certainties. They are permitted to punch me in the face, the victim feels in numb surprise and concludes in just as numb certainty: they will do with me what they want. Whoever would rush to the prisoner's aid—a wife, a mother, a brother, or friend—he won't get this far.

Not much is said when someone who has never been beaten makes the ethical and pathetic statement that upon the first blow the prisoner loses his human dignity. I must confess that I don't know exactly what that is: human dignity. One person thinks he loses it when he finds himself in circumstances that make it impossible for him to take a daily bath. Another believes he loses it when he must speak to an official in something other than his native language. In one instance human dignity is bound to a certain physical convenience, in the other to the right of free speech, in still another perhaps to the availability of erotic partners of the same sex. I don't know if the person who is beaten by the police loses human dignity. Yet I am certain that with the very first blow that descends on him he loses something we will perhaps temporarily call "trust in the world."

Trust in the world includes all sorts of things: the irrational and logically unjustifiable belief in absolute causality perhaps, or the likewise blind belief in the validity of the inductive inference. But more important as an element of trust in the world, and in our context what is solely relevant, is the certainty that by reason of written or unwritten social contracts the other person will spare me—more precisely stated, that he will respect my physical, and with it also my metaphysical, being. The boundaries of my body are also the boundaries of my self. My skin surface shields me against the external world. If I am to have trust, I must feel on it only what I *want* to feel.

At the first blow, however, this trust in the world breaks down. The other person, *opposite* whom I exist physically in the world and *with* whom I can exist only as long as he does not touch my skin surface as border, forces his own corporeality on me with the first blow. He is on me and thereby destroys me. It is like a rape, a sexual act without the consent of one of the two partners. Certainly, if there is even a minimal prospect of successful resistance, a mechanism is set in motion that enables me to rectify the border violation by the other person. For my part, I can expand in urgent self-defense, objectify my own corporeality, restore the trust in my continued existence. The social contract then has another text and other clauses: an eye for an eye and a tooth for a tooth. You can also regulate your life according to that. You *cannot* do it when it is the other one who knocks out the tooth, sinks the eye into a swollen mass, and you yourself suffer on your body the counter-man that your fellow man became. If no help can be expected, this physical overwhelming by the other then becomes an existential consummation of destruction altogether.

The expectation of help, the certainty of help, is indeed one of the fundamental experiences of human beings, and probably also of animals. This was quite convincingly presented decades ago by old Kropotkin, who spoke of "mutual aid in nature," and by the modern animal behaviorist Lorenz. The expectation of help is as much a constitutional psychic element as is the struggle for existence. Just a moment, the mother says to her child who is moaning from pain, a hot-water bottle, a cup of tea is coming right away, we won't let you suffer so! I'll prescribe you a medicine, the doctor assures, it will help you. Even on the battlefield, the Red Cross ambulances find their way to the wounded man. In almost all situations in life where there is bodily injury there is also the expectation of help; the former is compensated by the latter. But with the first blow from a policeman's fist, against which there can be no defense and which no helping hand will ward off, a part of our life ends and it can never again be revived.

Here it must be added, of course, that the reality of the police blows must first of all be accepted, because the existential fright from the first blow quickly fades and there is still room in the psyche for a number of practical considerations. Even a sudden joyful surprise is felt; for the physical pain is not at all unbearable. The blows that descend on us have above all a subjective spatial and acoustical quality: spatial, insofar as the prisoner who is being struck in the face and on the head has the impression that the room and all the visible objects in it are shifting position by jolts; acoustical, because he believes to hear a dull thundering, which finally submerges in a general roaring. The blow acts as its own anesthetic. A feeling of pain that would be comparable to a violent toothache or the pulsating burning of a festering wound does not emerge. For that reason, the beaten person thinks roughly this: well now, that can be put up with; hit me as much as you want, it will get you nowhere.

It got them nowhere, and they became tired of hitting me. I kept repeating only that I knew nothing, and therefore, as they had threatened, I was presently off, not to the army-administered Brussels prison, but to the "Reception Camp Breendonk," which was controlled by the SS. It would be tempting to pause here and to tell of the auto ride from Brussels to Breendonk through twenty-five kilometers of Flemish countryside, of the wind-bent poplars, which one saw with pleasure, even if the shackles hurt one's wrists. But that would sidetrack us, and we must quickly come to the point. Let me mention only the ceremony of driving through the first gate over the drawbridge. There even the Gestapo men had to present their identification papers to the SS guards, and if, despite all, the prisoner had doubted the seriousness of the situation, here, below the watchtowers and at the sight of the submachine guns, in view of the entrance ritual, which did not lack a certain dark solemnity, he had to recognize that he had arrived at the end of the world.

Very quickly one was taken into the "business room," of which I have already spoken. The business that was conducted here obviously was a flourishing one. Under the picture of Himmler, with his cold eyes behind the pince-nez, men who wore the woven initials SD on the black lapels of their uniforms went in and out, slamming doors and making a racket with their boots. They did not condescend to speak with the arrivals, either the Gestapo men or the prisoners. Very efficiently they merely recorded the information contained on my false identity card and speedily relieved me of my rather inconsiderable possessions. A wallet, cuff links, and my tie were confiscated. A thin gold bracelet aroused derisive attention, and a Flemish SS man, who wanted to appear important, explained to his German comrades that this was the sign of the partisans. Everything was recorded in writing, with the precision befitting the occurrences in a business room. Father Himmler gazed down contentedly onto the flag that covered the rough wooden table, and onto his people. They were dependable.

The moment has come to make good a promise I gave. I must substantiate why, according to my firm conviction, torture was the essence of National Socialism—more accurately stated, why it was precisely in torture that the Third Reich materialized in all the density of its being. That torture was, and is, practiced elsewhere has already been dealt with. Certainly. In Vietnam since 1964. Algeria 1957. Russia probably between 1919 and 1953. In Hungary in 1919 the Whites and the Reds tortured. There was torture in Spanish prisons by the Falangists as well as the Republicans. Torturers were at work in the semifascist Eastern European states of the period between the two World Wars, in Poland, Romania, Yugoslavia. Torture was no invention of National Socialism. But it was its apotheosis. The Hitler vassal did not yet achieve his full identity if he was merely as quick as a weasel, tough as leather, hard as Krupp steel. No Golden Party Badge made of him a fully valid representative of the Führer and his ideology, nor did any Blood Order or Iron Cross. He had to *torture*, destroy, in order to be great in bearing the suffering of others. He had to be capable of handling torture instruments, so that Himmler would assure him his Certificate of Maturity in History; later generations would admire him for having obliterated his feelings of mercy.

Again I hear indignant objection being raised, hear it said that not Hitler embodied torture, but rather something unclear, "totalitarianism." I hear especially the example of Communism being shouted at me. And didn't I myself just say that in the Soviet Union torture was practiced for thirty-four years? And did not already Arthur Koestler. . . ? Oh yes, I know, I know. It is impossible to discuss here in detail the political "Operation Bewilderment" of the postwar period, which defined Communism and National Socialism for us as two not even very different manifestations of one and the same thing. Until it came out of our ears, Hitler and Stalin, Auschwitz, Siberia, the Warsaw Ghetto Wall and the Berlin Ulbricht Wall were named together, like Goethe and Schiller, Klopstock and Wieland.[6] As a hint, allow me to repeat here in my own name and at the risk of being denounced what Thomas Mann once said in a much attacked interview: namely, that no matter how terrible Communism may at times appear, it still symbolizes an idea of man, whereas Hitler-Fascism was not an idea at all, but depravity. Finally, it is undeniable that Communism could de-Stalinize itself and that today in the Soviet sphere of influence, if we can place trust in concurring reports, torture is no longer practiced. In Hungary a Party First Secretary can preside who was himself once the victim of Stalinist torture. But who is really able to imagine a de-Hitlerized National Socialism and, as a leading politician of a newly ordered Europe, a Röhm follower who in those days had been dragged through torture? No one can imagine it. It would have been impossible. For National Socialism—which, to be sure, could not claim a single idea, but did possess a whole arsenal of confused, crackbrained notions—was the only political system of this century that up to this point had not only practiced the rule of the antiman, as had other Red and White terror regimes also, but had expressly established it as a principle. It hated the word "humanity" like the pious man hates sin, and that is why it spoke of "sentimental humanitarianism." It exterminated and enslaved. This is evidenced not only by the corpus delicti, but also by a sufficient number of theoretical confirmations. The Nazis tortured, as did others, because by means of torture they wanted to obtain information important for national policy. But in addition they tortured with the good conscience of depravity. They martyred their prisoners for definite purposes, which in each instance were exactly specified. Above all, however, they tortured because they were torturers. They placed torture in their service. But even more fervently they were its servants.

When I recall those past events, I still see before me the man who suddenly stepped into the business room and who seemed to count in Breendonk. On his field-gray uniform he wore the black lapels of the SS, but he was addressed as "Herr Leutnant." He was small, of stocky figure, and had that fleshy, sanguine face that in terms of popular physiognomy would be called "gruffly good-natured." His voice crackled hoarsely, the accent was colored by Berlin dialect. From his wrist there hung in a leather loop a horsewhip of about a meter in length. But why, really, should I withhold his name, which later became so familiar to me? Perhaps at this very hour he is faring well and feels content with his healthily sunburned self as he drives home from his Sunday excursion. I have no reason not to name him. The Herr Leutnant, who played the role of a torture specialist here, was named Praust. P-R-A-U-S-T. "Now it's coming," he said to me in a rattling and easygoing way. And then he led me through the corridors, which were dimly lit by reddish bulbs and in which barred gates kept opening and slamming shut, to the previously described vault, the bunker. With us were the Gestapo men who had arrested me.

If I finally want to get to the analysis of torture, then unfortunately I cannot spare the reader the objective description of what now took place; I can only try to make it brief. In the bunker there hung from the vaulted ceiling a chain that above ran into a roll. At its bottom end it bore a heavy, broadly curved iron hook. I was led to the instrument. The hook gripped into the shackle that held my hands together behind my back. Then I was raised with the chain until I hung about a meter over the floor.

In such a position, or rather, when hanging this way, with your hands behind your back, for a short time you can hold at a half-oblique through muscular force. During these few minutes, when you are already expending your utmost strength, when sweat has already appeared on your forehead and lips, and you are breathing in gasps, you will not answer any questions. Accomplices? Addresses? Meeting Places? You hardly hear it. All your life is gathered in a single, limited area of the body, the shoulder joints, and it does not react; for it exhausts itself completely in the expenditure of energy. But this cannot last long, even with peoples who have a strong physical constitution. As for me, I had to give up rather quickly. And now there was a crackling and splintering in my shoulders that my body has not forgotten until this hour. The balls sprang from their sockets. My own body weight caused luxation; I fell into a void and now hung by my dislocated arms, which had been torn high from behind and were now twisted over my head. Torture, from Latin *torquere,* to twist. What visual instruction in etymology! At the the same time the blows from the horsewhip showered down on my body, and some of them sliced cleanly through the light summer trousers that I was wearing on this twenty-third of July 1943.

It would be totally senseless to try and describe here the pain that was inflicted on me. Was it "like a red-hot iron in my shoulders," and was another "like a dull wooden stake that had been driven into the back of my head"? One comparison would only stand for the other, and in the end we would be hoaxed by turn on the hopeless merry-go-round of figurative speech. The pain was what it was. Beyond that there is nothing to say. Qualities of feeling are as incomparable as they are indescribable. They mark the limit of the capacity of language to communicate. If someone wanted to impart his physical pain, he would be forced to inflict it and thereby become a torturer himself.

Since the *how* of pain defies communication through language, perhaps I can at least approximately state *what* it was. It contained everything that we already ascertained earlier in regard to a beating by the police: the border violation of my self by the other, which can be neither neutralized by the expectation of help nor rectified through resistance. Torture is all that, but in addition very much more. Whoever is overcome by pain through torture experiences his body as never before. In self-negation, his flesh becomes a total reality. Partially, torture is one of those life experiences that in a milder form present themselves also to the consciousness of the patient who is awaiting help, and the popular saying according to which we feel well as long as we do not feel our body does indeed express an undeniable truth. But only in torture does the transformation of the person into flesh become complete. Frail in the face of violence, yelling out in pain, awaiting no help, capable of no resistance, the tortured person is only a body, and nothing else beside that. If what Thomas Mann described years ago in *The Magic Mountain* is true, namely, that the more hopelessly man's body is subjected to suffering, the more physical he is, then of all physical celebrations torture is the most terrible. In the case of Mann's consumptives, they still took place in a state of euphoria; for the martyred they are death rituals.

It is tempting to speculate further. Pain, we said, is the most extreme intensification imaginable of our bodily being. But maybe it is even more, that is: death. No road that can be travelled by logic leads us to death, but perhaps the thought is permissible that through pain a path of feeling and premonition can be paved to it for us. In the end, we would be faced with the equation: Body = Pain = Death, and in our case this could be reduced to the hypothesis that torture, through which we are turned into body by the other, blots out the contradiction of death and allows us to experience it personally. But this is an evasion of the question. We have for it only the excuse of our own experience and must add in explanation that torture has an indelible character. Whoever was tortured, stays tortured. Torture is ineradicably burned into him, even when no clinically objective traces can be detected. The permanence of torture gives the one who underwent it the right to speculative flights, which need not be lofty ones and still may claim a certain validity.

I speak of the martyred. But it is time to say something about the tormentors also. No bridge leads from the former to the latter. Modern police torture is without the theological complicity that, no doubt, in the Inquisition joined both sides; faith united them even in the delight of tormenting and the pain of being tormented. The torturer believed he was exercising God's justice, since he was, after all, purifying the offender's soul; the tortured heretic or witch did not at all deny him this right. There was a horrible and perverted togetherness. In present-day torture not a bit of this remains. For the tortured, the torturer is solely the other, and here he will be regarded as such.

Who were the others, who pulled me up by my dislocated arms and punished my dangling body with the horsewhip? As a start, one can take the view that they were merely brutalized petty bourgeois and subordinate bureaucrats of torture. But it is necessary to abandon this point of view immediately if one wishes to arrive at an insight into evil that is more than just banal. Were they sadists, then? According to my well-founded conviction, they were not sadists in the narrow sexual-pathologic sense. In general, I don't believe that I encountered a single genuine sadist of this sort during my two years of imprisonment by the Gestapo and in concentration camps. But probably they *were* sadists if we leave sexual pathology aside and attempt to judge the torturers according to the categories of, well, the *philosophy* of the Marquis de Sade. Sadism as the dis-ordered view of the world is something other than the sadism of the usual psychology handbooks, also other than the sadism interpretation of Freudian analysis. For this reason, the French anthropologist Georges Bataille will be cited here, who has reflected very thoroughly on the odd Marquis. We will then perhaps see not only that my tormentors lived on the border of a sadistic philosophy but that National Socialism in its totality was stamped less with the seal of a hardly definable "totalitarianism" than with that of *sadism.*

For Georges Bataille, sadism is to be understood not in the light of sexual pathology but rather in that of existential psychology, in which it appears as the radical negation of the other, as the denial of the social principle as well as the reality principle. A world in which torture, destruction, and death triumph obviously cannot exist. But the sadist does not care about the continued existence of the world. On the contrary: he wants to nullify this world, and by negating his fellow man, who also in an entirely specific sense is "hell" for him, he wants to realize his own total sovereignty. The fellow man is transformed into flesh, and in this transformation he is already brought to the edge of death; if worst comes to worst, he is driven beyond the border of death into Nothingness. With that the torturer and murderer realizes his own destructive being, without having to lose himself in it entirely, like his martyred victim. He can, after all, cease the torture when it suits him. He has control of the other's scream of pain and death; he is master over flesh and spirit, life and death. In this way, torture becomes the total inversion of the social world, in which we can live only if we grant our fellow man life, ease his suffering, bridle the desire of our ego to expand. But in the world of torture man exists only by ruining the other person who stands before him. A slight pressure by the tool-wielding hand is enough to turn the other—along with his head, in which are perhaps stored Kant and Hegel, and all nine symphonies, and the World as Will and Representation—into a shrilly squealing piglet at slaughter. When it has happened and the torturer has expanded into the body of his fellow man and extinguished what was his spirit, he himself can then smoke a cigarette or sit down to breakfast or, if he has the desire, have a look in at the World as Will and Representation.

My boys at Breendonk contented themselves with the cigarette and, as soon as they were tired of torturing, doubtlessly let old Schopenhauer be. But this still does not mean that the evil they inflicted on me was banal. If one insists on it, they were bureaucrats of torture. And yet, they were also much more. I saw it in their serious, tense faces, which were not swelling, let us say, with sexual-sadistic delight, but concentrated in murderous self-realization. With heart and soul they went about their business, and the name of it was power, dominion over spirit and flesh, orgy of unchecked self-expansion. I also have not forgotten that there were moments when I felt a kind of wretched admiration for the agonizing sovereignty they exercised over me. For is not the one who can reduce a person so entirely to a body and a whimpering prey of death a god or, at least, a demigod?

But the concentrated effort of torture naturally did not make these people forget their profession. They were "cops," that was their metiér and routine. And so they continued asking me questions, constantly the same ones: accomplices, addresses, meeting places. To come right out with it: I had nothing but luck, because in regard to the extorting of information our group was rather well organized. What they wanted to hear from me in Breendonk, I simply did not know myself. If instead of the aliases I had been able to name the real names, perhaps, or probably, a calamity would have occurred, and I would be standing here now as the weakling I most likely am, and as the traitor I potentially already was. Yet it was not at all that I opposed them with the heroically maintained silence that befits a real man in such a situation and about which one may read (almost always, incidentally, in reports by people who were not there themselves). I talked. I accused myself of invented absurd political crimes, and even now I don't know at all how they could have occurred to me, dangling bundle that I was. Apparently I had the hope that, after such incriminating disclosures, a well-aimed blow to the head would put an end to my misery and quickly bring on my death, or at least unconsciousness. Finally, I actually did become unconscious, and with that it was over for a while—for the "cops" abstained from awakening their battered victim, since the nonsense I had foisted on them was busying their stupid heads.

It was over for a while. It still is not over. Twenty-two years later I am still dangling over the ground by dislocated arms, panting, and accusing myself. In such an instance there is no "repression." Does one repress an unsightly birthmark? One can have it removed by a plastic surgeon, but the skin that is transplanted in its place is not the skin with which one feels naturally at ease.

One can shake off torture as little as the question of the possibilities and limits of the power to resist it. I have spoken with many comrades about this and have attempted to relive all kinds of experiences. Does the brave man resist? I am not sure. There was, for example, that young Belgian aristocrat who converted to Communism and was something like a hero, namely in the Spanish civil war, where he had fought on the Republican side. But when they subjected him to torture in Breendonk, he "coughed up," as it is put in the jargon of common criminals, and since he knew a lot, he betrayed an entire organization. The brave man went very far in his readiness to cooperate. He drove with the Gestapo men to the homes of his comrades and in extreme zeal encouraged them to confess just everything, but absolutely everything, that was their only hope, and it was, he said, a question of paying any price in order to escape torture. And I knew another, a Bulgarian professional revolutionary, who had been subjected to torture compared to which mine was only a somewhat strenuous sport, and who had remained silent, simply and steadfastly silent. Also the unforgettable Jean Moulin, who is buried in the Pantheon in Paris, shall be remembered here. He was arrested as the first chairman of the French Resistance Movement. If he had talked, the entire Résistance would have been destroyed. But he bore his martyrdom beyond the limits of death and did not betray one single name.

Where does the strength, where does the weakness come from? I don't know. One does not know. No one has yet been able to draw distinct borders between the "moral" power of resistance to physical pain and "bodily" resistance (which likewise must be placed in quotation marks). There are more than a few specialists who reduce the entire problem of bearing pain to a purely physiological basis. Here only the French professor of surgery and member of the Collège de France, René Leriche, will be cited, who ventured the following judgment: "We are not equal before the phenomenon of pain," the professor says.

> One person already suffers where the other apparently still perceives hardly anything. This has to do with the individual quality of our sympathetic nerve, with the hormone of the parathyroid gland, and with the vasoconstrictive substances of the adrenal glands. Also in the physiological observation of pain we cannot escape the concept of individuality. History shows us that we people of today are more sensitive to pain than our ancestors were, and this from a purely physiological standpoint. I am not speaking here of any hypothetical moral power of resistance, but am staying within the realm of physiology. Pain remedies and narcosis have contributed more to our greater sensitivity than moral factors. Also the reactions to pain by various people are absolutely not the same. Two wars have given us the opportunity to see how the physical sensitivities of the Germans, French, and English differ. Above all, there is a great separation in this regard between the Europeans on the one hand and the Asians and Africans on the other. The latter bear physical pain incomparably better than the former. . . .

Thus the judgment of a surgical authority. It will hardly be disputed by the simple experiences of a nonprofessional, who saw many individuals and members of numerous ethnic groups suffering pain and deprivation. In this connection, it occurs to me that, as I was able to observe later in the concentration camp, the Slavs, and especially the Russians, bore physical injustice easier and more stoically than did, for example, Italians, Frenchmen, Hollanders, or Scandinavians. As body, we actually are not equal when faced with pain and torture. But that does not solve our problem of the power of resistance, and it gives us no conclusive answer to the question of what share moral and physical factors have in it. If we agree to a reduction to the purely physiological, then we run the risk of finally pardoning every kind of whiny reaction and physical cowardice. But if we exclusively stress the so-called moral resistance, then we would have to measure a weakly seventeen-year old gymnasium pupil who fails to withstand torture by the same standards as an athletically built thirty-year old laborer who is accustomed to manual work and hardships. Thus we had better let the question rest, just as at that time I myself did not further analyze my power to resist, when, battered and with my hands still shackled, I lay in the cell and ruminated.

For the person who has survived torture and whose pains are starting to subside (before they flare up again) experiences an ephemeral peace that is conducive to thinking. In one respect, the tortured person is content that he was body only and because of that, so he thinks, free of all political concern. You are on the outside, he tells himself more or less, and I am here in the cell, and that gives me a great superiority over you. I have experienced the ineffable, I am filled with it entirely, and now see, if you can, how you are going to live with yourselves, the world, and my disappearance. On the other hand, however, the fading away of the physical, which revealed itself in pain and torture, the end of the tremendous tumult that had erupted in the body, the reattainment of a hollow stability, is satisfying and soothing. There are even euphoric moments, in which the return of weak powers of reason is felt as an extraordinary happiness. The bundle of limbs that is slowly recovering human semblance feels the urge to articulate the experience intellectually, right away, on the spot, without losing the least bit of time, for a few hours afterward could already be too late.

Thinking is almost nothing else but a great astonishment. Astonishment at the fact that you had endured it, that the tumult had not immediately led also to an explosion of the body, that you still have a forehead that you can stroke with your shackled hands, an eye that can be opened and closed, a mouth that would show the usual lines if you could see it now in a mirror. What? you ask yourself—the same person who was gruff with his family because of a toothache was able to hang there by his dislocated arms and still live? The person who for hours was in a bad mood after slightly burning his finger with a cigarette was lacerated here with a horsewhip, and now that it is all over he hardly feels his wounds? Astonishment also at the fact that what happened to you yourself, by right was supposed to befall only those who had written about it in accusatory brochures: torture. A murder is committed, but it is part of the newspaper that reported on it. An airplane accident occurred, but that concerns the people who lost a relative in it. The Gestapo tortures. But that was a matter until now for the somebodies who were tortured and who displayed their scars at antifascist conferences. That suddenly you yourself are the Somebody, is grasped only with difficulty. That, too, is a kind of alienation.

If from the experience of torture any knowledge at all remains that goes beyond the plain nightmarish, it is that of a great amazement and a foreignness in the world that cannot be compensated by any sort of subsequent human communication. Amazed, the tortured person experienced that in this world there can be the other as absolute sovereign, and sovereignty revealed itself as the power to inflict suffering and to destroy. The dominion of the torturer over his victim has nothing in common with the power exercised on the basis of social contracts, as we know it. It is not the power of the traffic policeman over the pedestrian, of the tax official over the taxpayer, of the first lieutenant over the second lieutenant. It is also not the sacral sovereignty of past absolute chieftains or kings; for even if they stirred fear, they were also objects of trust at the same time. The king could be terrible in his wrath, but also kind in his mercy; his autocracy was an exercise of authority. But the power of the torturer, under which the tortured moans, is nothing other than the triumph of the survivor over the one who is plunged from the world into agony and death.

Astonishment at the existence of the other, as he boundlessly asserts himself through torture, and astonishment at what one can become oneself: flesh and death. The tortured person never ceases to be amazed that all those things one may, according to inclination, call his soul, or his mind, or his consciousness, or his identity, are destroyed when there is that cracking and splintering in the shoulder joints. That life is fragile is a truism he has always known—and that it can be ended, as Shakespeare says, "with a little pin." But only through torture did he learn that a living person can be transformed so thoroughly into flesh and by that, while still alive, be partly made into a prey of death.

Whoever has succumbed to torture can no longer feel at home in the world. The shame of destruction cannot be erased. Trust in the world, which already collapsed in part at the first blow, but in the end, under torture, fully, will not be regained. That one's fellow man was experienced as the antiman remains in the tortured person as accumulated horror. It blocks the view into a world in which the principle of hope rules. One who was martyred is a defenseless prisoner of fear. It is fear that henceforth reigns over him. Fear—and also what is called resentments. They remain, and have scarcely a chance to concentrate into a seething, purifying thirst for revenge.

NOTES

5. Janos Kadar; installed as head of Hungary's "Revolutionary Workers' and Peasants' Government" after the Soviets crushed the 1956 October uprising.

6. Friedrich Gottlieb Klopstock (1724–1803); the initiator of German poetic Irrationalism and *Erlebnisdichtung* ("poetry of experience"). Christoph Martin Wieland (1773–1813); together with Lessing, the outstanding representative of the German Enlightenment and a forerunner of German classicism.

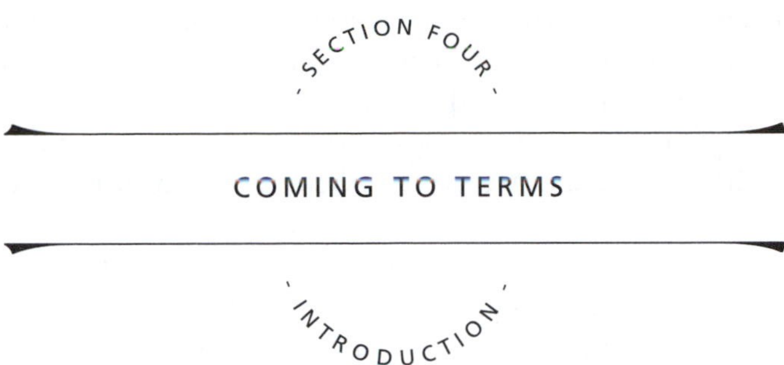

Section Four

COMING TO TERMS

Introduction

Hundreds of years ago, the great English poet Alexander Pope wrote of "this long disease, my life." As diagnoses, treatments, and prognoses become more sophisticated, and as some of our most dreaded conditions become chronic rather than acute and terminal, the experience of living with disease has become more complex for patients and those close to them. The experience of illness is shared by families, and sometimes legions of professionals. Patients turn to sources of information outside of their immediate caregivers. Treatments have their own consequences; intimate human relationships bear witness to the strains of survival, remissions, duration without cure. In fiction, drama, poetry, and the protean form of the memoir, patients and those who care about them give expression to the new world of living with—and not always quickly dying of—serious illness. Since medicine itself has become so successful, failure to tame every disease, especially the failure to conquer mental illness and despair, carries new pain for the survivors and mourners.

What all the works in this section have in common is their exploration of the time—often long and full of complexity—after the catastrophe, the diagnosis, the rescue, or the death. For as many practitioners and patients come to know only in part and after struggle, most consequences of accident, illness, and disaster are lengthy and undramatic, often more demanding in their repetitiveness than are the critical moments surrounding the diagnosis or the onset of disease.

Perhaps the most difficult and disconcerting work in this section is Marianne Paget's "Performing the Text," a dramatic reading constructed from Paget's path-breaking examination of the absence of communication between doctor and patient. Paget worked as a sociologist examining mistakes in medicine; the repercussions of the missed diagnosis in her case study and in her life were devastating, and in her own case, fatal. Like other works in this section, Paget's chapter enacts the disruption of narrative. Similarly, the poems by Maxine Kumin, written after the death by suicide of her dear friend Anne Sexton, document the interruption of a long and intimate conversation. Sexton and Kumin used to leave their telephones off the hook as they worked, whistling to call one another back to the open line between them until they hung up, according to mutual agreement, at the end of each writing day.

The selections in this section are all, in a sense, afterwords, about the creation and recreation of meaning in lives disrupted by losses, failures, deaths. After the initial transgression or catastrophe, each figure in these poems, essays, and stories works to construct a meaningful future. And each employs a particular form to embody that continuing decision. For Kumin, poetry was the natural choice of memorial, even in "October, Yellowstone Park," when she announces that she will write no more poems about this subject. For Gwendolyn Brooks, much celebrated for her poems about urban African-American life and death, "the mother" speaks the long mourning for the aborted children preserved in memory, but excluded from life.

The preservation of memory and the slow rediscovery of feeling, the unique trajectory of mourning and returning to life, are charted in formal as well as emotional terms. Often the written pieces begin from a point of numbness and work towards new intimations of feelings: empathy, acceptance, grief long buried from everyday light. The spare acknowledgment of feeling bad that comes through from the translations of Wislawa Symborska's poems epitomizes the honest assessments of the pieces in this section.

Lorrie Moore's acclaimed and acutely observed short story, "People Like That Are the Only People Here," concludes this section; it could as well enrich other parts of this anthology, and it has been reprinted in full and in part many times since its original publication in *The New Yorker.* Finding the way to integrate the unimaginable into the life of a parent—the sudden brush with the mortality of a child—is a task not willingly entered upon by any writer. But the work of literature to give form to the formless and to shape the apparently endless present into a narrative of past, present, and future, is exemplified by this final selection in this section: "Coming to Terms."

THE WORK OF TALK

MARIANNE A. PAGET

NOTE FROM THE EDITOR [MARJORIE L. DEVAULT]: In the previous chapter, Paget reports on the performance based on Emilie Beck's adaptation of her research article (Paget 1983a) and discusses her desire to write her own script, adapting the same analysis somewhat differently. Her script appears in this chapter.

One of the ironies of performance in the social sciences is that it can enter our official discourses—our books and journals—only through its written traces. A script on a page can give only a suggestion of the immediacy and embodiedness of performance—the very features that make it distinctive in our professional world. Paget's script is not easy to read, since it imports onto the stage the technical and analytic language of a particular mode of discourse analysis. In addition, the script presents conversation between the physician and patient in a form close to actual talk, including false starts, hesitations, and interruptions. Paget made some concessions to ease of delivery and understanding, particularly in translating from the microscopically detailed transcription of speech in her article into language somewhat easier to read. However, she was committed to preserving the attention to speech and the analytic language that she considered central to her project in human science.

As presented here, the script can be read in several different ways. It can be read for the content of the analysis, though for this purpose it is no doubt easier to read the research article that was its source. It can also be read for Paget's deepened interpretation of this medical encounter. In the creation of characters, the assignment of dialogue, and the addition of stage directions, she made decisions intended to communicate understandings of this encounter beyond those that can be easily expressed in written text alone. Most important, in my view, is the fact that the script can be performed. It can be read aloud, individually or in groups, and it can be staged—and these are the ways it will achieve fullest expression.

CAST

1st Narrator	1st Physician	1st Patient	Death
2nd Narrator	2nd Physician	2nd Patient	

1st Nar: They met three times in the early months of 1972 in a large, university-affiliated clinic to discuss her medical problems. Each of their encounters was ambiguous and unresolved. Each encounter exuded misunderstandings.

2nd Nar: Their talk was awry with disagreements, odd semantic constructions, radical breaks and shifts in discourse topics, and allusions to an operation that were not clarified.

1st Nar: The central tension of their talk was his assessment:

1st Phy: that her basic health was good and that the problem was her "nerves."

1st Pat: But throughout their meetings, she reported a number of minor and serious symptoms that challenged his assessment.

1st Nar: The stretch of talk that follows and others from the same series of interviews will be used to examine the speaking practice of physicians, particularly their practices of questioning patients.

2nd Nar: A diagnosis is not just an abstract thing connected with a nomenclature and a theory of disease entities,

2nd Phy: although it is that, too.

2nd Nar: It is not just a term on a medical chart or a record,

2nd Pat: although an infinite number can be found there.

2nd Nar: A diagnosis is a feature of the organization of talk, and its production is continuously realized in that talk.

1st Nar: This analysis will focus on questioning practices because these practices often construct the meaning of a patient's illness.

1st Phy: I want you to sit straight. No, sit facing me.

(Silence)

Do you wear a hat by preference or are you having anything wrong with your scalp?

1st Pat: Oh, I'm, I'm . . . I wear it because it's cold but I, uh, I, I . . . my scalp is a little bit . . . my scalp is getting all abrasions on it for some crazy reason or other.

1st Phy: Well, let me just have a look. Take it off just for a second.

1st Pat: Look at that . . . look at this, this . . . I can't even . . . I can't even bleach my hair. I don't know . . . I don't know if they're still there but last week it was all red. It was—

1st Phy: No, it looks pretty clean.

1st Pat: Yeah, that's what my barber just—

1st Phy: There's a little bit of dandruff there but that's about all.

1st Pat: Yeah.

1st Phy: All right, put your hat down.

1st Pat: My husband thinks—

1st Phy: You'll be more comfortable without it.

1st Nar: In this excerpt, which opens the first of three encounters, this physician introduces a topic with a compound question.

2nd Nar: "Do you wear a hat by preference or are you having anything wrong with your scalp?"

2nd Pat: He has apparently observed that this patient,

1st Pat: a woman in her mid-forties,

2nd Pat: is wearing both a frock, in preparation for an exam, and a hat.

1st Nar: The topic,

1st Pat: her hat and scalp,

1st Nar: is explored through a series of turns at talk in which each participant responds to the other's utterances.

2nd Pat: She answers both his initial questions.

1st Nar: "I'm, I'm . . . I wear it because it's cold"

1st Pat: is her response to his first question, and

2nd Nar: "But I, uh, I, I . . . my scalp is a little bit . . . my scalp is getting all abrasions on it for some crazy reason or other"

1st Phy: is her response to his second question.

2nd Phy: Her response is complex because it projects an act.

2nd Nar: Implicitly, it requests that he examine her scalp,

1st Phy: and it is heard that way.

2nd Pat: The physician responds. He both says,

1st Nar: "Well, let me just have a look"

1st Phy: and looks.

2nd Phy: His looking is captured in their talk's silence of almost two seconds,

2nd Pat: in his assessment, "No, it looks pretty clean,"

1st Pat: with which she agrees,

2nd Pat: and in his related observation that "There's a little bit of dandruff there,"

1st Pat: with which she also agrees.

2nd Nar: This discourse topic comes to its close with his request that she put her hat down and with his connected politeness,

2nd Phy: "You'll be more comfortable without it."

Death: His next request introduces a new topic. "Now let me see your throat."

(Pause)

1st Nar: The excerpt is a microparadigm of the pattern of their talk, for he continuously directs their talk.

2nd Nar: Through questions and other "requests" for action,

2nd Pat: and sometimes through commands,

2nd Nar: he introduces, develops, and dissolves discourse topics.

2nd Phy: Questions are, in fact, "requests" for action. They are used to carry on interactional activities, such as

2nd Nar: clarifying,

1st Nar: assessing,

2nd Nar: complaining,

1st Nar: and explaining.

2nd Nar: Abrupt breaks or shifts often appear in their discourse, and the physician, too, initiates these shifts and breaks.

1st Pat: She helps develop their talk by responding to his questions and his other "requests" and,

2nd Pat: sometimes, by suggesting and expressing her own concerns.

1st Pat: But often he ignores her concerns,

2nd Nar: which also contributes to the developing discontinuities in the movement of their talk.

Death: The exchange continues:

1st Phy: Now let me see your throat.

(Silence)

Uh, have the teeth been removed that were in question?

1st Pat: No. My mouth is driving me crazy. In fact when I sleep with my head over here or my head inclined on the side m-my whole mouth hurts.

1st Phy: Well, I would hate to have

1st Pat: Ohhh

1st Phy: them remove any more teeth without being sure that they

1st Pat: Ahhh

1st Phy: were the cause of something.

1st Pat: Oh, I know it but what am I gonna do?

1st Phy: Well, let's look straight . . .

(Silence)

1st Pat: His utterance,

2nd Phy: "Well, I would hate to have them remove any more teeth without being sure that they were the cause of something"

1st Nar: is representative of the abrupt shifts that occur in their talk.

1st Pat: His utterance does not develop her reply,

2nd Pat: "My mouth is driving me crazy."

1st Pat: He does not ask how long her mouth has been bothering her, how often it happens, or when she last saw a dentist.

2nd Phy: Instead, he shifts ground.

2nd Nar: The utterance contains an unmarked pronoun

1st Nar: "them"

2nd Nar: which has no previous referent in their talk, and suggests that

1st Nar: "them"

2nd Nar: may have removed teeth unnecessarily.

1st Nar: A discourse analyst must continuously confront ambiguities that arise in the highly contextual features of talk and its unfolding ellipses.

2nd Pat: In the previous exchange

2nd Phy: “them”

1s Phy: is a reference to unknown dentists who removed some of her teeth,

1st Pat: which this physician noticed while examining her mouth.

2nd Pat: His insinuation that some of her teeth may have been removed unnecessarily is the first of several insinuations about her past care.

1st Nar: His use of unmarked pronouns will recur.

1st Pat: She hears the suggested uncertainty about the appropriateness of removing some of her teeth and responds

2nd Pat: “Oh, I know it but what am I gonna do?”

1st Phy: He replies with a command

Death: “Well, let's look straight.”

2nd Phy: The physician's failure to respond to her question again shows the discontinuities of their talk.

2nd Pat: And his impoliteness captures a pattern of dominance

1st Phy: His

2nd Pat: and subordination

1st Pat: Hers

2nd Pat: as it is being constituted in their conversation.

1st Nar: Throughout their exchanges, however unconnected his utterances are with what has gone before, they will be supported.

2nd Nar: Even when appearing with unmarked references like “them,” they will be developed. She will reply.

2nd Pat: Very often, however, her inquires will go unsupported and unclarified.

1st Nar: Politeness forms like

1st Phy.
& 1st Pat: “okay,” “yeah,”

1st Nar: and

1st Phy.
& 1st Pat: “thanks”

2nd Pat: occasionally follow responses to questions or other requests.

2nd Nar: They acknowledge a response.

2nd Pat: But politeness forms are frequently deleted from discourse.

1st Pat: They are almost entirely absent from the speaking practices of this physician in these encounters.

2nd Phy: Questioning patients is the most common method of acquiring information about illness.

2nd Nar: Questions create a pool of usable knowledge in responding to illness.

1st Nar: In an analysis of the talk of British general practitioners and their patients,

2nd Nar: Byrne and Long report that patient care takes place as a series of discourse exchanges that last on the average of eight minutes.

2nd Phy: They reviewed twenty-five hundred tapes.

2nd Nar: In eight minutes, physicians attempted to establish rapport,

2nd Pat: discover the reason for a patient's visit,

2nd Phy: verbally and physically examine the patient,

2nd Nar: discuss the patient's condition,

2nd Phy: establish a treatment plan,

1st Nar: and terminate the exchange.

2nd Nar: Questioning practices will be the focus of detailed attention here because of a discovered problem in the talk of this physician and patient.

1st Nar: This woman is a postoperative

All: (*whispered*) cancer

1st Nar: patient,

1st Pat: concerned about the spread of her cancer and about her survival.

1st Nar: Yet across their three encounters, her condition as a

All: (*whispered*) cancer

1st Pat: patient and her fear that her cancer would metastasize were never introduced as discourse topics.

1st Nar: Her condition became apparent in the course of a close analysis of their talk, including increasingly detailed transcriptions of their encounters.

2nd Phy: Oblique references to her recent surgery appeared in their first exchange:

1st Phy: "scar"

1st Pat: “tumor”

1st Phy: “surgery”

1st Pat: and “remaining kidney.”

1st Phy: The physician assessed her many symptoms and complaints,

1st Pat: her anxieties about what was happening to her body,

Death: and her fear of her death

1st Phy: as signs of a neurotic depression.

1st Pat: He continually assured her that her basic health was good and that the problem was her nerves.

2nd Pat: Instead of discussing her concerns about

All: (*whispered*) cancer

2nd Pat: they talked about a virus,

1st Phy: persistent pain in her mouth,

1st Pat: her teeth and gums,

2nd Nar: her nerves,

1st Nar: her visits to other physicians and to dentists,

1st Phy: medical procedures she has undergone in the past

2nd Pat: or may undergo,

1st Pat: medications that she is taking

2nd Pat: or might take,

1st Phy: plans for new tests,

2nd Phy: additional visits,

2nd Nar: her weight,

2nd Phy: consultations with other physicians for a cyst on her face,

2nd Pat: and eyeglasses.

2nd Phy: Medical audiences are able to hear the talk's oblique references to surgery as a “conversation” about a cancer operation. Especially important in confirming this impression are references to procedures that were undertaken three months earlier by another clinic where her surgery was performed,

1st Phy: among the procedures, an angiogram.

1st Nar: References to these procedures appear on the third tape.

2nd Nar: The existence of cancer was independently corroborated through questionnaires that were collected in the course of the original study and made available.

1st Nar: Because this woman's condition as a

All: (*whispered*) cancer

1st Nar: patient was never discussed,

1st Pat: her essential concern about its recurrence could not be addressed.

1st Nar: More fundamentally, her continued symptoms, persistent reports of pain, anxieties about her health and health care could not be referred or, at least as the discourse developed, were not referred to her experience of

All: (*whispered*) cancer.

2nd Phy: Both the referents to her

All: (*whispered*) cancer

2nd Phy: and the implications of the experience were lost in the discourse.

1st Pat: Instead, her symptoms were referred to her nerves.

2nd Pat: She was reassured that her basic health was good.

1st Nar: For example, the physician said,

2nd Phy: "I'm sure that your basic health is good,"

1st Nar: and

2nd Pat: "Well, you're eventually gonna have to be convinced of it or you won't be well."

Death: "You got to feel it deep down in so that your . . . you have a chance to recover completely."

1st Nar: Their exchanges became marked by her struggle to resist his diagnostic assessment that the problem was her nerves

1st Pat: and by her effort to clarify the meaning of her symptoms.

1st Nar: Because her condition as a

All: (*whispered*) cancer

1st Nar: patient was never addressed,

2nd Phy: we will explore its exclusion by following allusions and oblique references to it in their first encounter.

1st Phy: Each knew that she had

All: (*whispered*) cancer,

1st Pat: and each knew that the other knew,

1st Phy: and each also knew that these oblique references

1st Phy. & 1st Pat: recurred without achieving expression.

1st Nar: Attention will be given to how discourse topics are established and developed because, although this topic was not developed, many, many others were.

2nd Phy: Excerpts from the early phase of the first encounter will be used

1st Phy: because it is in the early phase, the physical examination phase, that the physician begins to formulate his diagnosis

1st Pat: that the problem is nerves.

1st Nar: An excerpt that stands as their first major exchange on the problem of her nerves will be presented.

2nd Nar: Preliminary exchanges, along the way of that assessment, will also be presented.

1st Nar: Then a second assessment of her health will be displayed.

2nd Phy: The unspoken topic,

All: (*whispered*) cancer,

1st Nar: hovers on the verge of expression in the questions she asks.

2nd Pat: Discontinuities in the discourse are noted throughout.

2nd Phy: These discontinuities continuously capture asymmetries in questioning and answering practices that shaped the meaning of her illness.

1st Pat: I'm one person . . . have so darned many *complaints* and not being anything . . . I mean, you know (*softly*) in the past few months . . .

1st Phy: Hold it.

(Silence)

There has to be some explanation but it doesn't . . .

(Silence)

it doesn't have to *be* a *disease* in order to organize . . .

1st Pat: Oh, I'm not looking for a *dire* disease, you know (*softly*) or anything like that. I'm not looking for anything.

(Silence)

1st Nar: In this exchange, he interrupts her, a characteristic discourtesy that will recur.

1st Phy: "Hold it,"

1st Pat: he commands.

1st Nar: The examination is captured in a silence, and he begins to speak while examining her:

2nd Phy: "There has to be some explanation but it doesn't . . ."

1st Nar: Again, the exam is captured in a silence, then

2nd Phy: "it doesn't have to *be* a *disease* . . ."

1st Nar: This is his first suggestion that a disease may not be the cause of her pains.

2nd Nar: It is a kind of initial offering and it will be followed by others.

1st Nar: It comes as an expansion of a developing discourse topic,

1st Pat: her many complaints,

1st Phy: and their not being anything.

2nd Phy: The physician's speech carries an emphasis on "be" and "disease," and emphasis is important in hearing.

1st Nar: It invokes special notice in the melody of talk.

2nd Phy: Such emphasis, here the elongation of sound, can be translated as "hear what I am saying under this accent, it doesn't have to *bee* a *diseasse*."

2nd Pat: Several of her own utterances carry accents:

1st Pat: "complaints" and "dire."

2nd Pat: She hears his emphasis and interrupts to say that she is not looking for a "*dire* disease."

1st Nar: Her speech continues very softly, "or anything like that."

2nd Pat: Her interruption signals her sensitivity to the idea of disease.

2nd Nar: It does not expand on the other part of his offering, that pain may not be caused by a disease.

1st Nar: Soon she will ask about the pain in the area of her scar.

1st Pat: (*Softly*) Oh, that hurt.

1st Phy: Where? Oh, that's in the scar.

1st Pat: Right in here.

1st Phy: Yeah.

1st Pat: Oh, is that in the scar?

1st Phy: That *is* the scar.

1st Pat: I . . . it is?

1st Phy: No that—

1st Pat: Is it, is that . . . I had . . . is that supposed to hurt like that from a—

1s Phy: It . . . occasionally it does for quite a while.

1st Pat: Ohhh.

1st Phy: That does not represent anything wrong. That's because when they make a scar as big as that it has to cut nerves.

1st Pat: Oh, it . . . but it didn't hurt me until this week.

1st Phy: Well,

1st Pat: Ahuh.

1st Phy: Let's see.

1st Pat: Ohhh.

1st Phy: Now breathe.

(Silence)

2nd Phy: This exchange refers to pain that is located in the course of his examination of her back.

Death: "Oh, that hurt." "Where? Oh, that's in the scar." "Oh, is that in the scar?" "That *is* the scar." "Is it, is that . . . I had . . . is that supposed to hurt like that from a—"

1st Nar: Her question is interrupted in its course, and its last component is lost.

2nd Pat: The physician assures her that occasionally such pain continues for "quite a while,"

Death: an ellipsis of "quite a while after an operation."

2nd Pat: "That"

1st Nar: he continues

2nd Pat: “does not represent anything wrong.”

2nd Nar: “Oh, it . . .”

1st Nar: she continues

2nd Nar: “but it didn’t hurt me until this week.”

1st Nar: “*But*” signals a disagreement with his assessment that “that does not represent anything wrong,” and that disagreement is developed in her statement

2nd Pat: “it didn’t hurt me until this week.”

1st Phy: His response, “Well,” is a token of his recognition that she has disagreed.

1st Pat: And her response “Ahuh,” reaffirms her position against his reservations.

1st Nar: These are small, delicate signs of a continuously developing conflict about what is wrong with her.

2nd Nar: He says,

2nd Phy: “Let’s see” and dissolves the topic in the exam.

1st Phy: How good is your wind? Can you carry bundles and walk up a hill without being short of breath or do you—

1st Pat: No, I can’t even climb up a flight of stairs without getting completely exhausted.

1st Phy: Now do you have any pain under this (*pause*) kidney?

1st Pat: (*Sniff*) Ahhh

1st Phy: There.

1st Pat: Not when you touch it but I’ve been having pain.

1st Phy: (*whistling*)

1st Pat: pain in that area.

1st Phy: Fine. You do have pain in this area. Well, that’s too soon, you see,

1st Pat: Oh yeah. Oh, *that* hurts. Right there.

1st Phy: that’s too soon to tell anything about that.

1st Pat: (*Loud exhalation*) Hhhh.

(*Silence*)

How about in here?

1st Phy: Tch, no, wait a sec. We’re gonna do that later.

1st Pat: Oh. Okay. Hhh.

2nd Pat: This excerpt also occurs while he is examining her back.

2nd Phy: It begins with two questions and introduces a new discourse topic, her breathing.

2nd Pat: She answers his questions.

2nd Phy: But her response is not acknowledged.

2nd Nar: Acknowledgment has two forms. A response may be acknowledged either explicitly with a token like "oh" or "yeah" or implicitly by developing the content of what has just been said.

1st Nar: For example, "How often do you experience exhaustion?" would constitute an implicit acknowledgment.

2nd Nar: Here, neither one form or the other occurs.

1st Nar: Instead of developing her reply

Death: that she can't climb a flight of stairs without becoming exhausted

1st Nar: the physician begins a new discourse topic,

2nd Phy: "Now do you have any pain under this (*pause*) kidney?"

1st Nar: His failure to develop a discourse topic he has introduced constitutes an inattention to the semantic sense of what she has said about her exhaustion.

2nd Pat: And his inattentions will recur.

2nd Phy: In recurring, they will leave some of her responses hovering without development.

1st Nar: Once again, the exam is captured in a silence. Then this patient says,

2nd Pat: "Ahh"

1st Nar: and he

2nd Phy: "There"

1st Nar: and she

2nd Pat: "Not when you touch it but I've been having pain in that area."

2nd Phy: He whistles across part of her statement and says,

1st Phy: "Fine,"

2nd Phy: then he summarizes, "You do have pain in this area."

2nd Pat: In close synchrony with the semantic sense of his summary, she says,

Death: "Oh, *that* hurts. Right there."

2nd Pat: He continues,

2nd Phy: "Well, that's too soon, you see, that's too soon to tell anything about that."

1st Pat: She exhales loudly.

Death: "Anything about that," of course, refers to the unspoken topic and to the possibility that her

All: (*whispered*) cancer

Death: may return.

2nd Pat: Her noticeable exhalation suggests that she has heard that it is too soon to tell.

1st Nar: The exam is again captured in a silence between them.

2nd Phy: The many silences that punctuate their talk during the physical exam suggest its preeminence as an activity; and the many characteristic interruptions that return their talk to the exam emphasize the exam's importance.

1st Phy: It is an activity in which his power is expressed.

2nd Pat: Next she suggests, "How about in here?"

2nd Phy: He "tchs" the beginning of his utterance in response, and says,

2nd Pat: "No, wait a sec. We're gonna do that later."

1st Nar: He will, over the course of their encounters, "tch" at the beginning of many utterances and "well" at the beginning of others. Both "tch" and "well" become ongoing tokens of his disapproval.

2nd Pat: In the course of the physical examination, he asks about her family.

2nd Phy: "Do you have any problems in your home with your . . . husband or your marriage or is that . . ."

1st Pat: This topic appears without previous reference in their talk.

2nd Pat: Although the question has no discourse history and comes without prefatory notice as a question, she responds to it, and to a number of related questions.

1st Pat: She repeatedly supports the development of discourse topics and activities, however unconnected they are.

Death: Here, his inquiry moves progressively away from her recent surgery.

1st Phy: Do you have any problems in your home with your . . . husband or your marriage or is that . . .

1st Pat: Ahh . . . No, I haven't actually had problems. My husband is quite . . . perturbed that I, uh . . . in the past . . . four or five months, that I'm not . . . getting any better. And you know, he's . . . (*softly*) I'm not a happy person to be with (*long pause*) but I, before that I hadn't, uh . . .

1st Phy: There were no problems before that?

1st Pat: Well, there were domestic p-problems (*pause*). I, uh . . .

1st Phy: Do you think you were having more than average problems or probably less?

(Silence)

1st Pat: Um (*pause*). Maybe I was having a bit more that the average person . . . not from the marriage itself . . . the marriage is a good marriage . . .

1st Phy: It isn't anything enough to threaten your marriage?

1st Pat: Right now I think it's getting so. If I don't get . . . something done about my physical condition . . . about my outlook, uh, I don't doubt but what—I . . . I, I want to feel better. I, I was a . . . very active person . . . had many interests and many hobbies and I loved to do things with the children and with my husband and . . . I, I still do but I find that I just haven't got the . . . stamina . . . to do it . . . which is crazy because I think I have when I start to do it . . . and then I just fall apart.

1st Phy: Now big breath.

(Silence)

1st Nar: The question on her family life, on problems in her home with her husband, or her marriage, is not fully formed. It contains an

2nd Phy: "or is that . . ."

1st Nar: and a pause of two seconds.

2nd Pat: She responds across the awkwardness of the question and its shape, and her response stumbles over its course.

Death: "Ahh . . . No, I haven't actually had problems. My husband is quite . . . perturbed that I, uh . . . in the past . . . four or five months, that I'm not . . . getting any better. And you know, he's . . . (*softly*) I'm not a happy person to be with."

1st Nar: The repeated hesitations in her speech here display reflection. Pauses occur within phrases and clauses as well as between them.

2nd Nar: For example, "My husband is quite . . . perturbed that I, uh . . . in the past . . ."

2nd Pat: "That"

1st Nar: in her utterance "but I, before that I hadn't, uh . . ."

2nd Pat: refers to the past four or five months.

1st Nar: He develops the topic:

1st Phy: "There were no problems before that?"

2nd Pat: "That" again occurs, but here it does not refer to the past four or five months.

2nd Phy: This physician is not probing the problems with which she and her family have lived in the two months before her operation and the three since:

1st Phy: He is probing the time before that.

1st Nar: She responds,

2nd Pat: "Well, there were domestic p-problems."

1st Nar: There is a pause, then

2nd Pat: "I, uh . . ."

1st Nar: and her talk falls away in silence.

2nd Phy: Her reticence here is noticeable and is strongly heard. What is less noticeable is the shift away from the past four or five months of her life to the months before them.

2nd Nar: While taking her blood pressure he asks,

2nd Pat: "Do you think you were having more than average problems or probably less?"

1st Nar: The talk now has moved entirely away from the most recent events in her life.

2nd Nar: The discourse topic developing is the problem of her marriage before her

All: (*whispered*) cancer

2nd Nar: operation,

1st Nar: not the problems that can be produced by that operation.

2nd Nar: The "or" in his question in this cycle is one of his regular speaking practices. He asks questions, often in the form of either/or, which forces a choice.

1st Pat: She stumbles on.

2nd Pat: Then, unexpectedly, he returns the discussion to the present with

1st Nar: "It isn't anything enough to threaten your marriage?"

1st Phy: "It" refers to what was before the past four or five months.

2nd Phy: He means what was before the past four or five months "isn't enough to threaten your marriage" now, is it?

2nd Pat: She responds, "Right now I think it's getting so."

1st Nar: Her response again stumbles on across a number of pauses and hesitations.

1st Pat: And it contains considerable feeling.

2nd Pat: No acknowledgment occurs.

1st Phy: "Now big breath," he says.

1st Nar: Across the talk's breaks, across the recurrent discontinuities in the development of topics, across the unmarked and unreferenced terms in his questions, she makes sense of what he says and asks.

1st Pat: But in ignoring her replies, he makes a kind of nonsense of her talk, for his responses to her replies often do not develop what she has said but dissolve her answers back into the exam.

2nd Phy: Her talk goes without exploration often:

2nd Pat: Her physical condition,

1st Pat: her exhaustion,

Death: her anxieties about her health

2nd Pat: hover without clarification or resolution.

2nd Nar: The microparadigm of the movement of their talk is captured recurrently in these excerpts.

1st Phy: The physician controls their discourse.

2nd Pat: His control inhibits expression of her concern about her experience of

All: (*whispered*) cancer.

1st Phy: Well, has it possibly occurred to you that with all the troubles that your . . . body has gone through that your nerves *have now got* to the point where they suffer and where you need help to get your nerves restored?

1st Pat: Uh . . . yes, I . . . I think I'm a bit nervous . . . I, I, I don't see what you mean.

1st Phy: I, ha, I don't, I didn't mean overtly nervous. I meant that, that . . .

1st Pat: No?

1st Phy: your nerves have suffered to the point that they could be producing some of these pains (*pause*) because *I* don't believe you've got a *new* tumor every *place* you have a new pain. I wouldn't think of it.

1st Pat: (*Interrupting*) I'm not looking for a new tumor. (*Pause*) No sir, I never said that.

1st Phy: (*Interrupting*) and I don't think—no, I know you didn't—and I don't think there's anything broken

1st Pat: Okay.

1st Phy: where you're having the pains. (*Pause*) I *do* think there were nerves cut where you have your scar.

1st Pat: (*Interrupting*) It's right there, right there.

(Silence)

1st Phy: "*Have now got*"

2nd Pat carries strong stress

2nd Phy: and it expresses, across the obliqueness of the form of this utterance,

2nd Pat: his assessment that her nerves have now gotten to the point where they suffer and need assistance.

1st Pat: She, again, and quite characteristically, answers his question

2nd Pat: "Yes"

1st Pat: and observes that she is a little nervous

1st Phy: and she continues,

2nd Pat: "I don't see what you mean."

1st Phy: He interrupts to say that he does not mean overtly nervous.

2nd Phy: He explains that her "nerves have suffered to the point that they could be producing some of these pains."

2nd Nar:	This is his most explicit communication of the functional basis of some pain.
1st Phy:	After a pause of a second, he adds,
2nd Phy:	"because *I* don't believe you've got a *new* tumor every *place* you have a new pain."
Death:	And he then adds softly,
2nd Phy:	"I wouldn't think of it."
1st Pat:	And, in its course, she hears his reference to a new tumor and says that she is not looking for a new tumor.
2nd Pat:	"No, sir, I never said that."
1st Phy:	He continues his assessment and,
2nd Pat:	hearing her response,
1st Phy:	he acknowledges that she never said that.
1st Nar:	The synchrony here and the semantic sense of their utterances across the interruptions are rare.
1st Phy:	Here, they each hear and acknowledge that they have heard the other,
1st Pat:	and each thus knows and understands that
1st Phy:	she "never said that"
1st Pat:	and that she
2nd Pat:	is "not looking for a new tumor."
1st Pat:	He acknowledges his understanding with "I know you didn't."
1st Phy:	She responds to his acknowledgment with "okay."
2nd Pat:	Her statement that she is not looking for a new tumor echoes an earlier response:
1st Pat:	That she is not looking for a dire disease.
2nd Pat:	And it comes with a "no sir" which somewhat sardonically suggests his power as it is continuously being realized in their exchanges.
2nd Phy:	His observation, "*I* don't believe you've got a *new* tumor every *place* you have a new pain" finds its sense as a reference to her
All:	(*whispered*) cancer
1st Pat:	as does her retort,

2nd Pat: "I'm not looking for a new tumor."

1st Nar: His expansions

2nd Phy: "I don't think there's anything broken where you're having the pains"

1st Nar: and

2nd Pat: "I *do* think there were nerves cut where you have your scar"

1st Nar: are clarifications of his point of view. And his reference to scar once again alludes to the incision for which the scar stands.

Death: "It's right there, right there"

1st Nar: follows along.

2nd Pat: She will often point to areas of pain.

1st Nar: The silence that follows signals the exam once again and suggests that he may be looking where she has pointed.

2nd Phy: It is important to remember that these excerpts are taken from the first encounter, which continued for more than fifteen more minutes, and that two additional exchanges occurred between this physician and patient.

1st Nar: Yet these excerpts are not intended as mere illustrations. They capture a conversation filled with misunderstandings.

2nd Phy: The meaning of this patient's illness is constructed by the physician as her symptoms and pains are separated from her experience of

All: (*whispered*) cancer

2nd Phy: and progressively connected with her nerves.

1st Pat: And her illness as nerves is continuously confirmed by her nervousness.

2nd Pat: More fundamentally, the meaning of her illness is continuously constructed in what he sees, asks, and hears.

1st Nar: The small increments of the construction of her illness take shape in the questions he asks and the discourse topics he develops,

2nd Pat: as well as in the questions he does not ask and the discourse topics he does not develop.

Death: The direction of his questioning is always away from her experience of

All: (*whispered*) cancer

Death: and their "talk" about her

All: (*whispered*) cancer

Death: always obscures her experience of

All: (*whispered*) cancer.

1st Nar: The unmentioned discourse topic that hovers is progressively disconnected from her anxiety,

2nd Nar: and her "complaint" finally comes to antedate her experience of

All: (*whispered*) cancer

2nd Nar: and be the "real" source of her symptoms.

1st Nar: Later he will say, for example,

1st Phy: "You've been through the . . . anxiety of having this complaint for so long without anybody finding a reason for it and then having a m-major surgery."

2nd Phy: All the while each knows that the other knows

1st Pat: that she has had

All: (*whispered*) cancer.

1st Nar: The physician's progressive formulation of the problem as a matter of nerves produces continuous tension and conflict between them and this, too, confirms her nervousness.

2nd Pat: The patient participates in the development of the discourse process by answering questions and, sometimes, by expressing her own concerns.

2nd Phy: Although not as an equal,

1st Pat: she contributes to the ongoing misunderstanding between them.

2nd Pat: She too speaks only of the scar and the tumor in their first encounter.

1st Pat: She is both afraid to express her fear of the spread of cancer and afraid to ignore the possibility.

2nd Pat: She tries furtively to discover how a clinician thinks, to catch the truth of her circumstances, across the unspoken fear between them.

2nd Nar: A final excerpt follows.

2nd Phy: In this exchange, the physician again says that he can find nothing wrong.

1st Pat: She begins to ask about the scar.

2nd Pat: Softly she says, "That's the scar?"

2nd Phy: and then a series of questions about her condition.

2nd Pat: "Do you think maybe the, um . . . do you think maybe this kidney is, is, uh . . . overloaded or something?"

Death: "Oh, they removed an adrenal gland."

1st Pat: "Hhh, I don't know. I'm thinking maybe it's a hormone deficiency or something."

Death: Two of her questions are interrupted in their course and the third seems not to have been correctly heard.

2nd Pat: All her questions refer to the impact of her operation on her health.

2nd Phy: He looks at the scar and inquires about the other end of it and says,

2nd Nar: "It's beautiful surgery."

1st Pat: She replies, "It was terrible."

1st Phy: Well . . . I feel *nothing* in your abdomen that's *wrong*.

(Silence)

I don't feel any arteries that are too big and I don't feel any lumps.

(Silence)

I know you're tender there.

(Silence)

1st Pat: (*softly*) That's the scar?

1st Phy: See, the scar is—

1st Pat: Do you think maybe the, um . . . do you think maybe this kidney is, is, uh . . . overloaded or something?

1st Phy: Oh no.

1st Pat: No?

1st Phy: Tch, no. We'll do . . . we can do tests to make sure of that.

(Silence)

1st Pat: Oh, they removed an adrenal gland—

1st Phy: (*Interrupting*) You have an excellent reserve—

1st Pat: they removed an adrenal—

1st Phy: you have a margin of safety in both of those glands that easily takes up—

1st Pat: Oh okay.

(Silence)

Hhh, I don't know. I'm thinking maybe it's a hormone deficiency or something.

1st Phy: Let me just look at the scar.

(Pause)

No, no, that's all right.

(Silence)

Ah, how . . .

(Silence)

how about this end of the scar?

1st Pat: He . . . that's . . . that's, right there. It's, it's right in there—

1st Phy: (*Interrupting*) It's beautiful surgery.

1st Pat: Tch, it was terrible.

(Silence)

2nd Nar: This analysis has focused on questioning practices because questions often introduce, develop, and dissolve topics.

1st Nar: Although this physician's questions introduced, developed, and dissolved many topics, one topic was ignored: this woman's experience of

All: (*whispered*) cancer.

2nd Phy: In their three exchanges on her medical problems, no question ever addressed her experience of

All: (*whispered*) cancer.

1st Nar: Although a number of her questions gained their sense as references to her experience of

All: (*whispered*) cancer

2nd Pat: her questions never led to the establishment of her experience of

All: (*whispered*) cancer

2nd Pat: as a discourse topic.

1st Nar: As the meaning of her experience of

All: (*whispered*) cancer

1st Nar: became lost in their talk, its significance, in connection with her symptoms and pains, also was lost.

1st Pat: The early establishment of a diagnostic assessment that the problem was her nerves, and her sense that there was something wrong, provoked continuous tensions between them.

2nd Pat: Furthermore, as already noted, her nervousness continuously confirmed his diagnosis that the problem was nerves.

2nd Nar: Discourse is both spoken and heard, and the interpretive sense conversationalists make of their evolving talk is carried not only in the movement of their talk on a series of discourse topics, but also in the semantic sense of what is said and heard.

1st Nar: The many discontinuities in their discourse, only a few of which have been reported here, suggest that he was not listening.

2nd Phy: Many of her replies were not clarified.

2nd Pat: And almost all of her answers were not acknowledged.

1st Nar: His interruptions suggest that what she said was not very important to his understanding.

2nd Phy: He relied continuously on his observations and his questioning strategies.

2nd Pat: And his questioning strategies did not clarify the meaning of her symptoms and pains but continuously confirmed his observations of her nervousness.

2nd Phy: Furthermore, he failed to remember that cancer is not merely a "thing" to be excised by a medical procedure.

1st Pat: He spoke to her as though she were an anatomical display.

Death: "Your nerves have now got to the point where they suffer."

2nd Phy: "You've got pretty good teeth and joints."

2nd Nar: "It's beautiful surgery."

1st Nar: Talk, when it is serious rather than casual, is as much as it is anything at all a labor of understanding,

2nd Phy: of listening and interpreting, of clarifying and acknowledging what has been said, and responding.

1st Nar: It is an interactionally constituted activity sustained by conversationalists.

2nd Nar: The form and substance of serious talk is shaped by a dialectic of questioning and answering,

2nd Phy: and requesting and responding,

2nd Pat: and explaining and responding.

2nd Nar: And, in its course, the dialectic of talk realizes the many asymmetries that constitute the dialectic.

1st Nar: It was their talk's pervasive tensions and disharmonies that puzzled me, the sharp contrast between what she said and what he heard.

2nd Nar: An impression of radical misunderstanding led to increasingly fine transcriptions of their talk,

1st Nar: for on the surface these tapes do not reflect the problems of a "post-operative"

All: (*whispered*) cancer

1st Nar: patient, they reflect the problems of a hypochondriacal woman of forty-five being assured recurrently that her health is good and that the problem is her nerves.

2nd Phy: In their second exchange, which occurred one month later, they discuss other physicians who have, in the past, also told her that the problem is her nerves.

2nd Pat: Some, she reports, suggested that without even bothering to examine her.

2nd Phy: One had given her Valium surreptitiously.

2nd Pat: And she said, angrily,

1st Pat: "The same thing is happening again."

2nd Phy: For although she was given Valium and told that the problem was her nerves, she also had a tumor.

1st Pat: "How do you explain that?"

(Pause)

Death: Her question goes unanswered.

1st Phy: Their talk focuses on a virus,

2nd Pat: her sore throat,

1st Phy: the pain in her mouth,

2nd Pat: her visits to dentists,

1st Pat: to other doctors,

2nd Phy:	medical procedures she has undergone
2nd Pat:	or may undergo,
1st Phy:	medications she has taken
2nd Pat:	or is taking.
1st Nar:	She complains of persistent back pain.
1st Pat:	And she says that she is afraid.
2nd Phy:	He assures her that her basic health is good.
Death:	Their third exchange occurred one month after the second.
2nd Phy:	Almost half their talk is about the pain in her mouth,
2nd Pat:	her dental care,
2nd Phy:	and the medications she has received from another physician,
1st Pat:	including Valium and Prednisone.
2nd Pat:	She complains that she is gaining weight and thinks that Prednisone is causing that.
2nd Phy:	Prednisone is a corticosteroid, producing many serious side effects.
Death:	It is most commonly used to control the pain of rheumatoid arthritis,
2nd Pat:	and, although she reported many pains, joint pain was not among them.
1st Pat:	She complains again of back and abdominal pain.
2nd Phy:	They discuss the possibility of X-rays,
2nd Pat:	and the kinds of X-rays and medical procedures she has undergone in the past.
1st Pat:	She says that she does not want to die.
1st Phy:	He reassures her that her health is good.
Death:	Once again, at the end of their third encounter, he tells her that the problem is her nerves.
2nd Phy:	This analysis has not investigated this physician's intentions.
1st Nar:	I suspect that he would not have chosen so cruel an outcome of his encounters with this patient.
1st Phy:	In good faith, he taped their meetings as a participant in a research study. He, therefore, was no longer aware of his manner.

2nd Phy: This analysis has, however, addressed the question of how their talk developed.

1st Nar: What this physician might have intended does not seem as relevant in understanding their discourse,

2nd Nar: as how their talk proceeded

2nd Phy: and how, as a series of turns at talk on discourse topics, it shaped the meaning of her illness.

1st Phy: It was not his intentions that shaped their discourse;

1st Pat: it was his questioning practices.

1st Phy: It was not his intentions that shaped the meaning of her illness;

2nd Pat: it was his inattentions.

Death: And, in any case, it is not the intentions of physicians that are at issue here;

1st Nar: it is how a discourse process expresses and realizes the work of medicine.

2nd Nar: For the work is in the talk and the talk is a realization of the work.

1st Phy: (*Beginning to laugh*) The discourse of physicians and patients is controlled by physicians who, in asking questions,

1st Nar: (*Laughing*) "request"

2nd Phy: (*Laughing*) that patients respond on specific topics.

1st Nar: (*Laughing*) And the development of discourse topics is also controlled by physicians, who, with each successive question or request, shape the meaning of what is said.

1st Phy: (*Laughing*) This physician reported his diagnosis on a questionnaire called

2nd Nar: (*Laughing*) "Physician Questionnaire Concerning Specific Patients."

1st Nar: (*Laughing*) It was as follows:

2nd Phy: (*Laughing*) "One: depression,

1st Phy: (*Laughing*) conversion symptom,

2nd Phy: (*Laughing*) "Two: status post-nephrectomy for a hypernephroma, 1971."

1st Phy: (*Laughing*) He also reported that he was certain of his diagnosis.

2nd Pat: (*Laughing*) This patient also answered a questionnaire.

1st Pat:	(*Laughing*) Like so many physicians,
1st Nar:	(*Laughing*) she said,
1st Pat:	(*Laughing*) this physician told her that there was nothing wrong when she had
All:	(*Laughing and whispering*) cancer.
1st Nar:	(*Laughing*) She also said that since their last exchange she had gone to another hospital where she was told
2nd Nar:	(*Laughing*) that she has
All:	(*Laughing and whispering*) cancer
1st Pat:	(*Laughing*) of the spine.
Death:	(*Laughing*) No further information is available on this woman and her search for care. (*Laughing*)

WITHOUT

DONALD HALL

we lived in a small island stone nation
without color under gray clouds and wind
distant the unlimited ocean acute
lymphoblastic leukemia without seagulls
or palm trees without vegetation
or animal life only barnacles and lead
colored moss that darkened when months did

hours days weeks months weeks days hours
the year endured without punctuation
february with ice winter sleet
snow melted recovered but nothing
without thaw although cold streams hurtled
no snowdrop or crocus rose no yellow
no red leaves of maple without october

no spring no summer no autumn no winter
no rain no peony thunder no woodthrush
the book was a thousand pages without commas
without mice oak leaves windstorms
no castles no plazas no flags no parrots
without carnival or the procession of relics
intolerable without brackets or colons

silence without color sound without smell
without apples without port to rupture gnash
unpunctuated without churches uninterrupted
no orioles ginger noses no opera no
without fingers daffodils cheekbones
the body was a nation a tribe dug into stone
assaulted white blood broken to shards

provinces invaded bombed shot shelled
artillery sniper fire helicopter gunship
grenade burning murder landmine starvation
the ceasefire lasted forty-eight hours
then a shell exploded in a market
pain vomit neuropathy morphine nightmare
confusion the rack terror the vise

vincristine ara-c cytoxan vp-16
loss of memory loss of language losses
pneumocystis carinii pneumonia bactrim
foamless unmitigated sea without sea
delirium whipmarks of petechiae
multiple blisters of herpes zoster
and how are you doing today I am doing

one afternoon say the sun came out
moss took on greenishness leaves fell
the market opened a loaf of bread a sparrow
a bony dog wandered back sniffing a lath
it might be possible to take up a pencil
unwritten stanzas taken up and touched
beautiful terrible sentences unuttered

the sea unrelenting wave gray the sea
flotsam without islands broken crates
block after block the same house the mall
no cathedral no hobo jungle the same women
and men they longed to drink hayfields no
without dog or semicolon or village square
without monkey or lily without garlic

ORINDA UPON LITTLE HECTOR PHILIPS

KATHERINE PHILIPS

Twice forty months of wedlock I did stay,
Then had my vows crown'd with a lovely boy,
And yet in forty days he dropt away,
O swift vicissitude of human joy.

I did but see him and he disappear'd,
I did but pluck the rose-bud and it fell,
A sorrow unforeseen and scarcely fear'd,
For ill can mortals their afflictions spell.

And now (sweet babe) what can my trembling heart
Suggest to right my doleful fate or thee,
Tears are my Muse and sorrow all my art,
So piercing groans must be thy elegy.

Thus whilst no eye is witness of my moan,
I grieve thy loss (Ah boy too dear to live)
And let the unconcernèd world alone,
Who neither will, nor can refreshment give.

An off'ring too for thy sad tomb I have,
Too just a tribute to thy early hearse,
Receive these gasping numbers to thy grave,
The last of thy unhappy mother's verse.

Katherine Philips's collected poems were published posthumously in 1667. This edition is from *The World Split Open: Four Centuries of Women Poets in England and America, 1552–1950,* edited by Louise Berkinow (New York: Random House, 1974).

THE MOTHER

GWENDOLYN BROOKS

Abortions will not let you forget.
You remember the children you got that you did not get,
The damp small pulps with a little or with no hair,
The singers and workers that never handled the air.
You will never neglect or beat
Them, or silence or buy with a sweet.
You will never wind up the sucking-thumb
Or scuttle off ghosts that come.
You will never leave them, controlling your luscious
  sigh,
Return for a snack of them, with gobbling mother-eye.

I have heard in the voices of the wind the voices of my
  dim killed children.
I have contracted. I have eased
My dim dears at the breasts they could never suck.
I have said, Sweets, if I sinned, if I seized
Your luck
And your lives from your unfinished reach,
If I stole your births and your names,
Your straight baby tears and your games,
Your stilted or lovely loves, your tumults, your
  marriages, aches, and your deaths,
If I poisoned the beginnings of your breaths,
Believe that even in my deliberateness I was not
  deliberate.

Originally published in *A Street in Bronzeville,* by Gwendolyn Brooks (New York: Harper and Brothers, 1945), 'the mother" is reprinted here by consent of Brooks Permissions.

Though why should I whine,
Whine that the crime was other than mine?—
Since anyhow you are dead.
Or rather, or instead,
You were never made.
But that too I am afraid
Is faulty: oh, what shall I say, how is the truth to be
said?
You were born, you had body, you died.
It is just that you never giggled or planned or cried.

Believe me, I loved you all.
Believe me, I knew you, though faintly, and I loved, I
loved you
All.

ON BEING ASKED TO WRITE A POEM IN MEMORY OF ANNE SEXTON

MAXINE KUMIN

The elk discards his antlers every spring.
They rebud, they grow, they are growing

an inch a day to form a rococo rack
with a five-foot spread even as we speak:

cartilage at first, covered with velvet;
bendable, tender gristle, yet

destined to ossify, the velvet sloughed off,
hanging in tatters from alders and scrub growth.

No matter how hardened it seems there was pain.
Blood on the snow from rubbing, rubbing, rubbing.

What a heavy candelabrum to be borne
forth, each year more elaborately turned:

the special issues, the prizes in her name.
Above the mantel the late elk's antlers gleam.

OCTOBER, YELLOWSTONE PARK

MAXINE KUMIN

How happy the animals seem just now,
all reading the sweetgrass text, heads down
in the great yellow-green sea of the high plains—
antelope, bison, the bull elk and his cows

moving commingled in little clumps, the bull
elk bugling from time to time his rusty screech
but not yet in rut, the females not yet in heat,
peacefully inattentive—the late fall

asters still blooming, the glacial creeks running clear.
What awaits them this winter—which calves will starve
to death or driven by hunger stray from the park
to be shot on the cattle range—they are unaware.

It is said that dumb beasts cannot anticipate
though for terror of fire or wolves some deep
historical memory clangs out of sleep
pricking them to take flight. As flight pricked the poet

dead seventeen years today, who for seventeen
years before that was a better sister
than any I, who had none, could have conjured.
Dead by her own hand, who so doggedly whined

at Daddy Death's elbow that the old Squatter
at last relented and took her in. Of sane mind
and body aged but whole I stand by the sign
that says we are halfway between the equator

and the North Pole. Sad but celebratory
I stand in full sun on the 45th parallel
bemused by what's to come, by what befell,
by how our friendship flared into history.

Fair warning, Annie, there will be no more
elegies, no more direct-address songs
conferring the tang of loss, its bitter flavor
as palpable as alum on the tongue.

Climbing up switchbacks all this afternoon,
sending loose shale clattering below,
grimly, gradually ascending to a view
of snowcaps and geysers, the balloon

of Old Faithful spewing, I hear your voice
beside me (you, who hated so to sweat!)
cheerfully cursing at eight thousand feet
the killers of the dream, the small-time advice-

laden editors and hangers-on. I've come
this whole hard way alone to an upthrust slate
above a brace of eagles launched in flight
only to teeter, my equilibrium

undone by memory. I want to fling
your cigarette-and-whiskey-hoarse chuckle
that hangs on inside me down the back wall
over Biscuit Basin. I want the painting

below to take me in. My world that threatened
to stop the day you stopped, faltered
and then resumed, unutterably altered.
Where wild fires crisped its hide and blackened

whole vistas, new life inched in. My map
blooms with low growth, sturdier than before.
Thus I abstain. I will not sing, except
of the elk and his harem who lie down in grandeur

on the church lawn at Mammoth Hot Springs,
his hat rack wreathed in mist. This year's offspring
graze in the town's backyards, to the dismay
of tenants who burst out to broom them away.

May the car doors of tourists slam, may cameras go wild
staying the scene, may the occasional
antelope slip in to the herd, shy as a child.
May people be ravished by this processional.

May reverence for what lopes off to the hills
at dusk be imprinted on their brain pans
forever, as on mine. As you are, Anne.
All of you hammered golden against the anvil.

PONIES GATHERING IN THE DARK

ANITA ENDREZZE

The house was a forest remembering itself. The pine trees that held up the walls dreamed of stars dwelling in their needles. Jointed, branched, rooted, the trees still listened to the wind. The oak floors gleamed from the generations of human oils, but they still grew into their immense lineage of light and matter. The air between the ancient trees whispered with spirit bees and dark small birds.

Even the iron that pierced the flesh of trees had a voice. It was deep, metallic, and sank heavily in the human dreams. At night, the iron spoke most eloquently, recognizing the kinship of darkness in sky and earth. The nails sang of geodes in the heart and the gathering of elemental forces only vaguely understood. When the iron sang, humans slept, troubled, their hands remembering the first iron. The spear, the knife, the sharp edge of death.

Under the house, the ancient continent measured the journey of clay animals: giant beaver, tiny horses, elk, intricately scaled snakes, vast bears that had clawed the horizon to shreds. There is the memory of ice animals walking into the sun, their bones crushed under the weight of frozen moons. And there is the tribe of obsidian, those sharp-headed old ones, who danced around fire, singing the hunt before iron.

Long ago, the beavers built their lodges here, when the marshes were thick with mud and sweet rushes. In the middle of winter, the oldest would tell about First Beavers, giant creatures that gnawed down trees the size of the night.

The marsh became meadow; wild horses ran into the thunder of their song. They pulled grass with their strong teeth and fertilized the young pines. Their foals stood weak-kneed under the slivers of moon that spiked the trees' hearts. The horses rode the back of life and their bones crumbled into the afterbirth.

From *Ploughshares* Spring 1994: 51–55. Reprinted by permission of the author.

A family of black bears lived in the hollow tree that fell from the sky. A female bear shaman growled healing ceremonies, cleansing the air with broken cedar and chanting the fire back into lightning.

Later, a medicine man walked into the forest of tall trees. He heard the spirit horses drumming their hooves in the earth. All the others of their tribe, those descendants of runaway thunder, would within a short time be rounded up, branded with hot iron, put to the rein, plow or wagon. Now, he only felt their leaving, south to hills of thick grass, and not their destiny. Only the deep belly breathing of the night horses brought out the clover smell of stars and taught the medicine man where to put his sweat lodge.

He circled a spot that spoke to him with the smooth tones of water and the rootlike dreams of animals. He cleared the brush, pulling up the grass with his strong old hands. He carried rocks which had once been polished by glacier and flood and then buried under gravel and sand. These round, rock ones danced themselves up to the rain again. Their tribe has two hundred thousand million words for themselves. And even though they have been born speckled, crystallized, pitted, brittle, they know they are still part of Grandmother Earth's medicine bag.

He carried those rocks to the fire pit. He cut down saplings and bent them down to the earth again, building a hut dark as the womb. The branches rooted into the spiritual earth. He made a fire and the rocks told the story of their molten beginnings and the wood danced away into the feathered wind. The rocks blackened and cracked, hissed and cooled, as he tossed barkfulls of water on them. Steam rose, hot and thick.

The medicine man was old. It was his last sweat. His arms were well-muscled, but his skin draped over his bones. That afternoon, he sweated where horses once snorted at coming storms.

He heard the slap of beaver tails. He felt an icy wind and saw a wavering image of a face. It was an old woman wrapped in long-furred hides. She wore a necklace of a single mammoth tooth. She smiled at him and then was gone. In the dark, what he saw was inside of him but came from beyond. He felt the bears' snuffling muzzles. He nursed at one fingerlike breast.

Hours later, he crawled out of the sweat lodge. The night was clear. He sensed some kind of structure all around him. The stars shone through a roof high as the trees. It was a house, he figured out, but whether it was a metaphor for the universe or something from the future, he didn't know. The house was filled with busy humans. The people breathed their moisture into the trees. They offered up their breaths and the branches leafed out into air. People had been born in the house, their umbilical cords stretched from the salty waters to the nodding trees with their embracing branches. Cradled in wood, they slept with wood at the top of their heads where the soul enters, to the bottom of their feet, which is also called sole, but meant for grounding. The forest rose pine-scented and the people slept until they opened the thick-planked door of their death.

But what astonished him most of all was that he knew they were his children. Their skins were pink, white, brown, golden. Their eyes were the color of rocks: jade, obsidian, slate, amber. Or else the color of trees: green, yellow, brown. Some even had eyes the color of sky, water, or thunder. And their hair was the color of iron, bear, fire.

He saw them playing, laughing, arguing. He watched them dreaming, the soft dust of meteors sifting down through the roof to cover their faces with cool fire, their calm hands luminous, reaching out.

* * * * *

He awoke with a start. He saw the last of his vision dissolve into the cold morning air. But it had been a twisted and spotted arm that had reached out from his dreams. It was an arm from reality. His people were dying. That was why he was here, to find a way into the heart of a plant, to dream a cure.

He got up, clearing his throat. It felt dry. He took a deep breath to cleanse his body. The air around him felt hot. He ran the edge of his hand across his forehead.

His people had always been healthy. Only one plant had been necessary per patient. Now, the sicknesses didn't respond to his medicine. He tried many plants, gathered them, dried them, pounded, seeped and boiled them. Nothing worked. He needed a new medicine, one strong enough to stop death.

He pulled out his medicine bundle from his pack. He unrolled it, the leather supple. Packets of herbs were bound neatly. In a small bag, he fingered the splinter of wood touched by lightning. He used it for lancing. His fingers were long; the pads on the fingers were sensitive to the variables of health and sickness in the human body. In his mind's eye, touching a healthy body was like running his fingers across a pond of water so clear you couldn't tell which was air and which was water.

He set aside a bundle of dried salmonberry bark. It was good for the stomach when you ate too much salmon. There were also bundles of dried leaves, stems, and roots of the stinging nettle. He used this for headaches, pain of childbirth, and the ache in the joints of old people. Finally he found the two packets he'd been looking for: dried strawberry leaves for a tea and twigs from willow to cool a fever.

He made himself tea. He would eat nothing. He would fast and sweat until he was given the new plant for healing. He sipped the tea slowly. He could feel power in this place, but he was beginning to be aware of a strange uneasiness.

He thought of his grandsons. They'd been angry, on edge. His granddaughters had set their jaws firmly, eyes hard and brittle. Their dreams were of fire and strange spotted humans. The medicine man pondered. When had the camp changed? Two moons ago? No, it was when the Ute trader came from the south.

The medicine man had held the wobbling head of an infant as she died. He had smoothed the white hair of an old man who had terrible sores on his body. The man was his cousin. The two had raced together across the meadows when they were young, tiptoed silently beneath the nesting herons, stood watch at the edge of camp. Now, his old friend was dead, along with fourteen others.

He got up and prepared for another sweat.

*****

Inside the lodge, the air was thick. He brewed the willow twigs in the water he'd used to make the steam. He felt the long fronds of willow trees growing down into the darkness, their leaves glowing like bright spears or flashing fish. He felt the heat taking away his flesh, so that his bones became twigs. He was a willow tree bent over rocks and water.

He waited for a vision. He hoped for a plant to save his people. He threw more water on the rocks. The steam rolled off in crushing waves of liquid heat. He felt his chest tighten.

He was the last hope. His knowledge of plants that helped the body was immense, but he needed a deeper vision. He waited, praying.

He didn't feel the ponies gathering in the dark, their hooves heavy and powerful. He didn't see the bears disappearing into their own shadows. He didn't see an old woman beckoning to him.

His hand clutched at his chest. He fell over, head striking the stones, the darkness taking him into itself.

Three nights later, a big storm came up from the west. It blew down the old tree over the silent, cold sweat lodge. The tree fell down on the bones of the old man, bones that became tiny spirit horses, and bones that bears used for dream medicines in their long winter sleep. And bones that flowered from plants gathered by the hands of spirits pure as tears.

CATHEDRAL

RAYMOND CARVER

This blind man, an old friend of my wife's, he was on his way to spend the night. His wife had died. So he was visiting the dead wife's relatives in Connecticut. He called my wife from his in-laws'. Arrangements were made. He would come by train, a five-hour trip, and my wife would meet him at the station. She hadn't seen him since she worked for him one summer in Seattle ten years ago. But she and the blind man had kept in touch. They made tapes and mailed them back and forth. I wasn't enthusiastic about this visit. He was no one I knew. And his being blind bothered me. My idea of blindness came from the movies, the blind moved slowly and never laughed. Sometimes they were led by seeing-eye dogs. A blind man in my house was not something I looked forward to.

That summer in Seattle she had needed a job. She didn't have any money. The man she was going to marry at the end of the summer was in officers' training school. He didn't have any money, either. But she was in love with the guy, and he was in love with her, etc. She'd seen something in the paper: HELP WANTED—*Reading to Blind Man,* and a telephone number. She phoned and went over, was hired on the spot. She'd worked with this blind man all summer. She read stuff to him, case studies, reports, that sort of thing. She helped him organize his little office in the county social-services department. They'd become good friends, my wife and the blind man. How do I know these things? She told me. And she told me something else. On her last day in the office, the blind man asked if he could touch her face. She agreed to this. She told me he touched his fingers to every part of her face, her nose—even her neck! She never forgot it. She even tried to write a poem about it. She was always trying to write a poem. She wrote a poem or two every year, usually after something really important had happened to her.

When we first started going out together, she showed me the poem. In the poem, she recalled his fingers and the way they had moved around over her face. In the poem, she talked about what she had felt at the time, about what went through her mind when the blind man touched her nose and lips. I can remember I didn't think much of the poem. Of course, I didn't tell her that. Maybe I just don't understand poetry. I admit it's not the first thing I reach for when I pick up something to read.

Anyway, this man who'd first enjoyed her favors, the officer-to-be, he'd been her childhood sweetheart. So okay. I'm saying that at the end of the summer she let the blind man run his hands over her face, said goodbye to him, married her childhood etc., who was now a commissioned officer, and she moved away from Seattle. But they'd kept in touch, she and the blind man. She made the first contact after a year or so. She called him up one night from an Air Force base in Alabama. She wanted to talk. They talked. He asked her to send him a tape and tell him about her life. She did this. She sent the tape. On the tape, she told the blind man about her husband and about their life together in the military. She told the blind man she loved her husband but she didn't like it where they lived and she didn't like it that he was a part of the military-industrial thing. She told the blind man she'd written a poem and he was in it. She told him that she was writing a poem about what it was like to be an Air Force officer's wife. The poem wasn't finished yet. She was still writing it. The blind man made a tape. He sent her the tape. She made a tape. This went on for years. My wife's officer was posted to one base and then another. She sent tapes from Moody AFB, McGuire, McDonnell, and finally Travis, near Sacramento, where one night she got to feeling lonely and cut off from people she kept losing in that moving-around life. She got to feeling she couldn't go it another step. She went in and swallowed all the pills and capsules in the medicine chest and washed them down with a bottle of gin. Then she got into a hot bath and passed out.

But instead of dying, she got sick. She threw up. Her officer—why should he have a name? he was the childhood sweetheart, and what more does he want?—came home from somewhere, found her, and called the ambulance. In time, she put it all on a tape and sent the tape to the blind man. Over the years, she put all kinds of stuff on tapes and sent the tapes off lickety-split. Next to writing a poem every year, I think it was her chief means of recreation. On one tape, she told the blind man she'd decided to live away from her officer for a time. On another tape, she told him about her divorce. She and I began going out, and of course she told her blind man about it. She told him everything, or so it seemed to me. Once she asked me if I'd like to hear the latest tape from the blind man. This was a year ago. I was on the tape, she said. So I said okay, I'd listen to it. I got us drinks and we settled down in the living room. We made ready to listen. First she inserted the tape into the player and adjusted a couple of dials. Then she pushed a lever. The tape squeaked and someone began to talk in this loud voice. She lowered the volume. After a few minutes of harmless chitchat, I heard my own name in the mouth of this stranger, this blind man I didn't even know! And then this: "From all you've said about him, I can only conclude—" But we were interrupted, a knock at the door, something, and we didn't ever get back to the tape. Maybe it was just as well. I'd heard all I wanted to.

Now this same blind man was coming to sleep in my house.

"Maybe I could take him bowling," I said to my wife. She was at the draining board doing scalloped potatoes. She put down the knife she was using and turned around.

"If you love me," she said, "you can do this for me. If you don't love me, okay. But if you had a friend, any friend, and the friend came to visit, I'd make him feel comfortable." She wiped her hands with the dish towel.

"I don't have any blind friends," I said.

"You don't have *any* friends," she said. "Period. Besides," she said, "goddamn it, his wife's just died! Don't you understand that? The man's lost his wife!"

I didn't answer. She'd told me a little about the blind man's wife. Her name was Beulah. Beulah! That's a name for a colored woman.

"Was his wife a Negro?" I asked.

"Are you crazy?" my wife said. "Have you just flipped or something?" She picked up a potato. I saw it hit the floor, then roll under the stove. "What's wrong with you?" she said. "Are you drunk?"

"I'm just asking," I said.

Right then my wife filled me in with more detail than I cared to know. I made a drink and sat at the kitchen table to listen. Pieces of the story began to fall into place.

Beulah had gone to work for the blind man the summer after my wife had stopped working for him. Pretty soon Beulah and the blind man had themselves a church wedding. It was a little wedding—who'd want to go to such a wedding in the first place?—just the two of them, plus the minister and the minister's wife. But it was a church wedding just the same. It was what Beulah had wanted, he'd said. But even then Beulah must have been carrying the cancer in her glands. After they had been inseparable for eight years—my wife's word, *inseparable*—Beulah's health went into a rapid decline. She died in a Seattle hospital room, the blind man sitting beside the bed and holding on to her hand. They'd married, lived and worked together, slept together—had sex, sure—and then the blind man had to bury her. All this without his having ever seen what the goddamned woman looked like. It was beyond my understanding. Hearing this, I felt sorry for the blind man for a little bit. And then I found myself thinking what a pitiful life this woman must have led. Imagine a woman who could never see herself as she was seen in the eyes of her loved one. A woman who could go on day after day and never receive the smallest compliment from her beloved. A woman whose husband could never read the expression on her face, be it misery or something better. Someone who could wear makeup or not—what difference to him? She could, if she wanted, wear green eye-shadow around one eye, a straight pin in her nostril, yellow slacks and purple shoes, no matter. And then to slip off into death, the blind man's hand on her hand, his blind eyes streaming tears—I'm imagining now—her last thought maybe this: that he never even knew what she looked like, and she on an express to the grave. Robert was left with a small insurance policy and half of a twenty-peso Mexican coin. The other half of the coin went into the box with her. Pathetic.

So when the time rolled around, my wife went to the depot to pick him up. With nothing to do but wait—sure, I blamed him for that—I was having a drink and watching the TV when I heard the car pull into the drive. I got up from the sofa with my drink and went to the window to have a look.

I saw my wife laughing as she parked the car. I saw her get out of the car and shut the door. She was still wearing a smile. Just amazing. She went around to the other side of the car to where the blind man was already starting to get out. This blind man, feature this, he was wearing a full beard! A beard on a blind man! Too much, I say. The blind man reached into the back seat and dragged out a suitcase. My wife took his arm, shut the car door, and, talking all the way, moved him down the drive and then up the steps to the front porch. I turned off the TV. I finished my drink, rinsed the glass, dried my hands. Then I went to the door.

My wife said, "I want you to meet Robert. Robert, this is my husband. I've told you all about him." She was beaming. She had this blind man by his coat sleeve.

The blind man let go of his suitcase and up came his hand.

I took it. He squeezed hard, held my hand, and then he let it go.

"I feel like we've already met," he boomed.

"Likewise," I said. I didn't know what else to say. Then I said, "Welcome. I've heard a lot about you." We began to move then, a little group, from the porch into the living room, my wife guiding him by the arm. The blind man was carrying his suitcase in his other hand. My wife said things like, "To your left here, Robert. That's right. Now watch it, there's a chair. That's it. Sit down right here. This is the sofa. We just bought this sofa two weeks ago."

I started to say something about the old sofa. I'd liked that old sofa. But I didn't say anything. Then I wanted to say something else, small-talk, about the scenic ride along the Hudson. How going *to* New York, you should sit on the right-hand side of the train, and coming *from* New York, the left-hand side.

"Did you have a good train ride?" I said. "Which side of the train did you sit on, by the way?"

"What a question, which side!" my wife said. "What's it matter which side?" she said.

"I just asked," I said.

"Right side," the blind man said. "I hadn't been on a train in nearly forty years. Not since I was a kid. With my folks. That's been a long time. I'd nearly forgotten the sensation. I have winter in my beard now," he said. "So I've been told, anyway. Do I look distinguished, my dear?" the blind man said to my wife.

"You look distinguished, Robert," she said. "Robert," she said. "Robert, it's just so good to see you."

My wife finally took her eyes off the blind man and looked at me. I had the feeling she didn't like what she saw. I shrugged.

I've never met, or personally known, anyone who was blind. This blind man was late forties, a heavy-set, balding man with stooped shoulders, as if he carried a great weight there. He wore brown slacks, brown shoes, a light-brown shirt, a tie, a sports coat. Spiffy. He also had this full beard. But he didn't use a cane and he didn't wear dark glasses. I'd always thought dark glasses were a must for the blind. Fact was, I wished he had a pair. At first glance, his eyes looked like anyone else's eyes. But if you looked close, there was something different about them. Too much white in the iris, for one thing, and the pupils seemed to move around in the sockets without his knowing it or being able to stop it. Creepy. As I stared at his face, I saw the left pupil turn in toward his nose while the other made an effort to keep in one place. But it was only an effort, for that eye was on the roam without his knowing it or wanting it to be.

I said, "Let me get you a drink. What's your pleasure? We have a little of everything. It's one of our pastimes."

"Bub, I'm a Scotch man myself," he said fast enough in this big voice.

"Right," I said. Bub! "Sure you are. I knew it."

He let his fingers touch his suitcase, which was sitting alongside our sofa. He was taking his bearings. I didn't blame him for that.

"I'll move that up to your room," my wife said.

"No, that's fine," the blind man said loudly. "It can go up when I go up."

"A little water with the Scotch?" I said.

"Very little," he said.

"I knew it," I said.

He said, "Just a tad. The Irish actor, Barry Fitzgerald? I'm like that fellow. When I drink water, Fitzgerald said, I drink water. When I drink whiskey, I drink whiskey." My wife laughed. The blind man brought his hand up under his beard. He lifted his beard slowly and let it drop.

I did the drinks, three big glasses of Scotch with a splash of water in each. Then we made ourselves comfortable and talked about Robert's travels. First the long flight from the West Coast to Connecticut, we covered that. Then from Connecticut up here by train. We had another drink concerning that leg of the trip.

I remembered having read somewhere that the blind didn't smoke because, as speculation had it, they couldn't see the smoke they exhaled. I thought I knew that much and that much only about blind people. But this blind man smoked his cigarette down to the nubbin and then lit another one. This blind man filled his ashtray and my wife emptied it.

When we sat down at the table for dinner, we had another drink. My wife heaped Robert's plate with cube steak, scalloped potatoes, green beans. I buttered him up two slices of bread. I said, "Here's bread and butter for you." I swallowed some of my drink. "Now let us pray," I said, and the blind man lowered his head. My wife looked at me, her mouth agape. "Pray the phone won't ring and the food doesn't get cold," I said.

We dug in. We ate everything there was to eat on the table. We ate like there was no tomorrow. We didn't talk. We ate. We scarfed. We grazed that table. We were into serious eating. The blind man had right away located his foods, he knew just where everything was on his plate. I watched with admiration as he used his knife and fork on the meat. He'd cut two pieces of meat, fork the meat into his mouth, and then go all out for the scalloped potatoes, the beans next, and then he'd tear off a hunk of buttered bread and eat that. He'd follow this up with a big drink of milk. It didn't seem to bother him to use his fingers once in a while, either.

We finished everything, including half a strawberry pie. For a few moments, we sat as if stunned. Sweat beaded on our faces. Finally, we got up from the table and left the dirty plates. We didn't look back. We took ourselves into the living room and sank into our places again. Robert and my wife sat on the sofa. I took the big chair. We had us two or three more drinks while they talked about the major things that had come to pass for them in the past ten years. For the most part, I just listened. Now and then I joined in. I didn't want him to think I'd left the room, and I didn't want her to think I was feeling left out. They talked of things that had happened to them—to them!—these past ten years. I waited in vain to hear my name on my wife's sweet lips: "And then my dear husband came into my life"—something like that. But I heard nothing of the sort. More talk of Robert. Robert had done a little of everything, it seemed, a regular blind jack-of-all-trades. But most recently he and his wife had had an Amway distributorship, from which, I gathered, they'd earned their living, such as it was. The blind man was also a ham radio operator. He talked in his loud voice about conversations he'd had with fellow operators in Guam, in the Philippines, in Alaska, and even in Tahiti. He said he'd have a lot of friends there if he ever wanted to go visit those places. From time to time, he'd turn his blind face toward me, put his hand under his beard, ask me something. How long had I been in my present position? (Three years.) Did I like my work? (I didn't.) Was I going to stay with it? (What were the options?) Finally, when I thought he was beginning to run down, I got up and turned on the TV.

My wife looked at me with irritation. She was heading toward a boil. Then she looked at the blind man and said, "Robert, do you have a TV?"

The blind man said, "My dear, I have two TV's. I have a color set and a black-and white thing, an old relic. It's funny, but if I turn the TV on, and I'm always turning it on, I turn on the color set. It's funny don't you think?"

I didn't know what to say to that. I had absolutely nothing to say to that. No opinion. So I watched the news program and tried to listen to what the announcer was saying.

"This is a color TV," the blind man said. "Don't ask me how, but I can tell."

"We traded up a while ago," I said.

The blind man had another taste of his drink. He lifted his beard, sniffed it, and let it fall. He leaned forward on the sofa. He positioned his ashtray on the coffee table, then put the lighter to his cigarette. He leaned back on the sofa and crossed his legs at the ankles.

My wife covered her mouth, and then she yawned. She stretched. She said, "I think I'll go upstairs and put on my robe. I think I'll change into something else. Robert, you make yourself comfortable," she said.

"I'm comfortable," the blind man said.

"I want you to feel comfortable in this house," she said.

"I am comfortable," the blind man said.

* * * * *

After she'd left the room, he and I listened to the weather report and then to the sports roundup. By that time, she'd been gone so long I didn't know if she was going to come back. I thought she might have gone to bed. I wished she'd come back downstairs. I didn't want to be left alone with the blind man. I asked him if he wanted another drink, and he said sure. Then I asked if he wanted to smoke some dope with me. I said I'd just rolled a number. I hadn't, but I planned to do so in about two shakes.

"I'll try some with you," he said.

"Damn right," I said. "That's the stuff."

I got our drinks and sat down on the sofa with him. Then I rolled us two fat numbers. I lit one and passed it. I brought it to his fingers. He took it and inhaled.

"Hold it as long as you can," I said. I could tell he didn't know the first thing.

My wife came back downstairs wearing her pink robe and her pink slippers.

"What do I smell?" she said.

"We thought we'd have us some cannabis," I said.

My wife gave me a savage look. Then she looked at the blind man and said, "Robert, I didn't know you smoked."

He said, "I do now, my dear. There's a first time for everything. But I don't feel anything yet."

"This stuff is pretty mellow," I said. "This stuff is mild. It's dope you can reason with," I said. "It doesn't mess you up."

"Not much it doesn't, bub," he said, and laughed.

My wife sat on the sofa between the blind man and me. I passed her the number. She took it and toked and then passed it back to me. "Which way is this going?" she said. Then she said, "I shouldn't be smoking this. I can hardly keep my eyes open as it is. That dinner did me in. I shouldn't have eaten so much."

"It was the strawberry pie," the blind man said. "That's what did it," he said, and he laughed his big laugh. Then he shook his head.

"There's more strawberry pie," I said.

"Do you want some more, Robert?" my wife said.

"Maybe in a little while," he said.

We gave our attention to the TV. My wife yawned again. She said, "Your bed is made up when you feel like going to bed, Robert. I know you must have had a long day. When you're ready to go to bed, say so." She pulled his arm. "Robert?"

He came to and said, "I've had a real nice time. This beats tapes, doesn't it?"

I said, "Coming at you," and I put the number between his fingers. He inhaled, held the smoke, and then let it go. It was like he'd been doing it since he was nine years old.

"Thanks, bub," he said. "But I think this is all for me. I think I'm beginning to feel it," he said. He held the burning roach out for my wife.

"Same here," she said. "Ditto. Me, too." She took the roach and passed it to me. "I may just sit here for a while between you two guys with my eyes closed. But don't let me bother you, okay? Either one of you. If it bothers you, say so. Otherwise, I may just sit here with my eyes closed until you're ready to go to bed," she said. "Your bed's made up, Robert, when you're ready. It's right next to our room at the top of the stairs. We'll show you up when you're ready. You wake me up now, you guys, if I fall asleep." She said that and then she closed her eyes and went to sleep.

The news program ended. I got up and changed the channel. I sat back down on the sofa. I wished my wife hadn't pooped out. Her head lay across the back of the sofa, her mouth open. She'd turned so that her robe had slipped away from her legs, exposing a juicy thigh. I reached to draw her robe back over her, and it was then that I glanced at the blind man. What the hell! I flipped the robe open again.

"You say when you want some strawberry pie," I said.

"I will," he said.

I said, "Are you tired? Do you want me to take up to your bed? Are you ready to hit the hay?"

"Not yet," he said. "No, I'll stay up with you, bub. If that's all right. I'll stay up until you're ready to turn in. We haven't had a chance to talk. Know what I mean? I feel like me and her monopolized the evening." He lifted his beard and he let it fall. He picked up his cigarettes and his lighter.

"That's all right," I said. Then I said, "I'm glad for the company."

And I guess I was. Every night I smoked dope and stayed up as long as I could before I fell asleep. My wife and I hardly ever went to bed at the same time. When I did go to sleep, I had these dreams. Sometimes I'd wake up from one of them, my heart going crazy.

Something about the church and the Middle Ages was on the TV. Not your run-of-the-mill TV fare. I wanted to watch something else. I turned to the other channels. But there was nothing on them, either. So I turned back to the first channel and apologized.

"Bub, it's all right," the blind man said. "It's fine with me. Whatever you want to watch is okay. I'm always learning something. Learning never ends. It won't hurt me to learn something tonight. I got ears," he said.

* * * * *

We didn't say anything for a time. He was leaning forward with his head turned at me, his right ear aimed in the direction of the set. Very disconcerting. Now and then his eyelids drooped and then they snapped open again. Now and then he put his fingers into his beard and tugged, like he was thinking about something he was hearing on the television.

On the screen, a group of men wearing cowls was being set upon and tormented by men dressed in skeleton costumes and men dressed as devils. The men dressed as devils wore devil masks, horns, and long tails. This pageant was part of a procession. The Englishman who was narrating the thing said it took place in Spain once a year. I tried to explain to the blind man what was happening.

"Skeletons," he said. "I know about skeletons," he said, and he nodded.

The TV showed this one cathedral. Then there was a long, slow look at another one. Finally, the picture switched to the famous one in Paris, with its flying buttresses and its spires reaching up to the clouds. The camera pulled away to show the whole of the cathedral rising above the skyline.

There were times when the Englishman who was telling the thing would shut up, would simply let the camera move around over the cathedrals. Or else the camera would tour the countryside, men in fields walking behind oxen. I waited as long as I could. Then I felt I had to say something. I said, "They're showing the outside of this cathedral now. Gargoyles. Little statues carved to look like monsters. Now I guess they're in Italy. Yeah, they're in Italy. There's paintings on the walls of this one church."

"Are those fresco paintings, bub?" he asked, and he sipped from his drink.

I reached for my glass. But it was empty. I tried to remember what I could remember. "You're asking me are those frescoes?" I said. "That's a good question. I don't know."

The camera moved to a cathedral outside Lisbon. The differences in the Portuguese cathedral compared with the French and Italian were not that great. But they were there. Mostly the interior stuff. Then something occurred to me, and I said, "Something has occurred to me. Do you have any idea what a cathedral is? What they look like, that is? Do you follow me? If somebody says cathedral to you, do you have any notion what they're talking about? Do you know the difference between that and a Baptist church, say?"

He let the smoke dribble from his mouth. "I know they took hundreds of workers fifty or a hundred years to build," he said. "I just heard the man say that, of course. I know generations of the same families worked on a cathedral. I heard him say that, too. The men who began their life's work on them, they never lived to see the completion of their work. In that wise, bub, they're no different from the rest of us, right?" He laughed. Them his eyelids drooped again. His head nodded. He seemed to be snoozing. Maybe he was imagining himself in Portugal. The TV was showing another cathedral now. This one was in Germany. The Englishman's voice droned on. "Cathedrals," the blind man said. He sat up and rolled his head back and forth. "If you want the truth, bub, that's about all I know. What I just said. What I heard him say. But maybe you could describe one to me? I wish you'd do it. I'd like that. If you want to know, I really don't have a good idea."

I stared hard at the shot of the cathedral on the TV. How could I even begin to describe it? But say my life depended on it. Say my life was being threatened by an insane guy who said I had to do it or else.

I stared some more at the cathedral before the picture flipped off into the countryside. There was no use. I turned to the blind man and said, "To begin with, they're very tall." I was looking around the room for clues. "They reach way up. Up and up. Toward the sky. They're so big, some of them, they have to have these supports. To help hold them up, so to speak. These supports are called buttresses. They remind me of viaducts, for some reason. But maybe you don't know viaducts, either? Sometimes the cathedrals have devils and such carved into the front. Sometimes lords and ladies. Don't ask me why this is," I said.

He was nodding. The whole upper part of his body seemed to be moving back and forth.

"I'm not doing so good, am I?" I said.

He stopped nodding and leaned forward on the edge of the sofa. As he listened to me, he was running his fingers through his beard. I wasn't getting through to him, I could see that. But he waited for me to go on just the same. He nodded, like he was trying to encourage me. I tried to think what else to say. "They're really big," I said. "They're massive. They're built of stone. Marble, too, sometimes. In those olden days, when they built cathedrals, men wanted to be close to God. In those olden days, God was an important part of everyone's life. You could tell this from their cathedral-building. I'm sorry," I said, "but it looks like that's the best I can do for you. I'm just no good at it."

"That's all right, bub," the blind man said. "Hey, listen. I hope you don't mind my asking you. Can I ask you something? Let me ask you a simple question, yes or no. I'm just curious and there's no offense. You're my host. But let me ask if you are in any way religious? You don't mind my asking?"

I shook my head. He couldn't see that, though. A wink is the same as a nod to a blind man. "I guess I don't believe in it. In anything. Sometimes it's hard. You know what I'm saying?"

"Sure, I do," he said.

"Right," I said.

The Englishman was still holding forth. My wife sighed in her sleep. She drew a long breath and went on with her sleeping.

"You'll have to forgive me," I said. "But I can't tell you what a cathedral looks like. It just isn't in me to do it. I can't do any more than I've done."

The blind man sat very still, his head down, as he listened to me.

I said, "The truth is, cathedrals don't mean anything special to me. Nothing. Cathedrals. They're something to look at on late-night TV. That's all they are."

It was then that the blind man cleared his throat. He brought something up. He took a handkerchief from his back pocket. Then he said, "I get it, bub. It's okay. It happens. Don't worry about it," he said. "Hey, listen to me. Will you do me a favor? I got an idea. Why don't you find us some heavy paper? And a pen. We'll do something. We'll draw one together. Get us a pen and some heavy paper. Go on, bub, get the stuff," he said.

So I went upstairs. My legs felt like they didn't have any strength in them. They felt like they did after I'd done some running. In my wife's room, I looked around. I found some ballpoints in a little basket on her table. And then I tried to think where to look for the kind of paper he was talking about.

Downstairs, in the kitchen, I found a shopping bag with onion skins in the bottom of the bag. I emptied the bag and shook it. I brought it into the living room and sat down with it near his legs. I moved some things, smoothed the wrinkles from the bag, spread it out on the coffee table.

The blind man got down from the sofa and sat next to me on the carpet.

He ran his fingers over the paper. He went up and down the sides of the paper. The edges, even the edges. He fingered the corners.

"All right," he said. "All right, let's do her."

He found my hand, the hand with the pen. He closed his hand over my hand. "Go ahead, bub, draw," he said. "Draw. You'll see. I'll follow along with you. It'll be okay. Just begin now like I'm telling you. You'll see. Draw," the blind man said.

So I began. First I drew a box that looked like a house. It could have been the house I lived in. Then I put a roof on it. At either end of the roof, I drew spires. Crazy.

"Swell," he said. "Terrific. You're doing fine," he said. "Never thought anything like this could happen in your lifetime, did you, bub? Well, it's a strange life, we all know that. Go on now. Keep it up."

I put in windows with arches. I drew flying buttresses. I hung great doors. I couldn't stop. The TV station went off the air. I put down the pen and closed and opened my fingers. The blind man felt around over the paper. He moved the tips of his fingers over the paper, all over what I had drawn, and he nodded.

"Doing fine," the blind man said.

I took up the pen again, and he found my hand. I kept at it. I'm no artist. But I kept drawing just the same.

My wife opened up her eyes and gazed at us. She sat up on the sofa, her robe hanging open. She said, "What are you doing? Tell me, I want to know."

I didn't answer her.

The blind man said, "We're drawing a cathedral. Me and him are working on it. Press hard," he said to me. "That's right. That's good," he said. "Sure. You got it, bub. I can tell. You didn't think you could. But you can, can't you? You're cooking with gas now. You know what I'm saying? We're going to really have us something here in a minute. How's the old arm?" he said. "Put some people in there now. What's a cathedral without people?"

My wife said, "What's going on? Robert, what are you doing? What's going on?"

"It's all right," he said to her. "Close your eyes now," the blind man said to me.

I did. I closed them just like he said.

"Are they closed?" he said. "Don't fudge."

"They're closed," I said.

"Keep them that way," he said. He said, "Don't stop now. Draw."

So we kept on with it. His fingers rode my fingers as my hand went over the paper. It was like nothing else in my life up to now.

Then he said, "I think that's it. I think you got it," he said. "Take a look. What do you think?"

But I had my eyes closed. I thought I'd keep them that way for a little longer. I thought it was something I ought to do."Well?" he said. "Are you looking?"

My eyes were still closed. I was in my house. I knew that. But I didn't feel like I was inside anything.

"It's really something," I said.

ASHES TO ASHES TO ASHES

RUTH NADELHAFT

Several months before his death, my father suffered one of his periodic attacks of angina; in pain and panicky, he chose to go to the hospital, insisting that I be with him in the examining room. My mother came along and worried in the waiting room. They were both hard of hearing by then, and he was especially fearful that he wouldn't be able to understand what the doctors had to tell him. Since we'd been to the hospital for this kind of thing repeatedly, I was not entirely absorbed in the experience. After the initial flurry of attention and tests, we had a long wait, and my father grew impatient.

He sat up on the gurney in a blue-and-white striped hospital bathrobe that made his light blue eyes even more vivid. His skin, always youthful, looked almost impossibly healthy for a man so sick. He was then well past eighty-four and would die within a year. "I'm running out of patience," he announced in a strong voice. Since his arrival at the hospital, when he had been feeling desperate, he had visibly taken on strength. His natural temperament was beginning to return.

"Try not to run out of patience before you run out of time," I replied. We sat there in silence for a few moments more. Then my father cleared his throat rather lengthily and loudly. He fixed me with a stern glance, and I stood up.

"Are you aware of my wishes in the event of my demise?" he asked.

I was astonished by his language, if not by the question. Everyone in my family speaks in complete sentences, and we do use a somewhat formal vocabulary, but this was way beyond our usual level.

" I think so," I replied. "You want to be cremated, right?"

"Yes, I do. But you may not know what I want done with my ashes."

It was true; I didn't. I looked expectantly at him.

"I wish my ashes to be kept until such time as your mother dies. Then I want them to be sprinkled in her coffin and buried with her."

From *The Maine Scholar* 11 (Autumn 1998): 75–89. By permission of the publisher.

I was aghast. "Does *she* know that?" I blurted out.

He didn't bother to answer. Clearly, this was as far as he had planned. His vision of my mother's body covered by my father's ashes was ludicrous. It seemed just one more example of the way in which my father attached himself to her, smothering what we saw as her natural strength and stamina with his neediness and self-absorbed demands. The nurse returned then, telling us that he was stable and could go home.

I remembered every word of the bizarre exchange, but I couldn't imagine when or how I would get to check this out with my mother. For as long as I could remember, my father had staked out dying first. We all agreed that he would never survive my mother's death, and she was more or less resigned to this order of things.

A few months later, my friend Peggy's father died. He was about my parents' age. I hated to bring this news to them; for years I had imagined that I could magically keep them from dying, or at least from thinking about it, if I didn't let the news of death come to them through me. But they'd find this one out even if I didn't tell them. Conversation with both my parents at the same time had become increasingly hazardous in the last couple of years; their hearing loss was not identical, and what one might hear the other might not. They both talked to me at once, and I often found myself shouting in two directions. Sometimes, when I walked into my own house, I realized that I was still shouting and I had to make a conscious effort to get back to a normal level of conversation.

Today, sitting on the couch near my mother and facing my father, I said, "Peggy's father died on Tuesday; there'll be a memorial service on Friday, and I'll drive down."

"How did he die? " my mother asked, putting down her book. My father rested yesterday's *New York Times* in his lap and leaned forward to hear my reply. "He died very easily and quickly," I said, "after taking the dog for a walk. Peggy said he sat back down in his chair, the way he always did, and then he just died. Her mother found him a few minutes later when she came down to make coffee."

"Was he buried? " she asked. "No," I said," he wanted to be cremated, and I'm pretty sure he wanted his ashes scattered at sea. He was an ardent sailor."

"That's what I'd like," my mother said decisively. "I'd like my ashes to be scattered at sea. What about you, Allie?" she asked expectantly, lifting her head toward him.

My father drew himself up. "I *had* an idea of what I wanted done with my ashes," he said loudly, looking directly at me, "but now, frankly, I no longer give a damn." He rattled the paper and opened it fully, completely shutting himself off from further conversation. My mother seemed perfectly composed, already planning the note she would write to Peggy. I decided to get out of there as quickly as possible. I felt I'd at least averted the horrible prospect of having to scatter my father over my mother someday and then bury both of them. For the moment I felt nothing but relief.

When my father did die—almost exactly six months after the achievement of his eighty-fifth birthday, and less than a month after my parents celebrated their sixtieth wedding anniversary—it was during a brief stay at the hospital when we all, including my father, thought that he was once again recovering from a combination of angina and the accumulation of fluid around his heart. I was lucky enough to spend time with him the evening before he died and later stopped by to tell my mother all the details of that conversation. "I'm damned tired Rooty," he had said, ready for what we thought would be a well-deserved sleep.

The next morning he was agitated and irritable; he had a heart attack while being bathed, and within minutes he was dead. The news reached me at work, and I raced directly to the hospital expecting to find my mother there. But she had phoned from home and had stayed there to await me. I cried "Oh, Shit," and got to her porch within a few minutes to find her ready to go to the hospital with me. My father had been left in his bed, in his hospital bathrobe, with his glasses on. While I waited at the desk, the staff made sure that my mother had as much time with him as she wanted. After some time, I joined her and took his hand. It was still warm. In his last years, my father's extremities, especially his feet, had been cold. But his hands, of which he had always been vain, were today warm enough that we could sit holding them and feel he was still with us.

Eventually my mother got to her feet, choked with tears. "Good-bye, Allie," she said. "I know you had to do this." Shaking her head, she walked steadily out of the room. I stopped to thank the people at the nurses' station who would make the arrangements to have my father's body moved down the street to the funeral home. As I caught up with my mother, she stopped and looked at me very directly. "You take care of everything," she said. "I don't want to have anything more to do with this." "Okay," I said. I wasn't sure exactly what I was agreeing to do, but I knew I'd do whatever it turned out to be.

My mother was adamant that there be no funeral or obituary. My brother arrived very late that night, flying across the country. Together we went to the funeral parlor to arrange for a pine box and a room for a few hours so that family members could say good-bye to my father. We had no trouble picking out the box, but then we were shown into a room with various containers for ashes. Nothing there seemed appropriate to me, and my brother was getting increasingly restless and truculent. The funeral director, not especially pushy, irritated my brother to no end. Since I would be receiving the ashes, I decided to put off this decision; the person working with us was visibly relieved when we left. My brother burst out in irritation once we got to the street. "I hate those guys," he said loudly. "They're leeches."

"They did a wonderful job here for our friend Howard, and they'll do the same for us. It's really okay," I assured him. He brushed me away. "Fine, fine," he said. "It's your town. You deal with them."

While my brother was off collecting his family, who had taken a later flight, I gathered the clothing my father would wear in his coffin and into the fires of the crematorium. While I walked around upstairs, my mother sat in her accustomed place at one end of the couch, reading under the light of the lamp my father had found for her. I had no trouble selecting the right clothing until I began to look for a tie. I knew my mother would want my father to be as carefully dressed as he always had been, though in his later years he had taken to putting together patterns that struck some of us as typical "old man" combinations. I couldn't find his ties, and my composure unraveled completely. I began to sob uncontrollably as I opened closets and drawers, coming upon his meticulously arranged underwear, heavy socks (for those terribly cold feet) and ironed, folded handkerchiefs. Finally I could spare my mother no longer and went to her, thrusting my tearstained face under the light. "I can't find his ties," I sobbed, "I can't find his ties." Her eyes filled with tears, but her voice was steady. "They're in the top drawer of the low dresser in the middle of the bedroom." She turned back to the book she was holding.

When my mother looked at my father the next afternoon, she noticed that there was no handkerchief folded in the breast pocket of his jacket where he had always kept a clean one when he went out. She wasn't reproachful when she told me; it was just a mark of her close attention. I felt a pang of regret that I'd left something out, but I reminded myself that I'd remembered a belt even though I'd known it wouldn't be visible. Sure enough, no one, not even my mother, checked to see if my father was wearing a belt. Unembalmed, without makeup of any kind, he looked as he had in later life: an attractive man with beautiful white hair, elegant features, and improbably but tastefully matched clothing. His hands, with their carefully groomed nails and strong tracing of veins, were lightly crossed on his jacket. I could hardly bear to stop touching him, though he was now quite cold. I folded his ear over, as my mother used to do. When I was a child, she used to call it "packing Allie's ears." We would fold his earlobe up and the top of his ear down to make a sort of earpocket. While our small family was still taking turns leaning over the casket, my mother told me that she was ready to go home and that she'd like me to take her. We walked out to the car, leaving the rest behind. They would close the room behind them when they were finished, and the morticians would get the body to the crematorium.

At home, my mother walked heavily to her spot on the couch. I sat in a chair, close to her, and held her hand. "Well," she said, "is that it? Is that all there is?" The tone of her voice was implacably demanding.

"Not to my way of thinking, " I said truthfully. She looked and waited. "I think people have souls," I said, "I think people have souls, and their souls live on after them. I think there's an oversoul." My mother showed no sign of accepting or rejecting what I was saying but nodded slightly to indicate both that she'd heard me and that this conversation, the only one we ever had in her lifetime about immortality, was at an end.

A few days later, the funeral parlor phoned to tell me that my father's ashes, the "cremains," had arrived. The ashes were in a cardboard box covered with heavy mailing paper; the name on the package was my father's. The box was heavier than it looked; it was about eight inches square. I carried it under my arm to the car, where

I put it on the front seat next to me. Sitting in the parking lot of the funeral home, I opened the flaps of the wrapping, then the flaps of the box; inside I found a bag made out of what seemed to be industrial weight plastic; light beige in color, with a heavy twist'em holding it closed. I opened the bag and rubbed my father's ashes gently between my fingers. They were more uneven than I had expected, and I could feel larger pieces lower in the bag. I retied the twist'em, wiped my hands clean on my jeans, then repacked the box and rearranged the wrapping.

I left the parking lot and went to teach my class before picking up my husband, Jerry. He opened the door and was about to get in when he noticed the box on the seat. "Is this your father?" he asked. I'd forgotten I had him with me. "Whoops," I said. "Why don't we put him in the back seat?" When we arrived home, I left my father on the bottom step of the stairs to the second floor. Soon I would move him to the desk upstairs in my study. Some time later, my daughter Erica and her husband, Scott, were staying with us. Scott went upstairs to do some work on my computer while I prepared supper. While I was at the sink, Erica appeared at my elbow. "Is that Grandpa on your study desk?" she asked. "Scott was a little unnerved."

"Yes," I answered, "it's Grandpa. Why don't you put the box on the floor if it'll be easier for Scott."

"Right," Erica said, "thanks Mom."

I realized that the ashes had generally been recognized as mine to deal with—or not—for the foreseeable future. My brother, when he left after spending a week with my mother, wanted no further discussion about the ashes or their disposal. My mother began to write letters to my father and was so deeply involved in her own grief that I knew better than to talk to her about the box that contained the physical remains of my father. I was perfectly comfortable with the ashes. I thought of them as my father and was glad to have them around. It turned out that Peggy's father had indeed requested that his ashes be scattered at sea, and they had done that as a family. But they all dearly loved sailing, and carrying out his wishes was natural for them. We had no family tradition except, perhaps, reading and exchanging books. My father had talked scornfully of people who needed the "crutch of religion"; in fact, our rare irritable exchanges, which hardly lasted long enough to be called arguments, were usually about religion. He did not have a speculative or introspective mind and had no patience for notions of spirituality. My confidence in the existence of a soul was entirely my own.

Between the time that my father died on November 11 and the date of her own death on April 22, my mother was desperately lonely and unhappy. She was not depressed, not a candidate for treatment or therapy. She was eighty-four years old and didn't want to live without my father. She worried about money, and feared the prospect of going into what she called "an old age home," despite my fervent assurances that we would never let that happen and that we could manage any financial crisis that might arise.

We realized over the course of those months that we had been wrong all along about the balance in my mother and father's relationship. My father had proclaimed his love for my mother constantly, and he had visibly suffered the few times that she was ill or in the hospital. He had claimed the right to die first, while clinging to whatever reduced life that was possible for him, on oxygen and restricted almost entirely to the house for the last month or so of this life. We had all imagined that my mother, who was stoic about pain and not at all interested in talking about her body, would resume her walks once my father was no longer keeping her confined to the house. We imagined that she would start planning her flower garden. We thought she would be eager to see the birth of Erica's baby, due in October and awaited from the first days in February when Erica realized she was pregnant. On every count we were wrong. These months without my father seemed endless to her. Once, when I sat down next to her on one of my daily visits, she looked up at me from under her reading lamp and said, "I could live a long, long time like this." Her tone seemed full of barely controlled desperation. I didn't say anything, just took her hand, heavily spotted and bruised with age, and held it. We looked somberly at one another. Long ago, and repeatedly, I had promised both my parents that I would never attempt to keep either of them alive. I now made that promise again. "I'll do whatever you want me to do," I said. She patted my hand absently. We sat in silence a while longer.

A few days later, we went to consult with Ellie Bruchey, a friend and lawyer, about my mother's finances; she was eager to give everything over to me, an arrangement that I knew would not be desirable. But she needed to work this out with Ellie, so I made it clear that I would accept whatever they thought was best for my mother. Eventually my mother decided to leave things as they were. We did get a durable power of attorney that she made out on my behalf. I insisted that she list my brother as well. It was hard for him to be so far away, and I wanted her to acknowledge his involvement, even if it were only symbolically. I thought she felt better once this document had been signed and witnessed, but I think now that she saw it as a step along her way to complete withdrawal.

My mother succeeded in dying on April 22, my brother's birthday. She had a terrible day on April 21, a day I can hardly bear to remember. It was a Thursday, and for many months afterward I relived the last Thursday of her life. I believed that eventually I would get through Thursdays more easily, and in time that has turned out to be true.

She was experiencing congestive heart failure that day, which took its usual form of increased difficulty in breathing. She came downstairs and tried to call the doctor, knowing she needed help, but the phone upstairs was off the hook. She thought her phone was broken and resigned herself to waiting all day for me to come by, as she knew I would, when I came home from school. Jerry was sick that day and off to the doctor, which kept him from looking in on her as he usually did. By the time I got to her house that afternoon, she was exhausted, desperate to get to the bathroom, wretched in every way. I helped her walk to the bathroom, called the doctor, and agreed to bring her immediately to the emergency room. Once there, with oxygen, she began to improve.

After she was admitted, I left to gather some of the things she wanted: her toilet articles, as she and my father referred to them; the daily *Times* crossword puzzle; the books she was currently reading. When I returned, she was completing the standard intake interview with a resident; a technician was drawing blood. "I take care of myself," my mother was saying. "My daughter takes me shopping and provides transportation for me. And . . ." she hesitated, considering the proper language for what she wanted to say next, ". . . a friend," she said firmly, "takes me to the Bangor Public Library every Tuesday." There followed a series of increasingly invasive questions about her physical habits and abilities, which I could see irritated my mother. Finally, the resident seemed to have finished, but before he could stand up my mother spoke again.

"There's one question you forgot to ask, young man," she said in her coldest and firmest voice.

"What's that?" he asked quickly, looking alarmed.

"You neglected to ask when I last had sexual intercourse." She pronounced every letter in each word, looking straight into his mortified face.

"Good for you!" exclaimed the technician.

The resident hurriedly gathered his folder and clipboard and left. The technician, smiling broadly, followed. I remained with my mother awhile, figuring out how to adjust the reading light and guiding her fingers to the switch so that she could manage it without calling anyone to help her. Wearing her glasses and a blue hospital bathrobe, which was not very different from the one she usually wore at home, and with the bedside table piled high with her books, tissues, and the crossword puzzle, she did not look frightened or out of place. I kissed her goodnight and told her that I would be back by noon the next day. She was clearly feeling better and seemed comfortable.

My mother died the next morning at about twenty after ten. She had just successfully completed some sort of respiratory exercise and seemed fine to the therapists who administered the test. A few minutes later, when one went back to look in on her, she was dead. For some reason, the hospital people couldn't find me and called Jerry at his office. I saw him approaching and began yelling at him for being out without a jacket on this cold morning; his hands were to his mouth, in a gesture characteristic of him when he is deeply moved, and I knew immediately what he had to tell me. "Is my mother dead?" I asked. "She just died," he said, taking me in his arms.

I have always imagined my mother looking at the clock, thinking about my plan to arrive at noon, and deciding to die right then, before I could get back to her. Though I had promised not to let anyone keep her alive, and I had every intention of keeping my promise, I think my mother took things into her own hands. Sometimes I think she did that to spare me, but mostly I think that she had her own imperatives which carried all the weight right then.

By the time we got to the hospital, unlike the experience we had with my father, my mother's body had been removed to the morgue. I insisted on seeing her. I had to convince the nursing staff who, I suppose, were afraid I'd faint or create some kind of scene. I assured them that I knew that they had done everything possible for my mother, since they clearly couldn't understand how she had died when they had been caring for her so closely. Eventually I got to see her. Someone pulled out the stainless steel drawer on which she lay, her body zipped into a dark body bag, I unzipped it and touched her face, her neck, whatever I could easily reach. Her body was chilly from the cooler, but there was still a little residual warmth. I slipped my hand under her bathrobe and felt her breasts, long, soft, and flat under my fingers. I realized that my mother's nipples were inverted, and at that moment, I thought how much she would dislike this touching and what I had just discovered, since she had never chosen to tell me this when we talked about bottle feeding and nursing so many years before. I took away my hands, kissed her good-bye, and zipped up the bag.

Defying what I believed would have been my mother's wishes, I wrote an obituary that mentioned my father's death in November and a few details of my mother's life. I knew there were people who had loved her and wished for some way to show their affection. We were present in the funeral parlor for a few hours so that friends could pay their respects; earlier, our family gathered, as it had for my father. I had chosen her clothes. For the last months of her life, she had worn my father's blue cardigan almost every day. She was wearing it in her pine box, and she would wear it into the fires. She wore her glasses (cleaned, as so often during her life, by Jerry). She had been rereading George Eliot's *Middlemarch*, so I placed it in her hands. Afterward, the funeral director returned her glasses, her wedding ring, and *Middlemarch* to me. Her ashes arrived a few days later. The box, I realized, was smaller and lighter than my father's. I now had both my parents in the form of cremains. I put them side by side on the corner of my desk in the study, thinking that pretty soon I would have to decide what to do with them.

I had tried over the years to prepare myself for my parents' deaths. I'd imagined, accurately as it turned out, how they were likely to die and how I would probably feel. Primarily, I knew I would feel loneliness. Now I felt it in full force. For the time being, we made no plans about the house, which was a virtual museum of my parents' lives and tastes. Now, with my brother back in Seattle, I settled into a routine of visiting my parents' house to take care of the plants and contemplate life without them. It was during this time that I began to understand what I came to call the specificity of grief.

My mother had always kept a record of her reading in a loose-leaf notebook. After my father's death, she had begun a second loose-leaf book, sort of a journal in the form of letters to my father. Before he flew back to Seattle, my brother had read through this journal; he left it behind for me. He took very few things from the house. When I visited the house to take care of the plants, I wandered from room to room, opening drawers, looking in the medicine cabinet, dusting various surfaces. I didn't look at my mother's journal for a while, nor did I examine her reading record. I sat at her accustomed spot on the couch, looking at the room as she had looked at it for so many years. Eventually, I opened her journal and began to read the letters. Almost immediately I regretted my action. What was clear from the first page to the last—the first was written right after my father's death and the last a day or two before her own—was the terrible nature of my mother's grief and her overwhelming desire not to live any longer. Without my father she found life unbearable. Though she recognized our desire to help, and mentioned us from time to time to tell my father what we were trying to do for her, we scarcely existed for her.

My mother loved my father, as he had loved her, single-mindedly. I knew myself to be a beloved child, regarded by each of my parents as the completion of their marriage, but I knew myself to be outside their immediate circle as well. Over the years, the narrow confines of my parents' life together had always included me but had never centered on me. In their last years, I was the privileged outsider in their domestic arrangement. I brought news of the outside world and shared their joint life almost entirely. Yet I had never for a moment lost sight of their absolute attention to one another. Like the rest of my family, I imagined that my mother's strength resided within her, independent of my father. The journal made it clear that she, at least, had never thought she existed outside of his love for her. Nor did she wish to, when he died.

In those months between my father's death and her own, she read, talked on the phone, shopped, and went to the library. She gave up attending concerts and never again entered the Maine Center for the Arts, but she listened to opera on the radio and continued to read the *New York Times* and do the daily crossword puzzle. To us, she seemed herself, but inside she was consumed by a loneliness so specific and focused that our presence could not penetrate it. The small part of her journal that I read made me writhe at the thought of those endless days as she had experienced them. If only she had known, I thought, how soon she would die, she might have been able to enjoy some of those final desperate months.

In late August, Jerry and I left for a long-awaited sabbatical year in New York, taking my parents' ashes with us to our city apartment. We have photographs of ourselves standing at the rear of our station wagon, its insides piled high with computers and last-minute choices, each of us holding a box of ashes. When we unpacked, I placed the boxes on the floor in the corner of our bedroom where I had a desk and a work space and could lean down and touch them without leaving my chair or my sabbatical work. On top of the boxes, I placed my mother's bottle of White Linen toilet water, the only scent she had used for many years. On rare occasions, I opened the bottle and sniffed the contents. It was less than half full, and I imagined my mother rationing it in the months before her death. Next to the bottle of toilet water I placed the little leather travel diary that I had given my father for a trip to Israel and Italy in 1968. He rarely wrote anything, and the travel diary petered out before the end of the trip, but what remains testifies to his delight in both the journey and the diary itself. Until I opened it after their deaths, I had forgotten about it, so I was surprised to find the dedication in my handwriting. Every now and then I would read a few lines of my father's hasty jottings and smile.

My parents had grown up together in Manhattan. In some ways, they had regarded their life in New Jersey, and then in Maine, as a sort of exile. Their ashes and the other bits of recollection seemed at home in our Manhattan apartment, in a neighborhood they would have enjoyed enormously. I was relieved to be with them out of Maine; for the moment, I felt less need to decide what should happen next with their ashes.

Not long after we settled in the city, we spent a day on an art excursion which took us to places we had never been before. The excursion began with a ride on the Roosevelt Island tram and took us to the Isamu Noguchi sculpture museum and then to a reclaimed site along the Queens side of the East River, a place called Socrates Sculpture Park. The moment we entered the park, I began to cry; I felt that here was where my parents' ashes should eventually come. The park, originally an industrial dumping ground, was created and is maintained by a loose coalition of artists, primarily sculptors. Pieces that have been sources of contention or that have been rejected by the neighborhoods for which they were constructed have found their way to this park. They can be touched, climbed on, sometimes walked into. I found the site immensely moving. Its history, its designation as a people's park, its position at the edge of an industrial wasteland directly across from the towers of Manhattan all made it feel like a home of sorts. That day I thought I could consider scattering at least part of my parents' ashes there.

Yet the ashes are still in the corner of the bedroom of our New York apartment, and I have yet to return to Socrates Sculpture Park. Nor have I looked seriously for containers for the ashes, either together or separately. Over the months and years since the deaths of my parents, I have carried out my responsibilities as they wished. Having been a cosigner for all the bank accounts and funds, I have cashed them in and divided the amounts equally with my brother. I sold the house and arranged for the furniture, which none of us wanted, to go to auction. With my brother and Jerry, I emptied the house. We all agreed that if we could have preserved it forever, we would have. Short of that, we broke it up and saw its contents scattered. I took very little; one painting, a companion piece to a seascape on our living room wall; my mother's copy of *Middlemarch*; a few pieces of clothing for Erica. Neither my brother nor I had especially liked my parents' tastes in china, glasses, or silverware. My parents themselves had not been accumulators; they had thrown or given away almost everything that was not in their daily use. I wasn't sure, taking their ashes to New York, that either of them would have understood or approved of my decision to keep them around.

Over these few years, I have discovered that a number of people I know are also keepers of their parents' ashes. Like me, other children puzzle over what to do next, if anything, with these mortal remains that have somehow ended up in their care. Conversations with these people illuminate an approach to the nature of grief itself, which has long puzzled me. At one stage of our evolving new relationship, my brother was impatient with my slow management of dissolving of our parents' small estate; he also professed himself mystified by "where I was" in my own grieving process. I think he found me remote, conventional, glib. Since I had anticipated so much of what became my deep loneliness and private loss, I didn't do much open grieving, either at the immediate moments of my parents' deaths or afterward. Except for that one burst of sobs, I never wept publicly again. I almost envied other members of my family, especially my daughter, who wept at the very mention of their names. Both my children repeatedly dreamt about their grandparents, while I have had exactly one dream in which my mother appeared, and then as a sort of minor character. For awhile after my mother's death, I thought that if I could just manage to grieve properly I might hallucinate her presence, or my father's, or at least manage to hear their voices. Though I think of my parents daily, I don't have visions of their presence, intimations of their nearness, or a sense of their continuing care for me. I experience them as irretrievably, irrevocably gone from me, and I miss them as much as I thought I would.

I tried to grieve for my parents in a way that I felt was authentic for me, and I realized along the way, especially from my brother's remarks, that my way didn't make a whole lot of sense to those around me. People tried to help me, as I had tried to help my mother, and I experienced them as she must have experienced me. Our granddaughter Sophie was born the autumn following my mother's death. We came home for the birth, and I was in the delivery room with Erica and Scott as Sophie came into the world. I was tremendously moved by the experience, but it was clear that what I had thought about myself over the years continued to be true even after grandchildren came into my life: I had greatly loved my own two children but had no particular desire to be with other babies.

The first November after the death of my parents, I made Thanksgiving dinner as I always had. I missed my parents as deeply as ever. Because Thanksgiving had always been marked by my father's stuffing and his pies, we all felt his absence especially, but for me there was no emotional change in the quality of my loneliness. Erica was particularly tender toward me at this time and, being a new mother, she tried to give me her greatest gift: Sophie. It was a maddening experience for me; I craved solitude to think of my parents, but I was constantly distracted and interrupted by the loving attention of others. At one point, I managed to sit down in a rocking chair, feeling as though my parents were on the other side of the wall, talking to one another. I felt that if I could sit quietly enough, listen intently enough, I might catch the murmur of their voices. At that moment, Erica gave me Sophie to hold, and a minute later Jerry came to capture the moment in a photograph. I knew then that for years to come that photograph would continue to record a moment of truth containing many layers, some of which would be known only to me. Sophie, in her striped knit cap, slept against my neck. I held her carefully, feeling a desperation I could not possibly share, describe, or express.

I felt that I would never get to mourn "properly." I craved time, space, and silence. Once my parents' house had been sold, I felt a hint of relief. Because I never had to enter it again, and I refused the new owners' kind invitations to see what they had done, I began to let myself remember it as it had been. I craved the opportunity to remember, just remember, without a schedule, without chronology, without comparison to anyone else's memory or feeling. I wanted my parents back—I still want them back—in a way that is entirely selfish and entirely specific.

As I went about my daily life, I carried on a sort of running undertone (what a jazz recording once referred to as a walking bass) which commented on the nature of my grief, my mourning process, and its place in the world. I read everything I could find about loss, death, and mourning. Nothing described what I was feeling or what I thought I had learned from my mother's experience. My routine was not disrupted. I neither gained nor lost weight, and my level of health seemed unaffected. I had moments of delight and joy, and I was certainly not any more conventionally spiritual or, for that matter, any less so. My belief in the existence of the soul remained as it had always been, a part of my sense of myself in the world. I missed my parents.

To my regret, but not to my surprise, I missed my mother more than my father for the first couple of years. My father's last years had been difficult for him, for us all; pain and physical misery had diminished him, and he had recognized this at the time. He had not liked his own condition—his incessant focus on trying to get more physically comfortable, his limited capacity to be interested in anything outside of himself. He had grown harder to love, and he knew it. During his last months, I'd had several conversations with my friend Peggy, whose father had also suffered from a number of ailments. We commiserated with one another about what our fathers were going through and about our own gathering misery at not being able to sustain the love we wanted to feel as they became harder to live with. We reassured one another about our intentions and, sometimes, about our behavior. But we knew we would feel remorse in the end, and remorse is what I felt now that both my parents were dead. I had done all that I could for my mother, without reservation, but I knew that I had been less than totally loving toward my father. Even that exchange about his ashes had amused me more than it should have. I had focused on the absurd picture of my mother sprinkled with the ashes of her late, and excessively self-absorbed husband. I had protected myself against his passionate demand to be heard. I had managed not to promise him something that, however ridiculous, he craved enough to request of me in the unforgiving light of an emergency room cubicle.

Now that they were both dead, I mourned them and my own lost condition as their daughter. Though I had to some extent become the parent of my parents, as many of us do, I had retained my role as their daughter; our three white heads clearly belonged together when we appeared at concerts or gatherings. I mourned my lost self as I mourned them, and my mourning was woven into the fabric of every day of my life.

By bringing the subject of my parents' ashes into conversation with friends and acquaintances, I kept them alive in relation to me. I discovered that many people felt as I did. Orphaned in our fifties, we recognized our good fortune in having had parents for so long. At the same time, we acknowledged that we had become used to having parents and being children. We referred to the ashes we had received by their titles: my mother, my dad, Papa. We told stories to one another about the arrival of the ashes, their texture, our inability to decide what to do with them. Should we share them with other family members? Did anyone besides us know who our parents had really been and where they should finally rest?

It seemed that all of us who'd had this experience cherished the ashes we'd received and were grateful to our parents for having chosen cremation. Each time I found myself in conversation with a friend about the death of a parent and the questions evoked by the box of ashes that came afterward, I discovered that the friendship moved to what seemed a new level of intimacy and regard. I had always found my parents fascinating and welcomed opportunities to talk about them with friends who took loving their parents for granted. Just as I'd felt free to rail about my children in conversation with my parents, because we all loved one another and knew we loved the children as well, now I found that I felt free to talk about my feelings with other people who, like me, had lost parents but found themselves the custodians of the ashes.

I was no closer to a solution to the problem of finding a permanent home for the ashes. I realized this when I became involved in writing a piece of fiction and contemplated a scene in which the main character sprinkled some of her parents' ashes in a place I'd considered for my parents. As I thought about the scene, I realized that what was appealing to me in fiction was still impossible for me in my life. I am not ready to give up what remains of my parents, what remains in my possession. I'm ready to talk about alternatives, and I'm ready to envision the scene in which someone like me tosses something like them onto the rocks, the grass, the air of a place they would have enjoyed visiting. But describing such a scene in fiction is as much as I'm ready for right now.

Missing my parents has become a regular part of what it means for me to be alive in the world. I see my life, in one visual metaphor, as a stream. I imagine the stream to have currents moving within it, varying in speed and temperature. In this stream of my life, immediate concerns eddy and ripple, but thoughts of my parents are usually slower and cooler currents, always flowing just a bit further below the surface. The image suggests that my parents continue to enrich my life, and I suppose they do. Yet what I am conscious of is a sense of tears always gathering but never spilling over.

I have discovered grief as a subject, a territory to explore, a terrain to investigate. Because I was attentive to my parents, in every sense of that word, I learned about their way of growing old, facing death, losing one another. I resolved to try and understand and, even when I couldn't understand, to foster their ways of facing death. My father's imagination, never glorious, shriveled in his final years; his desire to be scattered over my mother, to envelop her in his remains, testifies to his love and his fear, his belief that without her he would be nothing. Although I couldn't understand such a desire for non-differentiation, my mother's way of living on and dying soon after taught me to distinguish between my wishes and their reality.

I have come to believe that each person's grief expresses as unmistakably as a handprint the nature of the person who lives on—or chooses not to. The intricately designed rituals of religious observance may satisfy some of the needs of traditionally religious people. I suppose that, to the degree that people are comprised of their religious beliefs, they may find in ritual enough to illuminate much of the territory of grief. But I have learned enough about myself to know that the thoughtful prescriptions of religious ritual, often beautiful in their cadence and intentions, do not fulfill or replace my need to continue walking this still unfolding terrain.

From my mother, I learned about the specificity of grief, a notion that I continue to explore and expand. Not only do I miss them specifically, with a loneliness that cannot be addressed by the presence of others, but I discern a specificity in my own way of grieving. My way allows room for remembering, but it also allows room for attempting to forget. I have begun the work of embroidering over the obdurate suffering of my mother's last Thursday. I am embroidering a veil of memory, like a scrim, which allows me to preserve the memory but dim the light that plays upon it. I am turning down the glare of the emergency room, leaving my father and me bathed in a more tender light, recollecting a lifetime of love extended to him. I take comfort in the realization that the first writing I did about my parents was about my father; a poem crafted swiftly and surely about a moment in which we both delighted, a moment of poetry, snow, and a drive home together.

I imagine that those of us who are the keepers of our parents' ashes recognize the ambiguity of this gift. Those compact boxes in their layers of plastic, cardboard, and brown paper contain and do not contain our parents. We can run our fingers through them, sniff their dry smell of bone, recognize them as objects in the landscape of our daily lives. Patting the reassuring outlines of their containers, we can imagine the parents of our past, larger than life, without borders or boundaries, spilling over into the contours of our hearts. Safely and helplessly separated from the contents of these boxes, our distance allows us to contemplate our parents at last: manageable, contained, less than life-sized.

In the world that reappears to us daily, a world both with and without those whose ashes we contemplate, we begin to imagine separating from the remains. In conversation, in writing, in pictures behind our closed eyelids, we begin to consider the winds, the waters, the grasses to which we may someday be able to confide "our" ashes—or what we still think of, while we are contemplating them, as our ashes.

WISTERIA

LESLIE NYMAN

A shudder of resistance shivered through me as I ran toward the old brick hospital. November's icy rain had stripped the last of the wisteria from the vines covering the stone-gray building. In spring, when I began my nursing career, the smell of these purple flowers filled the air; now the chill dampness of late autumn drained scent and color into memory.

Cold winds pushed me into the lighted entry hall where my coworkers, Alma and Rosy, were already shaking off the chill.

"Ah, rain. No me le gusto, sí? I don't like esta noche."

Alma chattered "Spanglish," her concession to a common language, and Rosy ignored me with her usual benign indulgence. Even though we shared jokes, coffee and donuts, and complaints about hospital policies, Rosy closed herself off to me.

"Bad storm tonight." I fumbled for a pen and paper while Louise, the evening-shift nurse, paced around the small enclosure of her desk, chart rack, and medicine cabinet.

"The first storms of the season are always the worst. November sets a chill in my bones that doesn't leave until May." She pulled on her rubber overshoes. "Come on, let's get report started so I can go home to a hot tub."

Before sitting down, I turned on the hall light and the second set of office lights. "It feels creepy in here tonight."

"This place can spook you until you get used to it," she laughed. "Wait until you've been around fourteen years, like me. Nothing about this place bothers me anymore."

I aspired to Louise's cool professionalism. She possessed the emotional distance that I believed distinguished the most competent nurses. She reported on the patients' conditions like a child reciting a poem. The rhythm pulled the matter-of-fact words along.

From *Between the Heartbeats: Poetry and Prose by Nurses,* edited by Cortney Davis and Judy Schaefer (Iowa City: U of Iowa P, 1995): 139–44. Reprinted by permission of the author.

"Mr. Edwards' ulcer is worse today. Try to change his position every two hours tonight. Miss Wallace is going to the general hospital in the A.M. for a biopsy." She looked up as if to say *at last* but merely shook her head and continued her report. "Mary Cromer refused to eat again today. Maybe it's time for a feeding tube . . . or a psych consult. I left her doctor a note. John Kline . . . ," she broke the rhythm with a deep sigh. "John needed morphine twice on my time, twice on the day shift. He seems to be getting worse. The morphine barely holds him for four hours." She lit a cigarette. "Can you believe it, Janie? This is still a PRN order." Exhaling a cloud of smoke, she leaned toward me confidentially. "You know, I think his doctor is afraid John will get addicted if we give it around the clock. The poor guy probably doesn't have another month to go. I wish we could keep him comfortable." Crushing out the half-smoked cigarette, she stood abruptly. "Everyone else on the floor is stable. Come on, let's make rounds so I can get out of here."

I followed Louise in and out of the dim rooms as she made a final check at each bedside. I made notes of the bags, bottles, and tubes that were to occupy my hours. The rooms were populated with sleeping, groaning, babbling patients.

"Hey you, get me up! I've got to get . . . ouch, ouch."

"Now, now Betty, wherever do you have to get to at this hour?" Louise teased the shrunken, wrinkled lady in bed.

"Get away, girl," the old woman spit. "My leg hurts, my leg."

Louise and I freed Betty from the tangle of sheets. We moved pillows behind her back and between her knees, arranging her in a more comfortable position.

"There, isn't that better now, dear?" Louise cooed. As we left the room Louise told me, "Betty's getting crazier by the day. She's totally out of it. She talks all day to her dead husband, doesn't even recognize her son when he visits. I guess she keeps the day shift entertained." She shrugged. "Anyway, I hope you have a quiet night. I'm free at last."

Gray light, like evening fog, settled in the hospital corridors. Only the absence of darkness lightened the hallways. The rowdy storm outside rattled the window but did not disturb the palpable rhythm of the midnight quiet. It felt as if everyone was inhaling at the same time and slowly exhaling together.

At one A.M. rounds everyone was stable. Mr. Edwards had been turned on his side. Alma and Rosy cleaned up soiled patients, changed linens, added a needed blanket, and restrained a restless sleeper. I like the pace of the night shift as it moved through its hours with the steady ticking of the clock. My only concern was that someone would die. No one had ever died on my shift. I felt a combination of shame and eagerness as I stood over a faltering patient, hoping he or she would live until eight A.M. Death scared me. I had no experience with it and thought of it as something ugly, painful, and vaguely contagious.

"Help me, help me please," a small voice cried.

"There go Betty otra vez. I change her sheets, but it no calm her. She unhappy vieja." Alma snapped her gum.

I did not know what more I could offer. She had already been given her tranquilizer for the night. "Maybe I'll sit with her awhile," I said to Rosy. She nodded.

"Oh dear, I'm so afraid." Betty's voice shook.

"It's OK, you're safe," I reassured her, stroking her large gnarled hands. Long ago they must have been useful and perhaps lovely, but now the nails were yellowed and splintered. I wondered about the crooked tip of her index finger. It looked as if it had been broken and never set right.

"They've all left me. I'm all alone," she cried. "Oh Charles. He never would have let them do this to me. He never let me be alone so." The depth of her sigh caused a wheeze.

"What was Charles like?" I asked, knowing that by talking about him she might find solace.

"He was a good man. You know, a *real* man." Her thin voice pretended strength. "So handsome. All the other girls were jealous." Her eyes twinkled. "Yes, everyone looked up to him."

Before leaving the room I stroked her soft white hair. She had fallen back to what I hoped was a pleasant dream.

Wind and rain tapped a lullaby on the window panes. Three A.M. was always a difficult hour for me to keep my eyes open. I walked through the rooms, stopping at each bedside, wondering what the patients' lives had been before illness and age had wasted them. I made sure the bedrails were up and that everyone was breathing.

John Kline was awake.

"The pain's comin' in waves." A shadow of playfulness lingered about his mouth. "I'm waitin' ta see what crests with the next wave."

He stopped talking, eyes closed and lips taut. My fingertips resting on his wrist felt his pulse increase with the pain.

"No ship in sight. Send for the Marines. Suppose I could have my medicine now?"

It had been the required four hours since his last shot. "The Marines have landed," I whispered as I administered the morphine. Tomorrow the nurses could do battle with the doctor for more ammunition against John's pain.

A bedrail rattled in the next room. I found Betty half turned around in bed, mumbling to herself.

"Get me out of here! I want to see my Charles." A trace of anger flickered. "He'd get me out of here!" her gray eyes misted. "I don't know what happened." She slid back into confusion. "Joey used to be a good boy, but then Charles died and, I don't know. . . ." Her uncomprehending eyes looked at me. "Dear, do I know you? What's your name?"

"Janie. My name is Janie and I'm your nurse."

"My nurse?" She was indignant in an instant. "I don't need a nurse. I've always been the healthiest of all my sisters—Sadie, she's the sick one. What do I need a nurse for?"

"Betty, it's hard for you to walk, and your family wants you to be safe and cared for."

"I don't need to be taken care of," she snapped. "Joey's always helped me. It's only right. I looked after my mother 'til the day she died." Betty turned her face away from me. "It's not right, it's just not right." She lifted her big hands to reveal their emptiness. "But I can tell you one thing." Her steely eyes turned to me. "If Charles were here, things would be different. He'd tell you and your people to go to hell."

Pride slipped into weariness. Paper-thin eyelids closed. Her wheezing filled the room.

"Please, don't go yet." She placed her knobby hand over mine. "Oh mama," her tiny voice cracked.

The building shivered in the cold wind. I heard Rosy exclaim, "Lord, what a night!" from down the hall. Icy rain slamming into the sill startled Betty.

"Quick, answer the door. I wonder who that could be?"

"It's only the weather, that's all. A storm," I whispered.

"A storm? I didn't know. I must watch for Charles. My glasses. I can't see. Where are my glasses?"

I placed very smudged bifocals on her shrunken face. In the dim hospital light she looked like an owl—eyes wide open looking into the night.

"Now dear, help me to the window. I've got to get to the window. Charles will be home soon." She pulled up her knees to swing herself out of bed. Her ankle fell between the bars of the siderail.

I untied the knot she had made with her legs, the siderail, and the linens, and helped her to sit on the edge of the bed, the flat of my hand supporting her bent back. She felt like nothing more than a bundle of twigs.

"Let's sit here a moment and rest."

"I've rested enough," she growled, her heavy hand pressed into my knee for leverage as she stood. It was a slow shuffle to the window. I tried to surround her thin body with my arms, my feet close to her leaden steps as she dragged across the linoleum floor, filling the room with her whistle and wheeze. Fixing her magnified gray eyes on a point on the window, she drew nearer as if guided by an invisible pulley. Goosebumps crawled over my skin and my palms were sweating, but I held her up as we proceeded. I craned my neck back toward the door, hoping that Rosy or Alma would appear. I never should have let this happen, but Betty's insistence was stronger than my fear.

Her long crooked fingers clung to the windowsill like a bird to a branch. I supported her waist while she leaned forward to peer out.

"I can see him coming up the road." Her frail body tensed with excitement.

I looked out the window. It was a dark night; the branches blowing against the pane were barely visible.

Betty stared hard into the night. "Oh, he works so hard, that old guy," she whispered. Her voice lightened into a song, almost a laugh. "Quick, Joey, can you smell the wisteria? It's so sweet."

Then she sank, quickly, painlessly into my arms. I nearly dropped her I was so surprised. In the breath of the second that precedes a thought, I understood—death had relieved her. The complete stillness when her wheezing ceased scared me. I struggled to carry her now-heavy body to the bed.

Deafened by the pounding of my own heart, I ran to find Alma and Rosy.

"I shouldn't have let her out of bed! I knew it!" Tears showed my confusion. "This never happened to me before." I searched their faces for a suggestion of what to do.

"Janie, calm yourself." Alma wrapped her long arm around my shoulders. "She was una vieja." She shrugged. "She died, rest her soul in heaven. We will finish the colecciones and IV for you while you take care of business." When she kissed my cheek I smelled her flowery perfume that had not faded during the night.

"You know," I said to Rosy, whose eyes revealed compassion, "she said she saw her husband. That was all she seemed to want really. I'm sort of glad, if she saw him like that, you know, at the end."

Rosy's smile offered me a moment of comfort.

"I don't know, I don't know." I paced in a tight circle. "Am I responsible?"

"No, Janie, you didn't do nothing. The old lady died because it was God's will, not yours. That mean old lady is in everlasting peace right now. She's not a joke for nobody."

Rosy's words helped to calm me into reason. The necessary phone calls were made, the paperwork completed.

As dawn ignited the dark sky, the sounds of early risers could be heard. Old machines cranking their engines, doubtful people looking to see if they were still alive, and groaning as they realized they had awakened into their nightmare. I opened the window in Betty's room. The storm was ending. Wet earth perfumed the cold air. Winter was coming, but for a moment I could almost smell the wisteria.

PREMATURE ELEGY
(A SEQUENCE OF POEMS)

FLORENCE ELON

BEQUEST

"From now on, you must wear
my cashmere-lined gloves,"
Mother urges, giving away
her favorite possessions.
Like Lear. Leans back against
her Sunday bed rest—
top half of an overstuffed chair
with gilded studs along the sides
and shiny arms—
the throne of a hospital sheet.

"Look at yours . . ."—
acrylic-lined, or worse,
with runs, like deep trenches,
as if they'd weathered
fifty winters.

She strokes smooth leather palms,
backs, knuckles, fingers,
milking the udders
lovingly. Turns them inside out.
"See—double, triple seams,"
louder, triumphant,
"My gloves will last forever!"

From *Self-Made* by Florence Elon, published by Secker and Warburg (1984). Reprinted by permission of The Random House Group Ltd.

ROOM 9639

Small rectangular plate
taped to your door:
raised metal letters—name;
date of birth, dash, and space
placed in parentheses below.
I see you're two years older
than I'd been told.

Inside, the window's bottom pane
props your X-rays:
clouds and wings—white, grey, black—
collage, symmetrically arranged.
That baseball—core of a bomb-blast—
may be what "indicates a mass."

Dismissing them with a gesture
your hand trembles, sweeping across
the narrow bed; a breathy voice,
"Part of my room's décor."

Eyes wander above the X-rays, bordered
by net curtains drawn to the side,
and stop, daydreaming, hypnotized
by the window's middle register,
film strip, the city there:

dark wide ribbon, the East River
dotted with boats by white banks
locked in ice. Only
thick charcoal from barge stacks
and clothing factories on shore
erupts, blows everywhere—
over the next-door helicopter pad
lightly powdered with snow.

HOTHOUSE ART

Too early for visiting hours
yesterday, pacing up and down
not corridors but avenues
I saw red, gold, and blue awnings,
rainbow stalls in windows,
picked out the tightest white rosebuds

already overblown.
Bruised petals curl into edges
dropping on the commode
and straight-backed chair
beside your bed.

The only thing that flourishes
in this overheated box with its faint
ammonia smell
is the patient herself:

eyelids, bright blue
as this winter afternoon's
unseasonably sunny, cloudless sky;
lips like dolls' scarlet
matching the cheek's perfect circle—
the house beautician's
made you blush like a corpse.

BUSINESS AS USUAL

Leading the troop—
stepping briskly, to a drum-beat—
my own mother. Behind,
like crutches, some hold up
others: thin arms crooked
around stick-waists or bony
shoulders trying to prop
drooping bodies into straight lines.

Only one is absent, she boasts.
Her own neighbor across the hall
refused to leave his bed
when she tried to recruit him—
shut himself like a book
and turned his body to the wall.

The others are still drifting
down corridors that radiate
to the lit lounge: a slow
procession of flip-flop slippers
and faded pastel robes,
wings fluttering. Squeaks
of wheel-chairs; coughs like barks.

Around the circular ward lounge
window panes blur—
winter ice slipping
as it collides with heated indoor air.

Mother takes charge:
smooths a bedwetter's plastic
over the polished lounge table;
spreads last week's newspapers on top;
lines up scissors, paints, empty jars
in rows, like surgical instruments,
to make Christmas decorations
for ward windows and doors.

So many years ago, teaching school,
she'd coax small heads to bend over
cut-outs of gold and silver stars;
prod hands to wind tinsel
around cardboard evergreen trees,
each tier shaped like the A-line skirts
girls in her classroom wore.

Sometimes, she'd make fingers paint
red and white stripes on wood
for candy canes that looked so real
a few flame-tongues stuck out to lick
the paint—bright as the lips
and cheeks on those raised faces.

QUEEN OF THE WARD

Flat on her back—
caught flounder, flapping,
gasping for air—
five days after surgery
Mother wants to take charge
even of "the hall to death's door."

"Nurse, I want my sponge
now, not after the commercial."
From the bed, one thin hand stretches.
"You all treat me like shit!"

Bite my tongue. Zip my lip.
I sit by her bed
on the hard-backed chair; straighten
my spine against it—
at her request—a ruler's edge.

Years ago, it was she who sat
beside the hospital bed
where I lay, throat too sore to cry
after a tonsilectomy.
My arm reached out as she rose to go:
visitors not allowed to stay
overnight, even with a five-year-old.

She squeezed into a closet
full of smelly disinfectants and sheets;
all night, fetched fresh ice cubes
for the pack on my jaw,
water and strawberry sherbet
from the ward's common refrigerator.

Next morning, she was caught
by the chief nurse—freshly
starched uniform
crinkling sharply—bawling her out.
Mother pointed a forefinger—
"Last night, not one of you
checked if this child was breathing!"

THE PATIENT SPEAKS

"As punctually as my pills
or mushy meals wheeled in on carts
my daughter herself arrives
in high heels, carrying the best
bouquets of all my visitors: tight buds,
clean petals, stems like rods.

On that folding chair set up by my bed
she reads endlessly from Shakespeare—
Measure for Measure, Lear, the rest . . .
in her university voice
that doesn't sound like anybody real—
but when I speak up out loud
of what doctors and nurses do wrong here,
watch Ms. Finicky wince!

Well, I could tell her a thing or two
about Lear myself.
It's all stored in my nutshell:
ingratitude, a parent's hell,
far sharper than the surgeon's knife.

One evening after she pecked
my cheek good-bye
I turned the other; she was gone.
I slowly opened
the drawer of my commode
and fished out the penknife
Willy left there for peeling fruit.

Off with the heads
of all the flowers
in the bouquet she brought that day:
asters, daisies, pom-poms, roses.
I did it democratically,
lined them up, held the stems—
snip-snip, chop-chop
in one fell swoop."

POWWOW

The whole clan round
your hospital bed in bunches
like the flowers they bring:
heads drooping, wilted, crushed
from the endless subway haul.
Word of death calls the people
you hardly ever see.

Kid brother, gone for thirty years—
because he married a shiksa
and changed his family name,
his mourning parents and sisters
staged a mock funeral
and sat shiva for eight days—
dressed in a charcoal business suit,
balding, grey, stands by your bed,
magically risen from the dead.

"Be the lucky one in five,"
your son-the-medicine-man prays.
Flown in to work your cure
he calculates the chances in his head;
runs back and forth from room
to lab, trying to beat
your doctors to the biopsy
report—a sorcerer who knows
his way around. It's not by chance
you're in the premier hospital,
his alma mater.

Visiting twice a week
and always on call, your daughter
from the neighborhood
stands in the circle round your bed.
Some impulse to escape tugs at her legs,
pulling them up and forward, out the door,
through the lounge, into the elevator,
leaving behind the ritual grief
that weighs so heavily
in everybody else's air—
sweet reek of the aunts' perfumes
blending with talc and after shave.

REPORT FROM THE HOSPITAL

WISLAWA SZYMBORSKA

We used matches to draw lots: who would visit him.
And I lost. I got up from our table.
Visiting hours were just about to start.

When I said hello he didn't say a word.
I tried to take his hand—he pulled it back
like a hungry dog that won't give up his bone.

He seemed embarrassed about dying.
What do you say to someone like that?
Our eyes never met, like in a faked photograph.

He didn't care if I stayed or left.
He didn't ask about anyone from our table.
Not you, Barry. Or you, Larry. Or you, Harry.

My head started aching. Who's dying on whom?
I went on about modern medicine and the three violets in a jar.
I talked about the sun and faded out.

It's a good thing they have stairs to run down.
It's a good thing they have gates to let you out.
It's a good thing you're all waiting at our table.

The hospital smell makes me sick.

THE SUICIDE'S ROOM

WISLAWA SZYMBORSKA

I'll bet you think the room was empty.
Wrong. There were three chairs with sturdy backs.
A lamp, good for fighting the dark.
A desk, and on the desk a wallet, some newspapers.
A carefree Buddha and a worried Christ.
Seven lucky elephants, a notebook in a drawer.
You think our addresses weren't in it?

No books, no pictures, no records, you guess?
Wrong. A comforting trumpet poised in black hands.
Saskia and her cordial little flower.
Joy the spark of gods.
Odysseus stretched on the shelf in life-giving sleep
After the labors of Book Five.
The moralists
with the golden syllables of their names
inscribed on finely tanned spines.
Next to them, the politicians braced their backs.

No way out? But what about the door?
No prospects? The window had other views.
His glasses
lay on the windowsill.
And one fly buzzed—that is, was still alive.

You think at least the note must tell us something.
But what if I say there was no note—
and he had so many friends, but all of us fit neatly
inside the empty envelope propped up against a cup.

IN PRAISE OF FEELING BAD ABOUT YOURSELF

WISLAWA SZYMBORSKA

The buzzard never says it is to blame.
The panther wouldn't know what scruples mean.
When the piranha strikes, it feels no shame.
If snakes had hands, they'd claim their hands were clean.

A jackal doesn't understand remorse.
Lions and lice don't waver in their course.
Why should they, when they know they're right?

Though hearts of killer whales may weigh a ton,
in every other way they're light.

On this third planet of the sun
among the signs of bestiality
a clear conscience is Number One.

ASTONISHING THE BLIND

JACK HODGINS

I should have been practicing this afternoon, I should be getting dressed and ready to walk to the concert hall, but I have been sitting here for most of an hour with my hand by the phone, unable to pick it up. You'll have some explaining to do, I'm afraid, when you're asked "Has the daughter who lives in Europe called?" How will you explain that I haven't? This letter will likely not get to you for a week.

The clock in the Markt Platz should be striking six in the afternoon. Above it a rooster crows; beside it a guard blows his horn and Death turns his hourglass over again. Of course I can't hear or see this from my desk at the guest-house window, but I've been to this town before and can imagine all the activity whenever a glance at my watch coincides with the hour. Church bells clang at unexpected times all over town, slamming metal against metal like wild children competing with pots and pans.

Carl will assume I've called on behalf of us both. You remain something of a hero to him, Dad, though it's been three years since you were together and could encourage one another's outrageous opinions. If he were here, he would pick up the telephone, even dial the numbers for me, and hold the receiver to my ear. "Your father," he would announce with pleasure, as though he had conjured you up. But Carl did not come with me this time, though it is just a three-hour drive from our home. He travels enough already with his Euro-bureaucracy work.

Besides, he despises this town. He dislikes most of the towns in this country, even the one where we live, but he thoroughly dislikes this one because it is here that he was a student. He disapproves of the renewed popularity of fraternity houses, sponsored by leading citizens, with their rituals and fencing duels and their patriotic songs that make your blood run cold. He is convinced there are professors here, happily retired and still unpunished, who once practiced "German physics" in the name of science. He finds it amusing that his alma mater is playing host to his wife, putting her up in this comfortable guest house and allowing her to perform in the beautiful old hall, the *alte aula,* surrounded by famous murals. I have instructions not to let it go to my head.

Perhaps I have. I wish you could see the room where I performed last evening and will again tonight, in the original university building. Chandeliers hang from the ceiling, whose crossbeams have been decorated with hand-painted figures. Giant Gothic windows fill one wall with stained-glass circle patterns. And wide paintings decorate the other walls with the city's history. The audience sees, at my back, a file of indignant Dominican monks leaving the city, expelled by a prince who has decided to erect the world's first Protestant university on the very spot their monastery has occupied for centuries. The first professors taught their heresies from precisely where the piano and I challenge conventional approaches to Mozart.

I'd forgotten something Carl had told me about this town: the blind come here from all over the country to be trained, so they can get around and do everything the same as everyone else. This did not occur to me until I was standing at an intersection yesterday afternoon, waiting for a traffic light to change. All at once I saw blind people everywhere—not in groups or clusters, but going in various directions at various speeds. "I am in a city of the blind," I thought. I almost said it aloud, quite liking the notion, as if there were something magical about it. It was astonishing to see how quickly they moved, with their white canes swinging back and forth before them without quite touching the ground—electronic in some way, I imagine, like the sonar system of bats. They walked faster than I could, some of them, and with far more confidence. Nothing tentative, nothing apologetic. I saw one young woman run to catch a bus that was about to pull away. A tall man came from behind and skipped carefully around me in his hurry to cross the street.

Not surprisingly, there were quite a few of the blind in my audience last evening. I found myself grateful to them for coming, though this was silly of course since you don't need eyesight to enjoy Rachmaninoff or my favorite Beethoven sonatas. It occurred to me that they may have been trained to hear more critically, and more appreciatively, than anyone else in the room. I played in order to astonish them.

I can't see it from here, the old university building with that wonderful hall, though the view from this guest-house desk includes the castle at the top of the hill and a jumble of timbered fairy-tale houses spilling down the steep sides. Immediately before me is the *alter botanischer garten* with its neglected flower beds. Wild mustard grows up through the roses. Its grass has gone to seed—some of it deliberately, I understand, for the birds. Its garbage cans are overturned, its pathways littered with the green dung of free-roaming swans.

This afternoon I walked along the gravel pathways of this former botanical garden with my dear old teacher—you remember my speaking of Professor Mueller?—who arranged to be driven from his retirement home so he could hear me perform last night. He assured me that he'd been pleased with my performance. I think you would have been proud as well. Of course he noticed, and he let me know he'd noticed, that

I have not yet entirely mastered the art of risking originality—or rather, have not yet mastered it with confidence. I am still too North American, he says, after all these years—seventeen!

He must be in his eighties now. Like you, he walks with a cane to keep his balance. This may have been what prompted me to mention you, and to tell him that today, ten thousand miles away, you were about to celebrate your sixtieth wedding anniversary.

Tears came suddenly to his eyes. He lost his own wife years ago, I remember. A woman he'd adored. "Still together after sixty years!" he said. "A happy marriage, I hope."

"Very," I said on your behalf. "One of those lifelong romances we read about but don't often witness. My folks have been inseparable since they were children."

"Inseparable" was the word he repeated. In his mouth it was filled with wonder.

Of course, with that word between us, I was forced to consider the violence that can be done by time. What does it mean to be "still together" anyway? To be inseparable, as you know better than anyone else, does not after all exclude the possibility of separation.

I held the professor's arm as we passed along the shoreline of a pond, where mallards sunbathed amongst the tangled surface roots of a sawed-off trunk, and entered a shaded plantation of sturdy old trees.

"But you must wish you were there!" said my Professor Mueller, referring again to your anniversary.

I assured him you understood the difficulty, when I was so far away. "I fly home every August, and stay for one month. I can't afford to go twice."

"And the children?" he said.

"Always go with me. They're nearly teenagers now, yet they start counting the days in June, excited about seeing their grandparents again."

"And Carl?" His eyebrows have become grey caterpillars riding his brow. It was he who had introduced us, you remember, after my debut concert—a tall loose-limbed young man who came backstage with an arm-load of cornflowers.

"Carl used to go with me," I said. "But he hasn't always been free in the past few years."

"And is not with you here?"

I began to suspect this was not Professor Mueller at all who was quizzing me, but you in disguise. "He works hard all week," I said. "His weekends are precious. He has his own commitments."

When we had left the gardens and were walking back to the professor's hotel along a paved footpath that runs between a stream and the fence surrounding a nursing home, we came upon a woman I recognized from last night. She'd sat in the second row, and smiled throughout my performance in that secretive way that suggests some private satisfaction no one else could possibly share. It was she, more than the others, that I'd wanted to astonish with my playing.

She was not smiling now. Nor was she walking with the confidence and speed I have become accustomed to here. She poked nervously ahead of herself with her white stick, veering towards the edge of the pavement. When she found herself jabbing at grass, she stopped, and poked at everything around her, experimenting in order to set herself back on course.

I asked if there was something wrong, if we could help. She drew our attention to her cane, which had a sharp bend towards the bottom. "Someone running," she said. "Tripped over my cane and fell. We both fell."

There were smudges of dirt on the knees of her corduroy pants.

"Then he got up and handed it back to me and ran off!" she said. "Didn't even give his name. If he had, his insurance might have paid for a new one. As it is, I'll have to pay for it myself and I can't afford it."

Her voice suggested the entire world was at fault. But there was little I could do about it. Professor Mueller's walking stick had no more magic than her wounded one. I offered to see her to her destination but she declined. She would get there eventually, she said, though it was obvious she felt impotent and angry, reduced to the state of someone tapping along in a nineteenth century novel or an old black-and-white movie.

I suppose Carl would not have given up so easily. He would have insisted on accompanying the woman to the administration building, or the library, even if this annoyed her. He would have known who to call, where to make a report. He might have had advice for appealing to the guilty man's conscience—an ad in the paper, perhaps—whereas I have thought of such things only now.

And my dear professor, once we had rejected his walking stick as useless, had gone into a brooding silence, as blank and confused and helpless as the silent elderly patients we could see in their grassy pen behind the chain link fence.

I think of these people as the *alter leute* when I see them through the kitchen window of my guest-house rooms. Neglected grandfathers stare from benches onto that long quiet yard. Neglected grandmothers curl up on cots to receive the attentions of the sun. One bent man in a dark cardigan pushes a walker slowly past, nodding to those who sit with knees apart and eyes on the past, and later makes the return journey, nodding his greetings again to those who watch. It is a long building, six or seven stories tall. There must be hundreds of residents who never come out. Only once in my three days here have I seen a white uniform among those who risk the fresh air. And only once have I seen a visitor—a young woman talking with a white-haired man whose expression was one of silent puzzlement: Who are you and why have you suddenly appeared to yatter at me like this? "Your daughter," I imagine her saying. "Don't you remember me? Did you think I'd forgotten you?"

"Dear God," Professor Mueller said. He was looking through the fence at a pale dumpling of a woman who had been tied to a chair with the long cloth belt of a housecoat. She seemed to be looking back at him. "Those of us who are loved," he said, "can hardly imagine how much we have to be grateful for!"

Who do you have? I wanted to ask. I recall no children. Perhaps he meant grateful students who, unlike myself, live close enough to pay attention to him. Or neighbours who have grown attached.

I know if I were to dial this phone now you would answer before the first ring was completed, since at this time of day (midmorning for you) you will be installed beside the phone in your leather chair, watching out the window for someone (Richard, I imagine) to drive you to the hospital. I hope he will have flowers, and a cake, and perhaps even a few balloons.

Mom will be in her wheelchair now, I suppose, looking out at the view of the bay. Someone will have washed and set her beautiful salt-white hair. I hope they've put her in the dress that matches her blue eyes. I'm sure they have tried to make her understand there are reasons to be happy today. If only it were possible to help her recall, even briefly, what she must have felt as an excited bride! I should pick up this bloody instrument now, if only to remind you to take flowers. Thinking of such things was never one of your strengths. I wonder if you remember that it is the larger, gaudier, long-stemmed flowers she has always liked best. Tiger lilies, Shasta daisies, spikey mandarin orange dahlias. I have wired flowers myself, but flowers will mean more when they are delivered by someone whose face is at least familiar.

I remember that, one day last August, I left her room ahead of you, thinking, "There's next to nothing left of her. She's been slowly taken from us." But when I looked back through the doorway, you were bent over her bed, in danger of toppling forward upon her, but laughing, mock complaining, "My God, you're mushy today, woman!" Both of her hands came up to bring your face to hers for a kiss. Whatever else has been taken, she still knows who she loves in this world.

I will not phone the hospital. The last time I phoned the hospital, I was told she would have to be awakened, and for a conversation that would probably only confuse her. I knew that she wouldn't recognize my voice, she would have to pretend she knew who I was. Nor would she remember the conversation five minutes afterwards. While I, on the other hand, would be unable to think of anything else for the rest of the day.

Poor Professor Mueller worried about the blind woman all the way back to his hotel. "There must be something we might have done," he said, his caterpillar eyebrows tilting down with worry. He turned this way and that, as though searching for inspiration amongst the foyer furniture. "All three of us standing about, equally helpless! What good were *our* eyes, when we were needed?" He decided to be amused by this, a little. "We were of no more use to her than those poor deserted souls behind the terrible fence."

Before we parted, he lifted my hand to his lips. When I promised to report the incident of the damaged walking stick to university authorities, he looked up with relief, and, I think, surprise. Then, still holding my hand, he admonished me to risk failure tonight with a more European brand of confidence. He also asked me to pass on his good wishes to my parents. And of course, as well, to Carl.

At the moment Carl will be leaving the flat to keep an appointment of his own. The day will have been spent in household chores, in writing business letters, shopping for items I have asked him to buy, and arranging for a sitter so he may now step out with a sense of satisfaction to conduct his acts of betrayal.

They meet at the bridge. That's all that I know. I don't even know which bridge, though I imagine it is where you enter town from the south. In my mind, he waits at the north end of the wet grey concrete bridge, standing under his umbrella (it is almost certainly raining there, though perhaps I only wish it were raining), watching for her approach along the river bank.

I don't know where they will go. Perhaps back to her place, after a stroll through the park. Certainly not to our house. They will drive out into the country, and stop at a café along the riverfront, I suppose. Or they will drive all the way to the city to attend the cinema, or perhaps a recital in the concert hall. Because they are known as colleagues who sometimes must travel together for their work, they believe they have no reason to be circumspect. Does he imagine that my friends have no eyes?

So you see where I have brought myself with this letter that was meant to be a way of avoiding things. It should not be so difficult to pick up the telephone now and wish you a happy sixtieth anniversary. Dressed up and ready to go, you won't have the patience for a long-winded news report on my life. Long-distance charges being what they are, you won't expect it. With a little skill and some self-control we should be able to get through this without either of us wondering aloud what we mean.

But I have waited too long, as I suppose I'd intended, and you've already left for your lunch at Extended Care. I may mail this on my way to the concert hall, if I find a yellow postbox on the route, or I may try again to telephone afterwards. In the meantime, when I play the Beethoven this evening, it will be not only to offer consolation to the dispossesed monks at my backs, but also to salute the patience and fidelity of a lifelong love as I have witnessed it. And of course to astonish the blind.

PEOPLE LIKE THAT ARE THE ONLY PEOPLE HERE: CANONICAL BABBLING IN PEED ONK

LORRIE MOORE

A beginning, an end: there seems to be neither. The whole thing is like a cloud that just lands and everywhere inside it is full of rain. A start: the Mother finds a blood clot in the Baby's diaper. What is the story? Who put this here? It is big and bright, with a broken khaki-colored vein in it. Over the week-end, the baby had looked listless and spacey, clayey and grim. But today he looks fine—so what is this thing, startling against the white diaper, like a tiny mouse heart packed in snow? Perhaps it belongs to someone else. Perhaps it is something menstrual, something belonging to the Mother or to the Baby-sitter, something the Baby has found in a wastebasket and for his own demented baby reasons stowed away here. (Babies: they're crazy! What can you do?) In her mind, the Mother takes this away from his body and attaches it to someone else's. There. Doesn't that make more sense?

* * * * *

Still, she phones the clinic at the children's hospital. "Blood in the diaper," she says, and sounding alarmed and perplexed, the woman on the other end says, "Come in now."

Such pleasingly instant service! Just say "blood." Just say "diaper." Look what you get!

In the examination room, pediatrician, nurse, head resident—all seem less alarmed and perplexed than simply perplexed. At first, stupidly, the Mother is calmed by this. But soon, besides peering and saying "Hmmmm," the pediatrician, nurse, and head resident are all drawing their mouths in, bluish and tight—morning glories sensing noon. They fold their arms across their white-coated chests, unfold them again and jot things down. They order an ultrasound. Bladder and kidneys. "Here's the card. Go downstairs; turn left."

* * * * *

In Radiology, the Baby stands anxiously on the table, naked against the Mother as she holds him still against her legs and waist, the Radiologist's cold scanning disc moving about the Baby's back. The Baby whimpers, looks up at the Mother. *Let's get out of here,* his eyes beg. *Pick me up!* The Radiologist stops, freezes one of the many swirls of oceanic gray, and clicks repeatedly, a single moment within the long, cavernous weather map that is the Baby's insides.

"Are you finding something?" asks the Mother. Last year, her uncle Larry had had a kidney removed for something that turned out to be benign. These imaging machines! They are like dogs, or metal detectors: they find everything, but don't know what they've found. That's where the surgeons come in. They're like the owners of the dogs. "Give me that," they say to the dog. "What the heck is that?"

"The surgeon will speak to you," says the Radiologist.

"Are you finding something?"

"The surgeon will speak to you," the Radiologist says again. "There seems to be something there, but the surgeon will talk to you about it."

"My uncle once had something on his kidney," says the Mother. "So they removed the kidney and it turned out the something was benign."

The Radiologist smiles a broad, ominous smile. "That's always the way it is," he says. "You don't know exactly what it is until it's in the bucket."

"'In the bucket,'" the mother repeats.

The Radiologist's grin grows scarily wider—is that even possible? "That's doctor talk," he says.

"It's very appealing," says the Mother. "It's a very appealing way to talk." Swirls of bile and blood, mustard and maroon in a pail, the colors of an African flag or some exuberant salad bar: *in the bucket*—she imagines it all.

"The Surgeon will see you soon," he says again. He tousles the Baby's ringletty hair. "Cute kid," he says.

* * * * *

"Let's see now," says the Surgeon in one of his examining rooms. He has stepped in, then stepped out, then come back in again. He has crisp, frowning features, sharp bones, and a tennis-in-Bermuda tan. He crosses his blue-cottoned legs. He is wearing clogs.

The mother knows her own face is a big white dumpling of worry. She is still wearing her long, dark parka, holding the Baby, who has pulled the hood up over her head because he always thinks it's funny to do that. Though on certain windy mornings she would like to think she could look vaguely romantic like this, like some French Lieutenant's Woman of the Prairie, in all of her saner moments she knows she doesn't. Ever. She knows she looks ridiculous—like one of those animals made out of twisted party balloons. She lowers the hood and slips one arm out of the sleeve. The Baby wants to get up and play with the light switch. He fidgets, fusses, and points.

"He's big on lights these days," explains the Mother.

"That's okay," says the Surgeon, nodding toward the light switch. "Let him play with it." The Mother goes and stands by it, and the Baby begins turning the lights off and on, off and on.

"What we have here is a Wilms' tumor," says the Surgeon, suddenly plunged into darkness. He says "tumor" as if it were the most normal thing in the world.

"Wilms'?" repeats the Mother. The room is quickly on fire again with light, then wiped dark again. Among the three of them here, there is a long silence, as if it were suddenly the middle of the night. "Is that apostrophe *s* or *s* apostrophe?" the Mother says finally. She is a writer and a teacher. Spelling can be important—perhaps even at a time like this, though she has never before been at a time like this, so there are barbarisms she could easily commit and not know.

The lights come on: the world is doused and exposed.

"*S* apostrophe," says the Surgeon. "I think." The lights go back out, but the Surgeon continues speaking in the dark. "A malignant tumor on the left kidney."

Wait a minute. Hold on here. The Baby is only a baby, fed on organic applesauce and soy milk—a little prince!—and he was standing so close to her during the ultrasound. How could he have this terrible thing? It must have been *her* kidney. A fifties kidney. A DDT kidney. The Mother clears her throat. "Is it possible it was my kidney on the scan? I mean, I've never heard of a baby with a tumor, and, frankly, I was standing very close." She would make the blood hers, the tumor hers; it would all be some treacherous, farcical mistake.

"No, that's not possible," says the Surgeon. The light goes back on.

"It's not?" says the Mother. Wait until it's *in the bucket,* she thinks. Don't be so sure. *Do we have to wait until it's in the bucket to find out a mistake has been made?*

"We will start with a radical nephrectomy," says the Surgeon, instantly thrown into darkness again. His voice comes from nowhere and everywhere at once. "And then we'll begin with chemotherapy after that. These tumors usually respond very well to chemo."

"I've never heard of a baby having chemo," the Mother says. *Baby* and *Chemo,* she thinks: they should never even appear in the same sentence together, let alone the same life. In her other life, her life before this day, she had been a believer in alternative medicine. Chemotherapy? Unthinkable. Now, suddenly, alternative medicine seems the wacko maiden aunt to the Nice Big Daddy of Conventional Treatment. How quickly the old girl faints and gives way, leaves one just standing there. Chemo? Of course: chemo! Why by all means: chemo. Absolutely! Chemo!

The Baby flicks the switch back on, and the walls reappear, big wedges of light checkered with small framed watercolors of the local lake. The Mother has begun to cry: all of life has led her here, to this moment. After this, there is no more life. There is something else, something stumbling and unlivable, something mechanical, something for robots, but not life. Life has been taken and broken, quickly, like a stick. The room goes dark again so that the Mother can cry more freely. How can a baby's body be stolen so fast? How much can one heaven-sent and unsuspecting child endure? Why has he not been spared this inconceivable fate?

Perhaps, she thinks, she is being punished: too many baby-sitters too early on. (Come to Mommy! Come to Mommy-Baby-sitter!" she used to say. But it was a joke!) Her life, perhaps, bore too openly the marks and wigs of deepest drag. Her unmotherly thoughts had all been noted: the panicky hope that his nap would last longer than it did; her occasional desire to kiss him passionately on the mouth (to make out with her baby!); her ongoing complaints about the very vocabulary of motherhood, how it degraded the speaker ("Is this a poopie onesie! Yes, it's a very poopie onesie!"). She had, moreover, on three occasions used the formula bottles as flower vases. She twice let the Baby's ears get fudgy with wax. A few afternoons last month, at snacktime, she placed a bowl of Cheerios on the floor for him to eat, like a dog. She let him play with the Dust-buster. Just once, before he was born, she said, "Healthy? I just want the kid to be rich." A joke, for God's sake! After he was born she announced that her life had become a daily sequence of mind-wrecking chores, the same ones over and over again, like a novel by Mrs. Camus. Another joke, those jokes will kill you! She had told too often, and with too much enjoyment, the story of how the Baby had said "Hi" to his high chair, waved at the lake waves, shouted "Goody-goody-goody" in what seemed to be a Russian accent, pointed at his eyes and said "Ice." And all that nonsensical baby talk: wasn't it a stitch? "Canonical babbling," the language experts called it. He recounted whole stories in it—totally made up, she could tell. He embroidered; he fished; he exaggerated. What a card! To friends, she spoke of his eating habits (carrots yes, tuna no). She mentioned, too much, his sidesplitting giggle. Did she have to be so boring? Did she have no consideration for others, for the intellectual demands and courtesies of human society? Would she not even attempt to be more interesting? It was a crime against the human mind not even to try.

Now her baby, for all these reasons—lack of motherly gratitude, motherly judgment, motherly proportion—will be taken away.

The room is fluorescently ablaze again. The Mother digs around in her parka pocket and comes up with a Kleenex. It is old and thin, like a mashed flower saved from a dance; she dabs it at her eyes and nose.

"The Baby won't suffer as much as you," says the Surgeon.

And who can contradict? Not the Baby, who in his Slavic Betty Boop voice can say only *mama, dada, cheese, ice, bye-bye, outside, boogie-boogie, goody-goody, eddy-eddy,* and *car.* (Who is Eddy? They have no idea.) This will not suffice to express his mortal suffering. Who can say what babies do with their agony and shock? Not they themselves. (Baby talk: isn't it a stitch?) They put it all no place anyone can really see. They are like a different race, a different species: They seem not to experience pain the way *we* do. Yeah, that's it: their nervous systems are not as fully formed, and *they just don't experience pain the way we do.* A tune to keep one humming through the war. "You'll get through it," the Surgeon says.

"How?" asks the Mother. "How does one get through it?"

"You just put your head down and go," says the Surgeon. He picks up his file folder. He is a skilled manual laborer. The tricky emotional stuff is not to his liking. The babies. The babies! What can be said to console the parents about the babies? "I'll phone the oncologist on duty to let him know," he says, and leaves the room.

"Come here, sweetie," the Mother says to the Baby, who has toddled off toward a gum wrapper on the floor. "We've got to put your jacket on." She picks him up and he reaches for the light switch again. Light, dark. Peekaboo: where's baby? Where did baby go?

* * * * *

At home, she leaves a message—"Urgent! Call me!"—for the Husband on his voice mail. Then she takes the Baby upstairs for his nap, rocks him in the rocker. The Baby waves good-bye to his little bears, then looks toward the window and says, "Bye-bye, outside." He has, lately, the habit of waving good-bye to everything, and now it seems as if he senses an imminent departure, and it breaks her heart to hear him. *Bye-bye!* She sings low and monotonously, like a small appliance, which is how he likes it. He is drowsy, dozy, drifting off. He has grown so much in the last year, he hardly fits in her lap anymore; his limbs dangle off like a pieta. His head rolls slightly inside the crook of her arm. She can feel him falling backward into sleep, his mouth round and open like the sweetest of poppies. All the lullabies in the world, all the melodies threaded through with maternal melancholy now become for her—abandoned as a mother can be by working men and napping babies—the songs of hard, hard grief. Sitting there, bowed and bobbing, the Mother feels the entirety of her love as worry and heartbreak. A quick and irrevocable alchemy: there is no longer one unworried scrap left for happiness. "If you go," she keens low into his soapy neck, into the ranunculus coil of his ear, "we are going with you. We are nothing without you. Without you, we are a heap of rocks. We are gravel and mold. Without you, we are two stumps, with nothing any longer in our hearts. Wherever this takes you, we are following. We will be there. Don't be scared. We are going, too. That is that."

* * * * *

"Take Notes," says the Husband, after coming straight home from work, midafternoon, hearing the news, and saying all the words out loud—*surgery, metastasis, dialysis, transplant*—then collapsing in a chair in tears. "Take notes. We are going to need the money."

"Good God," cries the Mother. Everything inside her suddenly begins to cower and shrink, a thinning of bones. Perhaps this is a soldier's readiness, but it has the whiff of death and defeat. It feels like a heart attack, a failure of will and courage, a power failure: a failure of everything. Her face, when she glimpses it in a mirror, is cold and bloated with shock, her eyes scarlet and shrunk. She has already started to wear sunglasses indoors, like a celebrity widow. From where will her own strength come? From some philosophy? From some frigid little philosophy? She is neither stalwart nor realistic and has trouble with basic concepts, such as the one that says events move in one direction only and do not jump up, turn around, and take themselves back.

The Husband begins too many of his sentences with "What if." He is trying to piece everything together like a train wreck. He is trying to get the train to town.

"We'll just take all the steps, move through all the stages. We'll go where we have to go. We'll hunt; we'll find; we'll pay what we have to pay. What if we can't pay?"

"Sounds like shopping."

"I cannot believe this is happening to our little boy," he says, and starts to sob again. "Why didn't it happen to one of us? It's so unfair. Just last week, my doctor declared me in perfect health; the prostate of a twenty-year old, the heart of a ten-year-old, the brain of an insect—or whatever it was he said. What a nightmare this is."

What words can be uttered? You turn just slightly and there it is: the death of your child. It is part symbol, part devil, and in your blind spot all along, until, if you are unlucky, it is completely upon you. Then it is a fierce little country abducting you; it holds you squarely inside itself like a cellar room—the best boundaries of you are the boundaries of it. Are there windows? Sometimes aren't there windows?

* * * * *

The Mother is not a shopper. She hates to shop, is generally bad at it, though she does like a good sale. She cannot stroll meaningfully through anger, denial, grief, and acceptance. She goes straight to bargaining and stays there. How much? she calls out to the ceiling, to some makeshift construction of holiness she has desperately, though not uncreatively, assembled in her mind and prayed to; a doubter, never before given to prayer, she must now reap what she has not sown; she must assemble from scratch an entire altar of worship and begging. She tries for noble abstractions, nothing too anthropomorphic, just some Higher Morality, though if this particular Highness looks something like the manager at Marshall Field's, sucking a Frango mint, so be it. Amen. Just tell me what you want, requests the Mother. And how do you want it? More charitable acts? A billion starting now. Charitable thoughts? Harder, but of course! Of course! I'll do the cooking, honey; I'll pay the rent. Just tell me. *Excuse me?* Well, if not to you, to whom do I speak? Hello? To whom do I have to speak around here? A higher-up? A superior? Wait? I can wait. I've got all day. I've got the whole damn day.

The Husband now lies next to her in bed, sighing. "Poor little guy could survive all this, only to be killed in a car crash at the age of sixteen," he says.

The wife, bargaining, considers this. "We'll take the car crash," she says.

"What?"

"Let's Make a Deal! Sixteen Is a Full Life! We'll take the car crash. We'll take the car crash, in front of which Carol Merrill is now standing."

Now the Manager of Marshall Field's reappears. "To take the surprises out is to take the life out of life," he says.

The phone rings. The Husband gets up and leaves the room.

"But I don't want these surprises," says the Mother. "Here! You take these surprises!"

"To know the narrative in advance is to turn yourself into a machine," the Manager continues. "What makes humans human is precisely that they do not know the future. That is why they do the fateful and amusing things they do: who can say how anything will turn out? Therein lies the only hope for redemption, discovery, and—let's be frank—fun, fun, fun! There might be things people will get away with. And not just motel towels. There might be great illicit loves, enduring joy, faith-shaking accidents with farm machinery. But you have to not know in order to see what stories your life's efforts bring you. The mystery is all."

The Mother, though shy, has grown confrontational. "Is this the kind of bogus, random crap they teach at merchandising school? We would like fewer surprises, fewer efforts and mysteries, thank you. K through eight; can we just get K through eight?" It now seems like the luckiest, most beautiful, most musical phrase she's ever heard: K through eight. The very lilt. The very thought.

The Manager continues, trying things out. "I mean, the whole conception of 'the story,' of cause and effect, the whole idea that people have a clue as to how the world works is just a piece of laughable metaphysical colonialism perpetrated upon the wild country of time."

Did they own a gun? The Mother begins looking through drawers.

The Husband comes back into the room and observes her. "Ha! The Great Havoc that is the Puzzle of all Life!" he says of the Marshall Field's management policy. He has just gotten off a conference call with the insurance company and the hospital. The surgery will be Friday. "It's all just some dirty capitalist's idea of a philosophy."

"Maybe it's just a fact of narrative and you really can't politicize it," says the Mother. It is now only the two of them.

"Whose side are you on?"

"I'm on the Baby's side."

"Are you taking notes for this?"

"No."

"You're not?"

"No. I can't. Not this! I write fiction. This isn't fiction."

"Then write nonfiction. Do a piece of journalism. Get two dollars a word."

"Then it has to be true and full of information. I'm not trained. I'm not that skilled. Plus, I have a convenient personal principle about artists not abandoning art.

One should never turn one's back on a vivid imagination. Even the whole memoir thing annoys me."

"Well, make things up, but pretend they're real."

"I'm not that insured."

"You're making me nervous."

"Sweetie, darling, I'm not that good. I can't do this. I can do—what can I do? I can do quasi-amusing phone dialogue. I can do succinct descriptions of weather. I can do screwball outings with the family pet. Sometimes I can do those. Honey, I only do what I can. I do *the careful ironies of daydream.* I do *the marshy ideas upon which intimate life is built.* But this? Our baby with cancer? I'm sorry. My stop was two stations back. This is irony at its most gaudy and careless. This is a Hieronymus Bosch of facts and figures and blood and graphs. This is a nightmare of narrative slop. This cannot be designed. This cannot even be noted in the preparation for a design—"

"We're going to need the money."

"To say nothing of the moral boundaries of pecuniary recompense in a situation such as this—"

"What if the other kidney goes? What if he needs a transplant? Where are the moral boundaries there? What are we going to do, have bake sales?"

"We can sell the house. I hate this house. It makes me crazy."

"And we'll live—where again?"

"The Ronald McDonald place. I hear it's nice. It's the least McDonald's can do."

"You have a keen sense of justice."

"I try. What can I say?" She pauses. "Is all this really happening? I keep thinking that soon it will be over—the life expectancy of a cloud is supposed to be only twelve hours—and then I realize something has occurred that can never ever be over."

The Husband buries his face in his hands: "Our poor baby. How did this happen to him?" He looks over and stares at the bookcase that serves as the nightstand. "And do you think even one of these baby books is any help?" He picks up the Leach, the Spock, the *What to Expect.* "Where in the pages or index of any of these does it say 'chemotherapy' or 'Hickman catheter' or 'renal sarcoma'? Where does its say 'carcinogenesis'? You know what these books are obsessed with? *Holding a fucking spoon.*" He begins hurling the books off the night table and against the far wall.

"Hey," says the Mother, trying to soothe. "Hey, hey, hey." But compared to his stormy roar, her words are those of a backup singer—a Shondell, a Pip—a doo-wop ditty. Books, and now more books, continue to fly.

* * * * *

Take Notes.

Is *fainthearted* one word or two? Student prose has wrecked her spelling.

It's one word. Two words—*Faint Hearted*—what would that be? The name of a drag queen.

* * * * *

Take Notes. In the end, you suffer alone. But at the beginning you suffer with a whole lot of others. When your child has cancer, you are instantly whisked away to another planet: one of bald-headed little boys. Pediatric Oncology. Peed Onk. You wash your hands for thirty seconds in antibacterial soap before you are allowed to enter through the swinging doors. You put paper slippers on your shoes. You keep your voice down. A whole place has been designed and decorated for your nightmare. Here is where your nightmare will occur. We've got a room all ready for you. We have cots. We have refrigerators. "The children are almost entirely boys," says one of the nurses. "No one knows why. It's been documented, but a lot of people out there still don't realize it." The little boys are all from sweet-sounding places—Janesville and Appleton—little heartland towns with giant landfills, agricultural runoff, paper factories, Joe McCarthy's grave (alone, a site of great toxicity, thinks the Mother. The soil should be tested).

All the bald little boys look like brothers. They wheel their IVs up and down the single corridor of Peed Onk. Some of the lively ones, feeling good for a day, ride the lower bars of the IV while their large, cheerful mothers whiz them along the halls. *Wheee!*

* * * * *

The Mother does not feel large and cheerful. In her mind, she is scathing, acid-tongued, wraith-thin, and chain-smoking out on a fire escape somewhere. Beneath her lie the gentle undulations of the Midwest, with all its aspirations to be—to be what? To be Long Island. How it has succeeded! Strip mall upon strip mall. Lurid water, poisoned potatoes. The Mother drags deeply, blowing clouds of smoke out over the disfigured cornfields. When a baby gets cancer, it seems stupid ever to have given up smoking. When a baby gets cancer, you think, Whom are we kidding? Let's all light up. When a baby gets cancer, you think, Who came up with *this* idea? What celestial abandon gave rise to *this*? Pour me a drink, so I can refuse to toast.

The Mother does not know how to be one of these other mothers, with their blond hair and sweatpants and sneakers and determined pleasantness. She does not think that she can be anything similar. She does not feel remotely like them. She knows, for instance, too many people in Greenwich Village. She mail-orders oysters and tiramisu from a shop in SoHo. She is close friends with four actual homosexuals. Her husband is asking her to Take Notes.

Where do these women get their sweatpants? She will find out.

She will start, perhaps, with the costume and work from there.

She will live according to the bromides. Take one day at a time. Take a positive attitude. *Take a hike!* She wished that there were more interesting things that were useful and true, but it seems now that it's only the boring things that are useful and true. *One day at a time.* And *at least we have our health.* How ordinary. How obvious. One day at a time. You need a brain for that?

* * * * *

While the Surgeon is fine-boned, regal, and laconic—they have correctly guessed his game to be doubles—there is a bit of the mad, overcaffeinated scientist to the Oncologist. He speaks quickly. He knows a lot of studies and numbers. He can do the math. Good! Someone should be able to do the math! "It's a fast but wimpy tumor," he explains. "It typically metastasizes to the lung." He rattles off some numbers, time frames, risk statistics. Fast but wimpy: the Mother tries to imagine this combination of traits, tries to think and think, and can only come up with Claudia Osk from the fourth grade, who blushed and almost wept when called on in class, but in gym could outrun everyone in the quarter-mile fire-door-to-fence dash. The Mother thinks now of this tumor as Claudia Osk. They are going to get Claudia Osk, make her sorry. All right! Claudia Osk must die. Though it has never been mentioned before, it now seems clear that Claudia Osk should have died long ago. Who was she anyway? So conceited: not letting anyone beat her in a race. Well, hey, hey, hey: don't look now, Claudia!

The Husband nudges her. "Are you listening?"

"The chances of this happening even just to one kidney are one in fifteen thousand. Now given all these other factors, the chances on the second kidney are about one in eight."

"One in eight," says the Husband. "Not bad. As long as it's not one in fifteen thousand."

The Mother studies the trees and fish along the ceiling's edge in the Save the Planet wallpaper border. Save the Planet. Yes! But the windows in this very building don't open and diesel fumes are leaking into the ventilating system, near which, outside, a delivery truck is parked. The air is nauseous and stale.

"Really," the Oncologist is saying, "of all the cancers he could get, this is probably the best."

"We win," says the Mother.

"Best, I know hardly seems the right word. Look, you two probably need to get some rest. We'll see how the surgery and histology go. Then we'll start with chemo the week following. A little light chemo: vincristine and—"

"Vincristine?" interrupts the Mother. "Wine of Christ?"

"The names are strange, I know. The other one we use is actinomycin-D. Sometimes called 'dactinomycin.' People move the *D* around to the front."

"They move the *D* around to the front," repeats the Mother.

"Yup!" the Oncologist says. "I don't know why—they just do!"

"Christ didn't survive his wine," says the Husband.

"But of course he did," says the Oncologist, and nods toward the Baby, who has now found a cupboard full of hospital linens and bandages and is yanking them all out onto the floor. "I'll see you guys tomorrow, after the surgery." And with that, the Oncologist leaves.

"Or, rather, Christ *was* his wine," mumbles the Husband. Everything he knows about the New Testament, he has gleaned from the sound track of *Godspell.* "His blood was the wine. What a great beverage idea."

"A little light chemo. Don't you like that one?" says the Mother. "*Eine kleine* dactinomycin. I'd like to see Mozart write that one up for a big wad o'cash."

"Come here, honey," the Husband says to the Baby, who has now pulled off both his shoes.

"It's bad enough when they want to refer to medical science as 'an inexact science,'" says the Mother. "But when they start referring to it as 'an art,' I get extremely nervous."

"Yeah. If we wanted art, Doc, we'd go to an art museum." The Husband picks up the Baby. "You're an artist," he says to the Mother, with the taint of accusation in his voice. "They probably think you find creativity reassuring."

The Mother sighs. "I just find it inevitable. Let's go get something to eat." And so they take the elevator to the cafeteria, where there is a high chair, and where, not noticing, they all eat a lot of apples with the price tags still on them.

* * * * *

Because his surgery is not until tomorrow, the Baby likes the hospital. He likes the long corridors, down which he can run. He likes everything on wheels. The flower carts in the lobby! ("Please keep your boy away from the flowers," says the vendor. "We'll buy the whole display," snaps the Mother, adding, "Actual children in a children's hospital—unbelievable, isn't it?") The Baby likes the other little boys. Places to go! People to see! Rooms to wander into! There is Intensive Care. There is the Trauma Unit. The Baby smiles and waves. What a little Cancer Personality! Bandaged citizens smile and wave back. In Peed Onk, there are the bald little boys to play with. Joey, Eric, Tim, Mort, and Tod (Mort! Tod!). There is the four-year-old, Ned, holding his little deflated rubber ball, the one with the intriguing curling hose. The Baby wants to play with it. "It's mine. Leave it alone," says Ned. "Tell the Baby to leave it alone."

"Baby, you've got to share," says the Mother from a chair some feet away.

Suddenly, from down near the Tiny Tim Lounge, comes Ned's mother, large and blond and sweatpanted. "Stop that! Stop it!" she cries out, dashing toward the Baby and Ned and pushing the Baby away. "Don't touch that!" she barks at the Baby, who is only a Baby and bursts into tears because he has never been yelled at like this before.

Ned's mom glares at everyone. "This is drawing fluid from Neddy's liver!" She pats at the rubber thing and starts to cry a little.

"Oh my God," says the Mother. She comforts the Baby, who is also crying. She and Ned, the only dry-eyed people, look at each other. "I'm so sorry," she says to Ned and then to his mother. "I'm so stupid. I thought they were squabbling over a toy."

"It does look like a toy," agrees Ned. He smiles. He is an angel. All the little boys are angels. Total, sweet, bald little angels, and now God is trying to get them back for himself. Who are they, mere mortal women, in the face of this, this powerful and overwhelming and inscrutable thing, God's will? They are the mothers, that's who. You can't have him! they shout every day. You dirty old man! *Get out of here! Hands off!*

"I'm so sorry," says the Mother again. "I didn't know."

Ned's mother smiles vaguely. "Of course you didn't know," she says, and walks back to the Tiny Tim Lounge.

* * * * *

The Tiny Tim Lounge is a little sitting area at the end of the Peed Onk corridor. There are two small sofas, a table, a rocking chair, a television and a VCR. There are various videos: *Speed, Dune,* and *Star Wars.* On one of the lounge walls there is a gold plaque with the singer Tiny Tim's name on it: his son was treated once at this hospital and so, five years ago, he donated money for this lounge. It is a cramped little lounge, which, one suspects, would be larger if Tiny Tim's son had actually lived. Instead, he died here, at this hospital and now there is this tiny room which is part gratitude, part generosity, part *fuck-you.*

Sifting through the videocassettes, the Mother wonders what science fiction could begin to compete with the science fiction of cancer itself—a tumor with its differentiated muscle and bone cells, a clump of wild nothing and its mad, ambitious desire to be something: something inside you, instead of you, another organism, but with a monster's architecture, a demon's sabotage and chaos. Think of leukemia, a tumor diabolically taking liquid form, better to swim about incognito in the blood. George Lucas, direct that!

Sitting with the other parents in the Tiny Tim Lounge, the night before the surgery, having put the Baby to bed in his high steel crib two rooms down, the Mother begins to hear the stories: leukemia in kindergarten, sarcomas in Little League, neuroblastomas discovered at summer camp. "Eric slid into third base, but then the scrape didn't heal." The parents pat one another's forearms and speak of other children's hospitals as if they were resorts. "You were at St. Jude's last winter? So were we. What did you think of it? We loved the staff." Jobs have been quit, marriages hacked up, bank accounts ravaged; the parents have seemingly endured the unendurable. They speak not of the *possibility* of comas brought on by the chemo, but of the *number* of them. "He was in his first coma last July," says Ned's mother. "It was a scary time, but we pulled through."

Pulling through is what people do around here. There is a kind of bravery in their lives that isn't bravery at all. It is automatic, unflinching, a mix of man and machine, consuming and unquestionable obligation meeting illness move for move in a giant even-steven game of chess—an unending round of something that looks like shadowboxing, though between love and death, which is the shadow? "Everyone admires us for our courage," says one man. "They have no idea what they're talking about."

I could get out of here, thinks the Mother. I could just get on a bus and go, never come back. Change my name. A kind of witness relocation thing.

"Courage requires options," the man adds.

The Baby might be better off.

"There are options," says a woman with a thick suede headband. "You could fall apart."

"No, you can't. Nobody does. I've never seen it," says the man. "Well, not *really* fall apart." Then the lounge falls quiet. Over the VCR someone has taped the fortune from a fortune cookie. "Optimism," it says, "is what allows a teakettle to sing though up to its neck in hot water." Underneath, someone else has taped a clipping from a summer horoscope. "Cancer rules!" it says. Who would tape this up? Somebody's twelve-year-old brother. One of the fathers—Joey's father—gets up and tears them both off, making a small wad in his fist.

There is some rustling of magazine pages.

The Mother clears her throat. "Tiny Tim forgot the wet bar," she says.

Ned, who is still up, comes out of his room and down the corridor, whose lights dim at nine. Standing next to her chair, he says to the Mother, "Where are you from? What is wrong with your baby?"

* * * * *

In the tiny room that is theirs, she sleeps fitfully in her sweatpants, occasionally leaping up to check on the Baby. This is what the sweatpants are for: leaping. In case of fire. In case of anything. In case the difference between day and night starts to dissolve, and there is no difference at all, so why pretend? In the cot beside her, the Husband, who has taken a sleeping pill, is snoring loudly, his arms folded about his head in a kind of origami. How could either of them have stayed back at the house, with its empty high chair and empty crib? Occasionally the Baby wakes and cries out, and she bolts up, goes to him, rubs his back, rearranges the linens. The clock on the metal dresser shows that it is five after three. Then twenty to five. And then it is really morning, the beginning of this day, nephrectomy day. Will she be glad when it's over, or barely alive, or both? Each day this week has arrived huge, empty, and unknown, like a spaceship, and this one especially is lit a bright gray.

"He'll need to put this on," says John, one of the nurses, bright and early, handing the Mother a thin greenish garment with roses and teddy bears printed on it. A wave of nausea hits her; this smock, she thinks, will soon be splattered with—with what?

The Baby is awake but drowsy. She lifts off his pajamas. "Don't forget, *bubeleh,*" she whispers, undressing and dressing him. "We will be with you every moment, every step. When you think you are asleep and floating off far away from everybody, Mommy will still be there." If she hasn't fled on a bus. "Mommy will take care of you. And Daddy, too." She hopes the Baby does not detect her own fear and uncertainty, which she must hide from him, like a limp. He is hungry, not having been allowed to eat, and he is no longer amused by this new place, but worried about its hardships. Oh, my baby, she thinks. And the room starts to swim a little. The Husband comes in to take over. "Take a break," he says to her. "I'll walk him around for five minutes."

She leaves but doesn't know where to go. In the hallway, she is approached by a kind of social worker, a customer-relations person, who had given them a video to watch about the anesthesia: how the parent accompanies the child into the operating room, and how gently, nicely the drugs are administered.

"Did you watch the video?"

"Yes," says the Mother.

"Wasn't it helpful?"

"I don't know," says the Mother.

"Do you have any questions?" asks the video woman. "Do you have any questions?" asked of someone who has recently landed in this fearful, alien place seems to the Mother an absurd and amazing little courtesy. The very specificity of a question would give a lie to the overwhelming strangeness of everything around her.

"Not right now," says the Mother. "Right now, I think I'm just going to go to the bathroom."

When she returns to the Baby's room, everyone is there: the surgeon, the anesthesiologist, all the nurses, the social worker. In their blue caps and scrubs, they look like a clutch of forget-me-nots, and forget them, who could? The Baby, in his little teddy-bear smock, seems cold and scared. He reaches out and the Mother lifts him from the Husband's arms, rubs his back to warm him.

"Well, it's time!" says the Surgeon, forcing a smile.

"Shall we go?" says the Anesthesiologist.

What follows is a blur of obedience and bright lights. They take an elevator down to a big concrete room, the anteroom, the greenroom, the backstage of the operating room. Lining the walls are long shelves full of blue surgical outfits. "Children often become afraid of the color blue," says one of the nurses. But of course. Of course! "Now, which one of you would like to come into the operating room for the anesthesia?"

"I will," says the Mother.

"Are you sure?" asks the Husband.

"Yup." She kisses the Baby's hair. "Mr. Curlyhead," people keep calling him here, and it seems both rude and nice. Women look admiringly at his long lashes and exclaim, "Always the boys! Always the boys!"

Two surgical nurses put a blue smock and a blue cotton cap on the Mother. The Baby finds this funny and keeps pulling at the cap. "This way," says another nurse, and the Mother follows. "Just put the Baby down on the table."

In the video, the mother holds the baby and fumes are gently waved under the baby's nose until he falls asleep. Now, out of view of camera or social worker, the Anesthesiologist is anxious to get this under way and not to let too much gas leak out into the room generally. The occupational hazard of this, his chosen profession, is gas exposure and nerve damage, and it has started to worry him. No doubt he frets about it to his wife every night. Now he turns the gas on and quickly clamps the plastic mouthpiece over the baby's cheeks and lips.

The Baby is startled. The Mother is startled. The Baby starts to scream and redden behind the plastic, but he cannot be heard. He thrashes. "Tell him it's okay," says the nurse to the Mother.

Okay? "It's okay," repeats the Mother, holding his hand, but she knows he can tell it's not okay, because he can see not only that she is still wearing that stupid paper cap but that her words are mechanical and swallowed, and she is biting her lips to keep them from trembling. Panicked, he attempts to sit. He cannot breathe; his arms reach up. *Bye-bye, outside.* And then, quite quickly, his eyes shut; he untenses and has fallen not *into* sleep but aside to sleep, an odd, kidnapping kind of sleep, his terror now hidden someplace deep inside him.

"How did it go?" asks the social worker, waiting in the concrete outer room. The Mother is hysterical. A nurse has ushered her out.

"It wasn't at all like the filmstrip!" she cries. "It wasn't like the filmstrip at all!"

"The filmstrip? You mean the video?" asks the social worker.

"It wasn't like that all! It was brutal and unforgivable."

"Why that's terrible," she says, her role now no longer mis-informational but janitorial, and she touches the Mother's arm, though the Mother shakes it off and goes to find the Husband.

* * * * *

She finds him in the large mulberry Surgery Lounge, where he has been taken and where there is free hot chocolate in small Styrofoam cups. Red cellophane garlands festoon the doorways. She has totally forgotten it is as close to Christmas as this. A pianist in the corner is playing "Carol of the Bells," and it sounds not only unfestive but scary, like the theme from *The Exorcist.*

There is a giant clock on the far wall. It is a kind of porthole into the operating room, a way of assessing the Baby's ordeal—forty-five minutes for the Hickman implant; two and a half hours for the nephrectomy. And then, after that, three months of chemotherapy. The magazine on her lap stays open at a ruby-hued perfume ad.

"Still not taking notes," says the Husband.

"Nope."

"You know, in a way, this is the kind of thing you've *always* written about."

"You are really something, you know that? This is life. This isn't a 'kind of thing.'"

"But this is the kind of thing that fiction is: it's the unlivable life, the strange room tacked onto the house, the extra moon that is circling the earth unbeknownst to science."

"I told you that."

"I'm quoting you."

She looks at her watch, thinking of the Baby. "How long has it been?"

"Not long. Too long. In the end, maybe those're the same things."

"What do you suppose is happening to him right this second?"

Infection? Slipping knives? "I don't know. But you know what? I've gotta go. I've gotta just walk a bit." The Husband gets up, walks around the lounge, then comes back and sits down.

The synapses between the minutes are unswimmable. An hour is thick as fudge. The Mother feels depleted; she is a string of empty tin cans attached by wire, something a goat would sniff and chew, something now and then enlivened by a jolt of electricity.

She hears their names being called over the intercom. "Yes? Yes?" She stands up quickly. Her words have flown out before her, an exhalation of birds. The piano music has stopped. The pianist is gone. She and the Husband approach the main desk, where a man looks up at them and smiles. Before him is a xeroxed list of patients' names. "That's our little boy right there," says the Mother, seeing the Baby's name on the list and pointing at it. "Is there some word? Is everything okay?"

"Yes," says the man. "Your boy is doing fine. They've just finished with the catheter, and they are moving on to the kidney."

"But it's been two hours already! Oh my God, did something go wrong? What happened? What went wrong?"

"Did something go wrong?" The Husband tugs at his collar.

"Not really. It just took longer than they expected. I'm told everything is fine. They wanted you to know."

"Thank you," says the Husband. They turn and walk back toward where they were sitting.

"I'm not going to make it." The Mother sighs, sinking into a fake leather chair shaped somewhat like a baseball mitt. "But before I go, I'm taking half this hospital out with me."

"Do you want some coffee?" asks the Husband.

"I don't know," says the Mother. "No, I guess not. No. Do you?"

"Nah, I don't, either, I guess," he says.

"Would you like a part of an orange?"

"Oh, maybe, I guess, if you're having one." She takes an orange from her purse and just sits there peeling its difficult skin, the flesh rupturing beneath her fingers, the juice trickling down her hands, stinging the hangnails. She and the Husband chew and swallow, discreetly spit the seeds into Kleenex, and read from photocopies of the latest medical research, which they begged from the intern. They read, and underline, and sigh and close their eyes, and after some time, the surgery is over. A nurse form Peed Onk comes down to tell them.

"Your little boy's in recovery right now. He's doing well. You can see him in about fifteen minutes."

* * * * *

How can it be described? How can any of it be described? The trip and the story of the trip are always two different things. The narrator is the one who has stayed home, but then, afterward, presses her mouth upon the traveler's mouth, in order to make the mouth work, to make the mouth say, say, say. One cannot go to a place and speak of it; one cannot both see and say, not really. One can go, and upon returning make a lot of hand motions and indications with the arms. The mouth itself, working at the speed of light, at the eye's instructions, is necessarily struck still; so fast, so much to report, it hangs open and dumb as a gutted bell. All that unsayable life! That's where the narrator comes in. The narrator comes with her kisses and mimicry and tidying up. The narrator comes and makes a slow, fake song of the mouth's eager devastation.

It is a horror and a miracle to see him. He is lying in his crib in his room, tubed up, splayed like a boy on a cross, his arms stiffened into cardboard "no-no's" so that he cannot yank out the tubes. There is the bladder catheter, the nasal-gastric tube, and the Hickman, which, beneath the skin, is plugged into his jugular, then popped out his chest wall and capped with a long plastic cap. There is a large bandage taped over his abdomen. Groggy, on a morphine drip, still he is able to look at her when, maneuvering through all the vinyl wiring, she leans to hold him, and when she does, he begins to cry, but cry without motion or noise. She has never seen a baby cry without motion or noise. It is the crying of an old person: silent, beyond opinion, shattered. In someone so tiny, it is frightening and unnatural. She wants to pick up the Baby and run—out of there, out of there. She wants to whip out a gun: *No-no's, eh? This whole thing is what I call a no-no.* Don't you touch him! she wants to shout at the surgeons and the needle nurses. Not anymore! No more! No more! She would crawl up and lie beside him in the crib if she could. But instead, because of all his intricate wiring, she must lean and cuddle, sing to him, songs of peril and flight: "We gotta get out of this place, if it's the last thing we ever do. We gotta get out of this place . . . there's a better life for me and you."

Very 1967. She was eleven then and impressionable.

The Baby looks at her, pleadingly, his arms splayed out in surrender. To where? Where is there to go? Take me! Take me!

* * * * *

That night, postop night, the Mother and Husband lie afloat in the cot together. A fluorescent lamp near the crib is kept on in the dark. The Baby breathes evenly but thinly in his drugged sleep. The morphine in its first flooding doses apparently makes him feel as if he were falling backward—or so the Mother has been told—and it causes the Baby to jerk, to catch himself over and over, as if he were being dropped from a tree. "Is this right? Isn't there something that should be done?" The nurses come in hourly, different ones—the night shifts seem strangely short and frequent. If the baby stirs or frets, the nurses give him more morphine through the Hickman catheter, then leave to tend to other patients. The Mother rises to check on him in the low light. There is gurgling from the clear plastic suction tube coming out of his mouth. Brownish clumps have collected in the tube. What is going on? The Mother rings for the nurse. Is it Renee or Sarah or Darcy? She's forgotten.

"What, what is it?" murmurs the Husband, waking up.

"Something is wrong," says the Mother. "It looks like blood in his N-G tube."

"What?" The Husband gets out of bed. He, too, is wearing sweatpants.

The nurse—Valerie—pushes open the heavy door to the room and enters quietly. "Everything okay?"

"There's something wrong here. The tube is sucking blood out of his stomach. It looks like it may have perforated his stomach and that now he's bleeding internally. Look!"

Valerie is a saint, but her voice is the standard hospital saint voice: an infuriating, pharmaceutical calm. It says, Everything is normal here. Death is normal. Pain is normal. Nothing is abnormal. So there is nothing to get excited about. "Well now, let's see." She holds up the plastic tube and tries to see inside it. "Hmmm," she says. "I'll call the attending physician."

Because this is a research and teaching hospital, all the regular doctors are at home sleeping in their Mission-style beds. Tonight, as is apparently the case every weekend night, the attending physician is a medical student. He looks fifteen. The authority he attempts to convey, he cannot remotely inhabit. He is not even in the same building with it. He shakes everyone's hands, then strokes his chin, a gesture no doubt gleaned from some piece of dinner theater his parents took him to once. As if there were an actual beard on that chin! As if beard growth on that chin were even possible! *Our Town! Kiss Me Kate! Barefoot in the Park!* He is attempting to convince, if not to impress.

"We're in trouble," the Mother whispers to the Husband. She is tired, tired of young people grubbing for grades. "We've got Dr. 'Kiss Me Kate,' here."

The Husband looks at her blankly, a mix of disorientation and divorce.

The medical student holds the tubing in his hands. "I don't really see anything," he says.

He flunks! "You don't?" The Mother shoves her way in, holds the clear tubing in both hands. "That," she says. "Right here and here." Just this past semester, she said to one of her own students, "If you don't see how this essay is better than that one, then I want you just to go out into the hallway and stand there until you do." Is it important to keep one's voice down? The Baby stays asleep. He is drugged and dreaming, far away.

"Hmmm," says the medical student. "Perhaps there's a little irritation in the stomach."

"A little irritation?" The Mother grows furious. "This is blood. These are clumps and clots. This stupid thing is sucking the life right out of him!" Life! She is starting to cry.

They turn off the suction and bring in antacids, which they feed into Baby through the tube. Then they turn the suction on again. This time on low.

"What was it on before?" asks the Husband.

"High," says Valerie. "Doctor's orders, though I don't know why. I don't know why these doctors do a lot of the things they do."

"Maybe they're . . . not all that bright?" suggests the Mother. She is feeling relief and rage simultaneously: there is a feeling of prayer and litigation in the air. Yet essentially, she is grateful. Isn't she? She thinks she is. And still, and still: look at all the things you have to do to protect a child, a hospital merely an intensification of life's cruel obstacle course.

* * * * *

The Surgeon comes to visit on Saturday morning. He steps in and nods at the Baby, who is awake but glazed from the morphine, his eyes two dark unseeing grapes. "The boy looks fine," the Surgeon announces. He peeks under the Baby's bandage. "The stitches look good," he says. The Baby's abdomen is stitched all the way across like a baseball. "And the other kidney, when we looked at it yesterday face-to-face, looked fine. We'll try to wean him off the morphine a little, and see how he's doing on Monday." He clears his throat. "And now," he says, looking about the room at the nurses and medical students, "I would like to speak with the Mother, alone."

The Mother's heart gives a jolt. "Me?"

"Yes," he says, motioning, then turning.

She gets up and steps out into the empty hallway with him, closing the door behind her. What can this be about? She hears the Baby fretting a little in his crib. Her brain fills with pain and alarm. Her voice comes out as a hoarse whisper. "Is there something—"

"There is a particular thing I need from you," says the Surgeon, turning and standing there very seriously.

"Yes?" Her heart is pounding. She does not feel resilient enough for any more bad news.

"I need to ask a favor."

"Certainly," she says, attempting very hard to summon the strength and courage for this occasion, whatever it is; her throat has tightened to a fist.

From inside his white coat, the surgeon removes a thin paperback book and thrusts it toward her. "Will you sign my copy of your novel?"

The Mother looks down and sees that it is indeed a copy of a novel she has written, one about teenaged girls.

She looks up. A big, spirited grin is cutting across his face. "I read this last summer," he says, "and I still remember parts of it! Those girls got into such trouble!"

Of all the surreal moments of the last few days, this, she thinks, might be the most so.

"Okay," she says, and the Surgeon merrily hands her a pen.

"You can just write 'To Dr.—Oh, I don't need to tell you what to write."

The Mother sits down on a bench and shakes ink into the pen. A sigh of relief washes over and out of her. Oh, the pleasure of a sigh of relief, like the finest moments of love;

has anyone properly sung the praises of sighs of relief? She opens the book to the title page. She breathes deeply. What is he doing reading novels about teenaged girls, anyway? And why didn't he buy the hardcover? She inscribes something grateful and true, then hands the book back to him.

"Is he going to be okay?"

"The boy? The boy is going to be fine," he says, then taps her stiffly on the shoulder. "Now you take care. It's Saturday. Drink a little wine."

* * * * *

Over the weekend, while the Baby sleeps, the Mother and Husband sit together in the Tiny Tim Lounge. The Husband is restless and makes cafeteria and sundry runs, running errands for everyone. In his absence, the other parents regale her further with their sagas. Pediatric cancer and chemo stories: the children's amputations, blood poisoning, teeth flaking like shale, the learning delays and disabilities caused by chemo frying the young, budding brain. But strangely optimistic codas are tacked on—endings as stiff and loopy as carpenter's lace, crisp and empty as lettuce, reticulate as a net—ah, words. "After all that business with the tutor, he's better now, and fitted with new incisors by my wife's cousin's husband, who did dental school in two and a half years, if you can believe that. We hope for the best. We take things as they come. Life is hard."

"Life's a big problem," agrees the Mother. Part of her welcomes and invites all their tales. In the few long days since this nightmare began, part of her has become addicted to disaster and war stories. She wants only to hear about the sadness and emergencies of others. They are the only situations that can join hands with her own; everything else bounces off her shiny shield of resentment and unsympathy. Nothing else can even stay in her brain. From this, no doubt, the philistine world is made, or should one say recruited? Together, the parents huddle all day in the Tiny Tim Lounge—no need to watch *Oprah.* They leave Oprah in the dust. Oprah has nothing on them. They chat matter-of-factly, then fall silent and watch *Dune* or *Star Wars,* in which there are bright and shiny robots, whom the Mother now sees not as robots at all but as human beings who have had terrible things happen to them.

* * * * *

Some of their friends visit with stuffed animals and soft greetings of "Looking good" for the dozing baby, though the room is way past the stuffed-animal limit. The Mother arranges, once more, a plateful of Mint Milano cookies and cups of take-out coffee for guests. All her nutso pals stop by—the two on Prozac, the one obsessed with the word penis in the word *happiness,* the one who recently had her hair foiled green. "Your friends put the *de* in *fin de siècle,*" says the husband. Overheard, or recorded, all marital conversation sounds as if someone must be joking, though usually no one is.

She loves her friends, especially loves them for coming, since there are times they all fight and don't speak for weeks. Is this friendship? For now and here, it must do, and is, and is, she swears it is. For one, they never offer impromptu spiritual lectures about death, how it is part of life, its natural ebb and flow, how we all must accept that, or other such utterances that make her want to scratch out some eyes. Like true friends, they take no hardy or elegant stance loosely choreographed from some broad perspective. They get right in there and mutter "Jesus Christ!" and shake their heads. Plus, they are the only people who not only will laugh at her stupid jokes but offer up stupid ones of their own. What do you get when you cross Tiny Tim with a pit bull? A child's illness is a strain on the mind. They know how to laugh in a fluty, desperate way—unlike the people who are more her husband's friends and who seem just to deepen their sorrowful gazes, nodding their heads with Sympathy. How exiling and estranging are everybody's Sympathetic Expressions! When anyone laughs, she thinks, Okay! Hooray: a buddy. In disaster as in show business.

Nurses come and go; their chirpy voices both startle and soothe. Some of the other Peed Onk parents stick their heads in to see how the Baby is and offer encouragement.

Green Hair scratches her head. "Everyone's so friendly here. Is there someone in this place who isn't doing all this airy, scripted optimism—or are people like that the only people here?"

"It's Modern Middle Medicine meets the Modern Middle Family," says the Husband. "In the Modern Middle West."

Someone has brought in take-out lo mein, and they all eat it out in the hall by the elevators.

* * * * *

Parents are allowed use of the Courtesy Line.

"You've got to have a second child," says a different friend on the phone, a friend from out of town. "An heir and a spare. That's what we did. We had another child to ensure we wouldn't off ourselves if we lost our first."

"Really?"

"I'm serious."

"A formal suicide? Wouldn't you just drink yourself into a lifelong stupor and let it go at that?"

"Nope. I knew how I would do it even. For a while, until our second came along, I had it all planned."

"What did you plan?"

"I can't go into too much detail, because—Hi, honey!—the kids are here now in the room. But I'll spell out the general idea: R-O-P-E."

* * * * *

Sunday evening, she goes and sinks down on the sofa in the Tiny Tim Lounge next to Frank, Joey's father. He is a short, stocky man with the currentless, flatlined look behind the eyes that all the parents eventually get here. He has shaved his head bald in solidarity with his son. His little boy has been battling cancer for five years. It is now in the liver, and the rumor around the corridor is that Joey has three weeks to live. She knows that Joey's mother, Heather, left Frank years ago, two years into the cancer, and has remarried and has another child, a girl named Brittany. The Mother sees Heather here sometimes with her new life—the cute little girl and the new, young, full-haired husband who will never be so maniacally and debilitatingly obsessed with Joey's illness the way Frank, her first husband, was. Heather comes to visit Joey, to say hello and now good-bye, but she is not Joey's main man. Frank is.

Frank is full of stories—about the doctors, about the food, about the nurses, about Joey. Joey, affectless from his meds, sometimes leaves his room and comes out to watch TV in his bathrobe. He is jaundiced and bald, and though he is nine, he looks no older than six. Frank has devoted the last four and a half years to saving Joey's life. When the cancer was first diagnosed, the doctors gave Joey a 20 percent chance of living six more months. Now here it is, almost five years later, and Joey's still here. It is all due to Frank, who, early on, quit his job as vice president of a consulting firm in order to commit himself totally to his son. He is proud of everything he's given up and done, but he is tired. Part of him now really believes things are coming to a close, that this is the end. He says this without tears. There are no more tears.

"You have probably been through more than anyone else on this corridor," says the Mother.

"I could tell you stories," he says. There is a sour odor between them, and she realizes that neither of them has bathed for days.

"Tell me one. Tell me the worst one." She knows he hates his ex-wife and hates her new husband even more.

"The worst? They're all the worst. Here's one: one morning, I went out for breakfast with my buddy—it was the only time I'd left Joey alone ever; left him for two hours is all—and when I came back, his N-G tube was full of blood. They had the suction on too high, and it was sucking the guts right out of him."

"Oh my God. That just happened to us," said the Mother.

"It did?"

"Friday night."

"You're kidding. They let that happen again? I gave them such a chewing-out about that!"

"I guess our luck is not so good. We get your very worst story on the second night we're here."

"It's not a bad place, though."

"It's not?"

"Naw. I've seen worse. I've taken Joey everywhere."

"He seems very strong." Truth is, at this point, Joey seems like a zombie and frightens her.

"Joey's a fucking genius. A biological genius. They'd given him six months, remember."

The Mother nods.

"Six month is not very long," says Frank. "Six months is nothing. He was four and a half years old."

All the words are like blows. She feels flooded with affection and mourning for this man. She looks away, out the window, out past the hospital parking lot, up toward the black marbled sky and the electric eyelash of the moon. "And now he's nine," she says. "You're his hero."

"And he's mine," says Frank, though the fatigue in his voice seems to overwhelm him. "He'll be that forever. Excuse me," he says, "I've got to go check. His breathing hasn't been good. Excuse me."

* * * * *

"Good news and bad," says the Oncologist on Monday. He has knocked, entered the room, and now stands there. Their cots are unmade. One wastebasket is overflowing with coffee cups. "We've got the pathologist's report. The bad news is that the kidney they removed had certain lesions, called 'rests,' which are associated with a higher risk for disease in the other kidney. The good news is that the tumor is stage one, regular cell structure, and under five hundred grams, which qualifies you for a national experiment in which chemotherapy isn't done but your boy is monitored with ultrasound instead. It's not all that risky, given that the patient's watched closely, but here is the literature on it. There are forms to sign, if you decide to do that. Read all this and we can discuss it further. You have to decide within four days."

Lesions? Rests? They dry up and scatter like M&M's on the floor. All she hears is the part about no chemo. Another sigh of relief rises up in her and spills out. In a life where there is only the bearable and the unbearable, a sigh of relief is ecstasy.

"No chemo?" says the Husband. "Do you recommend that?"

The Oncologist shrugs. What casual gestures these doctors are permitted! "I know chemo. I like chemo," says the Oncologist. "But this is for you to decide. It depends how you feel."

The Husband leans forward. "But don't you think that now that we have the upper hand with this thing, we should keep going? Shouldn't we stomp on it, beat it, smash it to death with the chemo?"

The Mother swats him angrily and hard. "Honey, you're delirious!" She whispers, but it comes out as a hiss. "This is our lucky break!" Then she adds gently, "We don't want the Baby to have chemo."

The Husband turns back to the Oncologist. "What do *you* think?"

"It could be," he says, shrugging. "It could be that this is your lucky break. But you won't know for sure for five years."

The Husband turns back to the Mother. "Okay," he says. "Okay."

* * * * *

The Baby grows happier and strong. He begins to move and sit and eat. Wednesday morning, they are allowed to leave, and leave without chemo. The Oncologist looks a little nervous. "Are you nervous about this?" asks the Mother.

"Of course I'm nervous." But he shrugs and doesn't look that nervous. "See you in six weeks for the ultrasound," he says.

The Baby smiles, even toddles around a little, the sun bursting through the clouds, an angel chorus crescendoing. Nurses arrive. The Hickman is taken out of Baby's neck and chest; antibiotic lotion is dispensed. The Mother packs up their bags. The Baby sucks on a bottle of juice and does not cry.

"No chemo?" says one of the nurses. "Not even a *little* chemo?"

"We're doing watch and wait," says the Mother.

The other parents look envious but concerned. They have never seen any child get out of there with his hair and white blood cells intact.

"Will you be okay?" asks Ned's mother.

"The worry's going to kill us," says the Husband.

"But if all we have to do is worry," chides the mother, "every day for a hundred years, it'll be easy. It'll be nothing. I'll take all the worry in the world if it wards off the thing itself."

"That's right," says Ned's mother. "Compared to everything else, compared to all the actual events, the worry is nothing."

The Husband shakes his head, "I'm such an amateur," he moans.

"You're both doing admirably," says the other mother. "Your baby's lucky, and I wish you all the best."

The Husband shakes her hand warmly. "Thank you," he says. "You've been wonderful."

Another mother, the mother of Eric, comes up to them. "It's all very hard," she says, her head cocked to one side. "But there's a lot of collateral beauty along the way."

Collateral beauty? Who is entitled to such a thing? A child is ill. No one is entitled to any collateral beauty!

"Thank you," says the Husband.

Joey's father, Frank, comes up and embraces them both. "It's a journey," he says. He chucks the Baby on the chin. "Good luck, little man."

"Yes, thank you so much," says the Mother. "We hope things go well with Joey." She knows that Joey had a hard, terrible night.

Frank shrugs and steps back. "Gotta go," he says. "Good-bye!"

"Bye," she says, and then he is gone. She bites the inside of her lip, a bit tearily, then bends down to pick up the diaper bag, which is now stuffed with little animals; helium balloons are tied to its zipper. Shouldering the thing, the Mother feels she has just won a prize. All the parents have now vanished down the hall in the opposite direction. The Husband moves close. With one arm, he takes the Baby from her; with the other, he rubs her back. He can see she is starting to get weepy.

"Aren't these people nice? Don't you feel better hearing about their lives?" he asks.

Why does he do this, form clubs all the time; why does even this society of suffering soothe him? When it comes to death and dying, perhaps someone in this family ought to be more of a snob.

"All these nice people with their brave stories," he continues as they make their way toward the elevator bank, waving good-bye to the nursing staff as they go, even the Baby waving shyly. *Bye-bye! Bye-bye!* "Don't you feel consoled, knowing we're all in the same boat, that we're all in this together?"

But who on earth would want to be in this boat? the Mother thinks. This boat is a nightmare boat. Look where it goes: to a silver-and-white room, where, just before your eyesight and hearing and your ability to touch or be touched disappear entirely, you must watch your child die.

Rope! Bring on the rope.

"Let's make our own way," says the Mother, "and not in this boat."

Woman Overboard! She takes the Baby back from the Husband, cups the Baby's cheek in her hand, kisses his brow and then, quickly, his flowery mouth. The Baby's heart—she can hear it—drums with life. "For as long as I live," says the Mother, pressing the elevator button—up or down, everyone in the end has to leave this way—"I never want to see any of these people again."

* * * * *

There are the notes.

Now where is the money?

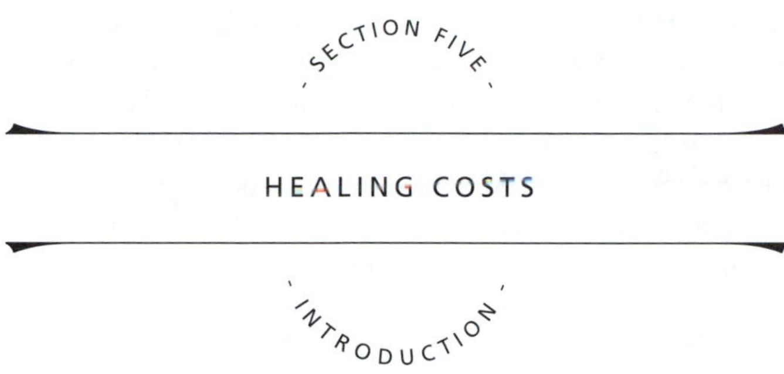

SECTION FIVE

HEALING COSTS

INTRODUCTION

This last section, devoted to the many kinds of costs associated with giving care, is of necessity more capacious and inclusive than any other section. It is enriched by the contributions of caregivers working and writing inside and outside the institutions of health care. The voices of those who examine themselves as professionals, acknowledging their fallibility as well as their exhilaration, their lapses, and their delights, provide proof of the value of language and of forms of literature as means for experiencing these costs as well as describing them. Again and again, caretakers turn to literary forms for their own sake as much as for the sake of others: capturing the ways of patients, the waywardness of imperfect understanding, laying bare the costs of denying care all depend on the power of literature itself.

One chapter from Marion Deutsche Cohen's extraordinarily candid account of her family's long experience with her husband's progressive multiple sclerosis appears in this section. But the full title of Cohen's volume (she is also a published poet and a teacher and scholar in the field of mathematics) makes clear the importance of the whole book—*dirty details: the days and nights of a well spouse.* Caring for those who suffer, whether acutely or chronically, takes a heavy toll. Those who care professionally struggle to preserve their equilibrium, sometimes at the apparent expense of their empathetic humanity. Those who care for family members or friends bear a heavy and difficult burden as well. An aspect of care, explored centuries ago by the great poet John Milton, concerns the individual's need to make something of illness or disability, to care for the new person, one's own self, who may come into existence through affliction; Milton shows this form of caring in his sonnet on his blindness. Large and powerful works which resist excerpting testify to this long-standing human responsibility; some of them are described in a final section recommending such works for all interested readers. In perhaps the most resonant recent investigation of the complexity of attempting to care, Anne Fadiman, in *The Spirit Catches You and You Fall Down,* brings readers into the troubling encounter between Hmong culture and Western medicine as both attempt to care for a stricken Hmong child.

In this section, contemporary issues about caring—the psychic, ethical, and financial assignment of resources—are addressed in works both recent and more distant in time. The special concerns of nurses receive close attention from Louisa May Alcott and Walt Whitman, both nurses in the American Civil War. The terrible responsibility for allocating scarce resources engages readers now who encounter Henri Barbusse's pre-World War One fable, "The Eleventh," which within a few poetic pages, encapsulates all the ethical implications of allocating care to some and not to all.

The still-evolving relations of doctors and nurses in their dealings with one another, with professional hierarchies, and with the larger world of health care administration inform the prizewinning work by Peter Baida, "A Nurse's Story," whose author died before it was selected as the year's best short story for the 1999 O. Henry Awards. In her volume of brief and evocative essays, *Kitchen Table Wisdom: Stories That Heal,* Rachel Naomi Remen, herself a doctor, illuminates the loneliness that those who try to heal may experience. Doctors, nurses, and companions speak candidly and movingly of the realities known to those who care. And in a remarkable book from almost half a century ago, Jan de Hartog documents the struggles, alienation, and piercing insight of workers, volunteers, and patients in a segregated hospital in the American South. In all these selections, the writers testify to the human costs and benefits of health care.

ADMISSION, CHILDREN'S UNIT

THEODORE DEPPE

Like the story of St. Lawrence that repelled me
when I heard it in high school, how he taught
his disciples to recognise the smell
of sin, then sent them in pairs through the Roman Empire,
separating good from evil, brother from brother.
Scrap of legend I'd forgotten until, interviewing a woman,
I drew my breath in and smelled
her, catching a scent that was there, then not there.

She said her son set fire to his room,
she'd found him fanning it with a comic, and what
should she have done? Her red hair
was pulled back in a braid, she tugged at its flames,
and what she'd done, it turns out, was hold her son
so her boyfriend could burn him with cigarettes.
The details didn't, of course, come out at first,
but I sensed them. The boy's refusal to take off his shirt.
His letting me, finally, lift it to his shoulders
and examine the six wounds, raised, ashy, second
or third degree, arranged in a cross.

Silence in the room, and then the mother blaming
the boyfriend, blaming the boy himself.
I kept talking to her in a calm voice, straining
for something I thought I smelled beneath
her cheap perfume, a scent—how can I describe this?—
as if something not physical had begun to rot.

I'd like to say all this happened when I first started
to work as a nurse, before I'd learned not to judge
the parents, but this was last week, the mother was crying,
I thought of handing her a box of tissues, and didn't.

When the Romans crucified Lawrence,
he asked Jesus to forgive him for judging others.
He wept on the cross because he smelled his own sin.

Sullen and wordless, the boy got up, brought his mother
the scented, blue Kleenex from my desk,
pressed his head into her side. Bunching
the bottom of her sweatshirt in both hands,
he anchored himself to her. Glared at me.
It took four of us to pry him from his mother's arms.

THE ELEVENTH

HENRI BARBUSSE

The Master, who had a pale head with long marble-like hair, and whose spectacles shone in solemnity, came to a standstill on his morning round opposite my little table at the door of Room 28, and condescended to announce to me that I was henceforth appointed to let in the ten poor people who every month were admitted to the hospitality of the House. Then he went on, so tall and so white among the assiduous flock of students that they seemed to be carrying a famous statuette from room to room.

I stammered the thanks which he did not hear. My 25-year-old heart felt a happy pride in reflecting that I had been chosen to preside in one of the noblest traditions of the House in which, a humble assistant, I was wandering lornly among wealthy invalids.

On the first day of every month the luxurious palace-hospital became the paradise of ten vagabonds. One of its outer doors was opened to admit the first ten who came, whoever they were, wherever they had fallen from or escaped. And for a whole month these ten human derelicts enjoyed the entire hospitality of the comfortable institution, just as much so as the Master's most valuable patients, as much as the arch-dukes and multi-millionaires. For them, too, were the lofty halls whose walls were not only white, but glistening, the huge corridors like covered streets, which in summer or in winter had the coolness or the mildness of spring. For them also, the immense garden beds set among green velvet, like bunches of flowers so enlarged by magic that one walked among them. For them equally, the outer walls, far off but impassable, which shield one against wide-open Space, against rambling roads, against the plains which come to an end no more than the sky. For thirty days the refugees busied themselves only with doing nothing, only worked when they ate, and were no longer afraid of the unknown or of the coming day. They who were remorseful learned to forget things, and they who were bereaved, to forget people.

When by chance they met each other, they simply had to turn their heads away hurriedly. There was not in all the House, by order of the Master, a mirror in which they would have found their bad dream again. At the day's end came the dormitory, peaceful as a cemetery, a nice cemetery, where one is not dead, where one waits—where one lives, but without knowing it.

At eight o'clock on the first day of the following month all ten of them went away, cast back into the world one by one, as into the sea. Immediately after, ten others entered, the first ten of the file which, since the night before, had been washed up against the wall of the house as upon the shores of an island. The first ten, no more, no less, no favours, no exceptions, no injustices; one rule only—they who had already been were never again admitted. The arrivals were asked nothing else—not even for the confession of their names.

And on the first day of the month, as soon as nine o'clock had sounded, exactly together from the Anglican church and the Catholic chapel of the House, I opened the little Poor-door.

A crowd of beings was massed against the door-wing and the wall. Hardly had the former turned in the shadow when the tattered heap rushed forward as though sucked in.

My helper had to throw himself forward to enforce a little order upon the greedy invasion. We had to detach by force, to tear away from the mass each one of the besiegers, who were pressed side by side and elbow to elbow, fastened to each other like fantastic friends. The eight entered, the ninth, the tenth.

And then the door was quickly closed, but not so quickly that it prevented me from seeing, only a step from me, him upon whom it closed, the eleventh, the unlucky one, the accursed.

He was a man of uncertain age; in his grey and withered face lack-lustre eyes floated. He looked at me so despairingly that he seemed to smile. The touch of that extraordinary disappointment made me start, of that face that was mute as a wound. I glimpsed in a flash—the time that the door took to shut—all the effort he had made to get there, even if too late, and how much he too deserved to come in!

Then I busied myself with the others; but a few minutes later, still affected by the distress I had read on the face of the outcast, I half opened the door to see if he were still there. No one. He and the three or four others—uncertain rags that had fluttered behind him—had gone to the four winds of heaven, carried away along the roads like dead leaves. A little shiver went through me, a shiver almost of mourning for the conquered.

At night, as I was falling asleep, my thoughts went again to them, and I wondered why they stayed there till the last moment, they who arrived only when ten had already taken their places at the door. What did they hope for? Nothing. Yet they were hoping all the same, and therein was a mean miracle of the heart.

We had reached the month of March. On the last day of the old month, towards nightfall, a rather frightened murmur crept from the side of the high road, close to the door. Leaning over a balcony, I could make men out there, stirring like insects. These were the supplicants.

The next morning we opened to these phantoms whom the magical story of the house had called across the world, who had awakened and unburied themselves from the lowest and most awful of depths to get there. We welcomed the ten who first came forward; we were obliged to drive back into life the eleventh.

He was standing, motionless, and offering himself from the other side of the door. I looked at him, and then lowered my eyes. He had a terrible look, with his hollow face and lashless eyelids. There breathed from him a reproach of unbearable artlessness.

When the door divided us forever, I regretted him, and should have liked to see him again. I turned towards the others, swarming in gladness on the flagstones, almost with resignation, wondering at my own firm conviction that the other, sooner than these, ought to have come in with us.

And it was so every time. Every time I became more indifferent to the crowd of admitted and satisfied, and devoted my gaze still more to him who was refused salvation. And every time he seemed to me the most pitiable case, and I felt that I was myself smitten in the person of the one condemned.

In June, it was a woman. I saw her understand and begin to cry. I trembled as I furtively scanned her; to crown all, the weeper's eyelids were blood-red as wounds.

In July, the appointed victim was incomparably regrettable by reason of his great age; and no living being was so compassionable as he who was repulsed the month after, so young was he. Another time, he who had to be snatched from the group of the elect besought me with his poor hands, encircled with the remains of frayed linen, like lint. The one whom Fate sacrificed the following month showed me a menacing fist. The entreaty of the one made me afraid, and the threat of the other pitiful.

I could almost have begged his pardon, the "eleventh" of October. He drew himself up stiffly; his neck was wrapped high in a grayish tie that looked like a bandage; he was thin, and his coat fluttered in the wind like a flag. But what could I have said to the unfortunate who succeeded him thirty days later? He blushed, stammered a nervous apology, and withdrew after bowing with tragic politeness—piteous remnant of an earlier lot.

And thus a year passed. Twelve times I let in the vagrants whom the stones had worn out, the workmen for whom all work was hopeless, the criminals subdued. Twelve times I let in some of those who clung to the stones of the wall as on to reefs of the sea coast. Twelve times I turned others away, similar ones, whom I confusedly preferred.

An idea beset me—that I was taking part in an abominable injustice. Truly there was no sense in dividing all those poor folk like that into friends and enemies. There was only one arbitrary reason—abstract, not admissible; a matter of a figure, a sign. At bottom, this was neither just nor even logical.

Soon I could no longer continue in this series of errors. I went to the Master, and begged him to give me some other post, so that I should not have to do the same evil deed again every month.

BAPTISM BY ROTATION

MIKHAIL BULGAKOV

As time passed in my country hospital, I gradually got used to the new way of life.

They were braking flax in the villages as they had always done, the roads were still impassable, and no more than five patients came to my daily surgery. My evenings were entirely free, and I spent them sorting out the library, reading surgical manuals and spending long hours drinking tea alone with the gently humming samovar.

For whole days and nights it poured with rain, the drops pounded unceasingly on the roof and the water cascaded past my window, swirling along the gutter and into a tub. Outside was slush, darkness and fog, through which the windows of the *feldsher's* house and the kerosene lantern over the gateway were no more than faint, blurred patches of light.

On one such evening I was sitting in my study with an atlas of topographical anatomy. The absolute silence was only disturbed by the occasional gnawing of mice behind the sideboard in the dining-room.

I read until my eyelids grew so heavy that they began to stick together. Finally I yawned, put the atlas aside and decided to go to bed. I stretched in pleasant anticipation of sleeping soundly to the accompaniment of the noisy pounding of the rain, then went across to my bedroom, undressed and lay down.

No sooner had my head touched the pillow than there swam hazily before me the face of Anna Prokhorova, a girl of seventeen from the village of Toropovo. She had needed a tooth extracting. Demyan Lukich, the *feldsher*, floated silently past holding a gleaming pair of pincers. Remembering how he always said "suchlike" instead of "such" because he was fond of a high-falutin' style, I smiled and fell asleep.

About half an hour later, however, I suddenly woke up as though I had been pinched, sat up, stared fearfully into the darkness and listened.

Someone was drumming loudly and insistently on the outer door and I immediately sensed that those knocks boded no good.

From *A Country Doctor's Notebook*. Trans. Michael Glenny. London: Harvil, 1975.

Then came a knock on the door of my quarters.

The noise stopped, there was a grating of bolts, the sound of the cook talking, an indistinct voice in reply, then someone came creaking up the stairs, passed quietly through the study and knocked on my bedroom door.

"Who is it?"

"It's me," came the reply in a respectful whisper. "Me, Aksinya, the nurse."

"What's the matter?"

"Anna Nikolaevna has sent for you. They want you to come to the hospital as quickly as possible."

"What's happened?" I asked, feeling my heart literally miss a beat.

"A woman has been brought in from Dultsevo. She's having a difficult labour."

"Here we go!" I thought to myself, quite unable to get my feet into my slippers. "Hell, the matches won't light. Ah well, it had to happen sooner or later. You can't expect to get nothing but cases of laryngitis or abdominal catarrh all your life."

"All right, go and tell them I'm coming at once!" I shouted as I got out of bed. Aksinya's footsteps shuffled away from the door and the bolt grated again. Sleep vanished in a moment. Hurriedly, with shaking fingers, I lit the lamp and began dressing. Half past eleven. . . . What could be wrong with this woman who was having a difficult birth? Malpresentation? Narrow pelvis? Or perhaps something worse. I might even have to use forceps. Should I send her straight into town? Out of the question! A fine doctor he is, they'll all say. In any case, I have no right to do that. No, I really must do it myself. But do what? God alone knows. It would be disastrous if I lost my head—I might disgrace myself in front of the midwives. Anyway, I must have a look first; no point in getting worried prematurely. . . .

I dressed, threw an overcoat over my shoulders, and hoping that all would be well, ran to the hospital through the rain across the creaking duckboards. At the entrance I could see a cart in the semi-darkness, the horse pawing at the rotten boards under its hooves.

"Did you bring the woman in labour?" I asked the figure lurking by the horse.

"Yes, that's right . . . we did, sir," a woman's voice replied dolefully.

Despite the hour, the hospital was alive and bustling. A flickering pressure-lamp was burning in the surgery. In a little passage leading to the delivery room Aksinya slipped past me carrying a basin. A faint moan came through the door and died away again. I opened the door and went into the delivery room. The small, whitewashed room was brightly lit by a lamp in the ceiling. On a bed alongside the operating table, covered with a blanket up to her chin, lay a young woman. Her face was contorted in a grimace of pain and wet strands of hair were sticking to her forehead. Holding a large thermometer, Anna Nikolaevna was preparing a solution in a graduated jug, while Pelagea Ivanovna was getting clean sheets out of the cupboard. The *feldsher* was leaning against the wall in a Napoleonic pose. Seeing me, they all jerked into life. The pregnant woman opened her eyes, wrung her hands and renewed her pathetic, long drawn-out groaning.

"Well now, what seems to be the trouble?" I asked, sounding confident.

"Transverse lie," Anna Nikolaevna answered promptly as she went on pouring water into the solution.

"I see-ee," I drawled, and added, frowning: "Well, let's have a look. . . ."

"Aksinya! Wash the doctor's hands!" snapped Anna Nikilaevna. Her expression was solemn and serious.

As the water flowed, rinsing away the lather from my hands, reddened from scrubbing, I asked Anna Nikolaevna a few trivial questions, such as when the woman had been brought in, where she was from. . . . Pelagea Ivanovna's hand turned back the blanket, I sat down on the edge of the bed and began gently feeling the swollen belly. The woman groaned, stretched, dug her fingers into her flesh and crumpled the sheet.

"There, there, relax . . . it won't take long," I said as I carefully put my hands to the hot, dry, distended skin.

The fact was that once the experienced Anna Nikolaevna had told me what was wrong, this examination was quite pointless. I could examine the woman as much as I liked, but I would not find out any more than Anna Nikolaevna knew already. Her diagnosis was, of course, correct: transverse lie. It was obvious. Well, what next?

Frowning, I continued palpating the belly on all sides and glanced sidelong at the midwives' faces. Both were watching with intense concentration and their looks registered approval of what I was doing. But although my movements were confident and correct, I did my best to conceal my unease as thoroughly as possible.

"Very well," I said with a sigh, standing up from the bed, as there was nothing more to be seen from an external examination. "Let's examine her internally."

Another look of approval from Anna Nikolaevna.

"Aksinya!"

More water flowed.

"Oh, if only I could consult Döderlein now!" I thought miserably as I soaped my hands. Alas, this was quite impossible. In any case, how could Döderlein help me at a moment like this? I washed off the thick lather and painted my fingers with iodine. A clean sheet rustled in Pelagea Ivanovna's hands and, bending down over the expectant mother, I began cautiously and timidly to carry out an internal examination. Into my mind came an involuntary recollection of the operating theatre in the maternity hospital. Gleaming electric lights in frosted-glass globes, a shining tiled floor, taps and instruments a-glitter everywhere. A junior registrar in a snow-white coat is manipulating the woman, surrounded by three intern assistants, probationers, and a crowd of students doing their practicals. Everything bright, well ordered and safe.

And there was I, all on my own, with a woman in agony on my hands and I was responsible for her. I had no idea, however, what I was supposed to do to help her, because I had seen childbirth at close quarters only twice in my life in a hospital, and both occasions were completely normal. The fact that I was conducting an examination was of no value to me or to the woman; I understood absolutely nothing and could feel nothing of what was inside her.

It was time to make some sort of decision.

"Transverse lie . . . since it's a transverse lie I must . . . I must. . . ."

"Turn it round by the foot," muttered Anna Nikolaevna as though thinking aloud, unable to restrain herself.

An older, more experienced doctor would have looked askance at her for butting in, but I am not the kind to take offense.

"Yes," I concurred gravely, "a podalic version."

The pages of Döderlein flickered before my eyes. Internal method. . . . Combined method. . . . External method. . . . Page after page, covered in illustrations. A pelvis; twisted, crushed babies with enormous heads . . . a little dangling arm with a loop on it.

Indeed I had read it not long ago and had underlined it, soaking up every word, mentally picturing the interrelationship of every part of the whole and every method. And as I read it I imagined that the entire text was being imprinted on my brain forever.

Yet now only one sentence of it floated back into my memory:

"A transverse lie is a wholly unfavorable position."

Too true. Wholly unfavorable both for the woman and for a doctor who only qualified six months ago.

"Very well, we'll do it," I said as I stood up.

Anna Nikolaevna's expression came to life.

"Demyan Lukich," she turned to the *feldsher,* "get the chloroform ready."

It was a good thing that she had said so, because I was still not certain whether the operation was supposed to be done under anesthesia or not! Of course, under anesthesia—how else?

Still, I must have a look at Döderlein. . . .

As I washed my hands I said:

"All right, then . . . prepare her for anesthesia and make her comfortable. I'll be back in a moment; I must just go to my room and fetch some cigarettes."

"Very good, doctor, we'll be ready by the time you come back," replied Anna Nikolaevna.

I dried my hands, the nurse threw my coat over my shoulders and without putting my arms into the sleeves I set off for home at a run.

In my study I lit the lamp and, forgetting to take off my cap, rushed straight to the bookcase.

There it was—Döderlein's *Operative Obstetrics.* I began hastily to leaf through the glossy pages.

> ". . . version is always a dangerous operation for the mother. . . ."

A cold shiver ran down my spine.

> "The chief danger lies in the possibility of a spontaneous rupture of the uterus. . . ."

Spon-tan-e-ous. . . .

> "If in introducing his hand into the uterus the obstetrician encounters any hindrances to penetrating to the foot, whether from lack of space or as a result of a contraction of the uterine wall, he should refrain from further attempts to carry out the version. . . ."

Good. Provided I am able, by some miracle, to recognize these "hindrances" and I refrain from "further attempts," what, might I ask, am I then supposed to do with an anaesthetized woman from the village of Dultsevo?

Further:

> "It is absolutely impermissible to attempt to reach the feet by penetrating behind the back of the fetus. . . ."

Noted.

> "It must be regarded as erroneous to grasp the upper leg, as doing so may easily result in the fetus being revolved too far; this can cause the fetus to suffer a severe blow, which can have the most deplorable consequences. . . ."

"Deplorable consequences." Rather a vague phrase, but how sinister. What if the husband of the woman from Dultsevo is left a widower? I wiped the sweat from my brow, rallied my strength and disregarded all the terrible things that could go wrong, trying only to remember the absolute essentials: what I had to do, where and how to put my hands. But as I ran my eye over the lines of black print, I kept encountering new horrors. They leaped out at me from the page.

> ". . . in view of the extreme danger of rupture . . ."
> ". . . the internal and combined methods must be classified as among the most dangerous obstetric operations to which a mother can be subjected . . ."

And the grand finale:

> ". . . with every hour of delay the danger increases . . ."

That was enough. My reading had borne fruit: my head was in a complete muddle. For a moment I was convinced that I understood nothing, and above all that I had no idea what sort of version I was going to perform: combined, bi-polar, internal, external. . . .

I abandoned Döderlein and sank into an armchair, struggling to reduce my random thoughts to order. Then I glanced at my watch. Hell! I had already spent twenty minutes in my room, and they were waiting for me.

> ". . . with every hour of delay . . ."

Hours are made up of minutes, and at times like this the minutes fly past at insane speed. I threw Döderlein aside and ran back to the hospital.

Everything there was ready. The *feldsher* was standing over a little table preparing the anesthetic mask and the chloroform bottle. The expectant mother already lay on the operating table. Her ceaseless moans could be heard all over the hospital.

"There now, be brave," Pelagea Ivanovna muttered consolingly as she bent over the woman, "the doctor will help you in a moment."

"Oh, no! I haven't the strength. No . . . I can't stand it!"

"Don't be afraid," whispered the midwife. "You'll stand it. We'll just give you something to sniff, and then you won't feel anything."

Water gushed noisily from the taps as Anna Nikolaevna and I began washing and scrubbing our arms bared to the elbow. Against a background of groans and screams Anna Nikolaevna described to me how my predecessor, an experienced surgeon, had performed versions. I listened avidly to her, trying not to miss a single word. Those ten minutes told me more than everything I had read on obstetrics for my qualifying exams, in which I had actually passed the obstetrics paper "with distinction." From her brief remarks, unfinished sentences and passing hints I learned the essentials which are not to be found in any textbooks. And by the time I had begun to dry the perfect whiteness and cleanliness of my hands with sterile gauze, I was seized with confidence and a firm and absolutely definite plan had formed in my mind. There was simply no need to bother any longer over whether it was to be a combined or bi-polar version.

None of these learned words meant anything at that moment. Only one thing mattered: I had to put one hand inside, assist the version with the other hand from outside and without relying on books but on common sense, without which no doctor is any good, carefully but firmly bring one foot downwards and pull the baby after it.

I had to be calm and cautious yet at the same time utterly decisive and unfaltering.

"Right, off you go," I instructed the *feldsher* as I began painting my fingers with iodine.

At once Pelagea Ivanovna folded the woman's arms and the *feldsher* clamped the mask over her agonized face. Chloroform slowly began to drip out of the dark yellow glass bottle, and the room started to fill with the sweet nauseous odor. The expressions of the *feldsher* and midwives hardened with concentration, as though inspired. . . .

"Haaa! Ah!" The woman suddenly shrieked. For a few seconds she writhed convulsively, trying to force away the mask.

"Hold her!"

Pelagea Ivanovna seized her by the arms and lay across her chest. The woman cried out a few more times, jerking her face away from the mask. Her movements slowed down, although she mumbled dully:

"Oh . . . let me go . . . ah. . . ."

She grew weaker and weaker. The white room was silent. The translucent drops continued to drip, drip, drip on to the white gauze.

"Pulse, Pelagea Ivanovana?"

"Firm."

Pelagea Ivanovna raised the woman's arm and let it drop: as lifeless as a leather thong, it flopped on to the sheet. Removing the mask, the *feldsher* examined the pupil of her eye.

"She's asleep."

* * * * *

A pool of blood. My arms covered in blood up to the elbows. Bloodstains on the sheets. Red clots and lumps of gauze. Pelagea Ivanovna shaking and slapping the baby, Aksinya rattling buckets as she poured water into basins.

The baby was dipped alternately into cold and hot water. He did not make a sound, his head flopping lifelessly from side to side as though on a thread. Then suddenly there came a noise somewhere between a squeak and a sigh, followed by the first weak, hoarse cry.

"He's alive . . . alive . . ." mumbled Pelagea Ivanovna as she laid the baby on a pillow.

And the mother was alive. Fortunately nothing had gone wrong. I felt her pulse. Yes, it was firm and steady; the *feldsher* gently shook her by the shoulder as he said:

"Wake up now, my dear."

The bloodstained sheets were thrown aside and the mother hastily covered with a clean one before the *feldsher* and Aksinya wheeled her away to the ward. The swaddled baby was borne away on his pillow, the brown, wrinkled little face staring out from its white wrapping as he cried ceaselessly in a thin, pathetic whimper.

Water gushing from the taps of the sluice. Anna Nikolaevna coughed as she dragged hungrily at a cigarette.

"You did the version well, doctor. You seemed very confident." Scrubbing furiously at my hands, I glanced sidelong at her: Was she being sarcastic? But no, her expression was a sincere one of pride and satisfaction. My heart was brimming with joy. I glanced round at the white and bloodstained disorder, at the red water in the basin and felt that I had won. But somewhere deep down there wriggled a worm of doubt.

"Let's wait and see what happens now," I said.

Anna Nikolaevna turned to look at me in astonishment.

"What can happen? Everything's all right."

I mumbled something vague in reply. What I had meant to say was to wonder whether the mother was really safe and sound, whether I might not have done her some harm during the operation . . . the thought nagged dully at my mind. My knowledge of obstetrics was so vague, so fragmentary and bookish. What about a rupture? How would it show? And when would it show—now or, perhaps, later? Better not talk about that.

"Well, almost anything," I said. "The possibility of infection cannot be ruled out," I added, repeating the first sentence from some textbook that came into my mind.

"Oh, tha-at," Anna Nikolaevna drawled complacently. "Well, with luck nothing of that sort will happen. How could it, anyway? Everything here is clean and sterile."

It was after one o'clock when I went back to my room. In a pool of light on the desk in my study lay Döderlein open at the page headed "Dangers of Version." For another hour after that, sipping my cooling tea, I sat over it, turning the pages. And an interesting thing happened: all the previously obscure passages became entirely comprehensible, as though they had been flooded with light; and there, at night, under the lamplight in the depth of the countryside I realized what real knowledge was.

"One can gain a lot of experience in a country practice," I thought as I fell asleep, "but even so one must go on and on reading, reading . . . more and more. . . ."

WHAT THE NURSE LIKES

CORTNEY DAVIS

I like looking into patients' ears
and seeing what they can never see.

It's like owning them.

I like patients' honesty—
they trust me with simple things:
  They wake at night and count heartbeats.
  They search for lumps.

I am also afraid.

* * * * *

I like the way women look at me
and feel safe.
Then I lean across them
and they smell my perfume.

I like the way men become shy.
Even angry men bow their heads
when they are naked.

* * * * *

I like lifting a woman's hair
to place stethoscope to skin,
the way everyone breathes differently—

the way men make suggestive groans
when I listen to their hearts.

From *Between the Heartbeats: Poetry and Prose by Nurses,* edited by Cortney Davis and Judy Schaefer (Iowa City: University of Iowa Press, 1994): 49–51. Reprinted by permission of the author.

I like eccentric patients:
Old women who wear purple knit hats
and black eyeliner. Men
who put makeup over their age spots.

* * * * *

I like talking about patients
as if they aren't real, calling them
"the fracture" or "the hysterectomy."

It makes illness seem trivial.

I like saying
You shouldn't smoke!
You must have this test!

I like that patients don't always
do what I say.

* * * * *

I like the way we stop the blood,
pump the lungs,
turn hearts off and on with electricity.

I don't like when it's over
and I realize

I know nothing.

* * * * *

I like being the one to give bad news;
I am not embarrassed by grief.

I like the way patients gather their hearts,
their bones, their arms and legs
that have spun away momentarily.

At the end of the gathering they sigh
and look up.

* * * * *

I like how dying patients become beautiful.

Their eyes concentrate light. Their skin
becomes thin and delicate as fog.
Nothing matters anymore
but sheets, pain, a radio, the time of day.

*****

I like watching patients die.

First they are living,
then something comes up from within
and moves from them.

They become vacant and yet
their bodies are heavy
and sink into the sheets.

I like how emptiness is seen first
in the eyes, then in the hands.

*****

I like taking care of patients
and I like forgetting them,

going home and sitting on my porch
while they stand away from me
talking among themselves.

I like how they look back
when I turn their way.

THE HOSPITAL

JAN DE HARTOG

How to describe the rapture of mercy? Like love, it is a state of ecstasy, universal and incommunicable, presenting itself to each individual in an utterly exclusive way. Compassion in action is as deeply emotional and all-transforming as love; it takes over your life, pervades your thoughts, makes your other activities and preoccupations seem secondary to that one overpowering urge: to help the helpless, to dispel darkness.

Even as I write this, I find it acutely embarrassing. I reached intellectual maturity in an age that was obsessed by the compulsion to debunk the sublime. Irrevocably conditioned by the intellectual tradition in which I grew up, I still have an instinctive sensation of truth only when a noble act is unmasked as the effect of ignoble subconscious causes. My life long, the words "charity" and "love" have been suspect, whereas the words "repression" and "libido" inspired confidence. I know, objectively, that a group of present-day analysts explaining the adult activities of Jesus as the outcome of his pre-adolescent predilection for anal eroticism is as grotesque as a group of their colleagues in the Middle Ages trying to determine how many angels could be comfortably seated on a needle's point. Subjectively, because I am part of a generation that must forever mistrust the sublime, I am ready to be convinced by psychoanalysts but never by theologians. So I am prepared to believe an analysis of my compulsion to go back into those little dark wards to mess with the sick and the dying as sublimated lust, and will forever refute the taint of saintliness. At the same time, I am sure that the patients in the Emergency Room did not care whether I helped them on the bedpan or gave them a bedbath out of fecal voyeurism or a thirst for beatification, as long as I did it kindly and expertly. And while I was on the floor I myself could not care less.

From that first day on, the hospital became my prime concern, my life. Even during my work at the University, my lectures, my hours of research and preparation, part of me was preoccupied with patients left behind, tasks to be finished, techniques of nursing to be mastered, bureaucratic obstacles to be circumvented. At first, I went one day a week, then two, finally I took on as many odd hours as I could spare, which amounted to my virtually holding down two jobs, one at the University, one in the hospital.

I began to feel I was getting familiar with the work when I began to sort out all those bewildering initials: IV bottles for Intra Venous feeding, DOA Room for Dead On Arrival, BP for Blood Pressure, EKG for Electrocardiogram, OB for Obstetrics ward, Pedi for Pediatrics, GYN for Gynecological Section, OR for Operating Room, LVN for Licensed Vocational Nurse (a practical nurse with one year's training), and DT'S for Delirium Tremens. The more familiar with the work I became, the more hours I spent at it. The end result was that I spent very little time at home.

It was a lucky circumstance that Marjorie became afflicted by the same compulsion. She and Priscilla had managed, after weeks of dutiful typing behind a desk in OB, to overcome the suspicion of the supervisor of the Newborn Nursery by never failing to turn up at the appointed hour, never complaining, yet making it plain that they sat there in Mrs. Willoughby's mother hubbards only in order to wangle their way into the nursery to help with the babies. Then, one night, the supervisor called on them because one of the nurses had failed to turn up and there were nearly eighty newborn babies to be fed and changed. Once inside the nursery, they stayed there, be it clandestinely. Marjorie became as engrossed in the new arrivals as I in the weary travelers at the other end of the road of life.

A surprising result of my working there was that very soon I no longer stopped to consider whether conditions in the hospital were normal or abnormal, acceptable or unacceptable; to look after the patients in Observation became my sole job and the challenge was so overwhelming that it excluded all abstract considerations. The most critical shortage in the hospital, I discovered, was the lack of staff. This had as a first effect the dissociation of the individual from the team. To ask someone else to do something for you cost more time than to do it yourself, and before you knew it you were a lone wolf. Anything that put itself between you and your objective, whether you were on your way with a bedpan to the hopper or going to the laundry to wheedle blankets out of them or scrounging for pillow slips, of which there was an eternal shortage, your instinctive reaction was to sidestep it and sneak past. This went for obstacles of every kind, but mainly for people. When faced with a shortage of pillow slips you could improvise by using sheets; if you found a drainage set had broken down you took another, and if that one turned out to be broken down too you got a third; but when you got into a conflict with a person, it was going to be time-consuming unless you managed to fade away while the other was bawling you out. And we had some powerful bawlers in Emergency.

There were, first of all, the doctors. Four of them made up the staff for each shift: a surgical resident, a medical resident and two interns. At nighttime and during weekends these were supplemented by more interns and medical students; on Saturday nights there occasionally were as many as a dozen doctors about. Even so, the Emergency Room turned out to be understaffed during those peak periods.

All doctors, even the residents, were young. The chief resident in charge of the Emergency Room, whom we rarely saw, could not be older than in his early thirties. He was an unapproachable young man, called in whenever there was a conflict, never to view a case. He always turned up in either shirtsleeves or a jacket, never in a white coat. I had no idea what kind of man he was, but in his impersonal remoteness he became identified in my mind with the prevailing attitude of the doctors toward their patients. All patients, regardless of age or sex, were addressed by their first name, or failing that by "Buddy" or "Honey." On principle, so it seemed, no one was called "Mister" or "Miss" by the doctors. The entire medical staff of the hospital was furnished by Baylor University, so this was perhaps a ruling imposed by the school. But in practice of the Emergency Room it set a tone of callousness. As most of the doctors were Texans or Southerners, they already had a paternalistic attitude at best toward the Negro patients delivered into their care; under the pressure of their overwhelming numbers, this attitude deteriorated in many cases into contempt.

After my first weekend in Emergency, I could understand why that was so. I saw, to my incredulous astonishment, the place that I had known for two days as a busy clinic, with the occasional interruption of a Shock Room case after a car accident or a shooting, change into a slaughterhouse. I had never seen anything like it, I had not even known that anything like this went on anywhere in the world. Around seven o'clock on Friday night the ambulances started to arrive screaming at the entrance in ever-increasing numbers, disgorging a writhing load of bleeding humanity. Car wrecks, stabbings, shootings, suicides, bottle fights, muggings, abortions, rapings, delirium tremens—within an hour the corridor was choked with stretchers, all the tables in the Suture Rooms were occupied, the rooms themselves jammed with additional stretchers. A dozen doctors tried frantically to keep up with the ever-mounting number of wounds waiting to be sewn up; by ten o'clock there was not a free stretcher left in the whole hospital, all the beds in Observation were occupied with moaning, wailing, cursing or unconscious bodies, most of them ditched there in a hurry, fully dressed, by running orderlies. Additional stretchers were jammed between the beds as the tide of violence and trauma mounted to its peak around two o'clock in the morning.

By then, the place was a chaos. The floors were slippery with blood and vomit, littered with soiled linen, dropped instruments, discarded bottles of Novocaine, torn gloves, paper wrappers of sterile gauze flats and the blood-soaked flats themselves, dropped regardless after the litter baskets had started to overflow. There had been no time to clean the stretchers between patients; blood-soiled mattresses had been flipped over and hastily covered with another sheet, as long as there were sheets. After that they were not even turned over any more; each man lay in the blood of his predecessor. It was a battlefield, monstrous and unimaginable; my overriding emotion was, in the end, an incredulous horror at what human beings could do to one another. Muggings, knifings, mutilations—the night had been a spine-chilling procession of viciousness and cruelty.

As the majority of the victims were Negro, it was asking too much of young Southern white males, already preconditioned by a tradition of racial superiority, to regard the screaming, cursing, vicious creatures whose sprees of bestial brutality ended on the blood-soaked tables in the Emergency Room at dead of night as their brothers, or even as human beings. To remain impervious to the obscene abuse with which some of the raving patients reacted to being strapped down on table or stretcher to have their wounds sewn up became a triumph of mature, humane detachment. To hear oneself accused of criminally assaulting one's own mother while trying to patch up the results of subhuman brutality and not to slap the foul-mouthed bastard in the teeth made the young white physician feel like a paragon of patience, while to deaden the bastard's laceration with an injection of Novocaine before suturing it, so as not to cause him any pain, became an act of unworldly saintliness.

After my first experience of the weekly slaughter I understood why some of the doctors could not bring themselves to define their male Negro patients as "men" but consistently referred to them as "bucks." This word even had a connotation of good-natured indulgence; when the going got really rough, they referred to them as "slobs," "toads," or "spooks." Understaffed, underequipped, taunted by bureaucratic bottlenecks in supplies and housekeeping, their contempt became dignity, their very presence an act of charity.

It was, of course, so they told themselves, a necessary part of their education. The Emergency Room at J.D. was the best school in suturing a man could have in peacetime. Nowhere in the South, with the possible exception of New Orleans, could a young physician expect such a generous and constant supply of stabbed, shot, fractured, lacerated, burnt and otherwise insulted living tissue for this training; and only in that context could he let himself be taunted, defiled and spat upon by the very creatures whose suffering he tried to alleviate. To accord human status to these "toads" and "spooks" was incompatible with any civilized concept of humanity. The only way to accept them was to consider them purely as "cases."

The traumatic nights of those weekends and Christian holidays formed the key to the general attitude of the doctors toward their patients in ER and indeed the whole hospital. The very reasonableness of this communal attitude made a few solitary individuals among the residents and the interns even more impressive in their humanity.

There was, for instance, Dr. Miller, the Medical Resident in ER, a thin, stoop-shouldered, bespectacled young man in his late twenties, so gentle, patient and exhausted that he already had the shuffling gait of an old man. His high-domed forehead under the prematurely receding hair was constantly furrowed with a frown of concern. In a corner of the doctor's desk stood a forgotten cookie tin containing sandwiches, candy bars and an apple, prepared by his wife, whom he must have promised solemnly every morning that he would eat it, between meals, whenever he had a chance. He never did; usually he remembered only at the last moment to take the tin with him when he left at the end of his shift, and distributed its contents among the patients in Observation so as to take it home empty. He was a man of infinite kindness and compassion. As Medical Resident he mainly looked after patients from the Emergency Clinic, but when the usual bloodbath during the weekends became hectic he was there, suturing with the rest. My first Saturday night would have been a night in hell if he had not been there, tranquil and gentle amidst the gore and the obscenities. I was running from room to room, breaking open new suture trays, setting them up, filling the little cups with Mecressin, Creomycin and Novocaine and the irrigation basins with saline. In every room, in the corridor, even in the passage to Observation, doctors were calling angrily for 3-0 Nylon, 4-0 Silk, 3-0 Plain, 6-0 Dermalon, sterile flats, sterile towels, hemostats; it was a madhouse of disjointed, frenetic activity. In the midst of it all sat Dr. Miller, suturing with infinite care the laceration in the forehead of a woman injured in a car wreck. He worked with such delicate tenderness that his sewing of her wound was gentler than the way her husband threw on her prostrate body the clean dress that he had gone home to fetch. During the week, battered and buffeted by an unending stream of human misery, visibly wilting toward the end of each grueling shift, his patience and concern with each individual patient acquired the stature of saintliness. At the end of my third day I was present in the room where he found himself confronted with an eighty-nine-year-old woman, blind and deaf, who had been delivered early that morning by a Negro orderly from one of the unspeakable private nursing homes that proliferated all over the city. The orderly had left her in the hall without registering her; when he called back to collect her at midnight he refused to wait while she was seen by a doctor; she had stayed in the waiting room overnight and all next day. It was this harassed old creature, stunned and insulted by inhumanity and neglect, that Dr. Miller found himself faced with that night. Both he and she were utterly exhausted, but undefeated; the result was a weird stage dialogue.

"How old are you, Miss Evans?"

"One fifteen Fraternity Drive."

"HOW OLD?"

"Hattie. Hattie Evans."

"HOW OLD?"

"Don't shout. I can hear. Her name was Fran, Francis Holmes. She has been dead sixty-nine years, what do you want her name for? I have a pain on the top of my head. Why don't you look at it?"

"Where in your head?"

A resigned sigh. "One hundred and fifteen Fraternity Drive. It's a nursing home."

A resigned sigh. "How am I supposed to find out what's ailing an eighty-nine-year-old woman who is both blind and deaf? Let's put her in a bed. I'll have to work her up completely, sometime tonight." As he left, he shyly patted her shoulder, unforgettable gesture of unity in defeat.

During the first days, Dr. Miller did not quite know how to approach me, which bothered me as much as it did him. The unspoken load was finally lifted from our minds when he proffered his lunch tin one day, saying, "Please, Mr. Volunteer, take the candy bar. I couldn't eat another bite."

I accepted it gratefully, realizing what it symbolized, although I couldn't eat another bite either. We had just come out of the Shock Room, where we had been attending, with half a dozen others, to a Negro girl whose leg had been severed by a train. The surgical resident had completed the severance; Mrs. Kowalski had taken a paper bag, written on it in prim nurses' handwriting: FANNY BACKUS, ONE SHOE WITH FOOT, put the foot inside, folded it shut and bidden me take it to the front desk. When I showed the bag to the normally unbending ladies of Reception, they screamed, asked furiously if I had gone crazy, and told me to take it out of there and to the Morgue, where it belonged.

I had never been to the Morgue before, though I had passed its door several times on my way through the basement to the laundry. Occasionally I had seen a stretcher waiting outside, with a still form covered by a sheet. This was the first time I had opened the door, after knocking on it absurdly and waiting for an answer. As I opened it, a strong smell of formaldehyde and a blast of icy cold hit me with unnerving force. In the half light, I saw a cellar-like room with concrete walls and floor. A stretcher with a man-sized steel tray on it stood in the middle of the floor, empty but for a pool of blood. In the corner I saw a heavily insulated door behind which, so I realized, lay the real Morgue, next to it a stack of paper bags, with names written on them. I added my bag to the stack; as I did so I read on one of them, "Hood, Albert," and a number. Where had I heard that name before? Then I saw, in my memory, the old man sitting up on his stretcher in the corridor that first day, his feet black with necrosis, his deformed hand clutching a dirty aspirin; and I heard Mrs. Judd's cheerful voice, "Hey, Mr. Hood! How are you? What brings you to us this time?"

I hastily closed the door and crossed the hall, to lean over the Dutch door of the laundry room and call, "Hello there! Anything for Emergency?" I knew that the women in the white aprons and old-fashioned maids' caps would shake their heads and shout over the noise of machinery, "No, nothing!" for I had collected a full trolley an hour before. I did it only to fill my lungs with the smell of clean linen, and because the head laundress was a jolly, bare-armed person whose grin and bawdy wink never failed to cheer me.

Mrs. Kowalski, the head nurse who had sent me off to the reception desk with that gruesome bag, knowing full well what the result would be, seemed to fit in much better with the prevailing attitude in ER than Mrs. Judd. She was an immensely capable nurse, on her feet without respite for the full eight hours of her shift; but at first sight one would never expect her to do a stroke of work as she had without any doubt the sexiest walk in the building. She never actually walked, let alone ran; she strolled with a sinuous, subtly seductive gait that went well with her flaming red bouffant hair, her striking black eyes and her Junoesque figure. But it went not at all with the broken-down stretchers full of desolate humanity, the benches crowded with wheezing, gasping asthma sufferers, the old, sagging beds with the drunk, the delirious, the dying and the dead in the darkness of the Observation wards. The way she applied tourniquets, put in IV's, took blood pressures or prepped a patient in the Shock Room was impressive in its perfectly controlled, casual craftmanship. But to see her deal with any patients other than those in shock or convulsions was chilling, because of her cold, detached objectivity. She disturbed me deeply when, for the first time, I witnessed her reaction to a spine-tingling scream of torment from the darkness of the Observation Ward. There was no reaction whatever; I was sure she had not heard it, or she would not be sitting there like that, it had raised the hair on the nape of my neck.

"Mrs. Kowalski," I ventured. "I believe someone is calling in there. . . ."

She answered, without looking up from the record she was reading, with that mincing drawl of sensual boredom, "Oh, I always ignore their first call, Mr. de Hartog."

One of the doctors, sitting next to her at the desk, said casually, "If you ask me, that was his last."

"All right, Mr. de Hartog," Mrs. Kowalski said, acidly and precisely, closing the record and slipping it back into its box with a somehow provocative gesture. "Why don't you go and have a look at Mr. Borkus and see what he wants this time?" Then she got up and strolled away, riveting the gaze of all males in sight, old and young, sick and healthy, on the fascinating double motion of her magnificent behind.

I had, on one early and embarrassing occasion, come out of Observation and asked her, "Mrs. Kowalski, is the lady in the corner with the broken arm allowed liquids?" She had calmly finished what she was writing, then slowly raised her eyes and fixed me with a gaze so mortifying that I felt like beating a retreat even before she asked, with that veiled seductive voice that carried a mile, "What lady with a broken arm are you referring to, Mr. de Hartog?"

I said, "Well, the lady in the corner. The one with the splint, I mean. . . ."

She gazed at me pensively, but the disturbing thing was that she was gazing at my upper lip, as if trying to determine what I would look like with a mustache. Then she said, in the breathless silence she had by then created, "I hear you are a writer, Mr. de Hartog. Is that so?"

I muttered, "Yes, but. . . ."

"Well, Mr. de Hartog," she said, charmingly, "one of these days I am going to write a book about *you.* That is not a splint the lady is wearing, that is an IV board." She gave me a small smile, turned back to her writing and added, as an afterthought, "And patients with IV's are, as a rule, not allowed liquids."

It must have been more than forty years ago that I had last blushed; not since my schooldays had I felt such powerless hatred, mixed with equally powerless admiration, for any woman alive. The outrageous circumstance was that I was old enough to be her father, although she inspired me with unfatherly thoughts. After that incident, whenever she spied me in any situation other than carrying a fainted patient or running with a stack of bedpans like a waiter, she would call me with that infuriating inflection of polite condescension of which she had the infernal secret, and ask me to do something that always turned out to be slightly degrading, even for the lowest form of human life in the Emergency Room. "Oh, Mr. de Hartog, the intercom has broken down; would you please stand at the entrance to the corridor and call through the names to the patients in the waiting room as the doctors ask for them?" Or "Mr. de Hartog, Housekeeping has gone to lunch and we have, in Suture Room Number Two, that overweight lady with explosive diarrhea. Could you do something about her, with a sheet perhaps?" I would not have minded either assignment had they been given me by anyone else; but she managed, by her very tone, to make the prospect of my bellowing names between the hall and the waiting room sound entertaining, while the idea of a middle-aged intellectual nervously trying to do something about an overweight lady with explosive diarrhea with a sheet, seemed to promise a *corrida* hilarious enough to attract a crowd.

The difference between Mrs. Judd and Mrs. Kowalski was typified in the way they administered an injection. Mrs. Judd, victim of compassion and afflicted with a sense of identification, would announce to the patient, as she rubbed the spot on his arm, "Now you're going to feel just a little pinprick, nothing at all." But the very fact of her personal concern made her prediction sound dire; when she gave the shot it would invariably result in a squeal, occasionally some patient with a natural talent for the stage would carry his theatrical reaction to the point of passing out. Mrs. Kowalski always made a point of talking to someone else while she was rubbing her victim's arm for the injection. "Oh, Mr. de Hartog, I hate to bother you with this, but would you mind having a look at the patients' toilet in Observation? I believe there's someone in there who hasn't come out for a number of hours." The mouth of her prey would fall open at this; while he or she stood gaping at me with a growing mental picture of what awaited me when I opened the door of the patients' toilet, Mrs. Kowalski would give the arm a sharp little blow with the side of her hand, like cops on TV who know karate. Her patient would swing round, crying, "Hey, listen! What do you think you are doing?" By then he had received his injection; the only drawback was that people afterward would stubbornly maintain they had *not* had their tetanus shot.

Mrs. Kowalski could perform technical feats of nursing that would have dazzled an audience in the days of vaudeville. She could change the sheets of a bed with a two-hundred-pound unconscious patient in it faster than two male orderlies combined, and she would emerge from this record performance with not a hair out of place, her face unflushed, her lips puckered in that small supercilious pout of boredom that could irritate her subordinates to screaming point, and reduce raving lunatics to performing lambs, producing their specimen cartons of urine submissively, on command. I disliked her heartily, until one day, when I happened to be the only one around, she asked me to help her restrain a deluded white woman who was screaming abuse in the Observation Ward. The moment the woman saw the red-headed pin-up enter her distorted field of vision, she began to screech insults at her. "You little nigger prostitute!" she screamed. "I saw you, you filthy slut! I saw you with those niggers, behind the diner!" Mrs. Kowalski frowned; I expected her to silence the poor soul expertly. To my amazement she stepped quietly back into the shadows, but stayed around to see whether I would need any help. The woman calmed down; when I joined her in the shadows, Mrs. Kowalski said, "This is a sad place, Mr. de Hartog. We have a great responsibility, haven't we?" Then she strolled away languidly, without waiting for my answer.

One of the people I liked best in Emergency was an elderly vocational nurse called Mrs. Birdland. She was an angelic woman, who ministered to the sick and the lonely in Observation with the soothing fussiness of a grandmother. She was probably no great shakes at the finer technical aspects of nursing, but she richly made up for any lack she might have had in that direction by giving each of her patients the feeling of being individually cared for. Mrs. Kowalski, her black eyes flashing Wagnerian lightning, would always manage to bag the scurrying, short-legged form of the fleeing Mrs. Birdland with a thunderbolt, whenever she had done something wrong. "Mrs. Birdland!" she would call, with the carrying power of the Last Trump. "Could you give me the vital signs of the gentleman in bed number nine again, please? According to your treatment sheet he is dead." The gentleman in No. 9 would, more likely than not, be happily asleep behind his curtain, soothed into slumber at last by Mrs. Birdland's homely ministrations. It seemed a shame to have him waked up from his first sleep by his ministering angel in a high state of fluster, fussing with inflatable cuffs, pressure gauges and stethoscopes in which, so she once confided to me, her eyes round with alarm, she sometimes heard music as she tried to listen to the pulse beat in the crease of a patient's arm. I liked working with Mrs. Birdland, but she was often pulled to other parts of the hospital by the Nursing Office during moments of calm in Emergency. On those occasions I was left alone with Miss Jennie, the Negro cleaning woman.

Miss Jennie had taught me how to fold sheets fresh from the laundry to the proper format before stacking them on the shelves in Observation. She was the only one who folded them that way; during other shifts they were flung onto the shelves by the armful by whoever happened to stop by to grab a few out of the trolley. She made me refold them, regulation fashion, and when it came to making beds she was harder to satisfy than a sergeant major. When I had made a bed on which, mysteriously, the bottom sheet seemed to be longer on one side than it was on the other, she would look at me with incredulous exasperation from under her rabbit-eared scarf, mop in hand, and cry, "How come you are so stupid?" I could never think of a satisfactory answer, so she would command, "Take it off and start all over again! And if again it don't work, go on doing it until I come back. When you think you're through, you can start stacking sheets."

I was not the only one she bossed around; she did the same to the interns in the bunkroom to which she had the key. But she could do no wrong, as far as I was concerned, after I heard her say on my second day in Observation, as I stood helpless between two beds and their gruesome contents, each one of them expiring, "Every time I come through here, I pray for them." It had seemed, at that moment, as if she were the only one in the building who cared about the two poor wretches in that horrible little dark ward. I discovered, as time went on, that she was the only one who could really cope with the worst of the damned, who sometimes lay in the far corner, raving obscenely, spitting in the face of death. I once found, when I arrived, in the back of the second ward, an old naked hallucinating tramp, dying in a tangle of soaked sheets and torn trousers, his wrists and ankles tied to the bed frame, cursing like a madman. When I tried to cover him with a sheet, he cried, "Goddammit, leave me alone! Goddammit, that hurts!" While I stood there, at a loss, he went on cursing and rambling. "I claim the six rings!" he cried. "They were promised to me! Those rings are mine!" Then he started to curse again, in an empty litany of obscenity. Suddenly I heard a voice say with quiet indignation, "You should not blaspheme; you should ask God to forgive you." I looked and saw Miss Jennie stand behind me, mop in hand, her glasses shimmering bleakly in the darkness. It seemed a harsh thing to say to a dying man, but suddenly the old tramp cried, "Yes, God, forgive me! . . . God, forgive me, Goddammit, Goddammit . . ." But even as he went on cursing, I had the uncanny feeling that she had done something for him that no one else could have done.

John Rivers, the orderly who had so brusquely stopped me during my first day in Emergency, when I had been about to give Mr. Hood a cup of water for his aspirin, was rarely seen in Observation; his stomping ground was the treatment section. I started out with a feeling of instinctive hostility towards him; in a way he truly integrated me by this feeling: he was the first man I cordially detested despite the fact that he was a Negro. After a few weeks I came to change my opinion of him under the pressure of a growing, reluctant admiration; to see him at work filled me with envy. Also, he knew more about Shakespeare than most of my students, not to mention myself, and the fact that he would, at particularly tense moments in the Shock Room when things hovered on the brink of chaos, calmly and rather pedantically quote the Bard was, so I discovered, part of his mastery of his profession. As time went on, I saw many a medical student saved from embarrassment by his tacit and poker-faced help. When, for instance, a tenderfoot asked with the superciliousness of insecurity for the wrong type of suture to go with the laceration he was about to sew up, John Rivers would say, "Yes, doctor," and drop the right one on his tray. He never committed the error of taste of making this a secret understanding; he managed to help with such aloofness that most students actually believed they had profited from a mistake on his part.

My most vivid memory of him is dated Christmas Eve, 1962, in Emergency. It was, without doubt, the most gruesome night of my life thus far. All through that night he was a tower of strength, impeccably correct, maddeningly unaffected, and seemingly untiring. When, at last, we were ready to hand over the nightmare of Hieronymus Bosch to the seven-to-three shift, we made one more round together to see if all was well. It wasn't; it was like daybreak on a battlefield. But it was the best we could do.

I remember him standing in the doorway to the courtyard, by the admissions desk: the hall filled with stretchers and litters, the air rank with the smell of sickness, the wailing of the damned a haunting litany at this dawn of Christmas Day. For a moment I stood there, overwhelmed by the horrendous notion that all this was hopeless, that it would never change. Then I felt a hand on my shoulder, and I looked up, and that was the first time I saw John Rivers smile."Come," he said, opening the door. "Absent thee from felicity awhile."

* * * * *

Between the extremes of the jolly women and our young friend who was never seen again, each of the volunteers had his own personal reaction. We had arranged to meet for worship in the middle of the morning in a lecture room on the second floor, between the Nursing Office and the Operating Rooms. There, surrounded by a blackboard with mathematical formulas and charts of the internal organs of the human body, we put up a circle of chairs and sat down. We arrived singly and in pairs; after about ten minutes, we were all there, including Lucille. I was preoccupied when I sat down in the circle, thinking about our young friend who had fled and the others who seemed to be having a hard time; but the moment I closed my eyes something unexpected happened. I was at once gathered in by what obviously was a communal sense of tranquility, a stillness that I had never before experienced in meeting. It was, I felt sure, shared by all of us. I realized that this was what I had been searching for, hoping for when I had sat in our previous dreary meetings, isolated in glumness. Suddenly a voice among us spoke, softly and hesitatingly but in great anguish. It was one of our women. "I don't think I can go on with this," she said. "It is all so terrible, so ghastly. I am so clumsy at it, so bad. I wish I could go on, but I am afraid that I am totally unsuited for this work. I wish God would give me guidance."

After she had spoken, we sat in silence for a while, with that sense of peace and light growing among us; then another voice spoke, one of our men. "When I want to drive a nail into the wall," he said, "and I can't find a hammer, I use my shoe. I know a shoe is totally unsuited for the work I am trying to make it do, but it is all I have available. Maybe God has the same problem, sometimes. Maybe he uses us to drive in this nail for lack of a hammer. All we can do is trust Him, and hope that He won't hit His thumb."

I had never realized that you could laugh in meeting for worship, and this was the most luminous, the most radiant meeting I had ever attended. We rose with deep gratitude toward the old, weighty Friends who had insisted that we hold our meeting for worship inside the hospital. They had been right. After that meeting, none of us thought of giving up the work.

During the weeks that followed, we went to meeting inside the hospital every Sunday morning in the midst of our work. Every time that radiant, luminous stillness gathered us in. No one spoke any more; all those later meetings were completely silent. To the outsider we were just a circle of people, sitting in silence for half an hour and then getting up and dispersing. But the Houston Meeting, that once had been the dullest we knew, had become the most inspiring. It no longer mattered whether we met in a circle, facing a blank wall or standing in a row. It had nothing to do with seating arrangements or noisy kids upstairs. It had to do with the fact that, for a few moments of stillness, we returned together to the source of our faith in the midst of practice.

A WOMAN'S WAR

FRANK T. VERTOSICK, JR.

While she was berrying
She bore that child . . .
And sprang forward, screaming
To terrify that child

–from an Alaskan Indian birth poem

"Breathe. Breathe. Breathe."

I repeated this mantra again and again as my wife fought to maintain her composure. Writhing in the throes of her increasingly ferocious uterine contractions, she labored with our first daughter as I watched, powerless to assist her. As chief neurosurgical resident of a large medical center, I could barely find a few idle hours in a day to sleep let alone participate in weekly Lamaze classes. One of our friends who had training as a Lamaze instructor gave us a crash course in natural childbirth techniques a few days earlier, but that brief exposure proved of little use in the heat of the moment. My wife wanted to deliver without anesthesia, the so-called "natural" way. Unfortunately, neither of us knew what we were doing and her pain soon spiraled out of control.

I sat slouched in an unpadded metal chair. That chair was a torture device; I was convinced that the OB nurse forced me to sit in it so that I, too, could suffer. My wife squirmed in her sweaty bed as I squirmed in that sweaty chair, two anxious people locked in a slow, joyless dance. I longed for the old days, when dads-to-be smoked and paced in the waiting room far removed from the drama of the birthing suite.

"Breathe!" I yelled again, but I didn't understand what these exhortations were supposed to accomplish. Telling a woman on the verge of passing out from hyperventilation to breathe is like leaning over the *Titanic*'s tilting deck rail and screaming, "Drown!" to those bobbing in the sea. What else can they do?

She calmed down as each contraction ended, but her anticipation of pain magnified with each successive spasm of her impatient womb. Hours passed and she grew dreadfully weary, her face moist and gray like the mask of someone approaching death. I had seen the same look many times before, the expression of a body pushed to its physiologic limit, and this appearance frightened me. The painless intervals grew shorter and the contractions lengthened, the normal progression of advancing labor. She wanted desperately to hang on and complete the "natural" process of birthing, but she finally realized that this pain could not continue. About seven hours into her labor, an anesthesiologist arrived at our request and inserted an epidural catheter into her back, a thin tube placed near the nerves of the lumbar spine. An infusion of spinal narcotic immediately deadened the pelvic area and uterus. Without the violent effects of pain to drive it forward, her labor slowed down slightly, but things eventually came to fruition with the birth of a screaming infant girl.

Because epidural anesthesia produces no sedation, my wife was still able to cooperate fully with the delivery. She didn't see the actual birth (my large head blocked her view of the mirror, a fact I'm not permitted to forget even ten years later), but she managed to hold her new child immediately. Both mother and child were bright and alert. In my wife's case, abandoning natural birth in favor of an epidural block did nothing to harm the birthing experience. In fact, the spinal narcotics enhanced it; by sparing my wife hours of agony, the epidural catheter allowed her to meet her new daughter in a rested and refreshed state. Emily proved to be a normal, healthy child and my wife recovered quickly and without problems. What more could anyone ask of childbirth?

Noneless, my wife harbored twinges of doubt concerning her performance, as if her first labor, although successful in outcome, was marred by some measure of personal failure because it was not natural in the strictest sense of the word. I, too, felt guilty about the epidural block. I considered my wife's plea for anesthesia to be my fault, not hers. After all, I hadn't made time in my schedule to learn how to coach a natural childbirth correctly, even though she had asked me to do so on numerous occasions. I wasn't prepared to do my part to assist her, to talk her through the ordeal without resorting to drugs and needles.

Looking back on that event of years ago, I'm somewhat mystified over this guilt. What's so bad about a comfortable labor and delivery, even one that required medical technology? In the historical scheme of things, I did nothing wrong. Prior to this century, childbirth was rarely a team sport. In those instances when expectant mothers needed the assistance of others, they sought out experienced women, not nervous and useless fathers.

Men view childbirth only as a process that produces their children. To women, of course, it's more—much more. Childbirth is a profound ritual teeming with spiritual and biological significance. Pain appears to play an indispensable role in that ritual. In the words of Helen Chasin:

Screwed on this centripetal ache, I fix on pain
and breathe it like an element.

Pain is, as Chasin observes, elemental in the process of childbirth. Just as pain and death are inseparable, so too are pain and birth. A dense layer of suffering envelops our corporeal world, and all souls wishing to enter or leave must push their way through it at their own peril.

Curiously, few people question the wisdom of using medical technology to cause painless death, yet many question the wisdom of using the same technology to achieve painless birth. Society considers the great number of cancer patients who die in great pain as an abject failure of the modern physician, yet each day women around the globe scream and pant their way through hours of unending labor rather than seek artificial pain relief. I find this odd. Why reject the natural agonies of cancer and embrace the natural agonies of childbirth? True, labor pain is brief, at most a day or two in duration, but it's also extreme. In quantitative ratings of pain severity, the pain of a first labor exceeds cancer pain by a considerable margin and falls just shy of the pain of limb amputation sans anesthesia. Why endure such torment willingly? No rational person would want to have a leg cut off without benefit of modern painkilling technique, yet thousands of women pay money to learn how to avoid anesthesia during childbirth. The pain of birth is no different from any other pain . . . or is it?

The introduction of general anesthesia into the birthing process in 1847 by James Young Simpson touched off a firestorm of controversy that burns to the present day. One camp argues that birth should be as painless as possible, even if relief comes in the form of drugs, nerve blocks, even general anesthesia; the opposing camp contends that childbirth should be free of all undue medical interference despite the great suffering such freedom imposes on the mother. What drives this strange controversy? Is the resistance to pharmacological pain control during the birthing process a cultural phenomenon, akin to the New Age fads of crystal energy and pyramid power, or does the desire for natural birth derive from some primitive neurological urge to feel the pain of creation? Scholars have been struggling to decipher the strange symbiosis between pain and the birthing process for centuries. They've made progress, but mysteries surrounding the psychology and physiology of childbirth pain still abound.

The trauma required for the creation of new life varies widely in the biological realm. The most primitive cellular lifeforms, including protozoans, fungi, and bacteria, literally rip themselves in two. Oak trees, on the other hand, silently drop their acorns to the ground. Fish, birds, reptiles, amphibians, and a few mammal species (for example, the platypus) lay eggs, a comparatively painless process as far as we can judge. Viruses don't even bother with their own reproduction, choosing instead to have other living things do it for them.

Most mammals, however, resort to the ancient single-cell strategy of tearing their bodies apart. Creating a large, complex mammal like the human infant from a single ovum is an arduous and nutritionally demanding process—too demanding to occur independent of the mother's body in some self-contained egg. Pea-brained chickens may be grown in this way; building a brainy human in like fashion would require so much nutrient yolk that the resulting egg would be the size of a small automobile.

Most fetal mammals must therefore stay tethered to their mother's bloodstream throughout development. So intertwined are their circulatory systems that mother and child function as one organism until the moment of separation. Once gestation is complete, the mother's body extrudes the child and their mutual bond divides in a torrent of fluid and blood. Our warm and gentle feelings about childbirth are misguided. In humans, the process is a thing of terror and violence. A woman's genitals and pelvic floor stretch to the breaking point and beyond. The vagina and rectum can be torn irreparably, the pelvic bones separated, the bladder smashed. The muscular uterus spasms with such vehemence that the child can be ejected like a missile. The first child I delivered as a medical student hit me in the chest and almost knocked the wind out of me (the child, fortunately, was unharmed). There is little gentle about this process.

Comedienne Joan Rivers once said that the stretching of genital skin needed to yield a baby can be simulated by grabbing the lowerlip and yanking it over the top of the head. She meant to be funny, but her analogy actually understates the situation. Given these rapid distortions of anatomy, it's no wonder labor and delivery are so painful, particularly for first-time mothers. Nevertheless, it remains more than a little mysterious that a process so essential to the procreation of our species should be such a fearful and agonizing experience.

As I've argued previously, natural selection doesn't bother with mercy unless it facilitates our survival and procreation. Nature doesn't protect us against cancer pain because cancer isn't a threat to our species. There's been no evolutionary impetus to produce painless cancers. In the case of childbirth, however, mercy should prevail since there's a very good Darwinian impetus for painless childbirth; the more childbirth hurts, the less inclined mothers will be to have children. This is especially true for human beings. Thanks to our huge brains, we have an excellent memory for pain and can devise complex strategies to avoid it.

In fact, we're so intelligent that we can avoid painful experiences we've seen but haven't personally experienced. Cows, for example, won't be put off by a barbed-wire fence simply because they've witnessed other cows getting tangled in it. They have to experience the pain firsthand. But in humans, watching a single painful childbirth might frighten an entire community of women out of bearing children. This isn't a theoretical concern. I have known more than one woman who opted not to have a child because of their fear of childbirth, and this in the age of anesthesia. One can only imagine the inhibitory fear of childbirth in the preanesthetic era.

Thus, it seems in our best interest as a species for our childbirth to be a pleasurable experience. After all, isn't that why sexual intercourse feels so good, to encourage us to make babies? Why gratify us at one end of gestation and torture us at the other? Yet nature shows women no mercy during childbirth.

Why?

* * * * *

I suspect that this lack of mercy wasn't intentional. There must have been great evolutionary pressures to reduce the misery of childbirth, but perhaps there wasn't enough time to do so. Consider the case of spinal disc disorders. As discussed previously, our rapid conversion from small-headed quadripeds to big-headed bipeds forced our spines to do things they weren't designed to do. The basic architecture of vertebrates evolved over hundreds of millions of years and was built to carry weight evenly distributed over a horizontal posture. In less than a million years, the same design was subsequently forced upright and, even worse, made to carry a mammoth head perched on its apex. With insufficient time to adapt the old spinal technology to this new posture, evolution sentenced us to the miseries of spinal pain.

It was a calculated trade-off: evolution balanced the benefits of unencumbered forelimbs against the sporadic incapacity produced by failing spines. The fact that our planet currently crawls with countless human bodies proves that this trade-off was worthwhile. Given another hundred million years, nature might yet work out the kinks in our spines, but, until then, we're stuck with jerry-rigged technology that has yet to keep pace with the demands placed on it.

Painful childbirth is a similar casualty of humankind's rapid entrance onto biology's stage. Our large head size evolved over an even shorter period of time than our erect posture. We know, for example, that the earliest bipeds still looked like pinheads compared to modern humans. As this rapid cranial expansion took place, female pelvic anatomy, like the spine, was confronted with the difficult task of adapting old technology to radical new uses. A birth canal designed to pass large litters of small, streamlined animals now had to accommodate the passage of one or two bulbous-headed progeny. It could be done, of course, but it was going to hurt.

There wasn't much that natural selection could do to prevent the escalation of childbirth pain caused by the expanding human head, certainly not in a scant fifty thousand generations. The only feasible ways to do this would be to give women a massive pelvis or to render the pelvis and genitals permanently anesthetic. Neither would be tenable. Creating permanently insensate genitals or an outsized pelvis simply to ameliorate a half dozen transiently painful experiences didn't make survival sense. As such, women are stuck with their painful ordeal, at least until natural selection comes up with a better solution in another million years or so.

The extreme stress placed on the birth canal during the passage of a human fetus has another unfortunate consequence: Childbirth became dangerous. Death during labor and delivery is relatively rare in all animals save humans. Prior to the advent of modern obstetrics, childbirth claimed the lives of three out of every hundred laboring mothers. Over multiple births, mothers in the premodern era had a significant lifetime risk of death, although our prodigious survival proves that our big heads were worth the risk.

Jared Diamond, in his book *The Third Chimpanzee,* postulates that the great dangers of human childbirth account for another misery unique to human females: menopause. Human females are fertile for about thirty years—less than one half of their natural life spans. While fertility declines somewhat with age in all mammals, including human men, only human women shut down their reproductive systems completely many years before they die. Diamond considers menopause a protective reflex. Women older than fifty may not be capable of withstanding childbirth. Moreover, the long period of a human child's vulnerability makes a mother's survival essential to the survival of her children. In short, she's simply too valuable to risk in never-ending cycles of pregnancy and childbirth. The human reproductive system allows each woman a limited opportunity to have children and then shields her from further risk. The relative period of infertility that occurs when new mothers are breastfeeding also protects the new infant from quickly losing a mother to a new pregnancy.

As I watched my wife strain to expel my daughter that night, I wasn't concerned about the survival of my species, only about her survival and the survival of our daughter. My wife in her bed and me in my chair, we both were witness to the steep price demanded by nature for the honor of being Homo sapiens—thinking man.

* * * * *

Childbirth pain isn't entirely unique to humans. The cramping of uterine contractions and the painful dilation of cervix and vagina affects most mammals, except, perhaps, the egg-laying platypus and marsupials like the kangaroo, which gives birth to tiny fetuses that then crawl into the mother's pouch to complete their final gestation. Any veterinarian can relate tales of difficult labors in horses, cows, and other beasts. Nevertheless, severe and frequent birthing pains seem limited to primates like us. In a 1985 study of pregnant monkeys and apes, over three quarters of laboring mothers exhibited signs of severe distress, including grimacing and writhing during labor and crying out during delivery, suggesting that our primate cousins also suffer during childbirth. Since we have the largest heads of any primates, our females suffer the most.

* * * * *

Because the size of our heads makes a painful childbirth unavoidable, nature came up with three tricks to compensate for the chilling effect that childbirth pain might exert on human reproductive behaviors. The first trick has already been mentioned: the joy of sex. Although we have a long memory for pain, we're also notorious for doing fun things despite the sorry consequences that will follow later. We get drunk fully aware of the hangover awaiting us the next day. We play that yearly volleyball game at the family reunion even though we know we won't be able to move for three days. A close friend of mine is allergic to shrimp, but he enjoys the crustaceans so much he still eats them and accepts that he will be sicker than a dog hours later. Since sex comes ahead of shrimp on the average person's "to do" list, it's no wonder that the consequences of childbirth may have little impact on the rate of impregnation.

The second trick is biochemical. Late in pregnancy the rising levels of endogenous narcotic substances known as endorphins increase the expectant mother's tolerance of pain. The hormone relaxin also softens the pelvic tissues, permitting easier deformation of the pelvic outlet during birth. How much these hormones increase the mother's actual comfort is debatable, but these changes show that the female body is trying to ameliorate the pain as best it can.

The final trick is much sneakier: silent ovulation. A female is fertile for only a few days following the release of a fresh ovum. In most mammals, the female undergoes visible changes in appearance and behavior during her fertile window. She becomes sexually aggressive and indiscriminate in her mating; her genitals may swell or change color and she may emit odors signaling her fertility. The human female, save for feeling an occasional mild pain caused by the rupture of a ripe ovarian follicle, remains oblivious to her ovulation. In fact, so silent is human ovulation that the timing of ovum release relative to the menstrual cycle wasn't deciphered by endocrinologists until 1930. Studies of sexual intercourse frequency during the menstrual cycle further suggest that couples have no clear knowledge of the time of maximum fertility; thus, there appears to be no covert signs of ovulation either—no subliminal body language, no chemical cues.

In *The Third Chimpanzee,* Diamond postulates that silent ovulation, like menopause, is also a biological phenomenon mandated by our hazardous and painful births. If ovulation were obvious, Diamond's argument goes, clever women would quickly learn to avoid intercourse during their fertile period, thereby enjoying the pleasures of sex without the consequences of pregnancy and childbirth. Silent ovulation makes this natural birth control impossible.

In addition to biological adaptations like pleasurable intercourse and silent ovulation, we have also developed cultural methods for hiding the pain of childbirth from impressionable young females. In his controversial study of human behavior, *The Naked Ape,* zoologist Desmond Morris popularized the idea that cultural practices often derive from biological necessity. In the spirit of Morris, I propose that childbirth rituals reflect the biological necessity of minimizing the negative impact of childbirth pain. Women throughout history and in diverse societies often sought to give birth alone or with the aid of older (and often post-menopausal) women. Granted, solitary birth is not uncommon among mammals, but humans are exquisitely social beings who usually seek out the sympathy of others in times of acute distress. Although solitude also makes good hygienic sense, it also keeps the birthing experience "in the closet." Childless women can't fear what they don't know.

In crowded civilizations like Japan where isolation is nearly impossible, women developed an immense stoicism during childbirth. This stoicism gave rise to the myth that childbirth pain itself is a modern cultural phenomenon. Early proponents of "natural childbirth" (including Grantly Dick-Read, the obstetrician who coined the phrase in the 1930s) believed that "primitive" cultures (more correctly, "nonwhite" cultures) were immune to labor pain entirely. "Primitives," as such women were called, simply dropped their children in the fields as effortlessly as having a bowel movement. "The primitive," Dick-Read wrote in his 1933 monograph "Natural Childbirth," "knows that she will have little trouble when her child is born."

In Dick-Read's paradigm, childbirth pain is an invention of pampered, out-of-shape white Europeans and could be cured by stripping them of their high society softheadedness. If they could only emulate their brown and yellow sisters, things would go easier for them. This sounds a tad racist, and it is. But then, there's more than a little racism in the early theories of childbirth pain. Dick-Read felt that "primitives" (a definition that included some fairly advanced cultures) don't think about their labors and so develop no fear and experience no tension or pain. The unstated implication is that these women are too simpleminded to be frightened or hurt by anything. Some early authors even considered childbirth pain the bane of women who mate outside of their "own kind." George Engelmann, in his excellent history of obstetrics published in 1882, writes that labor pain is worse when a woman is trying to deliver a "half-breed," perhaps, he speculates, because the size and shape of the child doesn't mesh with her pelvic anatomy.

In the final analysis, the idea that childbirth pain is a product of modern civilization is, in a word, hogwash. In Genesis, a document thousands of years old, God warns the fallen Eve that she and her descendants will give birth in pain. The Bible later favorably compares the courage of women in labor to the courage of men in battle. Clearly, ancient cultures were well aware of childbirth's difficulties. In 1945 C. S. Ford studied the pain of birth in sixty-four so-called "primitive" cultures and concluded that "the popular impression of childbirth in primitive societies as painless and easy is definitely contraindicated in our cases. As a matter of fact, it is often prolonged and painful."

Although pain itself isn't influenced by culture, expression of pain clearly depends upon cultural biases. A Japanese woman may display no outward signs of discomfort during labor, but when asked to fill out a questionnaire afterwards, she will rate pain severity the same as women of European descent. Childbirth stoicism in crowded civilizations may serve the same purpose that solitude does in more rural societies, namely, to protect impressionable young women from learning the truth about labor's trials and tribulations. If you can't scream where no one hears you, don't scream at all.

If this all seems far-fetched, remember that very small influences on reproductive behavior can cause significant perturbations in a species over thousands of generations. Had labor been treated as a public event throughout our history, there's little doubt certain females would be put off by the experience. This might have introduced an undesirable selection bias into the human genome. We don't know what common traits the birth-aversive women might have shared, traits that would have been selected out of the general population.

Could the simple acts of holding one's tongue during uterine contractions or going alone into the bushes to deliver a child have had any great impact on our species? Maybe not. But then, the reproduction of animals often hinges on seemingly silly things like the performance of an intricate dance, the sweetness of a song, or the coloration of a tail feather. Minuscule variations in mating behaviors can alter interbreeding in a way that redirects the course of the species' development.

* * * * *

Which brings us back to the controversy between the two camps, one favoring medical pain control and the other a natural labor and delivery. If biological factors might drive behaviors like stoicism and isolation during birthing, could such factors also drive a woman's yearning to give birth the old-fashioned way, under her own control and in her own blessed pain?

So far I've only mentioned the negative aspects of labor pain. Like other forms of pain, the pain of childbirth may be a double-edged sword, possessing both good and bad aspects. Women who have endured a particularly grueling labor may question whether there was any kernel of "good" in the experience, but labor pain may indeed serve a purpose.

Return to the title of my introduction: "The Megaphone of God." For the purposes of this discussion, childbirth pain may be better termed the Megaphone of Baby. After my wife had her epidural, the labor slowed. Without the driving effect of pain, a woman's mental focus on the urgent task at hand may wander. Labor is a dangerous time. With each uterine contraction, the blood flow through the placenta becomes compromised. As the baby descends into the birth canal, the head is deformed, literally squashed. None of these derangements has any lasting consequences provided they don't go on too long. Escalating pain forces the mother to pay attention and drive the event to completion as quickly as possible.

Tribes in northern Russia had a curious custom. During difficult labors, husband and wife had to discuss details of their sexual affairs with others. This unpleasantness presumably stimulated both parties to keep the labor, and conversation, as short as possible. Pain may play the same role: speed. The mother knows what she must do to end the pain—deliver the baby. Like the caller on a rowing team, the pain yells through its megaphone for her to keep stroking toward the finish line.

This isn't just idle speculation on my part. The need for a rapid labor and the role that pain plays in hurrying labor along have been known for centuries. Some cultures took to threatening or frightening the baby hurriedly out of the womb. The Alaskan poem at the beginning of this chapter speaks of terrifying the child, a common theme. Klamath Indian mothers told their infants that a rattlesnake was crawling into the womb to bite them if they didn't come out. Pahute mothers fasted during the final month of gestation in the belief that the child could be starved out, like starving a woodchuck from its den. Other cultures sought to increase a mother's pain in hopes of shortening labor. Russians of northern Asia used herbs believed to heighten pain sensitivity, while the Kazak of central Asia were more brutal: they held a woman's hand to a fire to keep labor moving. In the Philippines midwives placed wooden planks across the woman's abdomen and applied direct pressure to the womb. Notice that none of these maneuvers took the mother's comfort into consideration. Speed, not pain control, was the goal.

Plant remedies were common, but once again they were used for enhancing speed, not comfort. The ancient Mexicans routinely used the civapacthi plant to stimulate uterine contractions, much as modern obstetricians use the uterine stimulant oxytocin. A variety of other oxytocin-like herbs have been employed throughout the world. Some cultures used plants in a mechanical fashion by inserting dry leaves into the cervix. As the leaves soaked up uterine secretions, they expanded and dilated the cervix, again speeding labor.

With the advent of general anesthesia in the last century, physicians could now eliminate the pain of labor entirely. In doing so, they also slowed labor. This spurred the creation of a new device: the forceps, a pair of spoonlike metal instruments that allowed the obstetrician to reach into the birth canal and yank out the recalcitrant child. They did the job, but not without problems. Babies are designed to be pushed out of the vagina, not pulled out. Improperly or aggressively used, forceps could fracture the skull, harm the facial nerves (causing facial paralysis), even break the poor child's neck. Surely this isn't how nature intended children to be born—rudely pulled from a sedated or unconscious mother.

The obvious absurdity of this form of delivery helped spur a return to natural birthing practices in the middle part of this century. However, the man most responsible for popularizing natural childbirth, Grantly Dick-Read, advocated anesthesia-free birth for stranger reasons. In his 1944 book *Childbirth without Fear,* Dick-Read wrote: "The pain of labor, and its initiating cause, fear, extend their evil influence into the very roots of our social structure. They corrupt the minds and bodies of successive generations and bring distress and calamity where happiness and prosperity are the reward of a simple physiological performance." Dick-Read felt that natural childbirth created a primal force he called "motherlove," which could, in proper quantity, cure all the world's ills, from poverty to disease. He described his work as "no longer an obstetric practice only, but a mission—no longer a pursuit, but a calling."

Dick-Read and the other major advocate of natural birth, Paris obstetrician Fernand Lamaze (who imported the Pavlovian methods of childbirth used in the Soviet Union), didn't see pain as a necessary force that could be controlled and harnessed for the good of mother and child, but viewed pain instead as an evil interloper, something that by rights didn't belong in the birthing process at all. Dick-Read saw labor pain as a manifestation of fear alone, with no physiological role whatsoever. Those who advocate natural childbirth today must remember that Dick-Read's original intent was not the *management* of labor pain, but the abolition of labor pain. In Dick-Read's paradigm, labor pain shouldn't exist at all.

Dick-Read's mystic outlook no doubt traces back to the origins of his beliefs about pain and the mind. During trench warfare of World War I, a shell-shocked Dick-Read learned his Eastern relaxation techniques from an Indian noncommissioned officer. Eventually he came to think of his methods as capable of changing world history; by restoring childbirth to its pristine, natural state, Dick-Read could purge the world of evil. Critics questioned why women had to spend so much time learning "natural " techniques like the Dick-Read and Lamaze methods when "natural childbirth" should be so instinctive.

And Dick-Read had numerous critics to be sure, including competitor Lamaze. He gave abuse out as quickly as it came in, too, dismissing Lamaze's methods as just another attempt by the Russians to take credit for everything, even Shakespeare. One of his biggest foes was the National Birthday Trust Fund, or NBTF, a private organization in his native England that advocated the use of anesthesia in childbirth and raised money to allow poor women to have the same access to medically assisted births as rich women enjoyed. The NBTF funded research into safer anesthetic techniques, taught midwives how to administer home anesthesia, successfully lobbied the British Parliament to repeal laws against the administration of anesthesia by midwives, and even distributed chloroform ampules for that purpose. Thanks to the NBTF, labor pain became politicized, a form of class warfare. Poor women suffered because they were poor. The NBTF wanted all women to have the "Princess drugs," as they called the narcotics given to Princess (now Queen) Elizabeth during her delivery of Prince Charles.

Gradually, however, natural birth advocates began to turn the tide. Dick-Read even got an endorsement from Pope Pius XII, who penned an encyclical about childbirth in 1957. Although any method of alleviating childbirth pain may be contrary to divine intent, mused the pope, he found nothing in Catholic doctrine prohibiting the use of Dick-Read's "English" approach, feeling it allowed a more "Christian Delivery" than Lamaze's "Russian" method. It was hard to imagine anything Christian emanating from the Soviet Union in the 1950s, a fact not lost on the Holy Father. The Pope awarded Dick-Read a silver medal for his work, apparently overlooking the physician's earlier claim that Christianity was one of the biggest sources of unnatural labor pain in the first place.

* * * * *

Although the teachings of men like Grantly Dick-Read were often misguided, their message has validity. Putting women to sleep and pulling out their babies with makeshift barbecue tongs had serious drawbacks. Moreover, their assertion that women can be prepared mentally and physically for the rigors of childbirth in such a way that it becomes a tolerable and satisfying experience for them, even without drugs or needles, has also proven correct. For our second child, my wife and I completed full Lamaze training, and that labor went smoothly and without anesthetic help. Of course, second children tend to be easier than the first, but I was convinced that the preparation we received was indispensable. Maybe it was just a mental thing—but then, pain is often just a mental thing. Even my chair felt more comfortable.

The natural route shouldn't be carried to extremes. Techniques such as epidural anesthesia, caudal blocks, and even cesarean section may be necessary to provide a comfortable and safe delivery. Each case must be handled individually, and no woman should feel guilty about how she performs during labor. She should use whatever tools she has at her disposal to survive the experience unscathed. The only option my immigrant grandmother had was natural childbirth, and it yielded her a son paralyzed and brain-injured by a botched home delivery.

* * * * *

There's one other reproductive pain women endure: menstruation. Menstruation is truly a uniquely human pain—I can find no reference to menstrual discomfort in other animals. As in the case of childbirth, menstrual cramps have been dismissed as a modern manifestation, the complaining of weak women. Once again, the historical record contradicts this. The Koran calls menstruation "a hurt" and that's about as succinct a description as any. The ancient physician and anatomist Galen notes the pain of menstruation; he postulated that women menstruate because they are so idle most of the time they have to shed the excess sweat and blood that men routinely work off. I doubt Galen makes the National Organization for Women's top ten list of admired men.

The pain derives from the uterine spasms and hormonal surges that occur normally during the monthly menstrual cycle. These symptoms may, like migraine, help steer sexual intercourse to the middle part of the cycle, where fertility is greatest. If so, then add menstruation to the list of things we can blame on our big heads.

Stop and consider all of the possible consequences of our outsized brains. It certainly makes childbirth hazardous and painful, so hazardous that the female reproductive period must be abruptly terminated (menopause). Painful childbirth, in turn, could also account for the pleasurable sensation of intercourse, and explain why our ovulation is so silent—we have to be teased or duped into going through the experience of childbirth. This silent ovulation means that we have no period of heat like animals, so we have to be nudged into having sexual intercourse at the right time. Since the days before, during, and after menstruation are precisely the wrong time, women suffer a variety of ailments—migraines, cramps, mood swings—that make intercourse the last thing on their minds. We also developed social taboos concerning sex and menstruation, in some cultures to the point of labeling menstruating women unclean, unholy, even dangerous. The bumper sticker that reads "I have PMS and a gun, any questions?" shows that the "dangerous" label still lingers.

Dysmenorrhea—incapacitating menstrual cramps—and other chronic pelvic pain in women (including pain from endometriosis, sexually transmitted illnesses, and pelvic pain of unknown origin) exact an alarming toll on society, considering that these are nonlethal conditions. A study in the United Kingdom found that nearly 1 percent of all health care dollars spent in 1991 went toward menstrual disorders and female pelvic pain. Including lost time from work, dysmenorrhea is a billion dollar problem. Dysmenorrhea usually responds well to oral contraceptives used in conjunction with over-the-counter analgesics. But there is no cure for this condition, which carries the appropriate nickname "the curse."

* * * * *

While reading about birth customs, I was most impressed by one practice by the Aztecs of ancient Mexico. An Aztec woman who died in labor was buried with full military honors as a war hero and her family granted a pension. The Aztecs saw birth as "the woman's war" and, having seen it myself many times, I agree. It represents a woman's life-and-death struggle with her child, herself, and her species. For my brain to be large enough to write these pages, my mother and her mother before her had to wage that war. In birth, we see a courage equal to that shown by Christ in Gethsemane, the courage to face an almost unbearable ordeal simply because it is what must be done. The Aztecs practiced human sacrifice and played soccer with human heads, but their reverence for women should be a model for those of us who live in a more "enlightened" age.

MYSTERY AND AWE

RACHEL NAOMI REMEN

In the corner of the basement of the brownstone where my Uncle Frank lived and had his medical offices, there was a battered wardrobe closet made of heavy cardboard. On Saturday mornings when I was quite small, I often played down there by myself, waiting for my father, who worked as my uncle's X-ray technician. One day, more out of boredom than curiosity, I struggled to open the wardrobe door. The hinges had rusted. Inside, hanging from a hook, was a human skeleton.

I was pleased. After examining it for a long time and admiring the beautiful shapes and ivory softness of its bones and the brass pins which cleverly held them together, I discovered that by standing on a chair I could lift it off the hook and bring it out. It was not very heavy. For a long time it became my playmate, my guest at endless tea parties, the confidant of my secrets. Thinking back, I realize how strange a picture this must have made, but it did not seem odd at the time. Or frightening.

At about this same time, I suffered from a repetitive series of night terrors centered on the dumbwaiter, a common feature of hallways in the apartment houses of the forties. The dumbwaiter was designed for lifting groceries five or six stories from the lobby of the building or lowering garbage to the incinerator in the basement. It was a box that moved up and down a vertical shaft and was operated manually by a rope-and-pulley system. Most of the time when one opened the door, the dumbwaiter box was at the floor of whatever neighbor above or below had most recently used it. My mother would reach into the blackness of the shaft and pull on the ropes until the wooden box appeared.

The black emptiness of the shaft terrified me and for a long time I dreamed of it almost nightly. I was certain that the blackness was alive and that some night it would escape its hiding place and get me. I could not sleep unless a light was on. The night terrors went on until an elevator was installed in the building and the dumbwaiter shaft was sealed up. These fears were a prominent part of the fabric of my life back then. I would tell the skeleton about them during our tea parties. The known was far more comfortable than the unknown, even then.

As a physician, I was trained to deal with uncertainty as aggressively as I dealt with disease itself. The unknown was the enemy. Within this worldview, having a question feels like an emergency; it means that something is out of control and needs to be made known as rapidly, efficiently, and cost-effectively as possible. But death has taken me to the edge of certainty, to the place of questions.

After years of trading mystery for mastery, it was hard and even frightening to stop offering myself reasonable explanations for some of the things that I observed and that others told me, and simply take them as they are. "I don't know" had long been a statement of shame, of personal and professional failing. In all of my training I do not recall hearing it said aloud even once.

But as I listened to more and more people with life-threatening illness tell their stories, not knowing simply became a matter of integrity. Things happened. And the explanations I offered myself became increasingly hollow, like a child whistling in the dark. The truth was that very often I didn't know and couldn't explain, and finally, weighted down by the many, many instances of the mysterious which are such an integral part of illness and healing, I surrendered. It was a moment of awakening.

For the first time, I became curious about the things I had been unwilling to see before, more sensitive to inconsistencies I had glibly explained or successfully ignored, more willing to ask people questions and draw them out about stories I would have otherwise dismissed. What I found out in the end was that the life I had defended as a doctor as precious was also Holy.

I no longer feel that life is ordinary. Everyday life is filled with mystery. The things we know are only a small part of the things we cannot know but can only glimpse. Yet even the smallest of glimpses can sustain us.

Mystery seems to have the power to comfort, to offer hope, and to lend meaning in times of loss and pain. In surprising ways it is the mysterious that strengthens us at such times. I used to try to offer people certainty in times which were not at all certain and could not be made certain. I now just offer my companionship and share my sense of mystery, of the possible, of wonder. After twenty years of working with people with cancer, I find it possible to neither doubt nor accept the unprovable but simply to remain open and wait.

I accept that I may never know where truth lies in such matters. The most important questions don't seem to have ready answers. But the questions themselves have a healing power when they are shared. An answer is an invitation to stop thinking about something, to stop wondering. Life has no such stopping places, life is a process whose every event is connected to the moment that just went by. An unanswered question is a fine traveling companion. It sharpens your eye for the road.

As a freshman in medical school I had been randomly selected as class photographer and given a camera to take pictures for the yearbook. I took pictures for four years. At first I felt burdened by the responsibility, the need to carry the heavy camera with me to class, to remember to look at things. But in time, the camera caused me to see my ordinary surroundings far more clearly, to become aware of beauty around me in some very unlikely places. It had given me new eyes. A good question is like that Zeiss.

In some fairy tales there is a magic word which has the power to undo the spell that has imprisoned someone and free them. When I was small, I would wait anxiously until the prince or the princess stumbled on the formula and said the healing words that would release them into life. Usually the words were some sort of nonsense like "Shazam." My magic words have turned out to be "I don't know."

Freedom

I was just beginning my private practice as a counselor to people with cancer when a patient of mine died. He was young, a forty-year old engineer with cancer of the pancreas. He was referred to me by his oncologist, who said, "Look, I've run out of treatment. I'm willing to talk to him, but I really have nothing more to offer him." Knowing this doctor to be a kind man, I realized that he simply did not know that he had anything other than his expertise that might be of value to his patient. So I said that I would be willing to talk to this man for whom there was no further treatment.

Shortly afterwards, we started our sessions. Richard was a reserved man, very tall and gaunt. He was always carefully and impeccably dressed. The clothing he wore was made to fit the much larger man he once was. I was struck, as I often am when people are this sick, by the iron will that keeps them going. He had refused my offer to visit him at his home, insisting that he would come to my office. Later his family told me that it took him more than two hours to dress himself. Refusing their help, he would put on one shoe, then rest, then struggle with the other.

We did four or five sessions together in all. We talked about many things: about his symptoms and his bitterness over what had befallen him, about his feelings of isolation from the people around him, about opening communications with his family. Once or twice, his family came and we all talked and it helped.

One day as he came in he asked me if I would write him a prescription. "Are you in pain?" I asked, my heart sinking. Had his complex regime of pain control lost its effectiveness? It was all we had. He shook his head. "No," he said. "I'm just anxious all the time. I haven't been able to sleep for two nights. I just lie there. Can you give me something?"

I said that I could and asked him if he had any idea what was causing this. "You've been through so much," I told him. "Why now?"

He had no idea.

Had he been having dreams? "Just the one," he told me. In it a ravenous beast was pursuing him. He had not been able to see it but had simply known that it was there. He had awakened, sweating, but he could not remember anything more. I waited for him to continue but he had not made a connection between the dream and what he was feeling.

"Perhaps we should revisit that dream," I suggested. "It may help us to understand." He nodded his agreement. I suggested then that he close his eyes, take a few deep breaths, and let me know when he felt ready to begin. When he signaled his readiness, I asked him to imagine himself back in his dream. This proved surprisingly easy for him. In his imagination, he started to run. In the next ten or fifteen minutes I did everything I knew to help bring him into another relationship with the beast that was pursuing him, to free him of being its prey. Nothing worked. "Become invisible," I suggested.

"It can see me."

"Hide behind something."

"It knows where I am."

"Talk to it."

"It won't answer me." As it gained on him, his anxiety grew.

As it became clear that he would not be able to evade the beast, I began to ask him questions about it. He still could not see it and continued to run, but gradually his answers helped him to know a great deal more about it. He told me that it was irresistible and merciless. There was no negotiating with it. It was "inevitable." But it was not evil. He was very clear about that. In fact, he said it seemed to him to be natural. After some time I said to him, "You know, Richard, you have tried everything. Maybe the only thing left for you to do is to allow it to eat you."

I had expected him to object, to talk about the things he was attached to, the people he would leave behind, but he immediately moved in this direction and imagined himself overtaken. For a while things became intense; Richard sat with his eyes closed, weeping, sweating, and shaking so forcefully I could hear his chair rocking. He seemed far too frail for this and I began to doubt the wisdom of this thing. But slowly the shaking stopped, and he grew calm. Gradually the room became deeply still and in the stillness I had the impression of sunlight, but I knew it was almost five o'clock. Suddenly I remembered the little boy with leukemia who had seemed to know he was going home. I could see him clearly, sitting cross-legged on his bed pillow and smiling at me.

Richard seemed completely relaxed and at peace. So was I. We sat there together for a while and then he said softly, "There is light, there is only Light. I am Light." We sat for a while longer, and then he opened his eyes and said, "Hey, I don't feel anxious at all. That was great, Doctor." The session was over and he left. I had forgotten to give him a prescription for tranquilizers and he had not reminded me.

I was still new to this sort of counseling and for the next three or four days I kept thinking about the session. Intellectually, I suspected that Richard's anxiety had something to do with what Freud calls the fear of Non-Being. But Richard's dream experience seemed different, similar to some other things I had recently read about near-death experience, things that were not yet in the medical literature.

Finally, I called Richard at home and told him I had been thinking about him. "How are you doing?" In a conversational and pleasant voice, he told me that he was doing much worse. He started to describe his new symptoms, yet he seemed calm about these very major physical changes. I pointed this out to him. "Yes, I feel different. That was a helpful session."

"How are you spending your time?"

"Just thinking about things."

"What sort of things?"

He laughed. "Crazy ideas."

"Tell me one."

And he told me that the day before, he had been lying in bed, thinking about getting up, and suddenly out of the corner of his eye he had become aware of some sort of a barrier or a wall just behind him. As he noticed it, he realized that he had always known it was there but he had never seen it before. I encouraged him to say more. "Well, I know I'm here on this side of it. But at the same time, I know I'm on the other side of it too. I don't know what that means. Do you?"

"No," I said.

"Well, I think about it a lot and it makes me feel good. It gives me that same feeling I had in your office. Sort of peaceful and joyful."

"That's a good feeling to have," I told him.

"Yes," he said.

There was a silence and very softly he started to laugh and hung up the phone. Two or three days later, I heard that he had died. I like to think he died a little differently than he might have. I like to think that, but I don't know. I can still hear his laugh.

The Question

For the last ten years of his life, Tim's father had Alzheimer's disease. Despite the devoted care of Tim's mother, he had slowly deteriorated until he had become a sort of walking vegetable. He was unable to speak and was fed, clothed, and cared for as if he were a very young child. As Tim and his brother grew older, they would stay with their father for brief periods of time while their mother took care of the needs of the household. One Sunday, while she was out doing the shopping, the boys, then fifteen and seventeen, watched football as their father sat nearby in a chair. Suddenly, he slumped forward and fell to the floor. Both sons realized immediately that something was terribly wrong. His color was gray and his breath uneven and rasping. Frightened, Tim's older brother told him to call 911. Before he could respond, a voice he had not heard in ten years, a voice he could barely remember, interrupted. "Don't call 911, son. Tell your mother that I love her. Tell her that I am all right." And Tim's father died.

Tim, a cardiologist, looked around the room at the group of doctors mesmerized by this story. "Because he died unexpectedly at home, the law required that we have an autopsy," he told us quietly. "My father's brain was almost entirely destroyed by this disease. For many years, I have asked myself, 'Who spoke?' I have never found even the slightest help from any medical textbook. I am no closer to knowing this now than I was then, but carrying this question with me reminds me of something important, something I do not want to forget. Much of life can never be explained but only witnessed."

What is the Sound of One Hand Clapping?

"For everything that happens in this world, children, there are two reasons: the good reason and the real reason." Mrs. Mullins, my fourth grade teacher, was a salty lady and many of her remarks were as cynical as this one. Often her class was too young to understand her meaning, and fearful of missing something important, I had written some of them down. Two decades later I found this one in a notebook in my own childish scrawl. I was a young physician, pretty cynical myself by then, and I chuckled at my old teacher's assessment of the deviousness of the world and assumed that one of the two reasons was false. Now, almost five decades later, I suspect actually both are true.

At the heart of every story is Mystery. The reasons we attribute to events may be far different from their true cause. Often our first interpretation of events is quite different from our last reading of them. Mystery is a process, and so is our understanding of it.

The ability to seek and find meaning in life is based more than anything on the capacity to hold paradox and maintain an unblushing cognitive dissonance. The objective world and the subjective world lie one atop the other. Spiritual causality and immediate causality are often different yet occupy the same space, and so truth may be less a matter of either/or than both/and. So perhaps Mrs. Mullins was wiser than she knew. For everything that happens in this world there *are* two reasons: the good reason and the Real reason.

Consider the Zen practice of the koan, the question or problem posed by Zen masters to each other or by masters to students. The koan is a dilemma, a mystery which the rational mind cannot solve. By frustrating and thwarting our usual strategies of obtaining answers, knowing and understanding, it causes us to begin anew. The key to the resolution of a koan is a shift in the being of the student which allows for a new understanding of the question itself.

In presenting a koan, the teacher engages the student with mystery in a highly personal way. The student becomes intimate with the question, and sometimes struggles with it for a very long time. At first Zen students respond to the mystery much as we all do: with frustration, with outraged pride, with a sense of unfairness and victimhood, with self-pity, even with anger toward the teacher. None of this works. Having exhausted all these ways, we can begin to find the capacity for other ways and these new ways begin to change us. By putting the habitual mind into a place of stuckness, a sort of fruitful darkness, we may inadvertently step back into that fertile and pregnant place of not-knowing called in Zen "beginner's mind."

Mystery can present in very ordinary ways. I didn't always know this. In the early days of my counseling practice I had a remarkable woman as a client. A gifted artist and sculptor, she had gradually become addicted to alcohol. Many years ago, when she hit bottom, her four children were taken from her and given to her mother to raise. Eventually she went into treatment and with great personal strength began a long-lasting recovery and built a productive life of service.

Now in her early fifties, she carried a great deal of responsibility at work and had a lovely apartment of her own.

After several months of sessions, she seemed on the verge of living more openheartedly and I felt this could represent a profound healing for her. At the time, friends of mine were involved in a spiritual practice to open the heart. I called them and asked them to teach me the "heart meditation" which had been so helpful to them. During one of her next visits, I taught this meditation to her and went over it with her very carefully. It took the entire session, but I felt it had been worth it. I reminded her of the importance of doing the meditation every day. She said that she would.

A week later things seemed unchanged. I asked her if she was doing the heart meditation. Sheepishly she said that she had only done it once. So we spent the remainder of the session going over it again. The following week she returned anxious and distressed. I asked once again about the meditation. No, she had not done it at all. In annoyance she said that she was not really very interested in doing it, that there was another issue that was troubling her. She would rather talk about that than the heart meditation now.

In a shaky voice she told me that in the past few weeks a rat had invaded her apartment. She felt it was unclean, even vicious, and it upset her that such a thing could enter the beautiful space that she had so painstakingly created for herself. Despite the obvious importance of this to her and its possible symbolic value, I was frustrated. At the time, I had a very limited sense of the elegance of the spiritual and the many ways it may show itself. Talking about the heart was far more important to me and I thought this rat was in my way. With a sigh I said, "Tell me more."

She became increasingly upset as she talked. She had felt unable to personally set a trap, so she had asked her son if he would come and do this for her. He had but it hadn't helped. The rat still came nightly. The people at work had also tried to be helpful. One of the women had even brought some of the bait she had used when mice invaded her garage. That hadn't worked either. Finally, she had asked the super of the building to inspect her apartment. He had spent a morning covering over all the possible entry points he could find, but the rat was still there. By this time she was almost in tears. In my impatience, I hardly noticed.

"What have *you* done about it?" I asked her. It turned out that other than putting away the edibles she had not really done very much. Finally becoming attentive, I was struck by the number of other people who had become involved. Somewhat unkindly I pointed this out. "I think this is your rat," I told her. "It will probably be there until you personally do something about it." The minute the words were out I regretted them. They had been harsh and filled with judgment.

For a week I felt badly. I had been unsympathetic and caught up in my own agenda. But she returned for her next appointment, radiant. Encouraged and undaunted, I asked her if she had done the heart meditation. It had completely slipped her mind. But a lot had happened. She told me that when she left she had been so hurt and angry that she thought she would not come back. She had been angry for days. Then she had begun to wonder if there might be something to what I was saying. So she had gone to the hardware store to see if they had a trap that would not hurt the rat. She bought something called, unbelievably, a Hav-a-Hart trap, but couldn't bring herself to use it. Traps were "just not her thing." She had felt completely overwhelmed. "I'm just too *softhearted*," she told me. Finally it came to her that if it really was her rat, why, she could deal with it in her way. She had gone to the pound and found a kitten that no one wanted and brought it home. She had not seen the rat since.

Her eyes became wet. She had not had a pet since she was four, when her father had brought home a puppy. She had loved it. Her mother had told her she could have it if she took care of it herself. But four is far too young for that sort of thing. She had tried, but the puppy was too much for her. Her mother had a hot temper, especially when she was drinking. One day the puppy would not stop barking and whining and she could not understand what it wanted and calm it. Enraged, her mother had taken it into the bathroom and drowned it.

I was stunned. Softly she told me that she had always believed this was her fault, that she had not loved the puppy well enough. But the kitten was doing well, it was growing, and every day when she came home from work, it came to meet her and rub up against her legs and purr. Finally her tears overflowed. "It really is growing," she said. "Perhaps my love is enough now."

There are many ways to look at this story but it is certainly not a story about rats. The elegance with which life offers a woman who has never trusted her own love an opportunity to experience its power is breathtaking. I like to think of this also as a story about ultimate causality. My sense of timing was true . . . but I went astray in not looking at the events of her life for the ways in which her healing was already in process, in thinking that it was I who needed to open my client's heart. We may not always recognize the ways that healing starts in our lives. The beginning of a greater wholeness may look as different as an opportunity to meet new men, a rat in an immaculate apartment, an odd idea that just won't go away, or an experience that strains our sense of the ordinary to its limits. Collaboration with this process may require a respect for the mystery which is at the heart of all growth.

The resolution of a koan requires a certain trust of mystery, a faith that there is an answer which will come in time. Understanding often requires a retreat into inner stillness, a movement away from frustration toward an expectant listening, an openness to understanding paired with a willingness to go without understanding until you have become ready to receive it. When the answer and the seeker have grown toward one another the answer seems to emerge by itself. The resolution of a koan is usually obvious; it has been staring us in the face all along, but we have never seen it before. Once glimpsed, it is difficult to believe that we ever saw things another way, and indeed we will never see things in the old way again. Our eyes have been changed by the way in which we have met with the unknown.

Like good science, the resolution of a koan requires a trust in the larger pattern which underlies the happening that the mind does not understand, and the understanding which is gained is often accompanied by a deep appreciation of the elegance of that pattern, the intelligence of the nature of things. A sense of wonder. An appreciation of the very mystery which has frustrated us. A sense of belonging to it.

Many of the problems Life poses us are seemingly without solutions, much like the koans the Zen teacher presents to the student. Yet meaning and wisdom emerge from one of Life's stories much in the way that the resolution of a koan emerges. Awaiting this meaning is almost like awaiting a birth. After we live a story or hear a story we become pregnant with its meaning. Sometimes the pregnancy may take weeks or even years. Often over time, pregnant with one story, we may give birth to many meanings, each one deeper than the one before. Most of the best stories I have ever lived or been told are like this.

Certainly suffering and illness are koans. Life may itself be a koan. Those people who are able to meet with life the way a Zen student meets with a koan will be moved along a spiritual trajectory by events which reduce others to bitterness and defeat. Not only their physical body but the quality of their soul may be changed in the encounter.

In Darkness

Light in various forms is commonly regarded as symbolic of the energies of healing. Many self-help books use the sun in healing meditations and imageries. Those of my patients who have read these books have come to expect light to symbolize the source of their healing. But things are not always as we have come to expect and the mysterious may surprise us as it did these two men.

The first, a salesman, was referred by his physician because his denial of his disease made it difficult for him to take care of himself. Over and over again he would do foolhardy things like lifting heavy boxes soon after abdominal surgery and forgetting his medications when he traveled. Essential treatment had been delayed or even sabotaged several times and he had suffered a great deal of unnecessary illness because of this. Just prior to his visit, he had developed a drug toxicity and all but lost the strength in his right arm. During the three days it had taken him to notice this he continued to take the medication. He finally called his physician only when his wife pointed out to him that he was dropping things. His doctor had taken him off the offending medication. Frightened by the possibility of permanent damage to the nerve in his arm, he had agreed to seek counseling.

In our initial conversation, he described his cancer as "this black hole in the middle of my life that keeps pulling me in." When an image appears like this in the course of ordinary conversation, it is rarely random and may tell as much about a person's unconscious world, their deepest attitudes and beliefs, as the contents of their dreams. Without our knowing it, the dream-maker in us may whisper our secrets directly to others. Steve's choice of words suggested that he was using all of his strength to resist a pull, not to surrender to the force of the disease in his life. Perhaps for him, paying attention to his symptoms and taking prescribed medications came under the heading of surrender.

I called his attention to the picture in his words and suggested that it might be saying something important about himself and his life. Perhaps so much of his energy was being used up in resistance that it did not leave him a lot left over to live with. He nodded. I asked him what was in the hole. "Just darkness," he said simply. I invited him to explore this with me in his imagination, to allow himself to be pulled into the hole just to see what it was like.

He hesitated only for a moment. Then he closed his eyes and began to enter into his own image. He imagined himself pulled into the hole, into the darkness. The following comments are from my session notes. Each one is separated by several minutes of silence.

There is darkness. Big darkness. I am floating.
The darkness is very soft . . . gentle . . . It supports me.
I have no needs here . . . (Sighs)
I am tired.
I am at rest . . . totally at rest. Every cell is resting.
Every cell is open. I am filling up . . . filling up with life.
I could not fill up because I could not open up . . . let go.
I can open up in the darkness.
Life is everywhere.
Whatever happens, it will be okay . . . .

The second man, caught up in rage at his cancer and its treatment, responded to the question "What do you think may be needed for your healing?" with a terse "Nothing!" Taking his statement at face value, I asked him to describe "nothing" to me. "Unending darkness," he said. Commenting on the power of that image, I encouraged him to close his eyes and allow himself to experience it.

As his face became more and more relaxed, I asked him how he was feeling. Again, these comments from my session notes are each separated by several minutes of silence.

> There is darkness all around me . . . .
> I'm not falling. It holds me. I am held in darkness.
> Wrapped in darkness.
> The darkness is . . . soft . . . almost tender. (Sighs)
> It's safe here.
> I needed to feel safe. I haven't relaxed since I got the diagnosis. (Sighs again) I can rest.
> I am so tired.
> No pain here. No hunger. No need.

I encouraged him to let himself relax fully. Watching him, it was apparent that he had slipped into a light trance or doze. I covered him with a soft wool blanket that I keep in my office. After a while, he commented that he could hear a sound "like a great heartbeat." It was deeply comforting.

I encouraged him to lean up against it. To rest. Soon he began to weep softly, saying, "Mama, Mama."

Another patient with cancer, a woman, told me of a dream. She turns a corner on a familiar street and is suddenly confronted by a black-cloaked figure:

> I call out for help but there is no one. I am utterly alone with this dark figure. As I turn to flee, the cloak is thrown over me. I struggle but there is no one in the cloak, only darkness. It is black, totally black, but somehow I can see . . . not with my eyes . . . the blackness goes on forever. It is very quiet. Completely silent. Velvety. Soft. I am not falling. I am floating in endless darkness. Floating . . .
>
> I am free. There is no gravity. My body does not hurt anymore. (Long pause) The darkness is like love. It's very, very good in here. It takes me in exactly as I am. There's no judgment. I am not wrong. I . . . just am.

These patients and the many others who have had such experiences were taken by surprise by the power of their spontaneous imagery and its form. We often think of health and sickness as an expression of the goodness/evil polarity. Most languages reflect this identification. We say "I feel bad" when we feel sick and "I feel good" when we recover. Darkness and light are a further extension of this polarity: healing, as a function of the good, is associated with light, and sickness, as a function of evil, is associated with darkness.

Darkness has suffered bad press for millennia. Yet is it really so surprising that spontaneous healing imagery may present itself in this way? According to the traditions of alchemy, darkness was the necessary condition for purification and transformation. Alchemists put impure dross metals into a sealed flask, creating the perfect darkness required for the transformation into pure gold.

As light represents the archetype of masculine energy, darkness suggests the power of the feminine, and it makes an intuitive sense that the *experience* of healing may be associated with darkness. Darkness is a condition of the beginning. The body first comes into being in darkness. It is nurtured, as a seed, in darkness. Some people may find their healing in remembering the beginning.

Seeing around the Corner

My given name is Rachel. I was named after my mother's mother. For the first fifty years of my life, I was called by another name, Naomi, which is my middle name. When I was in my middle forties, my mother, who was at that time almost eighty-five, elected to have coronary bypass surgery. The surgery was extremely difficult and only partly successful. For days my mother lay with two dozen others in the coronary intensive-care unit of one of our major hospitals. For the first week she was unconscious, peering over the edge of life, breathed by a ventilator. I was awed at the brutality of this surgery and the capacity of the body, even in great age, to endure such a major intervention.

When she finally regained consciousness she was profoundly disoriented and often did not know who I, her only child, was. The nurses were reassuring. We see this sort of thing often, they told me. They called it Intensive Care Psychosis and explained that in this environment of beeping machines and constant artificial light, elderly people with no familiar cues often go adrift. Nevertheless I was concerned. Not only did Mom not know me but she was hallucinating, seeing things crawling on her bed and feeling water run down her back.

Although she did not seem to know my name, she spoke to me often and at length, mostly of the past, about her own mother who died before I was born and who was regarded as a saint by all who knew her. She spoke of the many acts of kindness which her mother had done without even realizing she was being kind. "*Che-sed,*" said my mother, using a Hebrew word which roughly translates as "loving kindness." The shelter offered to those who had none, the encouragement and financial support which helped others, often strangers, to win their dreams. She spoke of her mother's humility and great learning and of the poverty and difficulty of life in Russia which she remembered as a child. She recalled the abuses and hatreds the family experienced to which many others had responded with anger and her mother only with compassion.

Days went by and my mother slowly improved physically although her mental state continued to be uncertain. The nurses began correcting her when she mistook them for people from her past, insisting that the birds she saw flying and singing in the room were not there. They encouraged me to correct her as well, telling me this was the only way she might return to what was real.

I remember one visit shortly before she left the intensive care unit. I greeted her asking if she knew who I was. "Yes," she said with warmth. "You are my beloved child." Comforted, I turned to sit on the only chair in her room but she stopped me. "Don't sit there." Doubtfully I looked at the chair again. "But why not?"

"Rachel is sitting there," she said. I turned back to my mother. It was obvious that she saw quite clearly something I could not see.

Despite the frown of the special nurse who was adjusting my mother's IV, I went into the hall, brought back another chair, and sat down on it. My mother looked at me and the empty chair next to me with tenderness. Calling me by my given name for the first time, she introduced me to her visitor: "Rachel," she said. "This is Rachel."

My mother began to tell her mother Rachel about my childhood and her pride in the person I had become. Her experience of Rachel's presence was so convincing that I found myself wondering why I could not see her. It was more than a little unnerving. And very moving. Periodically she would appear to listen and then she would tell me of my grandmother's reactions to what she had told her. They spoke of people I had never met in the familiar way of gossip: my great-grandfather David and his brothers, my great-granduncles, who were handsome men and great horsemen. "Devils," said my mother, laughing and nodding her head to the empty chair. She explained to her mother why she had given me her name, her hope for my kindness of heart, and apologized for my father who had insisted on calling me by my middle name, which had come from his side of our family.

Exhausted by all this conversation, my mother lay back on her pillows and closed her eyes briefly. When she opened them again, she smiled at me and the empty chair. "I'm so glad you are both here now," she said. "One of you will take me home." Then she closed her eyes again and drifted off to sleep. It was my grandmother who took her home.

This experience, disturbing as it was for me at the time, seemed deeply comforting to my mother and became something I revisited again and again after she died. I had survived many years of chronic illness and physical limitation. I had been one of the few women in my class at medical school in the fifties, one of the few women on the faculty at the Stanford medical school in the sixties. I was expert at dealing with limitations and challenges of various sorts. I had not succeeded through *loving kindness.* Over a period of time I came to realize that despite my successes I had perhaps lost something of importance. When I turned fifty, I began asking people to call me Rachel, my real name.

Remembering the Sacred

In response to an invitation to remember a moment in the practice of medicine that might be considered a sacred experience, a seasoned neonatologist, the director of the neonatal unit at a large southern hospital, offered a group of colleagues this account. After weeks of struggle, her patient, a tiny premature baby, was dying despite everything that a state-of-the-art intensive care nursery could offer. It would not be long and it was time for the parents to say good-bye. With a heavy heart she called the baby's father and invited him to meet her at the hospital. The child's mother, distraught after weeks of uncertainty, now required medication. She had stopped visiting a few weeks ago. He would come alone, he said.

As she put down the phone she became aware of the beeping of the monitors and other machines and the bustle of the intensive care nursery and felt the need for some quiet to organize her thoughts while she waited for him to arrive. She went down the hall to the chapel, the only quiet place nearby, to be alone for a few minutes and find words to tell the young father that his little son was not going to make it.

Fifteen minutes later, as she was walking toward the visitors' waiting room, she found herself thinking that perhaps she should give the baby a trial with a certain drug. The thought surprised her, as this drug was not customarily used for the baby's problem, and she shook her head in annoyance. But the strange thought would not easily go away. She reviewed the baby's course with the father, assuring him that everything possible had been done and suggesting they go to the intensive care nursery together to say good-bye. As she looked at the sadness in his face, she found herself thinking, "After all, what does it matter?" and suggested that perhaps there was one more thing she could try, a drug not usually given for this condition, but which she was thinking of using now. She would like to have his permission to use it. He gave this readily and they went to the nursery together.

The baby appeared moribund. Embarrassed to make so unusual a request of the nurses, she prepared the injection and administered it herself. Together she and the father waited, standing on either side of the Isolette, watching the blue and gasping baby. There was no change. Wanting to give him a chance to be alone with his child for the last time, she left to do some paperwork. A few hours later, she looked into the unit and was surprised to see him still there. She approached the Isolette and found that the infant's tiny chest had slowed and his breathing was normal. Scarcely able to believe her eyes, she raised her head and found the father looking at her. Their eyes held for a long, wordless moment. This was the moment she had chosen to tell us about as a "sacred" moment. Recently these parents brought their child back to visit her. He is twelve years old.

The circle of physicians sat thinking about this for a while. Then the neonatologist began to describe the way in which she had dealt with this strange happening at the time. She has a very orderly and pragmatic mind, she told us, and it had disturbed her. She had tried to find an explanation for it so she could dismiss it. Gradually she became convinced that somewhere she had read or heard a preliminary report of research which mentioned the use of this drug for the baby's condition and this was why she had thought of it. She could not remember the journal or the meeting where she had gotten this information, but she became more and more certain that it was so. This allowed her to forget the whole thing.

About two years later, she read of a study of premature infants with severe respiratory distress who had been given this very drug and had recovered. The mystery was solved! Delighted, she called the researchers to ask where they had published their preliminary reports or presented their work in progress. She was stunned to discover that this article was the first time that the study had been written up or presented anywhere. It had just been too odd to talk about until the results were final. She told them then that she had an additional case.

In musing aloud about her personal reactions, she told us that she had clung to an explanation that would have allowed her to keep her familiar and comfortable sense of the way in which the world works. She had rejected the gift of awe once, so it had to be given to her again.

A second physician, a specialist in palliative care, talked about an experience he had while caring for a hospitalized young man who was dying of AIDS. Both the patient and his family were bitter, rejecting, and hostile despite his efforts to reach out to them. Finally giving up on it, he had simply delivered the best technical care he knew.

At three o'clock one morning he was called by the nurses, who informed him that his patient had died and asked him to come in to pronounce him dead and sign the death certificate. Remembering that he needed to be at rounds very early the next morning, he hastily threw clothes over his pajamas, and began driving to the hospital. As he drove down the darkened streets, he spontaneously looked up and saw the night sky as if for the first time. The darkness seemed a silent and holy emptiness without beginning or end. In this vastness, stars hung as countless pure points of radiance. He had never seen the night in this way and was filled with awe and a profound feeling of peace and gratitude. His intellect attempted to dismiss this as fanciful, pointing out the need to hurry and take care of business so as to be able to get up early the next day. But he stopped his car by the side of the road anyway, got out, and allowed the experience of awe to wash over him. In about fifteen minutes it receded and he drove on to the hospital under a sky that looked much the same as always. The experience had been brief, but powerful and surprisingly important to him although he couldn't say why.

Together the group of physicians considered what this experience may possibly have meant. Various interpretations were offered, but the one that stopped further conversation was that perhaps the patient, in passing onward, may have found a way to share his present perspective directly with his doctor as an apology and a parting gift. As one of the doctors put it, "Perhaps at the moment of death there is a reclaiming of wholeness . . . and that wholeness may pass very close to us."

Mystery

I was late for what was to be my last visit with my mother. Pushing through rush hour traffic, tired from a long day at the office, I stopped to buy her some flowers. It was seven in the evening and the florist had no purple irises, my mother's favorites, and little of anything else. Sympathizing with my distress, he offered me a bouquet of half-closed iris buds from his icebox, assuring me that they would open in a few hours. I took them and waited, irritated and impatient, as he wrapped them in green tissue. A strange-looking bouquet. Then I hurried on.

Carrying the flowers, I pushed through the heavy doors of the ward. A nurse was waiting there for me. "I'm so sorry," she said. My mother had died a short time before. Stunned, I allowed myself to be led to her room. She lay in her bed, seemingly asleep. Her hands were still warm. The nurse asked if there was anyone I wanted her to call. Numbly I gave her the numbers of some of my oldest friends and sat down to wait. It was peaceful and very still in the room. One by one my friends came.

Four days later I was three thousand miles away arranging for my mother's burial. It was an unseasonably hot spring and New York City was at its worst, muggy and uncomfortable. The funeral director was a person of sensitivity and kindness. Gently he went over the arrangements, assuring himself and me again of the details of my mother's wishes which we had discussed on the phone. Then he paused. "There was something that came from California with your mother. May I show you?" he asked. Together we walked down the corridor to where my mother lay in her closed pine coffin. Lying on the coffin lid, still in the twist of green tissue paper was the bouquet I had left in my mother's hospital room on her bed. But now the irises were in full bloom. I remember them still with great clarity, each one huge and vibrant, seemingly filled with a purple sort of light. They had been out of water for four days.

It would be easy indeed to dismiss this sort of experience, not to make a simple shift in perspective or find a willingness to suspend disbelief for a moment. Not to consider adding up the column of figures in another way and wonder. The willingness to consider possibility requires a tolerance of uncertainty. I will never know whether or not I was once for a moment in the presence of my Russian grandmother or if my mother used my final gift of flowers to make me a gift of her own, letting me know that there may be more to life than the mind can understand.

The Final Lesson

Sometimes the particulars of the way in which someone dies, the time, place, even the circumstances, may cause those left behind to wonder whether the event marks the healing of hidden patterns and personal issues, and answers for that person's certain lifelong questions. Death has been referred to as the great teacher. It may be the great healer as well. *Educare,* the root word of "education," means to lead forth the innate wholeness in a person. So, in the deepest sense, that which truly educates us also heals us.

The theory of karma suggests that life itself is in its essential nature both educational and healing, that the innate wholeness underlying the personality of each of us is being evoked, clarified, and strengthened throughout the challenges and experiences of our lifetime. All life paths may be a movement toward the soul. In which case our death may be the final and most integrating of our life's experiences.

When I met Thomas, he was over seventy, a family-practice physician who had been in solo practice for almost fifty years. Whole families, from grandparents to grandchildren, looked to him for help in their troubles, counted on his counsel, and called him their friend. He looked the part too, gray-haired, kindly, his body as spare and gnarled as an old oak.

At the time that we met, he had end-stage lung cancer. He could no longer get around without the constant flow of oxygen through a nasal catheter, and the previous month he had closed his medical practice. Until the last year he had never missed a day. An astute diagnostician, he had come because he knew he was dying. He proposed that we open a series of conversations about his life. He had done some reflection in recent years but felt that sharing the process at this point might be helpful in readying himself for death.

Thomas felt death to be an unqualified ending to life. Raised a Catholic, he had left the church early and embraced science as a way to bring order to the chaos of life. It had not failed him. Yet life had intrinsic value for him and he wished to examine and understand his own life and what it had meant.

It surprised me that a man this altruistic, compassionate, and reverent toward the life in others, this awed by the beauty of anatomy and physiology, held no religious or spiritual belief. Curious, I asked him about the circumstances under which he had decided to leave the church. Open and frank about other details of his long life, he was reticent in the extreme about this. He had left at sixteen over a specific happening. I never found out what it was.

Thomas had been a loner all his life. Never married, he had led a personal life that was solitary almost to the point of asceticism. Yet he was a connoisseur of beauty in all its forms, a patron of the arts, poetry, theater, music, ballet, and literature. His library held over a thousand books. Thomas's major commitment was to his medicine, his families and their needs, hopes, and dreams. His devotion to them was absolute.

Very early on in our discussions, I asked him how he saw his relationship to his patients. Looking at a small figurine of a shepherd with his flock that another patient had given me, he smiled. "Like that." We spent the next few weeks examining the nature of his work and what it had meant to him. The shepherd was a steward of the life in the flock, he protected them from danger, helped them to find nurture and fulfill themselves. He delivered their young. He found the strays and brought them back to the others.

Thomas told me many stories of his shepherding and the life of his flock. We examined these stories together, sharing our thoughts and perspectives. In the telling and the reflection, he seemed to be unfolding a much deeper sense of what his life had meant to others and what he had stood for. In these discussions, he often used an odd Victorian word: they "sheltered" with him. He was their safety, their support, their friend. He was there for them, constant, vigilant, and trustworthy. We discussed the yang or masculine principle of action and protection and the yin or feminine principle of acceptance and nurture and how these came together in the person of a shepherd. The symbol emerged as a symbol of wholeness.

All the while, he was becoming more and more ill, his breathing more labored. Eventually I raised the issue of his personal isolation. Who did he shelter with, who was the shepherd's shepherd? "No one," he said, the words holding more pain than he had expressed before. It became clear that he did not believe that there was a place of sheltering for himself. Shepherd though he was professionally, personally he had become separated from the flock, a nonparticipant, a lost person. He seemed unwilling to go much further with this.

Puzzled, I asked him to make up a story about a lost lamb, and haltingly he described a lamb that had been lost for so long that he could not even remember there was a flock. He had learned to survive by himself, to eat what was available, to hide from predators. "Does this lamb know that his shepherd is looking for him?" I asked. "No," he said, "the lamb had done something very bad and the shepherd had forgotten him."

"As a shepherd yourself, would you look for a lost lamb who had done something bad?" He seemed puzzled. I reminded him of the young patient from the projects he had told me about, the one he had taken on as a guardian from the juvenile courts, the girl who eventually went on to college. I asked him why he had gone after her and brought her home. "Why, she was one of mine," he said unhesitatingly. "Yes," I said. There was a small silence. Then he abruptly changed the subject, but I saw he was deeply affected by the thought that the bond between the shepherd and his sheep might lie beyond judgment and was deeper than he had previously thought.

We talked of many other things over the next months and gradually the image of the shepherd retreated to the back of my mind. We spoke of childhood and manhood and lost love, and the richness of seventy years of living became apparent to us both. It had been a good life.

Thomas was hospitalized once and his health continued to worsen. His oncologist had exhausted all treatment for his cancer and began to increase medications to ease his respiratory distress. Gradually he became too ill to come to the office and in the fall I began to see him at his home. Hospice was called and by the beginning of December he had become so short of breath that he could no longer speak. I sat with him and held his hand. Sometimes I would read him poetry or sing to him a little.

Somehow he kept hanging on. The hospice workers were surprised by his endurance. One of his nurses told me that she thought he was waiting for something. I thought perhaps she was right but I had no idea of what it could be. His brother had come from the East Coast to say good-bye and many of his patients had already visited and left cards and other expressions of their love.

On Christmas Eve I received a call from his nurse. Thomas had been in a coma all day and now he was having difficulty with his secretions. Would I come? As soon as I saw Thomas, I realized that he was dying. His breathing, always labored, had become shallow and intermittent. The nurse with him was young and seemed a little uncertain and so I invited her to stay as I talked to him. He did not respond in any way. We changed his sheets and made him more comfortable. Then we sat down together to wait. Gradually the space between his breaths lengthened and after a while his breathing stopped.

The young nurse seemed relieved. She called Thomas's brother, who had asked to be notified and who said that he would fly out the next day. He asked that she call the funeral director Thomas had chosen and she called him, too. She called his oncologist to sign the death certificate. There seemed nothing more to do. I stood for a time at the foot of Thomas's bed, thinking about him and wishing him well. Then I left.

It was dark and I had grown quite cold. Holding my keys in my pocket, I huddled into my coat and walked a little faster. I had almost reached my car when church bells throughout the city began ringing. For a moment I stopped, confused. Could they be ringing for Thomas? And then I remembered. It was midnight. The Shepherd had come.

THE WOUND-DRESSER

WALT WHITMAN

An old man bending I come among new faces,
Years looking backward resuming in answer to children,
Come tell us old man, as from young men and maidens that love me,
(Arous'd and angry, I'd thought to beat the alarum, and urge relentless war,
But soon my fingers fail'd me, my face droop'd and I resign'd myself,
To sit by the wounded and soothe them, or silently watch the dead;)
Years hence of these scenes, of those furious passions, these chances,
Of unsurpass'd heroes, (was one side so brave? The other was equally brave;)
Now be witness again, paint the mightiest armies of earth,
Of those armies so rapid so wondrous what saw you to tell us?
What stays with you latest and deepest? of curious panics,
Of hard-fought engagements or sieges tremendous what deepest remains?

O maidens and young men I love and that love me,
What you ask of my days those the strangest and sudden your talking recalls,
Soldier alert I arrive after a long march cover'd with sweat and dust,
In the nick of time I come, plunge in the fight, loudly shout in the rush of
successful charge,
Enter the captur'd works—yet lo, like a swift running river they fade,
Pass and are gone they fade—I dwell not on soldiers' perils or soldiers' joys,
(Both I remember well—many of the hardships, few the joys, yet I was content.)

But in silence, in dreams' projections,
While the world of gain and appearance and mirth goes on,
So soon, what is over forgotten, and waves wash the imprints off the sand,
With hinged knees returning I enter the doors, (while for you up there,
Whoever you are, follow without noise and be of strong heart.)

This version of "The Wound-Dresser" is from *Civil War Poetry: An Anthology,* edited by Paul Negri (Mineola: Dover, 1997): 91–93.

Bearing the bandages, water and sponge,
Straight and swift to my wounded I go,
Where they lie on the ground after the battle brought in,
Where their priceless blood reddens the grass the ground,
Or to the rows of the hospital tent, or under the roof'd hospital,
To the long rows of cots up and down each side I return,
To each and all one after another I draw near, not one do I miss,
An attendant follows holding a tray, he carries a refuse pail,
Soon to be fill'd with clotted rags and blood, emptied and fill'd again.

I onward go, I stop,
With hinged knees and steady hand to dress wounds,
I am firm with each, the pangs are sharp yet unavoidable,
One turns to me his appealing eyes—poor boy! I never knew you,
Yet I think I could not refuse this moment to die for you, if that would save you.

On, on I go, (open doors of time! open hospital doors!)
The crush'd head I dress, (poor crazed hand tear not the bandage away,)
The neck of the cavalry man with the bullet through and through I examine,
Hard the breathing rattles, quite glazed already the eye, yet life struggles hard,
(Come sweet death! be persuaded O beautiful death!
In mercy come quickly.)

From the stump of the arm, the amputated hand,
I undo the clotted lint, remove the slough, wash off the matter and blood,
Back on his pillow the soldier bends with curv'd neck and side falling head,
His eyes are closed, his face is pale, he dares not look on the bloody stump,
And has not yet look'd on it.
I dress a wound in the side, deep, deep,
But a day or two more, for see the frame all wasted and sinking,
And the yellow-blue countenance see.

I dress the perforated shoulder, the foot with the bullet-wound,
Cleanse the one with a gnawing and putrid gangrene, so sickening, so offensive,
While the attendant stands aside me holding the tray and pail.

I am faithful, I do not give out,
The fractur'd thigh, the knee, the wound in the abdomen,
These and more I dress with impassive hand, (yet deep in my breast a fire, a
burning flame.)

Thus in silence in dreams' projections,
Returning, resuming, I thread my way through the hospitals,
The hurt and wounded I pacify with soothing hand,
I sit by the restless all the dark night, some are so young,
Some suffer so much, I recall the experience sweet and sad,
(Many a soldier's loving arms about this neck have cross'd and rested,
Many a soldier's kiss dwells on these bearded lips.)

A NIGHT

LOUISA MAY ALCOTT

Being fond of the night side of nature, I was soon promoted to the post of night nurse, with every facility for indulging in my favorite pastime of "owling." My colleague, a black eyed widow, relieved me at dawn, we two taking care of the ward between us, like regular nurses, turn and turn about. I usually found my boys in the jolliest state of mind their condition allowed; for it was a known fact that Nurse Periwinkle objected to blue devils, and entertained a belief that he who laughed most was surest of recovery. At the beginning of my reign, dumps and dismals prevailed; the nurses looked anxious and tired, the men gloomy or sad; and a general "Hark!-from-the-tombs-a-doleful-sound" style of conversation seemed to be the fashion: a state of things which caused one coming from a merry, social New England town, to feel as if she had got into an exhausted receiver; and the instinct of self-preservation, to say nothing of a philanthropic desire to serve the race, caused a speedy change in Ward No. 1.

More flattering than the most gracefully turned compliment, more grateful than the most admiring glance, was the sight of those rows of faces, all strange to me a little while ago, now lighting up, with smiles of welcome, as I came among them, enjoying that moment heartily, with a womanly pride in their regard, a motherly affection for them all. The evenings were spent in reading aloud, writing letters, waiting on and amusing the men, going the rounds with Dr. P., as he made his second daily survey, dressing my dozen wounds afresh, giving last doses, and making them cozy for the long hours to come, till the nine o'clock bell rang, the gas was turned down, the day nurses went off duty, the night watch came on, and my nocturnal adventures began.

My ward was now divided into three rooms; and, under favor of the matron, I had managed to sort out the patients in such a way that I had what I called, "my duty room," my "pleasure room," and my "pathetic room," and worked for each in a

"A Night" is Chapter 4 of *Hospital Sketches*, written by Louisa May Alcott in 1863. This edition is from a BLS Publication (Carlisle, MA: Applewood Books, 1992).

different way. One, I visited, armed with a dressing tray, full of rollers, plasters, and pins; another, with books, flowers, games, and gossip; a third, with teapots, lullabies, consolation, and, sometimes, a shroud.

Wherever the sickest or most helpless man chanced to be, there I held my watch, often visiting the other rooms, to see that the general watchman of the ward did his duty by the fires and the wounds, the latter needing constant wetting. Not only on this account did I meander, but also to get fresher air than the close rooms afforded; for, owing to the stupidity of that mysterious "somebody" who does all the damage in the world, the windows had been carefully nailed down above, and the lower sashes could only be raised in the mildest weather, for the men lay just below. I had suggested a summary smashing of a few panes here and there, when frequent appeals to headquarters had proved unavailing, and daily orders to lazy attendants had come to nothing. No one seconded the motion, however, and the nails were far beyond my reach; for, though belonging to the sisterhood of "ministering angels," I had no wings, and might as well have asked for a suspension bridge, as a pair of steps, in that charitable chaos.

One of the harmless ghosts who bore me company during the haunted hours, was Dan, the watchman, whom I regarded with a certain awe; for, though so much together, I never fairly saw his face, and, but for his legs, should never have recognized him, as we seldom met by day. These legs were remarkable, as was his whole figure, for his body was short, rotund, and done up in a big jacket, and muffler; his beard hid the lower part of his face, his hat-brim the upper; and all I ever discovered was a pair of sleepy eyes, and a very mild voice. But the legs!—very long, very thin, very crooked and feeble, looking like gray sausages in their tight coverings, and finished off with a pair of expansive, green cloth shoes, very like Chinese junks with the sails down. This figure, gliding noiselessly about the dimly-lighted rooms, was strongly suggestive of the spirit of a beer-barrel mounted on cork-screws, haunting the old hotel in search of its lost mates, emptied and staved in long ago.

Another goblin who frequently appeared to me, was the attendant of "the pathetic room," who, being a faithful soul, was often up to tend two or three men, weak and wandering as babies, after the fever had gone. The amiable creature beguiled the watches of the night by brewing jorums of a fearful beverage, which he called coffee, and insisted on sharing with me; coming in with a great bowl of something like mud soup, scalding hot, guiltless of cream, rich in an all-pervading flavor of molasses, scorch and tin pot. Such an amount of good will and neighborly kindness also went into the mess, that I never could find the heart to refuse, but always received it with thanks, sipped it with hypocritical relish while he remained, and whipped it into the slop-jar the instant he departed, thereby gratifying him, securing one rousing laugh in the doziest hour of the night, and no one was the worse for the transaction but the pigs. Whether they were "cut off untimely in their sins," or not, I carefully abstained from inquiring.

It was a strange life—asleep half the day, exploring Washington the other half, and all night hovering, like a massive cherubim, in a red rigolette, over the slumbering sons of man. I liked it, and found many things to amuse, instruct, and interest me. The snores alone were quite a study, varying from the mild sniff to the stentorian snort, which startled the echoes and hoisted the performer erect to accuse his neighbor of the deed, magnanimously forgive him, and, wrapping the drapery of his couch about him, lie down to vocal slumber. After listening for a week to this band of wind instruments, I indulged in the belief that I could recognize each by the snore alone, and was tempted to join the chorus by breaking out with John Brown's favorite hymn:

"Blow ye the trumpet, blow!"

I would have given much to have possessed the art of sketching, for many of the faces became wonderfully interesting when unconscious. Some grew stern and grim, the men evidently dreaming of war, as they gave orders, groaned over their wounds, or damned the rebels vigorously; some grew sad and infinitely pathetic, as if the pain borne silently all day, revenged itself by now betraying what the man's pride had concealed so well. Often the roughest grew young and pleasant when sleep smoothed the hard lines away, letting the real nature assert itself; many almost seemed to speak, and I learned to know these men better by night than through any intercourse by day. Sometimes they disappointed me, for faces that looked merry and good in the light, grew bad and sly when the shadows came; and though they made no confidences in words, I read their lives, leaving them to wonder at the change of manner this midnight magic wrought in their nurse. A few talked busily; one drummer boy sang sweetly, though no persuasions could win a note from him by day; and several depended on being told what they had talked of in the morning. Even my constitutionals in the chilly halls possessed a certain charm, for the house was never still. Sentinels tramped round it all night long, their muskets glittering in the wintry moonlight as they walked, or stood before the doors, straight and silent, as figures of stone, causing one to conjure up romantic visions of guarded forts, sudden surprises, and daring deeds; for in these war times the hum drum life of Yankeedom has vanished, and the most prosaic feel some thrill of that excitement which stirs the nation's heart, and makes its capital a camp of hospitals. Wandering up and down these lower halls, I often heard cries from above, steps hurrying to and fro, saw surgeons passing up, or men coming down carrying a stretcher, where lay a long white figure, whose face was shrouded and whose fight was done. Sometimes I stopped to watch the passers in the street, the moonlight shining on the spire opposite, or the gleam of some vessel floating, like a white-winged sea-gull, down the broad Potomac, whose fullest flow can never wash away the red stain of the land.

The night whose events I have a fancy to record, opened with a little comedy, and closed with a great tragedy; for a virtuous and useful life untimely ended is always tragical to those who see not as God sees. My headquarters were beside the bed of a

New Jersey boy, crazed by the horrors of that dreadful Saturday. A slight wound in the knee brought him there; but his mind had suffered more than his body; some string of that delicate machine was over strained, and, for days, he had been re-living in imagination, the scenes he could not forget, till his distress broke out in incoherent ravings, pitiful to hear. As I sat by him, endeavoring to soothe his poor distracted brain by the constant touch of wet hands over his hot forehead, he lay cheering his comrades on, hurrying them back, then counting them as they fell around him often clutching my arm, to drag me from the vicinity of a bursting shell, or covering up his head to screen himself from a shower of shot; his face brilliant with fever; his eyes restless; his head never still; every muscle strained and rigid; while an incessant stream of defiant shouts, whispered warnings, and broken laments, poured from his lips with that forceful bewilderment which makes such wanderings so hard to overhear.

It was past eleven, and my patient was slowly wearying himself into fitful intervals of quietude, when, in one of these pauses, a curious sound arrested my attention. Looking over my shoulder, I saw a one-legged phantom hopping nimbly down the room; and, going to meet it, recognized a certain Pennsylvania gentleman, whose wound-fever had taken a turn for the worse, and, depriving him of the few wits a drunken campaign had left him, set him literally tripping on the light, fantastic toe "toward home," as he blandly informed me, touching the military cap which formed a striking contrast to the severe simplicity of the rest of his *undress* uniform. When sane, the least movement produced a roar of pain or a volley of oaths; but the departure of reason seemed to have wrought an agreeable change, both in the man and his manners; for, balancing himself on one leg, like a meditative stork, he plunged into an animated discussion of the war, the President, lager beer, and Enfield rifles, regardless of any suggestions of mine as to the propriety of returning to bed, lest he be court-martialed for desertion.

Any thing more supremely ridiculous can hardly be imagined than this figure, all draped in white, its one foot covered with a big blue sock, a dingy cap set rakingly askew on its shaven head, and placid satisfaction beaming in its broad red face, as it flourished a mug in one hand, an old boot in the other, calling them canteen and knapsack, while it skipped and fluttered in the most unearthly fashion. What to do with the creature I didn't know; Dan was absent, and if I went to find him, the perambulator might festoon himself out of the window, set his toga on fire, or do some of his neighbors a mischief. The attendant of the room was sleeping like a near relative of the celebrated Seven, and nothing short of pins would rouse him; for he had been out that day, and whiskey asserted its supremacy in balmy whiffs. Still declaiming, in a fine flow of eloquence, the demented gentleman hopped on, blind and deaf to my graspings and entreaties; and I was about to slam the door in his face, and run for help, when a second and saner phantom came to the rescue, in the likeness of a big Prussian, who spoke no English, but divined the crisis, and put an end to it, by bundling the lively monoped into his bed, like a baby, with an authoritative command to "stay put," which received added weight from being delivered in an odd conglomeration of French and German, accompanied by warning wags of a head decorated with a yellow cotton night cap, rendered most imposing by a tassel like a bell-pull. Rather exhausted by his excursion, the member from Pennsylvania subsided; and, after an irrepressible laugh together, my Prussian ally and myself were returning to our places, when the echo of a sob caused us to glance along the beds. It came from one in the corner—such a little bed!—and such a tearful little face looked up at us, as we stopped beside it! The twelve years old drummer boy was not singing now, but sobbing, with a manly effort all the while to stifle the distressful sounds that would break out.

"What is it, Billy?" I asked, as he rubbed the tears away, and checked himself in the middle of a great sob to answer plaintively:

"I've got a chill, ma'am, but I ain't cryin' for that, 'cause I'm used to it. I dreamed Kit was here, and when I waked up he wasn't, and I couldn't help it, then."

The boy came in with the rest, and the man who was taken dead from the ambulance was the Kit he mourned. Well he might, for, when the wounded were brought from Fredericksburg, the child lay in one of the camps thereabout, and this good friend, though sorely hurt himself, would not leave him to the exposure and neglect of such a time and place; but, wrapping him in his own blanket, carried him in his arms to the transport, tended him during the passage, and only yielded up his charge when Death met him at the door of the hospital which promised care and comfort for the boy. For ten days, Billy had burned or shivered with fever and ague, pining the while for Kit, and refusing to be comforted, because he had not been able to thank him for the generous protection, which, perhaps, had cost the giver's life. The vivid dream had wrung the childish heart with a fresh pang, and when I tried the solace fitted for his years, the remorseful fear that haunted him found vent in a fresh burst of tears, as he looked at the wasted hands I was endeavoring to warm:

"Oh! if I'd only been as thin when Kit carried me as I am now, maybe he wouldn't have died; but I was heavy, he was hurt worser than we knew, and so it killed him; and I didn't see him, to say good bye."

This thought had troubled him in secret; and my assurances that his friend would probably have died at all events, barely assuaged the bitterness of his regretful grief.

At this juncture, the delirious man began to shout; the one-legged rose up in his bed, as if preparing for another dart, Billy bewailed himself more piteously than before: and if ever a woman was at her wit's end, that distracted female was Nurse Periwinkle, during the space of two or three minutes, as she vibrated between the three beds, like an agitated pendulum. Like a most opportune reinforcement, Dan, the bandy, appeared, and devoted himself to the lively party, leaving me free to return to my post; for the Prussian, with a nod and smile, took the lad away to his own bed, and lulled him to sleep with a soothing murmur, like a mammoth humblebee. I liked that in Fritz, and if he ever wondered afterward at the dainties which sometimes found their way into his rations, or the extra comforts of his bed, he might have found a solution of the mystery in sundry persons' knowledge of the fatherly action of that night.

Hardly was I settled again, when the inevitable bowl appeared, and its bearer delivered a message I had expected, yet dreaded to receive:

"John is going, ma'am, and wants to see you, if you can come."

"The moment this boy is asleep; tell him so, and let me know if I am in danger of being too late."

My Ganymede departed, and while I quieted poor Shaw, I thought of John. He came in a day or two after the others; and, one evening, when I entered my "pathetic room," I found a lately emptied bed occupied by a large, fair man, with a fine face, and the serenest eyes I ever met. One of the earlier comers had often spoken of a friend, who had remained behind, that those apparently worse wounded than himself might reach a shelter first. It seemed a David and Jonathan sort of friendship. The man fretted for his mate, and was never tired of praising John—his courage, sobriety, self-denial, and unfailing kindliness of heart; always winding up with: "He's an out an' out fine feller, ma'am, you see if he aint."

I had some curiosity to behold this piece of excellence, and when he came, watched him for a night or two, before I made friends with him; for, to tell the truth, I was a little afraid of the stately looking man, whose bed had to be lengthened to accommodate his commanding stature; who seldom spoke, uttered no complaint, asked no sympathy, but tranquilly observed what went on about him; and, as he lay high upon his pillows, no picture of dying statesman or warrior was ever fuller of real dignity than this Virginia blacksmith. A most attractive face he had, framed in brown hair and beard, comely featured and full of vigor, as yet unsubdued by pain; thoughtful and often beautifully mild while watching the afflictions of others, as if entirely forgetful of his own. His mouth was grave and firm, with plenty of will and courage in its lines, but a smile could make it as sweet as any woman's; and his eyes were a child's eyes, looking one fairly in the face, with a clear, straightforward glance, which promised well for such as placed their faith in him. He seemed to cling to life, as if it were rich in duties and delights, and he had learned the secret of content. The only time I saw his composure disturbed, was when my surgeon brought another to examine John, who scrutinized their faces with an anxious look, asking of the elder: "Do you think I shall pull through, sir?" "I hope so, my man." And, as the two passed on, John's eye still followed them, with an intentness which would have won a truer answer from them, had they seen it. A momentary shadow flitted over his face; then came the usual serenity, as if, in that brief eclipse, he had acknowledged the existence of some hard possibility, and, asking nothing yet hoping all things, left the issue in God's hands, with that submission which is true piety.

The next night, as I went my rounds with Dr. P., I happened to ask which man in the room probably suffered most; and, to my great surprise, he glanced at John:

"Every breath he draws is like a stab; for the ball pierced the left lung, broke a rib, and did no end of damage here and there; so the poor lad can find neither forgetfulness nor ease, because he must lie on his wounded back or suffocate. It will be a hard struggle, and a long one, for he possesses great vitality; but even his temperate life can't save him; I wish it could."

"You don't mean he must die, Doctor?"

"Bless you, there's not the slightest hope for him; and you'd better tell him so before long; women have a way of doing such things comfortably, so I leave it to you. He won't last more than a day or two, at furthest."

I could have sat down on the spot and cried heartily, if I had not learned the wisdom of bottling up one's tears for leisure moments. Such an end seemed very hard for such a man, when half a dozen worn out, worthless bodies round him, were gathering up the remnants of wasted lives, to linger on for years perhaps, burdens to others, daily reproaches to themselves. The army needed men like John, earnest, brave, and faithful; fighting for liberty and justice with both heart and hand, true soldiers of the Lord. I could not give him up so soon, or think with any patience of so excellent a nature robbed of its fulfillment, and blundered into eternity by the rashness or stupidity of those at whose hands so many lives may be required. It was an easy thing for Dr. P. to say: "Tell him he must die," but a cruelly hard thing to do, and by no means as "comfortable" as he politely suggested. I had not the heart to do it then, and privately indulged the hope that some change for the better might take place, in spite of gloomy prophesies; so, rendering my task unnecessary.

A few minutes later, as I came in again, with fresh rollers, I saw John sitting erect, with no one to support him, while the surgeon dressed his back. I had never hitherto seen it done; for, having simpler wounds to attend to, and knowing the fidelity of the attendant, I had left John to him, thinking it might be more agreeable and safe; for both strength and experience were needed in his case. I had forgotten that the strong man might long for the gentle tendance of a woman's hands, the sympathetic magnetism of a woman's presence, as well as the feebler souls about him. The Doctor's words caused me to reproach myself with neglect, not of any real duty perhaps, but of those little cares and kindnesses that solace homesick spirits, and make the heavy hours pass easier. John looked lonely and forsaken just then, as he sat with bent head, hands folded on his knee, and no outward sign of suffering, till, looking nearer, I saw great tears roll down and drop upon the floor. It was a new sight there; for, though I had seen many suffer, some swore, some groaned, most endured silently, but none wept. Yet it did not seem weak, only very touching, and straightway my fear vanished, my heart opened wide and took him in, as, gathering the bent head in my arms, as freely as if he had been a little child, I said, "Let me help you bear it, John."

Never, on any human countenance, have I seen so swift and beautiful a look of gratitude, surprise and comfort, as that which answered me more eloquently than the whispered—

"Thank you, ma'am, this is right good! this is what I wanted!"

"Then why not ask for it before?"

"I didn't like to be a trouble; you seemed so busy, and I could manage to get on alone."

"You shall not want it any more, John."

Nor did he; for now I understood the wistful look that sometimes followed me, as I went out, after a brief pause beside his bed, or merely a passing nod, while busied with those who seemed to need me more than he, because more urgent in their demands. Now I knew that to him, as to so many, I was the poor substitute for mother, wife, or sister, and in his eyes no stranger, but a friend who hitherto had seemed neglectful; for, in his modesty, he had never guessed the truth. This was changing now; and, through the tedious operation of probing, bathing, and dressing his wounds, he leaned against me, holding my hand fast, and, if pain wrung further tears from him, no one saw them fall but me. When he was laid down again, I hovered about him, in a remorseful state of mind that would not let me rest, till I had bathed his face, brushed his bonny brown hair, set all things smooth about him, and laid a knot of heath and heliotrope on his clean pillow. While doing this, he watched me with the satisfied expression I so like to see; and when I offered the little nosegay, held it carefully in his great hand, smoothed a ruffled leaf or two, surveyed and smelt it with an air of genuine delight, and lay contentedly regarding the glimmer of the sunshine on the green. Although the manliest man among my forty, he said, "Yes, ma'am," like a little boy; received suggestions for his comfort with the quick smile that brightened his whole face; and now and then, as I stood tidying the table by his bed, I felt him softly touch my gown, as if to assure himself that I was there. Anything more natural and frank I never saw, and found this brave John as bashful as brave, yet full of excellencies and fine aspirations, which, having no power to express themselves in words, seemed to have bloomed into his character and made him what he was.

After that night, an hour of each evening that remained to him was devoted to his ease or pleasure. He could not talk much, for breath was precious, and he spoke in whispers; but from occasional conversations, I gleaned scraps of private history which only added to the affection and respect I felt for him. Once he asked me to write a letter, and as I settled pen and paper, I said, with an irrepressible glimmer of feminine curiosity, "Shall it be addressed to wife, or mother, John?"

"Neither, ma'am; I've got no wife, and will write to mother myself when I get better. Did you think I was married because of this?" he asked, touching a plain ring he wore, and often turned thoughtfully on his finger when he lay alone.

"Partly that, but more from a settled sort of look you have; a look which young men seldom get until they marry."

"I didn't know that; but I'm not so very young, ma'am, thirty in May, and have been what you might call settled this ten years. Mother's a widow, I'm the oldest child she has, and it wouldn't do for me to marry until Lizzy has a home of her own, and Jack's learned his trade; for we're not rich, and I must be father to the children and husband to the dear old woman, if I can."

"No doubt but you are both, John; yet how came you to go to war, if you felt so? Wasn't enlisting as bad as marrying?"

"No, ma'am, not as I see it, for one is helping my neighbor, the other pleasing myself. I went because I couldn't help it. I didn't want the glory or the pay; I wanted the right thing done, and people kept saying the men who were in earnest ought to fight. I was in earnest, the Lord knows! but I held off as long as I could, not knowing which was my duty. Mother saw the case, gave me her ring to keep me steady, and said 'Go': so I went."

A short story and a simple one, but the man and the mother were portrayed better than pages of fine writing could have done it.

"Do you ever regret that you came, when you lie here suffering so much?"

"Never, ma'am; I haven't helped a great deal, but I've shown I was willing to give my life, and perhaps I've got to; but I don't blame anybody, and if I was to do it over again, I'd do it. I'm a little sorry I wasn't wounded in front; it looks cowardly to be hit in the back, but I obeyed orders, and it don't matter in the end, I know."

Poor John! it did not matter now, except that a shot in front might have spared the long agony in store for him. He seemed to read the thought that troubled me, as he spoke so hopefully when there was no hope, for he suddenly added:

"This is my first battle; do they think it's going to be my last?"

"I'm afraid they do, John."

It was the hardest question I had ever been called upon to answer; doubly hard with those clear eyes fixed on mine, forcing a truthful answer by their own truth. He seemed a little startled at first, pondered over the fateful fact a moment, then shook his head, with a glance at the broad chest and muscular limbs stretched out before him:

"I'm not afraid, but it's difficult to believe all at once. I'm so strong it don't seem possible for such a little wound to kill me."

Merry Mercutio's dying words glanced through my memory as he spoke: "'Tis not so deep as a well, nor so wide as a church door, but 'tis enough." And John would have said the same could he have seen the ominous black holes between his shoulders; he never had, but, seeing the ghastly sights about him, could not believe his own wound more fatal than these, for all the suffering it caused him.

"Shall I write to your mother, now?" I asked, thinking that these sudden tidings might change all plans and purposes. But they did not; for the man received the order of the Divine Commander to march with the same unquestioning obedience with which the soldier had received that of the human one; doubtless remembering that the first led him to life, and the last to death.

"No, ma'am; to Jack just the same; he'll break it to her best, and I'll add a line to her myself when you get done."

So I wrote the letter which he dictated, finding it better than any I had sent; for, though here and there a little ungrammatical or inelegant, each sentence came to me briefly worded, but most expressive; full of excellent counsel to the boy, tenderly bequeathing "mother and Lizzie" to his care, and bidding him good bye in words the sadder for their simplicity. He added a few lines, with steady hand, and, as I sealed it, said, with a patient sort of sigh, "I hope the answer will come in time for me to see it;" then, turning away his face, laid the flowers against his lips, as if to hide some quiver of emotion at the thought of such a sudden sundering of all the dear home ties.

These things had happened two days before; now John was dying, and the letter had not come. I had been summoned to many death beds in my life, but to none that made my heart ache as it did then, since my mother called me to watch the departure of a spirit akin to this in its gentleness and patient strength. As I went in, John stretched out both hands:

"I knew you'd come! I guess I'm moving on, ma'am."

He was; and so rapidly that, even while he spoke, over his face I saw the grey veil falling that no human hand can lift. I sat down by him, wiped the drops from his forehead, stirred the air about him with the slow wave of a fan, and waited to help him die. He stood in sore need of help—and I could do so little; for, as the doctor had foretold, the strong body rebelled against death, and fought every inch of the way, forcing him to draw each breath with a spasm, and clench his hands with an imploring look, as if he asked, "How long must I endure this, and be still!" For hours he suffered dumbly, without a moment's respite, or a moment's murmuring; his limbs grew cold, his face damp, his lips white, and, again and again, he tore the covering off his breast, as if the lightest weight added to his agony; yet through it all, his eyes never lost their perfect serenity, and the man's soul seemed to sit therein, undaunted by the ills that vexed his flesh.

One by one, the men woke, and round the room appeared a circle of pale faces and watchful eyes, full of awe and pity; for, though a stranger, John was beloved by all. Each man there had wondered at his patience, respected his piety, admired his fortitude, and now lamented his hard death; for the influence of an upright nature had made itself deeply felt, even in one little week. Presently, the Jonathan who so loved this comely David, came creeping from his bed for a last look and word. The kind soul was full of trouble, as the choke in his voice, the grasp of his hand, betrayed; but there were no tears, and the farewell of the friends was the more touching for its brevity.

"Old boy, how are you?" faltered the one.

"Most through, thank heaven!" whispered the other.

"Can I say or do anything for you anywheres?"

"Take my things home, and tell them that I did my best."

"I will! I will!"

"Good bye, Ned."

"Good bye, John, good bye!"

They kissed each other, tenderly as women, and so parted, for poor Ned could not stay to see his comrade die. For a little while, there was no sound in the room but the drip of water, from a stump or two, and John's distressful gasps, as he slowly breathed his life away. I thought him nearly gone, and had just laid down the fan, believing its help to be no longer needed, when suddenly he rose up in his bed, and cried out with a bitter cry that broke the silence, sharply startling every one with its agonized appeal:

"For God's sake, give me air!"

It was the only cry pain or death had wrung from him, the only boon he had asked; and none of us could grant it, for all the airs that blew were useless now. Dan flung up the window. The first red streak of dawn was warming the grey east, a herald of the coming sun; John saw it, and with the love of light which lingers in us to the end, seemed to read in it a sign of hope of help, for, over his whole face there broke that mysterious expression, brighter than any smile, which often comes to eyes that look their last. He laid himself gently down; and, stretching out his strong right arm, as if to grasp and bring the blessed air to his lips in a fuller flow, lapsed into merciful unconsciousness, which assured us that for him suffering was forever past. He died then; for, though the heavy breaths still tore their way up for a little longer, they were but the waves of an ebbing tide that beat unfelt against the wreck, which an immortal voyager had deserted with a smile. He never spoke again, but to the end held my hand so close that when he was asleep at last, I could not draw it away. Dan helped me, warning me as he did so that it was unsafe for dead and living flesh to lie so long together; but though my hand was strangely cold and stiff, and four white marks remained across its back, even when warmth and color had returned elsewhere, I could not but be glad that, through its touch, the presence of human sympathy, perhaps, had lightened that hard hour.

When they had made him ready for the grave, John lay in state for half an hour, a thing which seldom happened in that busy place; but a universal sentiment of reverence and affection seemed to fill the hearts of all who had known or heard of him; and when the rumor of his death went through the house, always astir, many came to see him, and I felt a tender sort of pride in my lost patient; for he looked a most heroic figure, lying there stately and still as the statue of some young knight asleep upon his tomb. The lovely expression which so often beautifies dead faces, soon replaced the marks of pain, and I longed for those who loved him best to see him when half an hour's acquaintance with Death had made them friends. As we stood looking at him, the ward master handed me a letter, saying it had been forgotten the night before. It was John's letter, come just an hour too late to gladden the eyes that had longed and looked for it so eagerly! but he had it: for, after I had cut some brown locks for his mother, and taken off the ring to send her, telling how well the talisman had done its work, I kissed this good son for her sake, and laid the letter in his hand, still folded as when I drew my own away, feeling that its place was there, and making myself happy with the thought, that, even in his solitary grave in the "Government Lot," he would not be without some token of the love which makes life beautiful and outlives death. Then I left him, glad to have known so genuine a man, and carrying with me an enduring memory of the brave Virginia blacksmith, as he lay serenely waiting for the dawn of that long day which knows no night.

A NURSE'S STORY

PETER BAIDA

The pain in Mary McDonald's bones is not the old pain that she knows well, but a new pain. Sitting in her room in the Booth-Tiessler Geriatric Center, on the third floor, in the bulky chair by the window, Mary tries to measure this pain. She sits motionless, with a grave expression on her face, while the cheerless gray sky on the other side of the window slowly fades toward evening.

Mary McDonald knows what this pain comes from. It comes from a cancer that began in her colon and then spread to her liver and now has moved into her bones. Mary McDonald has been a nurse for forty years, she has retained the full use of her faculties, and she understands perfectly where this pain comes from and what it means.

* * * * *

"Union?" Eunice Barnacle says. "What do I want with a union?"

"Miss Barnacle," Mary McDonald says, looking at her from the chair by the window, "do you think you're paid what you're worth?"

Miss Barnacle is a lean, sharp-featured black woman in her middle twenties, with a straight nose, small teeth, wary eyes, and a straightforward manner, who joined the staff at Booth-Tiessler about a month ago. "This place can't afford to pay me what I'm worth," she says.

"That's certainly what they want you to believe, Miss Barnacle. May I ask a nosy question?"

"I suppose."

"What do they pay you, Miss Barnacle?"

"That's my business."

"Eight-fifty per hour. Is that about right, Miss Barnacle?"

Miss Barnacle, in her white uniform, turns pale. She has paused with her hand on the doorknob, looking over the neatly made bed to the chair where Mary McDonald is sitting. Pearl gray light falls on a walker near the chair. Mary McDonald's hands are closed in her lap, over a green-and-gold quilt. Her face is solemn.

"Do you think this place *knows* what you're worth, Miss Barnacle?"

* * * * *

A good death. That's what everyone wants.

Mary McDonald still remembers, from her first year as a nurse, well over forty years ago, a little old woman named Ida Peterson, with a tumor in her neck near the carotid artery. The call bell at the nurse's station rang, and Mary McDonald walked down the hall, opened the door, and was struck squarely in the face by something warm, wet, and red.

Blood from a ruptured artery gushed out of Mrs. Peterson's tracheotomy opening, out of an ulcerated site on her neck, out of her nose, out of her mouth. Mary was stunned. She saw blood on the ceiling, on the floor, on the bed, on the walls.

Mrs. Peterson had wanted to die a peaceful, dignified death, in the presence of her husband. She had wanted to die a "natural" death. Now, as the life poured out of her, she lifted her hand to wipe her nose and mouth. With wide eyes, she looked at the blood on her hand.

Ida Peterson had wanted a natural death, in the presence of her husband, and she was getting one, in the presence of Mary McDonald, a nurse she had known for five minutes.

Mrs. Peterson's blue, terrified eyes looked into Mary McDonald's eyes for the full fifteen minutes it took her to bleed to death. Her hand gripped Mary's hand. Mary did nothing. Her orders were to allow Mrs. Peterson to die a natural death.

Mary had never before seen an arterial bleed. She still remembers the splash of blood on her face when she stepped into Mrs. Peterson's room. She still remembers how long it took Mrs. Peterson to die. You wouldn't think that a little woman could have so much blood in her.

* * * * *

"They tell me you were some good nurse," Eunice Barnacle says, taking Mary's blood pressure.

"I'm still a good nurse," Mary McDonald says.

"They tell me you helped start the nurses' union, over at the hospital."

"Who tells you?"

"Mrs. Pierce."

"Ah."

"Mrs. Pierce says those were the days."

"Maybe they were."

Eunice loosens the blood pressure cup from Mary's arm. "Mrs. McDonald?"

"Yes?"

"That union—" Eunice hesitates, looking at the floor.

"What about it?" Mary says.

"You think it helped you?"

* * * * *

Booth's Landing is an unpretentious town with a population of nearly nine thousand, located among gently rolling hills on the east side of the Hudson River, fifty miles north of New York City. In every generation, for as long as anyone can remember, the Booths and the Tiesslers have been the town's leading families. The Booth family descends from the town's founder, Josiah Booth, a merchant of the Revolutionary War period whom local historians describe as a miniature version of John Jacob Astor. The Tiessler family descends from Klaus Tiessler, an immigrant from Heidelberg who in 1851 founded a factory that makes silverware.

"A nice town," people who live in Booth's Landing say, "A nice place to bring up a family." That's how Mary McDonald has always felt, and that's what she has always said when people ask her about the place.

In every generation, for as long as anyone can remember, one member of the Booth family has run the town's bank, and one member of the Tiessler family has run the silverware factory. The town also supports one movie theater, two sporting goods stores, two opticians, three auto repair shops, one synagogue, and nine churches. Most of the people who die in Booth's Landing were born there. Many have died with Mary McDonald holding their hands.

Oh, not so many, Mary thinks, pursing her lips. Not that she has kept count. Why would anyone keep count?

You can do worse than to live and die in a place like Booth's Landing. The air is fresh. The streets are clean and safe. The leading families have paid steady attention to their civic and philanthropic responsibilities. If you're sick in Booth's Landing, you go to the Booth-Tiessler Community Hospital. If you want to see live entertainment, you buy tickets for the latest show at the Booth-Tiessler Center for the Performing Arts. If you can no longer take care of yourself, you arrange to have yourself deposited in the Booth-Tiessler Geriatric Center.

At the Booth-Tiessler Community College, nearly fifty years ago, Mary McDonald fulfilled the requirements for her nursing degree. Now, sitting by her window on the third floor in the Geriatric Center, looking over the cherry tree in the yard below toward the river, with the odor of overcooked turnips floating up from the kitchen on the first floor, she finds her mind drifting over her life, back and forth, here and there, like a bird that hops from place to place on a tree with many branches.

* * * * *

"I've never been a troublemaker."

That was what Mary McDonald said to Clarice Hunter when Clarice asked her to help form a nurses' union at the Booth-Tiessler Community Hospital in 1965.

"Hon," Clarice Hunter said, "do you know what the nurses get paid in New York City?"

"I don't live in New York City," Mary said.

"You know what the nurses get paid in Tarrytown?"

"I don't live in Tarrytown."

"It's only ten minutes drive."

"Okay. What do they get paid in Tarrytown?"

Clarice told her.

"Holy moly," Mary McDonald said.

"Will you help me?" Clarice said.

"Clarice, don't pester me."

"You call this pestering?"

Mary did not answer.

"What's the problem, Mary?"

"I'm not a big believer in unions."

"Being a doormat—is that what you believe in?"

Mary pursed her lips.

"It's your Catholic upbringing," Clarice said.

"What about it?"

"Mary, they *programmed* you. They programmed you to bow down to authority."

No doubt about that, Mary thought. Call me Bended Knee.

"Mary, your help would mean a lot to us."

"I've never been a troublemaker."

* * * * *

"I don't think I'll ever make much money."

That was what George McDonald told Mary, a long time ago.

Well, George, you were right about that.

Mary was twenty-one when she met him, in 1948. She had just taken her first job at the hospital, as a nurse in the emergency room.

George was twenty-seven. In the Pacific, he had fought in the Battle of the Coral Sea and in the Battle of Midway.

The first time Mary saw him, George was helping his father carry a sofa up the stairs into the apartment his sister had rented, on Jefferson Street. Mary was friends with the sister, Eleanor, a nurse at the hospital.

He was a big man, six foot three, with hair the color of fresh corn and a big, boyish smile. The war had left him with a scar six inches long, an angry pink dent, on his left shin.

Mary herself was a heavyset young woman, with a figure that lacked curves. Even in her twenties, she looked as if she had been carved from a block of wood. As she aged, she looked as if she'd been carved from a larger block.

I was stout, not fat.

On their first date, George took Mary to see a movie called *Johnny Belinda.* Then they went over to Krieger's, the luncheonette on Main Street. Mary had a hot fudge sundae.

George taught at Booth's Landing High School. He played the clarinet. He thought he would be satisfied teaching music and living in Booth's Landing for the rest of his life.

"I guess I'm not too ambitious," he said.

On the second date, George took Mary on a picnic, in Dabney Park. After lunch he took her rowing. At the far end of the lake, they paused in the shadows under tall trees. Kiss me, Mary thought. George crossed his hands over his knees.

"I don't think I'll ever make much money," he said. "I've never cared much about it."

"There's more to life than money," Mary said.

On the third date, George took Mary to see a movie called *The Snake Pit.* Would you like to go to Krieger's for a sundae, he asked when it was over.

"I don't want a sundae," Mary said. "Let's go walk by the river."

She took his hand as they walked down Tremont Street. The night was cool. His fingers were as thick as cigars.

Six months later they were married.

Mary still remembered the way his fingers felt, laced in hers.

Thirty-nine years together. Three kids, all of them grown now and moved away. No other women in his life, no other men in hers.

He died of kidney failure in 1988. A man who rarely lost his temper, a father who taught his sons how to scramble eggs and his daughter how to throw a baseball, a small-town music teacher who loved the clarinet.

Oh, George, I miss you. You can't imagine.

Maybe you can.

* * * * *

"How you feeling today, Mrs. M?" Dr. Seybold says. He is a large man with a friendly face, pink skin, and paprika-colored hair. His breath smells of peppermint.

"Well enough, Tom. How you feeling?"

"I'm fine, ma'am. Thank you."

"How's your family?"

"My mother broke her toe."

"Broke her toe? How'd she do that?"

"Bowling."

"Dropped a bowling ball?"

"No. Dropped a coffee mug. She tried to hop away, but she couldn't hop fast enough."

"None of us hop as fast as we used to."

"That's the truth, Mrs. M."

"You tell her I hope she feels better. Don't forget."

Forty years ago, in the years before Tom Seybold was born, his mother had two miscarriages. Mary still remembers the look in Laura Seybold's eyes after the second one. She had carried the child for six months, the happiest months of her life, and when she lost it, her life went out of her eyes, the spring went out of her step, and for a full year she wandered through town with a bleak, dazed, shellshocked look on her face. Mary still remembers taking care of Laura Seybold during the three days she spent in the hospital after the Saturday night when she swallowed every pill in the house.

Tom Seybold puts his hand gently on Mary's shoulder.

"You sure you're feeling fine, Mrs. M?"

A coffee mug. Broke her toe with a coffee mug.

"Tom, how long have you known me?"

"As long as I can remember."

"May I ask you an honest question?"

"Why sure, Mrs. M."

"Considering I've got a colon cancer that's chewing up my liver, just how well do you expect me to feel?"

* * * * *

Meat loaf.

If this is Monday, that gray-brown slab on Mary McDonald's plate must be meat loaf.

"What I want to know is where the money goes," Lucy Heywood says. "We *pay.* It's not as if we don't pay."

"What I want to know," Penny Mack says, "is what happens to us when the money's all gone."

"Moneymoneymoneymoney," Roy Quigley says. "If I had a dollar for every day I've spent worrying about money, I'd be a rich man."

"I'm tired of meat loaf," Barbara Collins says.

"Did you read in the paper about Frank Sinatra?" Lucy Heywood says.

"You're not tired of meat loaf," Mary McDonald says.

"I am," Barbara Collins says. "I certainly am."

"What happened to variety shows?" Penny Mack says. "Remember Garry Moore?"

"That man has no shame," Lucy Heywood says.

"Garry Moore?"

"Sinatra."

"Did you see those photos of Princess Di?"

"Whatever happened to Carol Burnett?"

"You're not tired of meat loaf," Mary McDonald says, leaning toward Barbara Collins. "You're tired of life."

"I'm *not,*" Barbara Collins says, holding up a fork with a gravy-smeared piece of meat loaf on the end of it. "I'm *not* tired of life."

* * * * *

Mary McDonald's grandmother also died of colon cancer. *Also* is the word that comes into Mary's mind. Her grandmother died in 1957, or maybe 1958. If you lived long enough, Mary had noticed, you forget when things happened. The only years she remembered were the years her kids were born.

Mary's parents took her grandmother down to New York City, to Columbia Presbyterian, so a famous surgeon could operate. Mary could remember the look on the surgeon's face, after the operation, when he came into the room where Mary and her parents were waiting.

Mary sighs, sitting by the window in her room. Outside, in the yard below her window, a breeze stirs the leaves of the cherry tree. The sky is white today. Poor Grandma! The famous surgeon cut her open, looked inside, and sewed her up. Nothing he could do. Just as, nine months ago, a different surgeon had sewed up Mary.

My goose is cooked.

At Booth-Tiessler, in Grandma's final days, Clarice Hunter was the nurse on the day shift. Mary remembers her grandmother telling her how Clarice had bathed her, and combed her hair, and talked to her. Mary's grandmother was a plain-looking, plain-talking woman, with only an eighth-grade education, who expected nothing from life and generally got what she expected. But then, in the last days of her life, she got Clarice Hunter as her nurse.

"This woman is a jewel," Mary's grandmother said to Mary, while Clarice blushed. "This woman is a blessing."

"Just doing my job," Clarice said, checking Grandma's pulse.

At one o'clock in the morning on the night Mary's grandmother died, she insisted on seeing her family. The night nurse called Mary's parents, who came to the hospital with Mary.

"Where's Clarice?" Mary's grandmother said. "I want to see Clarice."

"It's the middle of the night," Mary said. "She'll be here in the morning."

"I need her *now,*" Mary's grandmother said, turning on Mary a look so fierce that Mary still remembered it.

Mary called Clarice, who came to the hospital at two in the morning. At three, Mary's grandmother fell asleep with her mouth wide open. At six, with a terrifying snort, she woke and died. Clarice helped the night nurse wash the body. Then she worked the day shift.

* * * * *

"Little stick," Eunice Barnacle says, leaning over. She pushes a tiny needle into a vein in Mary's hand. Blood flows back through the needle, into the tubing.

"Good shot," Mary said.

"Tell me about that strike. When was it?"

"1967."

"What was it made you want a union?"

"I didn't want one. Not at first."

"So what happened?"

* * * * *

At a sink, in the nurses' lavatory, Clarice Hunter is crying. The year is 1965, ten years after the death of Mary McDonald's grandmother. Mary is thirty-eight; Clarice is ten years older. Mary walks over to the sink and, carefully, puts one hand on her friend's shoulder.

"You okay?" Mary asks.

"I guess." Clarice blows her nose. "Thanks."

Mary waits.

"Mary?"

"Yes."

"They're driving me crazy. They're running me off my feet."

"They're running all of us, dear."

"But it's making me crazy, Mary. I lost my temper with Mrs. Grbeck, I nearly got into a fight with Mr. Palermo's daughter, and I forgot all about Mr. Howard's pain medicine. That poor man waited *fifty* minutes for his pain medicine."

"We're all rushing, Clarice. We're all making mistakes."

"Mary, I have *twenty* patients."

"I know, dear."

"I can't take care of twenty patients."

"I know, dear."

"Mary?"

"Yes."

"You know how hard a nurse has to work."

"Of course."

"What'll I do, Mary? I can't take care of twenty patients. I can't. I just *can't.*"

* * * * *

"How about you, Mary?"

In the nurses' lounge, back in 1965, that was the question Ruth Sullivan asked, a few days after Mary McDonald had found Clarice Hunter crying at the sink in the nurses' lavatory.

In three weeks, the nurses would vote on whether to form a union. Mary had always expected to vote no.

"I think maybe I'll vote yes," Mary said.

"You'll vote yes?"

"I think so. Maybe."

"I thought you didn't believe in unions."

"I don't, but I think—oh, I don't know. I think I changed my mind. Maybe."

It hadn't occurred to Mary McDonald that anyone would care how she voted. But if you talked to other nurses, you found out that Mary's opinion made a difference.

"I hear Mary McDonald's voting yes," a nurse would say.
"Really?"
"That's what I heard."
"I thought she didn't want a union."
"She changed her mind."
"Really?"
"That's what I heard."
The vote drew near. Arguments were made, pro and con. Tempers flared. In September 1965, the nurses voted in favor of a union.

* * * * *

In the nurses' lounge, Pam Ryder is leafing through a copy of *Family Circle* magazine.
"Well, it won't be long now," Eunice Barnacle says.
"What?" Pam Ryder says.
"Mrs. McDonald," Eunice Barnacle says.
"Poor woman," Pam Ryder says.
"She told me about that union, over at the hospital."
"We need one here," Pam Ryder says.
"You think so?"
"You don't?"
Eunice does not answer. Pam Ryder turns the page in her magazine. Eunice stirs her coffee.
"I know one thing," Eunice says.
Pam Ryder looks up, brushing a hair off her forehead.
"That union can't help her now," Eunice says.

* * * * *

"May I have this dance?"
Brad, her youngest, bends over Mary with his hand outstretched. Mary struggles to her feet. Brad takes her right hand with his left. His other hand settles on the small of her back. Barely moving, they dance.
In her chair, half dozing, Mary remembers that dance.
It was two months ago, on Mary's sixty-ninth birthday. All three of her children had come to Booth's Landing, with their families.
They know what's up.
George, Jr. offered, again, to take her to Chicago.
"I want to die here," Mary said.
"But Mother—"
"No but."
A gangling, loose-jointed, long-armed boy, a star athlete, George, Jr. had grown up to become an earnest, quiet-voiced man who dresses in rumpled suits. He's an attorney, but, of course, he can't win an argument with his mother. Who can? Though

he's tall and moves gracefully, he's no longer slim. His face has grown puffy. His belly bulges over his belt.

"George," Mary said, on her birthday two months ago. "You need to lose weight."

"Yes, Mother," George said. The look in his eyes told her how sad he was to see her dying.

Oh, George, I'm sorry I nagged you. But it's true, you *should* lose weight.

Jane came from Boston, with her two little girls, cute as could be, but bored, and who could blame them? They didn't understand why Mommy had dragged them to see their grandmother.

"Jane, you look tired."

"Mother, I'm a *nurse.* You know what that means."

Three years ago, Jane had a drinking problem. Now she's licked it—maybe.

But she bites her fingernails and smokes.

Jane, do you think I didn't notice?

Brad came all the way from Seattle, where he's worked for a decade. Everyone laughed again at the story about the phone call when he'd told his parents about the job.

"Microwhat?" Mary had said.

"Microsoft, Mother."

"You couldn't get a job with IBM?"

"Mother, I'm working for Bill Gates."

"Bill who?"

Mary turned a happy pink while Brad told the story.

"Look at Mom! Look at her face!"

Brad, my baby. That time when you ran full speed into the clothesline and busted your head open, and I held you while Dad drove us to the emergency room—I know you can't remember, but no one will ever love you the way I loved you on that ride to the hospital.

* * * * *

"Enough about me, Eunice. Tell me about yourself."

"I was born in Virginia, in Richmond," Eunice says. "My father was no good. My mother brought me up."

Outside, three black birds are flying toward the river.

"I don't like to talk about my family, Mrs. McDonald."

"That's all right. You don't have to."

Two days later, while Eunice gives Mary a back rub, the conversation resumes. The smell of rubbing alcohol makes Mary feel drowsy. Rain is drizzling from a bleak sky.

"My mother—she's in jail."

"Oh?"

"She had a boyfriend, Jethro, who beat her when he got drunk. So, about six years ago, Jethro got arrested, and she bailed him out. But then, when they got home, she killed him."

"Oh!"

"They gave her life in prison. I guess maybe they had to."

"Why did she bail him out?"

"That's the thing. She bought a shotgun. She bailed him out to kill him."

"Hmm."

"She's in Sing Sing. It's only thirty minutes drive. I visit every Sunday. You know what's funny?"

"What?"

"Sing Sing. It's in a town called Ossinning. I never knew that before."

Mary feels Eunice's fingers on her back.

"She's a good woman, my mother. But she did wrong. I know that."

Mary feels Eunice's fingers on her shoulder blades.

"That fellow Jethro, he pushed her too far."

George would give her a back rub, and then a front rub, and then—well, what's marriage for?

"My mother, she's only thirty-nine. She was sixteen when I was born."

* * * * *

A football, thrown with a perfect spiral, thrown forty yards through the gray November air, beneath a sky like the sky outside this minute, a football hurled forty yards and falling into the hands of the receiver, glancing over his shoulder at exactly the right moment, reaching up at exactly the right moment, making the catch, and sprinting into the end zone.

It was the winter of 1967. George, Jr. threw the football, Warren Booth Jr. caught, the Booth's Landing football team won the county championship, and life was as good as it gets.

Except for the strike.

The strike had begun in September, two years after the nurses organized their union.

What did the nurses want? That was the question that Richard Dill, a reporter on the Booth's Landing *Gazette,* asked Clarice Hunter, who was the head of the Strike Committee. Clarice told him.

Money.

Job security.

Some say in decisions relating to staffing levels.

No, no, no. That was what management said. So Mary McDonald, who never in her life, before or after the strike, ever voted for anyone but a Republican, found herself on a picket line.

* * * * *

Sister Rosa, the Executive Director, was a short, no-nonsense woman who made it her business to be seen, striding through the halls of Booth-Tiessler Community Hospital, waging war on dust, dirt, and disorder, encouraging nurses and nurses' aides, keeping doctors in line, looking for inefficiencies to eliminate, attacking problems, pushing for improvements.

"Mr. Dill," Sister Rosa said in the first interview that she gave after the strike began, "our nurses are wonderful, all our employees are wonderful, but we cannot let employees set their own salaries. We cannot let employees define the terms and conditions of employment. We cannot let employees set staffing levels."

Remembering, Mary McDonald sighs.

Oh, Sister Rosa, how I admired you! How I hated doing anything that might displease you. How I wanted you to *like* me. How I wanted to hear you say, "Good work, Mary. . . . Nice job, Mary."

"Mr. Dill, management must not run away from its responsibilities."

Five years before the strike, Mary McDonald worked with Sister Rosa on a project to improve the patient scheduling system in the radiation department. With Sister Rosa guiding the project, staff members collected and evaluated treatment time data. Then Sister Rosa designed a system that matched the time allotted for an appointment to the complexity of the treatment. A more flexible scheduling system was put in place. The result: a twenty percent decrease in patient waiting time, and a fifteen percent increase in physician and hospital revenue. Mary later used what she had learned from Sister Rosa to improve the patient scheduling system in the chemotherapy department.

"Mr. Dill, management must *manage.*"

* * * * *

One week before Thanksgiving. Outside, a nasty sky. Inside, the radiator clanks and rattles. Eunice has brought Mary McDonald a tiny white pill in a tiny white cup.

"You visiting your family for Thanksgiving, Mrs. McDonald?"

"No." Mary swallows her pill. "I'm too tired."

"Your family coming here?"

"They came for my birthday. That was enough. How about you, Eunice?"

"Guess I'll take my little girl to see my mom." Eunice has a daughter, three years old, in day care.

"That's nice." Mary looks at Eunice, who is looking at her watch while she checks Mary's pulse. Mary feels the pressure of Eunice's fingers—a nice feeling.

You're a good nurse, Eunice, but the two-year degree isn't enough. You should go back to school. Do it now, while you're young.

Mary hears those words in her head, but she does not say them aloud. Mary and Eunice often talk about Eunice's future, but Mary does not feel like talking today.

"I've got a new picture." Eunice opens her wallet, takes out a photo, and holds it out for Mary to see. The photo shows a bright-eyed little girl with twin pigtails sitting on a mechanical rocking horse, outside Tyler's Pharmacy.

"I heard from her daddy."

"Oh?"

"He lost his job, out in San Diego. Asked if I could send him some money."

Eunice is staring at the photo of her little girl.

"That man," Eunice says, shaking her head. "That man needs a brain transplant."

* * * * *

For six months, the nurses carried picket signs outside the hospital. Twenty nurses, on the picket line, every day and into the night. Mary still remembers the looks people gave them. Friendly looks, hostile looks, curious looks. She still remembers the sign she carried: TOGETHER WE WILL WIN.

The hospital hired a company that specialized in fighting strikes. The company flew in scab nurses. On the picket line, Mary sang: "UNION BUSTING, IT'S DISGUSTING."

In Booth's Landing, people took sides. Millie Tolliver said to Mary at a PTA meeting, "Mary, I'm surprised at you." Carl Usher, the plumber whose son took clarinet lessons from George, said, "Mrs. McDonald, I just don't see how you girls can walk out on your patients." In an interview on TV, Cheryl Hughes, a woman whom Mary had always liked, whose husband prepared Mary and George's tax returns, said, "If you ask me, it's an outrage. Let's just hope nobody dies. These women ought to be ashamed."

* * * * *

The web that connects people in a small town is more tightly spun than the web that exists in a large city. In Booth's Landing, the man who will write Mary McDonald's obituary for the local newspaper is the son of the reporter who covered the nurses' strike of 1967.

Richard Dill, the father, lives on the same floor as Mary McDonald at the Booth-Tiessler Geriatric Center. Richard Dill sees that Mary has lost twenty pounds in the last six months, sees that her step is weaker each time she comes out of her room, sees that she comes out less and less often, and sees that her skin grows paler and paler, grayer and grayer, with every week.

Watching Mary fade away, Richard Dill remembers her as a sturdy woman carrying her picket sign, thirty years ago. He remembers her twenty years ago, nursing his wife after her surgery.

Roger Dill, the son, sometimes sees Mary in the hall with her walker when he visits his father, and he nods amiably in her direction, but he does not remember the nurses' strike of '67 because he was only three years old when it took place. Roger Dill does not remember that, when he was six, Mary's daughter Jane was one of his camp counselors. He remembers the surgery his mother had when he was twelve, but he does not remember any of his mother's nurses.

"A nice boy," Mary thinks when she sees Roger Dill, though she merely nods as he walks with his father in the hall. Mary remembers Roger at the age of twelve, a skinny kid carrying a football helmet, visiting his mother in the hospital. Poor woman. What was her name? Jennifer. From a town called Mistletoe, in Mississippi. Mary taught her how to care for the colostomy bag that she needed after her surgery.

* * * * *

Two months into the strike, the hospital withdrew recognition of the union.

"Withdrew recognition?" Mary said to Clarice Hunter. "How can they do that?"

"They can't," Clarice Hunter said. "Not unless they've hired those scabs as permanent replacements."

"Sister Rosa wouldn't do that."

In fact, that was exactly what Sister Rosa had done.

"What'll we do?" Mary asked Clarice.

"We'll move into Phase Two."

Phase One: the nurses carried picket signs outside the hospital.

Phase Two: the nurses took their fight up to the top of Mountainview Drive.

Why Mountainview Drive? Because that was where Warren Booth, the Chairman of the Board, lived with his wife and children.

Mary McDonald remembers Warren Booth, with a big frown on his broad, well-scrubbed face, when he came down the driveway from his mansion to confront the strikers. She remembers the tone of his voice, and the look in his eyes, and the way his jaw worked, and the way he turned on his heel and strode back up the driveway and into the house.

George Jr. said: "But, *Mom,* don't you see what you're doing? I'm the *quarterback,* and Warren Jr. is my best receiver."

In Booth's Landing, back in 1967, the public schools were good enough that the son of the richest man in town and the son of George and Mary McDonald could go to the same school and play on the same football team.

"Mom, Warren's my *teammate.*"

"Yes, George, I understand. But out in the world, where I work—well, let's just say that Warren's dad isn't my teammate."

* * * * *

Frank Gifford.

"If Frank Gifford ever comes to town," George used to say, "I'll have to lock Mary away from him."

Well, George, you may have been right about that.

Mary and the Giants. Everybody who knew Mary McDonald knew about her love affair with the Giants.

She was a knowledgeable fan. When the announcer said that the Giants had gone into their "prevent defense," Mary would shout: "No! Not the prevent! Anything but the prevent!" She'd seen the Giants lose too many games when the prevent defense failed to prevent anything.

Her other great love was beer, the darker the better, "I can't stand that piss-colored beer," she would tell people. Once she discovered Guinness, she never drank anything else.

It's true. I could use one right now.

She didn't like games. She didn't like to travel. She didn't have any hobbies. What she really liked was—nursing.

That's also true. I loved it from day one.

She knew things that only nurses know. If you smell an unpleasant odor coming from a patient's urine drainage bag, add ten milliliters of hydrogen peroxide to the bag when you empty it. If a nasogastric feeding tube becomes clogged, use diet cola to flush it. If you need to remove oil-based paint that is close to a patient's eyes or mouth, use mineral water, not turpentine.

In the neighborhood where George and Mary lived, phone calls to physicians were rare. People called Mary first, and Mary told them what to do.

* * * * *

"So they hired permanent replacements," Eunice Barnacle said. "Then what?"

"What you have to remember," Mary said, "is that Booth-Tiessler is part of a chain of hospitals. And it's a chain of *Catholic* hospitals. That's why nuns run the place."

"What difference does it make who runs it?"

"A big difference. Maybe all the difference."

Most of the striking nurses also were Catholic. They didn't merely picket outside the hospital. They prayed:

> Give us this day our daily bread,
> And forgive us our trespasses,
> As we forgive those who trespass against us.

And they chanted:

> United we bargain,
> Divided we beg!

And they sang:

> I dreamed I saw Joe Hill last night,
> Alive as you and me. . . .

On TV in those days, in and around Booth's Landing, people saw nurses on strike, with their picket signs lowered and their heads bowed in prayer. When people remembered the strike, years later, what they remembered was nurses praying on the sidewalk outside the hospital.

"If the hospital hadn't been run by an order of nuns," Mary McDonald said to Eunice Barnacle, "I think we'd have lost. But we hit those nuns where it hurt. We appealed to their consciences."

The Sisters of Mercy—that's what the nuns were called. Somebody looked up their mission statement. It said that they were committed to act in solidarity with the poor, the weak, the outcast, the elderly, and the infirm.

On the chilliest day that winter, with her cheeks freezing and her breath visible in the air, Mary McDonald read the Sisters of Mercy mission statement out loud, while TV cameras rolled.

Then Beverly Wellstone began a fast. A nurse who had once been a nun, she was five feet tall, trim and intense, with bright blue eyes and cinnamon-colored hair. She fasted for thirty-three days, her eyes growing brighter and brighter as the flesh fell from her face. Other nurses fasted in support, usually for twenty-four or forty-eight hours. The TV cameras kept rolling.

"I am fasting in an effort to bring this strike to the attention of higher authorities," Beverly Wellstone said. The look in her eyes was the look you see in paintings, in the eyes of martyred saints.

Other strikers begged her to stop, but Beverly Wellstone declined with a nearly invisible movement of her parched lips.

"To represent the women on this picket line," Beverly Wellstone said, "is an honor and privilege I will never know again in my life."

A camera crew arrived from New York. One of the national networks had picked up the story. That night, millions of people learned about the striking nurses of Booth's Landing. From her cot in the basement of a local church, Beverly Wellstone whispered a few words about the role of faith in her life. Warren Booth Sr., entering the hospital for an emergency meeting of the Board, declined to comment. He looked haggard and distracted.

The next day, according to newspaper reports published later, a stranger arrived in Booth's Landing. Three days later, the strike was over.

* * * * *

"A stranger?" Eunice Barnacle said.

"An emissary of the Cardinal," Mary McDonald said.

"What did he do?"

"He carried a message to Sister Rosa."

"A message from the Cardinal?"

"Yes."

"Then what happened?"

"Talks resumed, but in a different spirit."

Eunice was leaning against the windowsill in Mary McDonald's room. The light that poured through the window from a clear winter sky made her skin shine. Mary

McDonald, as she told the story, was sitting up comfortably in bed, her back supported by two pillows set on end.

"So you won?" Eunice Barnacle said.

"The scab nurses were dismissed," Mary said. "The striking nurses were rehired. The effort to decertify the union was abandoned."

"You got the salary increase you wanted?"

"No. We got about half the increase we wanted. But we also got something we wanted for our patients."

"What was that?"

"More staff on the medical and surgical floors. For the next three years, after we signed that contract, we had the staff to give the kind of care we wanted to give."

* * * * *

Thirty thousand dollars—that was what Sister Margaret calculated that Booth-Tiessler Community Hospital would save annually by buying less expensive surgical gloves. Sister Margaret's expertise in materials management dazzled everyone who worked with her at Booth-Tiessler. It was an expertise she had honed in years of hard work under the eye of her mentor and predecessor, Sister Rosa, whom she had succeeded as Executive Director in 1984.

Sister Margaret had turned on her dictaphone, with the intention of dictating a memorandum on the subject of surgical gloves, when Sister Celia softly entered the office with the latest pile of papers and reports for Sister Margaret's in-box. Something in Sister Celia's eyes—a flicker that suggested the desire to speak—led Sister Margaret to lift her own eyes with an inquiring look.

"Mary McDonald died this morning," Sister Celia said.

"Ah." The word came out of Sister Margaret's mouth as a sigh. When Mary McDonald was transferred from the Geriatric Center to the hospital, three days ago, Sister Margaret had suspected that the end was near. Now, memories of Mary McDonald mixed in Sister Margaret's mind with the thought that the time had come to take another look at soap prices.

What Sister Margaret said, looking at Sister Celia, was simply: "A good nurse. . . . A *damned* good nurse." The word *damned* was pronounced with an emphasis that verged on audacity. Sister Margaret remembered the nurses' union, and the strike of 1967, and the look on Sister Rosa's face in the days after the Cardinal had sent his emissary to Booth's Landing. "Of course," Sister Margaret said, "we had our differences."

* * * * *

Roger Dill, at his old-fashioned desk in the old-fashioned offices of the Booth's Landing *Gazette,* took a long sip of coffee, paused to savor the warmth in his stomach, and typed: "Mary McDonald died at the Booth-Tiessler Nursing Home on December 16. She was sixty-nine."

Roger closed his eyes. When they opened, his fingers moved swiftly: "A graduate of Booth-Tiessler Community College, Mrs. McDonald worked for many years as a nurse at Booth-Tiessler Community Hospital. . . ."

Roger closed his eyes again. People of no great consequence died every week in Booth's Landing, and Roger Dill was required to write three to five paragraphs about them. It was not a task that he resented, but it was not one that excited or inspired him. How much could he say about a nurse he had never met?

"Mrs. McDonald is survived by three children. . . ."

Roger Dill suppressed a yawn and thought about the legs of his son's piano teacher. Even with coffee, he found that it was sometimes a challenge not to fall asleep with his fingers on the keyboard, the computer humming gently on his desk, and the conventional sentences taking shape in his head.

* * * * *

From his office on the top floor of the Booth's Landing Savings and Loan Association, a sturdy stone building at the intersection of Tremont and Main Streets, Warren Booth Jr. could see the blue shimmer of the Hudson, sweeping south, and, beyond it, the fields and meadows of New Jersey. Though it had rained a few hours ago, the day had brightened. Warren Booth allowed his gaze to linger on the river, beneath the sparkling blue of the midafternoon sky.

The Booth's Landing *Gazette* lay open on Warren Booth's desk. Looking out over the river, the town's leading banker found himself falling into a strangely agitated mood. Nearly thirty years had passed, yet he still remembered the days when nurses picketed his family's house, while he tried to prepare for the biggest football game of his life.

In those days, nothing in the world had seemed more important to Warren Booth than the Booth's Landing football team. George McDonald had been the team's quarterback. Warren had been the team's primary receiver. The team itself had been outstanding—the best that anyone could remember. Yet Warren remembered the winter of 1967 as a painful and confusing time, because a group of nurses, including George McDonald's mother, had made life miserable for Warren's father. Why? *Why?*

With an exasperated sigh, Warren Booth shifted in his chair. He had inherited not merely his father's position in life but also his attitudes on matters pertaining to civic and business affairs. The nerve! The nerve of those women. What great enterprise had they ever managed? What did they know about worldly affairs?

Something that resembled a grimace appeared on the face of Warren Booth. The fact that he himself had never managed any great enterprise did not occur to him. Those women had made Warren's father out to be some Scrooge, and the press, the damned press—well, better not to think about the press.

Warren Booth took a deep breath. He would send a condolence card to George McDonald, in Chicago. Yes, he would do that. Hell, he would go to the funeral. Why not? Go to the funeral. Pay his respects. See old George. . . . Talk with old

George? What would they say to one another? What could they possibly say to one another?

Sighing, Warren Booth leaned back in his chair, looked up at the ceiling, and closed his eyes. The look on his face was the look of a troubled man. He kept his eyes closed a long time.

Forget the funeral. Send a card.

* * * * *

Two blocks from the little red-brick apartment building where Eunice Barnacle lives, there is a park with swings and sliding boards and a jungle gym. Even in winter, on a sunny day, the park fills with children. With all the young voices squealing and shouting, and young feet running and jumping, it is as happy a place as you can find in Booth's Landing. This park is where Eunice Barnacle went, with her three-year-old daughter, on the day after Mary McDonald died.

It was a Saturday, bright and cold, with a sky completely white. Eunice pushed her daughter on a swing, then sat on a green wooden bench, apart from the other mothers, while her daughter played in the sandbox. After a while, another woman sat down near Eunice. The women talked for a time, and then they sat without talking for nearly half an hour. Then Eunice said:

"You know what we need, Carrie?"

"What?"

"A union."

"Union? What do we need with a union?"

"You think you're paid what you're worth?"

"Eunice, what's got into you?"

"Nothing."

"That woman brainwashed you."

"Nobody brainwashed me."

"You could get us in trouble, Eunice."

"We're already in trouble."

"Not me. I'm not in trouble."

"That's what you think."

To a little girl in a bulky red jacket, in the sandbox, Eunice yelled: "Coretta, sweetie, five more minutes."

"Mommy, *no!*"

"Five minutes, Coretta."

The woman on the bench next to Eunice folded her arms across her chest. She was wearing an orange scarf over a silver-gray coat. Eunice was wearing a white scarf over a crimson coat.

"I've never been a troublemaker," the woman said. "One thing I've learned in life, Eunice. You go looking for trouble, you'll find it."

Eunice did not answer. The sun had gone behind a cloud. A chill came into the air.

A month ago, Eunice recalled, she had asked Mary McDonald if the union had really helped her. The old woman had thought a long time before she said, "To tell the truth, it had its good points and its bad points. Like most things." Eunice had asked her to explain the good points and the bad points. "Some other time," the old woman had said. "I'm tired now."

But the subject had never come up again, so now Eunice did not know what Mary McDonald would have said.

"Coretta! Sweetie!" Eunice called.

"But *Mommy!*"

"Time to go, honey."

The child opened her mouth as if to wail, paused, closed her mouth, stood, held out her arms, and toddled toward Eunice.

"Let's go home, sweetie. Mommy's tired."

* * * * *

At Santino's Funeral Home, Nick Santino and Harry Orbit were preparing the body of Mary McDonald for its final resting place.

"Here's one I'm sorry to see," Nick Santino said.

"Oh?"

"Mary McDonald."

"You knew her?"

"A nurse. Took care of my mother, back when she was dying."

Mary's body lay on a porcelain embalming table, under a sheet. Nick paused, looking at the face of the dead woman. The eyes were closed, the skin was wrinkled and pale, the lips were crooked. A white thread, half an inch long, lay on the face below the left eye. Nick lifted off the thread.

Nick and Harry washed Mary's body with warm water and a soapy solution. They cleaned Mary's fingernails. Through a needle that Nick placed in the jugular vein, they drained the blood from Mary's body.

Harry inserted cotton in both nostrils, to hold the nose straight. Nick sewed Mary's lips shut.

A machine pumped embalming fluid into Mary's body. After the fluid had entered Mary's hands, Nick crossed them over her chest. He applied adhesive glue to hold her fingers together.

Nick paused, looking at Mary's face. A refrigerator hummed in a corner of the room.

"This woman took care of my mother," Nick said, looking down at her. "She took care of my mother like she was taking care of her own mother."

Nick shooed away a fly that was buzzing near Mary's cheek. He touched Mary's hair with a gloved hand. He looked at Harry.

"This woman washed my mother's feet," Nick said, with sudden intensity. "This woman cleaned my mother's toes with a toothbrush."

* * * * *

Mary McDonald, late in the last day of her life, fell into a sleep as deep as a child's sleep after an overactive day. Her eyes were closed, her head was tilted back, her lips were open, her breathing was steady, though not strong.

At one point a middle-aged woman in a nun's outfit came into the room, closing the door behind her. With a mild expression on her face and her hands crossed at her waist, the visitor stood looking down at the sleeping woman. Mary's eyes opened.

"Sister Rosa. How nice of you to visit."

"Don't mention it, dear. How are you?"

"Not long for this world, I'm afraid."

"Don't be afraid."

"No. I'm not."

"Have they given you something for pain, Mary?"

"Oh, yes. Thank God for morphine."

"I'll do that."

Mary thought for a moment, with a slightly puzzled expression on her face. Then she let the thought go.

"Sister Rosa?"

"Yes."

"When you died, *after* you died, was it—what you expected?"

"I'm not allowed to talk about that, dear."

"No, I guess not."

Mary closed her eyes again. She kept them closed for a long time. When she opened them again, the light in the room seemed different.

"Sister Rosa?"

"Yes, dear."

"Would you mind holding my hand?"

"Of course not, dear."

Sister Rosa put her hand on Mary's hand. The nun's hand was warm—warmer than Mary's, perhaps. Mary closed her eyes again, but opened them almost at once.

"There's something on my mind, Sister Rosa."

"What's that, dear?"

"The strike—you remember the strike?"

"Of course, dear."

"I hope you didn't take it the wrong way?"

"The wrong way, dear?"

"It wasn't about *you,* Sister Rosa. I hope you understand that."

"I do, dear."

"But the nurses—we couldn't let things go, the way they were going."

"I understand, dear."

"We couldn't roll over and die."

"Of course, dear. I understand."

"You do?"

"Mary, I'm *glad* you fought."

"You are?"

"Workers have to fight."

"You really think so?"

"The whole system depends on it."

"I'm not sure about that, Sister Rosa."

"Well, I am."

A sound came from the door, but no one was there. Sister Rosa looked at the door, then back at Mary.

"Would you like to see George?" Sister Rosa said.

"Is he here?"

"He's right outside."

"Could I see him?"

"Of course."

Mary closed her eyes. When she opened them, the light in the room was different. Sister Rosa had gone, but George had not come in. A woman in a white uniform was standing at the bedside, taking Mary's pulse. Mary felt the pressure of her fingers on her wrist.

"I'd like to see George," Mary said.

"George?"

From the foot of the bed, someone said: "That's her husband. My father."

"Jane?"

"I'm right here, Mom."

"How nice. I'm glad you've come, Jane."

"Me, too."

"Brad?"

Mary felt confused. The nurse let go of her wrist.

Mary looked on the other side of her bed. Brad was there, in a navy sweater, and George, Jr., in a rumpled suit, with his hand reaching into a bag of pretzels.

"You had a good sleep," Brad said.

George said, "I'm right here, Mom. We're all here with you."

Mary looked at him. His belly bulged over his belt.

"You need to lose weight, George."

"Yes, Mom. I know."

"Promise."

George withdrew his hand from the bag without a pretzel.

"I promise, Mom."

I can't help myself, George. A mother's a mother till her dying breath.

But where was *her* George? Sister Rosa had said he was here.

Out loud Mary said, "I don't want a sundae. Let's go walk by the river."

The woman in the white uniform went out of the room. Mary's children talked softly to one another. Mary listened for a while with her eyes closed. She could hear the voices, but the words escaped her. When she opened her eyes, her husband was standing by her bed. The smile on his face made Mary want to get up and throw her arms around his neck. He was young and tall, his hair was the color of fresh corn, his fingers were as thick as cigars, and he had his clarinet with him.

A SEPARATE SPECIES: RELATIONSHIPS WITH THE WORLD AND WITH OURSELVES

MARION DEUTSCHE COHEN

Well spouses often talk about how old friends no longer come around. They add that they no longer feel comfortable with old friends, and they can't make new friends because they never go anywhere. "We don't fit in with married couples," they continue, "nor are we exactly swinging singles." Saying things like this, some of them have tears in their eyes.

My own experience has been slightly different. While I have contended with some of that isolation, I have also had many good friends who have listened, if not understood. Moreover, many of my friendships have been enhanced by my being a well spouse; for example, a friend who just found out that her forty-two-year old husband might have Alzheimer's can turn to me for understanding. Some friendships have begun because of shared well-spouse experiences. A poet acquaintance became a friend when, at a chance meeting at the local drugstore, she mentioned that a lover of hers had died from complications of MS. A mother in the park has a husband who's manic depressive, so we always have long conversations.

However, one of my non-well-spouse friends recently confided that she had felt overawed by my circumstances. "Sometimes I find that I hesitate to share my own personal problems with you," she said. "I'm afraid they'll just pale in the light of yours." This friend did add, "You act in such a way that I usually don't feel that way."

Still, I join all well spouses in feeling some alienation from the world. Not only are we becoming a separate species from our ill spouses, we're becoming a separate species, period. Perhaps, to the rest of the world, *we're* the ones who are ill. The motto of the Well Spouse Foundation is, "When one is sick, two need help." In my book *The Level of Doorknobs* I talk about the "disabled family." Jeff's MS makes the entire household disabled.

I use the word *alienated* to describe how I've felt much of the time, although I have kept up many friendships, old and new . . . although I have been able to do nearly everything I've wanted to do, though maybe not as much of it as I've wanted . . . although being a well spouse has not kept me from writing, doing math, teaching, piano playing, singing, thrift shopping, and being a full-time stay-at-home mother . . . although I've connected up with the world in the way I've wanted to . . . although I feel satisfied that I've been able to contribute what I have in me to contribute . . . and although it does not sound as though I've been isolated or alienated.

Our experience simply is not that of most people. A well spouse does not view things the way a non-well spouse does. "In social situations," says Fern, "or with relatives, other people are in their various normal stages, and they have various normal news, like ski trips and marriages and stuff. What can I talk about? I can say, 'Well, I had a whole hour to myself last week.' It feels like nothing, compared to what other people do. It's when I get together with other people that I realize how different I am. At home I don't quite realize, I take my life pretty much for granted." Recall that Fern is a working person, a professional; she also has a wide range of friends and goes on weekend trips, probably as often as anybody else. Still, she has the feeling of being different; there is always that threat, that tendency toward anger, bitterness, and alienation.

What I felt was confused. I couldn't believe that society, which included my friends and relatives, was allowing our dire straits to continue. As an adult, I understood that my attitude was at least slightly nonsensical or unrealistic; still, I felt betrayed. And when people (usually acquaintances rather than friends) said things like "We all have our crosses to bear" or "We have to be strong," I was either too furious to say much or too furious to keep my mouth shut. On the other hand, when people had the right attitude, when they sympathized, when they said anything approaching "You really have had a hard life" or "You got a bum rap" or "Yes, we all have our crosses to bear but you definitely got more than your share," I sometimes got furious, too. Their words rubbed my situation in, made it all extra true, even felt mocking or sadistic. I heard behind their words, "Yes, we do know. We do know what you're going through. And we're letting it happen, anyway." At the very least I felt disappointed.

Now I think I know the answer to the question Why don't they rescue us? For the same reason we don't rescue our ill spouses.

Still, those two months I was down with a broken ankle, Jeff's brother could have come on a regular basis instead of just dropping in every once in a while, often when an attendant was there anyway. And Louise's husband could have said, "I'll be over to put him to bed every Tuesday and Thursday evening," instead of us having to call him all the time. My friends who were mothers could have said, "Tell Devin he can count on Jeremy and me coming by and taking him to the park every Monday." It would have taken some of the worry out of our lives if they had offered something regular, something we could count on more than once. We could have used an organized support system; I would have loved it if our friends had all gotten together and worked out some giant plan.

During that broken-ankle era only Aurelio came several times a week. In fact, overhearing me tantrum one evening, he boomed the welcome words, "Okay, I'm moving back in for awhile." Only Aurelio seemed to understand that in times of dire straits, everyone is responsible. During that broken-ankle period, it was only Aurelio from whom we didn't feel alienated.

Again, many people seemed to think our dire straits were just plain stress. "You can do it," they'd say. "You just *feel* like you can't." "It's beyond all that," is what well spouses say about those kinds of encounters. "It's just a whole different realm."

People who'd say, "I'm worried about you, Marion," or "I have a feeling you're not saying how bad things really are" were often those to whom I truly was not saying how bad things really were because they were not the people I confided in or who would listen if I did confide in them. Still, it felt like criticism. Or like that case worker who grabbed me to her, demanding I cry on her shoulder. It didn't feel like harsh criticism, just criticism. Or advice. But definitely not praise or acknowledgment. To any variant of "You're not saying how bad things really are," I'd sometimes quip, at least in my mind, "Oh, are you curious to know how bad things really are? Then buy my poetry books!"

But the hurt went deep. And suppose, I'd speculate, someone said, "Marion talks too much about how bad things are." Was anyone saying that? What did I want them to say? I wanted them to say, "She's expressing it exactly enough, just right, exactly how and how much she should, neither too little nor too much."

As always among friends, sometimes mine seemed to understand and then suddenly didn't. Sandy and I got together for dinner one evening after she'd just landed a great job that involved taking people out to expensive restaurants about twice a week on "the account." Three gorgeous, sensitive, passionate men had answered her ad in the *Philadelphia Magazine* personals, and none seemed to mind that she'd stipulated no sex because of fear of AIDS. "They're happy to just kiss," she told me. So I started telling her that if I were to decide to seek other men besides Jeff, or if (meaning when) Jeff died, I'd put an ad in the personals that would read something like: "My experiences include getting a Ph.D. in math, publishing nine poetry books, losing a full-term baby, gaining four full-term babies, and having a husband with MS. I'm very, very vulnerable but strong in ways you can't imagine." "And," I told Sandy, "I wouldn't just say no sex; I'd say no kissing."

"Oh," said Sandy, "you might surprise yourself."

Many well spouses have surprised themselves, and many haven't. Many, indeed, have been disappointed. Well spouses have a range of different feelings and needs concerning sex, or companionship, with people other than their ill spouses. Many are too tired, too taken up, too a lot of things, to be interested in sex or even companionship. The issue of extramarital affairs is not simple to a well spouse, and Sandy's comment felt presumptuous. It disturbed, upset, and alienated me. I was in no mood to be surprised, even by myself, and I felt very, very vulnerable.

I felt subtly alienated even from people who were helping us. During two of those broken-ankle weeks Verna from Blue Cross came in five hours a day. She cooked, cleaned, took Dev to the park, did anything I'd ask, and cheerfully. She was attentive, intelligent, and compassionate. But to me, compassion felt strangely nightmarish. It smacked of hospitals, blood, and nurses with strange ways. Maybe that's part of the definition of compassion, that it must come from strangers.

Doris, too, the tough, cheerful nurse who tended daily to Jeff's bedsore was smart, entertaining, and compassionate. But she was still a nurse. Still hospital. And full of instructions, though slightly apologetic, as to what I'd be responsible for once her two weeks were up.

Well, I thought, what can anybody do? Compassionate can't be the same thing as tender. Tender comes with knowing, with loving, with time. And right there, right then, all that was tender—meaning my husband and my children—was powerless.

* * * * *

The whole situation was alienating. In some sense, I was even alienated from my own home. I often didn't understand things. Big math Ph.D., I didn't know how to load the family camera or use the computer in Elle's room. And it was a while before I learned how to operate the VCR. I had neither the time nor the energy nor the interest. I had no room in my life for more skills, especially unpaid skills.

One midnight the doorbell rang, and I went to peek through the hole. It was no one I recognized. "Yes?" I called.

"It's the security guard," said the voice. "I'd like to talk to you."

I realized he was some stranger wanting money. I didn't know whether he planned to ask for it or just get it, but I had not opened, not come remotely close to opening, the door. Nevertheless for one small minute, my feeling was, "Oh, the security guard. Sure. Naturally. Come on in." For certainly, I thought, neighbors must have noticed how strange and suspicious our house and family were. The trike lift, the trikes themselves, Jeff never out, Aurelio always around, not to mention all the characters. "It's no surprise they're investigating," I thought. "It's no wonder they sent the security guard."

Sometimes I felt alienated from the community. On late dark nights, being out in the streets felt strange. One midnight, coming home from a well-spouse meeting, I found myself peeking ahead, and behind, buildings, porches, alleys. Patrolling, like our cat. Not believing that God or police or anything else would protect me. Believing, perhaps, that they would protect everyone *except* me. At the meeting a seventy-year-old woman had told us about "baby-duty" (that is, toilet); another seventy-year-old woman had talked about getting robbed by attendants; I had once again described nights and toilet. I'd gotten the feeling that no one is looking out for anyone.

The night that the police had come to our door and asked, "Were you screaming? Are you all right?" Suppose I had answered, "No, I'm not all right. I'm being raped and molested"? And then suppose I'd gone into detail about nights, lifting, and toilet? Would they have said, "Oh, we don't mean that kind of rape. We don't protect anyone from that kind of rape." (Just like Volunteers of America didn't have "that kind of volunteers.")

Walking along that street, I thought, "It's only a matter of time before I get raped. Not molested, but raped. And not that kind of rape, but actual rape. And then if one of the attendants actually did rape me, Jeff would somehow convince himself that it didn't happen, or that it was okay. Maybe I'd be convinced, too. After all, a good attendant is hard to find."

The rules are different, or feel different, when you're a well spouse. We're second- or third-class citizens, so naturally we feel alienated from the community. And we also feel alienated from all the smaller communities to which we belong based on our individual interests, beliefs, and circumstances. Our age group, for example, or our religious or choral group; the black community, gay community, home-schooling community. Being well spouses does not prevent but does complicate our memberships in our various niches.

Kathy's husband was totally paralyzed in a sports accident; her boys at the time were ages three and six. At the annual well-spouse convention she stood up and told us all, "When I was at my son's school play last week, I felt very alienated; I just was not like the other mothers." And my friend and neighbor Joy, whose husband is manic depressive, says, "When I talk with the other mothers at the park, I just can't relate; they talk about their problems like 'Jimmy won't take a nap' and 'Johnny won't eat his spinach' and to me those just don't seem like problems." Well-spouse mothers feel alienated from the community of mothers.

"In the work itself, everything's fine," says Fern of her job as a family therapist. "In fact, it's a real escape from my life at home, and it seems easy, compared to what I have to do at home. And if any of my clients have a situation where they're dealing with chronic illness, then—unless the situation is too similar to mine—my own experience helps. But at staff meetings, when everyone socializes a little before-hand, some people talk about personal stuff like 'My child was up at 2:00 a.m. last night.' Well, I can't say, 'My husband was up at 2:00, and at 3:00, and at 4:00, and I had to clean him up.' I can't say things like that. It would be too shocking, too distracting. It would take up too much time. So I'm alienated sometimes at work; I'm not normal."

As a feminist, I had always been careful not to play into the "woman as long sufferer" role. But I was suffering, and I was suffering long. I was not refusing to do nights, lifting, and toilet, and I was answering each and every "Mar!" I did understand that true feminism means being woman identified and doesn't preclude being a well spouse. But still, at times, I worried that my feminism might be at stake.

Jeff's illness naturally led to our family's involvement in the disability community, but that community does not always feel like my community. The disability movement is not the well-spouse movement. Disability advocates take into account the cause of care givers, but that's not their emphasis. Many well spouses have said, for example—and I can see the pain and hurt in their faces—that what solves the problem of sex and sexuality for disabled people is often quite inadequate for the partners of disabled people.

Also, my well-spouse poems are not always chosen for disability anthologies; often editors have said they want to stick with writers who are themselves disabled. "I am disabled," I have told them. "Anyone who does nights, lifting, and toilet is very definitely physically challenged." I understand that I am probably wrong, that my disability is not quite the same. But I have often felt disabled—and alienated from anyone who claimed I wasn't.

* * * * *

On one of my broken-ankle mornings four and a half years ago we received a phone call around 7:30 a.m. from our regular attendant. He wasn't going to be able to make it today; his ten-month-old son was in the hospital with a high fever. We were desperate. Jeff had to be at work by 1:00, to teach his first class of the semester. I hit the Resources for Living Independently list, which give names of four attendants at a time. The first guy I rang up asked what salary the service pays. I told him, and he screamed at me, "You're a real con artist. You're pocketing the money. I've been in this business a long time." I'm sure he would have gone on and on in that vein had I not hung up on him.

"How dare he talk to me like that?" I screamed to Jeff, shaking and sobbing. Although I soon calmed down, the experience brought home once again the awareness that I'd been forced to compromise. I never liked hiring housekeepers or taking taxis. I worried about being exploitive. And now I was forced to hire attendants, to appear horribly rich to non-white, non-middle class people, none of whom would know that we'd bought this huge center-city house with settlement money from a case involving the death of our two-day old daughter. I felt bourgeois and politically incorrect—I'd worked through the guilt, but this just wasn't my way.

Well spouses often feel weak, ineffective, and perhaps ashamed and guilt ridden. Our belief systems are often threatened. We're forced, or feel we're forced, to go against our beliefs, our habits, our life-styles, and our expectations. We can't or mayn't be good mothers, or good grandmothers, or good feminists, or good disability advocates; we can't keep in touch with certain friends, keep up with cultural events, or attend church or shul as often as we'd like or feel we should. We can't take jobs because we have to stay home and be care givers, or we *must* take jobs because we've lost our ill spouse's income.

We always believed we'd be "better" care givers when the time came. Or we were modest; we believed we'd never touch, dress, or undress our mates in front of others (meaning attendants). Like Arin as a young teenager, we believed the government would come to our aid; we believed in government and in health-care systems. We believed in our relatives and friends, that when the time came they would be there for us. We believed love conquers all.

I used to say, "People don't want solutions, only problems," and I prided myself on seeking and usually finding solutions to many of my problems, especially with respect to being a mother. Now I was stuck with a problem whose partial solutions, which I worked very hard to find, made little dent.

"If I didn't have this situation," says Fern, "I would be different." Indeed, how much of our selves has been taken from us? How much have our relationships with our very selves been undermined?

Friends would remark how tired I looked. If I was getting up twenty times a night, I must look tired. "But I *don't* look tired," I'd think. "In fact, just this morning that woman on the subway, who doesn't know I get up twenty times a night, was telling me how pretty I look—'alert,' she said, 'alive.'" I don't even feel tired, at least not today. Others can't help being swayed by their knowledge of our situation, and we can't help being swayed by what others say and think. Is there a typical care-giver image out there—a prejudice, a stereotype? And does it alienate us from ourselves?

Our houses are messy, or messier than they would be. I'd find whole pieces of shit in the laundry, because attendants can't or don't do toilet and washing at the same time. Our bodies, our selves—our houses, our selves. The people we associate with so much of the time are more downtrodden than they would be. Other ill people besides our spouses, other well spouses, attendants, especially the characters. Our lives in general are less in control than they would be.

So many variables can make for confusion. Where do our selves end and our situations begin? What is the connection between us and what is done to us? If you're so smart, why ain't you rich? applies to us less than If we're so smart, why are we barely even poor? If we're so well adjusted, if we've been through therapy and support groups, why aren't we in control of our lives?

Maybe we have a handle on it. Maybe, like Fern, and like me, we continually take stock and are able to keep up with this stock taking. Still, I have felt many times like a sucker, an enabler, a professional victim. How could anyone allow any man to do these things to her? No one, no molester, makes anyone do *toilet*. No wonder we feel weak.

On the other hand, society also calls us strong. Because we do nights, lifting, and toilet, we're viewed as strong, and sometimes it's assumed that we're strong in all ways. For example, do we only imagine that people who know we're well spouses don't open doors for us? If we have time to shop and may leave our homes, do we dress in practical clothes, where otherwise we might not? Do I like to create a "feminine" look with my long dresses and long hair to counteract that image? Is one of the reasons I kept having babies so I could be, if a "strong" woman, at least a woman?

Does strong sometimes translate into bossy or insensitive? Have we actually become bossy and insensitive? Do we wonder whether we've become that way? Do we bend over backwards not to be that way? If a care-giver stereotype exists, is it ever self-perpetuating?

The question What does everybody think of us? was, for me, never entirely answered, but well spouses generally agree that people don't think about us much at all. "All the attention is on my spouse. Out in the streets, everyone notices the person in the wheelchair, never the person pushing the wheelchair." That lament has been voiced countless times at well-spouse support-group meetings. In *Mainstay,* Maggie Strong calls it the "invisibility" of the well spouse.

I fought hard against invisibility. If anyone dared say, "It's so hard for him," I'd snap, "And it's also hard for me and the kids."

Eight years ago a neighbor asked, "Hi, Mar, how's Jeff?"

"Fine," I answered. "His wife just had a baby."

I related that incident in *The Level of Doorknobs,* and Maggie Strong later mentioned it in several of her presentations, in the well-spouse newsletter, and, so I heard one day from several friends and relatives, on Oprah Winfrey. That story has also gotten back to me at various well-spouse gatherings. Well spouses seem bolstered by hearing that kind of retort.

But I was not always so plucky. One Sunday—attendant's day off—Jeff had been calling "Mar!" with more than his usual frequency. All the phone calls had been for him (friends, physics colleagues, solar-energy contacts), and I had to help with most of them. At the end of the day I had finally had the opportunity to take a shower, because Jeff was in the midst of a long phone call, writing a physics paper with someone I'll call Stu. So I knew I wouldn't need to help him with another phone call and that he wouldn't need to call for me; his nose, for example, never itched while he was on the phone.

So I was in the shower, and just as I was beginning to truly rejuvenate Bret called up to me from downstairs. "Mom? The phone! It's for you."

Ah, finally! A call for me! Friend? I wondered. Student? Publisher? Although I wasn't quite dried off, I grabbed for that phone. (We had a phone in every room, including the bathrooms, to accommodate Jeff.)

"Marion? Hi!" said the voice. "This is Stu." The physicist Jeff had just been talking to. "Jeff told me to call back and ask for you. He was having trouble holding on to the receiver and he asked me to call back and ask for you because . . . well, he knew he wouldn't be able to answer and hold the receiver so. . . ."

My heart sank. My temper rose. I wished I could be inaudible as well as invisible. "Huh?" I said. "I'm in the shower; you'll have to wait." But no matter how long he waited, no matter how long *I* waited, I wouldn't be in the mood to help Jeff with that call from Stu. I had to do it without being in the mood. And I had to be (or had to feel as though I was) an accessory to the invisibility plot.

I had this same feeling whenever I walked down the street alone and I happened to pass another "disabled family." Especially if it was the husband in the trike and the wife and kids walking alongside him, I longed to say something; I longed to make contact. But I never did because, in order to make that contact, I needed Jeff and the trike and the kids with me. In those cases I felt invisible in the opposite way from the example with Stu; it was my care-giver identity I was being deprived of. I felt split. Indeed, when I wasn't with Jeff, I had what the disability movement calls "an invisible disability." And why, I wondered, didn't a disabled family ever pass by when Jeff and the kids were with me? Probably, I see now, because increasingly Jeff wasn't with me in the streets.

Less than a year ago, I felt strangely bitter over an incident that deprived me of my care-giver identity in another way. A bunch of us were playing *Therapy,* a kind of trivia game. I got the card that read: "Mary wakes up gradually, Sally wakes up suddenly. Who remembers her dreams better, Mary or Sally?"

"Aha!" I thought. "I wake up suddenly, or am awakened suddenly. And that dream life just slips away. I don't remember my dreams. But those few times when I wake up by myself, not by a jar, I wake up gradually and I have time to note each detail of my dream as I say good-bye to it, and I remember my dream well."

So I answered, "Mary. The one who wakes up gradually."

But the card was turned over, and it was Sally, the sudden awakener.

I felt betrayed, shortchanged. Insult had been added to injury. My experience and expertise at waking up suddenly had not paid off. Even when being a well spouse connects up with the world, it connects up wrong. Indeed, my life, and therefore my self, had not helped me; my well-spouse self had not helped me.

I was in a funny position, was how I often thought of it. The role it puts you in, is how my friend Nancy thought of it. It was a hard-to-peg role. To my husband I was wife, mother, master, servant, warden, prisoner, boss, secretary, know-it-all, captor, captive; I was mousy, strong, weak, and so on. They were roles I fought all the way.

ELEGY FOR IRIS

JOHN BAYLEY

JANUARY 1, 1997

Didn't Margaret Thatcher, at the mention of whose name Cloudy always starts barking, used to say there was no such thing as "society"? She didn't put it in quotes, of course: She knew what she meant. But her point wouldn't have been so obviously untrue if she had said there is no such thing as the "people," a word that today only achieves some sort of meaning if placed, whether accidentally or deliberately, in a given context. But "the people" are a fictitious body, invoked by politicians in the interest of democratic emotionalism, whereas "society" is still a neutrally descriptive word, making sense in any context. The only way "the people" can be contextualised is as "ordinary people," another purely emotive phrase which has just been used by the Archbishop of Canterbury in his New Year's speech on TV. Every "ordinary" person is, in fact, extraordinary, often grotesquely so, and in every sort of way.

I pondered such matters while making Iris her drink, after the Archbishop's speech. Important to make a routine of this. Around twelve o'clock or a little before. The drink itself slightly dishonest: a little drop of white wine, a dash of Angostura bitters, orangeade, a good deal of water. Iris likes it, and it has a soothing effect, making her sit watching TV for longer periods. Otherwise, she is apt to get up and stand with her back to the TV, fiddling incessantly with her small *objets trouvés*—twigs and pebbles, bits of dirt, scraps of silver foil, even dead worms rescued from the pavement on our short walks. She also puts water—sometimes her drink—on the potted plants by the window, which are now wilting under the treatment. But she never does this with a real drink, an alcoholic one. Sensible girl—her old fondness for bars still stands her in good stead.

FEBRUARY 20, 1997

Teletubbies. They are part of the morning ritual, as I try to make it. I have to insist a bit, as Alzheimer's now seems to have grown inimical to routines. Perhaps we all know by instinct that an adopted routine preserves sanity.

Just after ten, as part of the BBC 2 children's programme, the Teletubbies come on. One of the few things we can really watch together, in the same spirit. "There are the rabbits!" I say quite excitedly. One of the charms of this extraordinary programme is the virtual-reality landscape supplied: an area of sunlit grass—natural—dotted with artificial flowers, beside which the real rabbits hop about. The sky looks authentic as well, just the right sort of blue, with small white clouds. The Teletubbies have their underground house, neatly roofed with grass. A periscope sticks out of it. A real baby's face appears in the sky, at which I make a face myself, but Iris always returns its beaming smile.

The creatures emerge, four of them, in different coloured playsuits. How are they animated? What is inside their plump cloth bodies? The way they trot about and smile is almost obscenely natural, as are their grown-up male voices. Twiggy or something, Winky, Poo. . . . They trot about, not doing anything much, but while they are there, Iris looks happy, even concentrated.

This form of childishness is itself like virtual reality. We used to have a more genuine, spontaneous kind. It began, just before we were married, with a postcard of a very clueless-looking kitten putting its nose wonderingly round a door. Appropriately labelled "Ginger." Iris sent it to me, making a balloon on the front and writing in it, "Just coming." She became Ginger, and then Gunga.

"Haunted by Gunga," I teased her the other day, will be the title of the first section of my autobiography. She laughs and is pleased to be talked to that way, but I don't think she recognises the word anymore.

Something about the Teletubbies reminds me of going to see the bluebells in Wytham Wood. Since living in Oxford and finding out about this amenity, we have been to see them every year. Coming on them if the sun is shining has something of the beautiful dubiousness of Teletubby land. Can they be real? Do they really exist? They are in a thick and distant part of the wood, under dark conifers that stretch away downhill, and as they recede into darkness, they light up into their most intense colour. They vanish as if into a strange land where an endless dark blue lake begins. Close at hand, they look much more ordinary—greyish, purplish.

We stand and look at them. Last May, for the first time, Iris seemed not to take them in at all.

On the way there are real trees. Two gigantic sycamores, overpowering as a cathedral. But Iris has now a great fear of trees and I hurry her past them. I thought, This had better be the last time we come here.

As we got in the car, I said to her reassuringly, "Soon be back in Teletubby land."

But I don't think she remembered what Teletubbies were. I would quite like to be able to forget them myself.

The sense of someone's mind. Only now an awareness of it; other minds are usually taken for granted. I wonder sometimes if Iris is secretly thinking: How can I escape? What am I to do? Has nothing replaced the play of her mind when she was writing, cogitating, living in her mind? I find myself devoutly hoping not.

MARCH 1, 1997

When Iris's mother was taken to the mental hospital, we did not tell her where she was going. I had doped her, but the drive seemed interminable. As the nurse took her away, she looked back at us with a lost, unreproachful look.

The same look's on Iris's face when I manage to leave her for an hour with a friend.

Like school. Being left there. Probably such moments would not be so painful now if they hadn't started all those years ago at school, inside one's own ego.

I knew where I was going when I was taken to school. But being left there felt the same as the look on Iris's face, and her mother's. In fact, we retrieved her mother after she had been in the asylum a few weeks. Back again later. So it *was* like school.

Associations of that look. Seeing it, I remember the first little boy I met at school, after being left there. He was wizened, like a little old man, with a pale, leprous skin. I shrank from him, all the more because he was extremely friendly, confidential. He said, "Shall I tell you what my father told me? My father said it was the most important thing there was. He said, 'There is no difference at all between men and women. *Absolutely none at all.*'"

I regard the little boy with horror and fear. It all seemed part of this nightmarish new world of school. At the time, it seemed the worst thing I had ever heard, or was ever likely to hear.

* * * * *

Long piece in *London Review* on Iris's essay collection *Existentialists and Mystics.* The critic made a great thing of the contrast between Iris's views on the novel—the importance in it of free and independent individuals, character creations, *et cetera*—and her own practices in writing fiction, which instead of giving her characters "a free and realised life make them as unfree as pampered convicts." This has always interested me, too. In one way, it is an obviously true point; in a more important sense, it is irrelevant. For Iris makes a free world in her novels, which carries total conviction because it is like no other, and like no one else's. That is what matters, and that is why this world has such mesmeric appeal for all sorts of different people.

It is bound to be a tautology to talk about "freedom" in a novel, in which only the author is free to do as he likes. Pushkin, and Tolstoy following him, liked to emphasise that their characters "took charge," and that they were surprised by what they did, and by what happened to them. Once again, there is a kind of truth in that, but it won't really do. It is a cliché which novelists invent or repeat. What matters is whether the world created is both convincing and wholly *sui generis*, and here, of course, Pushkin and Tolstoy pass with top marks. So does Iris, in her own way.

I remember that time, years ago, when I was working on a study of Tolstoy, and Iris and I endlessly used to discuss the sort of perplexing questions that arise in the case of great novelists. I used to make the point that Tolstoy's greatest and least visible strength, or "freedom," was the cunning way he blended many different novel tactics when creating a character. At one moment, they behave, as if deliberately, like "people in a novel"; the next, they are suddenly like people we know, as inconsequential as people in life. They seem entirely themselves, as created characters, but the next moment they are behaving just as we might do, so that one can ask in a rather eerie and disquieting way, How does this writer know what I am like?

Tolstoy's people are both completely particular and completely general. At this point in my argument (such as it was), Iris used to look thoughtful. As a philosopher, she wanted to get things more clear than that; and I used to think that perhaps there was a real incompatibility between the philosophic mind and the simple undifferentiated muddle in which free characters and creation must move. Tolstoy, I felt, was not clearheaded at all; he merely picked up one thing and dropped another. Plato wouldn't have cared for that, or for Tolstoy—or for the novel generally.

Your characters, I used to tell her, have contingent aspects because you know that there are so many contingent things in life, and therefore the novel must have them, too. But contingency in some novels is not like that; it is glorious in itself and has no other purpose than to be itself. It's always funny, like the dog in *Two Gentlemen of Verona.*

"Is there a dog in *Two Gentlemen of Verona*?" she asked.

"I think so. I hope so, but I may have got the play wrong. Anyway, you see what I mean?"

Iris always, and as if indulgently, did see what I meant, though it didn't necessarily mean anything to her. We loved those conversations, usually over food or wine. Only for a few moments or minutes did they last, with the gramophone playing in the background. It all seemed funny, too. But I was surprised how much of what we touched on, all clarified and sharpened, is there in the essays collected in *Existentialists and Mystics,* superbly edited by Peter Conradi. Peter pointed out to me a lot of things about this collection, things which he said were like things in *The Characters of Love* and *Tolstoy and the Novel.* It hadn't struck me before, because those words between Iris and me, now vanished, just seem part of us both, although how that can be when our minds were so different—hers clear, mine muddled—remains a mystery.

We can still talk as we did then, but it doesn't make sense anymore, on either side. I can't reply in the way I used to do then, but only in the way she speaks to me now. I reply with the jokes or nonsense that still make her laugh. So we are still part of each other.

MARCH 30, 1997

The horrid wish, almost a compulsion at some moments, to show the other how bad things are. Force her to share the knowledge, relieve what seems my isolation.

I make a savage comment today about the grimness of our outlook. Iris looks relieved and intelligent. She says, "But I love you."

* * * * *

Iris surprised me when the radio was on and we were having lunch—toast, cheese, beetroot, and lettuce salad—by asking, "Why does he keep saying 'education'?" She sounded anxious. Anxiety and agitation are so much a part of her speech now, like the unending query "When are we going?" But lunch and supper are usually quite peaceful times. Trying to make everything as much a reassuring routine as possible. But now something on the radio has very much unreassured her. Government ministers say "education" so often. It ought to be a soothing word, even if a comparatively meaningless one.

It occurs to me that Iris is worried that it might mean something different now, which she has failed to grasp. In a sense, of course, that is true. It refers to skills with computers and such, which we know nothing about. But I think it is the frequency of the word in political speech that bothers her. It becomes like her own queries.

I try to say something about the importance of education, and everyone getting enough of it. Iris still looks anxious. "Do they read books?" I wonder whether education now chiefly means reading books, as it did when she was at school and college. Her coherence perturbs me. Normally now, sentences trail off, become deadlocked—start again in another place. Only anxiety queries complete themselves, and this seems to be one. I remember the kindly specialist at the hospital advising that another word suggested from outside can clear the circuit, as it were, temporarily allay the language anxiety. "It's a question of learning. I suppose. As we used to," I say. Her face does clear a little. *Learning* is not a word one hears much now, and certainly not *book learning. Education* has taken over. But *learning* is, or used to be, the more specific term.

> When land is sold and money spent,
> Then learning is most excellent.

The old rhyming proverb returns to my head—is it borne on the same mysterious circuitry that has failed in Iris's case?

* * * * *

"When are we going?"

"I'll tell you when we go."

Iris always responds to a jokey tone. But it is sometimes hard to maintain. Violent irritation possesses me and I shout out before I can stop myself, "Don't keep asking me when we are going!" Only a short time ago, it seems, this would have registered as a "tantrum," and the circuit would have visibly adjusted itself and responded with that mixture of amusement and forbearance, complete understanding, which survived as an automatic but infinitely welcome response. One notices that a lot of women respond to snappish husbands in public, and no doubt in private, too, with what Milton, describing Eve, tellingly refers to as "sweet austere composure." The opposite of understanding. Eve was the first to rail herself off in sex disapproval.

Iris never did that. She never got cross herself, and she never does now; but when I did so in the past, she would soothe me by a particular sort of reassurance, implying that I was most lovable and close to her when I was being angry, silly, or tiresome.

Now her face crumples into tears. I hasten to comfort her, and she always responds to comfort. We kiss and embrace now much more than we used to.

* * * * *

Often something that Iris says now, or a word she repeats, starts me off, too, on some more or less dotty train of association. I remember her mother with the early stages of Alzheimer's—not diagnosed or labeled then. She used to repeat a word in a touching way, as if it were a talisman or portent. If somebody said "journey" or "Baron's Court," where she lived, she would go on repeating it at intervals, and the same if someone happened to say "shandy" or "ham and cheese." Once the mind attends to this involuntary habit, it becomes a conscious one. I become aware that the word *learning* has been popping up at intervals in my mind, and so I play with it idly.

Significant, perhaps, that it is in some way a competitive word. A learned man stands out from his fellows, an educated man does not especially do so. Hence, *education* is a more okay word, something we can all have if the government goes about it the right way. It used to be normal to try to shine, to have read some book or books that others had not, to be able to quote. Lord Birkenhead, or someone like that, proclaimed in the thirties—was it in Oxford?—that there were still "plenty of glittering prizes for the sharp sword." The comment was adapted, ironically, by Auden in his poem "Oxford," so attitudes to that sort of thing must already have been changing. If prizes are given now, they must be given to all—in theory at least.

It's a relief in a way that things have changed. The atmosphere of "learning" is always tiresome, can be oppressive. Even my dear Barbara Pym, whose novels I am so fond of, must have been awful when she was young, and all her set, too, because they were always trying to dazzle with clever remarks, or by neatly capping quotations. Innocent enough, and rather charming in her early novels, but it must have been fatiguing in life. Socially speaking, people thought they had to try in those days.

Iris is a great contrast with all that. When young, she was already formidably learned, but I'm sure it never showed. Perhaps considered unsuitable for serious women to show it? Male dons certainly vied with each other, and I remember disliking it while trying to keep up with it. Nowadays, Common Room conversation is blessedly untaxing. But does "learning" require some sort of overt display, like a bird's feathers, to show how important it still is, or should be? It would have been thought odd if Prime Minister Blair had proclaimed his new government's policy to have been "learning, learning, learning," instead of "education, education, education." In spite of its competitive nature, learning is ideally an end itself, and no government particularly wants to encourage that, or to pay for it, either.

APRIL 15, 1997

Moving from stage to stage. How many are there? How many will there be? I used to dread Iris's moment of waking, because the situation seemed to strike her then in full force, at least for a minute or two. Reassuring noises, so far as possible, and then she would go back to sleep, and I would sit beside her, reading or typing. The sound of it seemed to help as reassurance. Iris's greed for sleep had something desperate about it, and yet she slept, and still sleeps, so easily and so long in the morning that it was a great mutual comfort. Lying beside me, she is like an athlete who had passed on the torch to a back-up member of the relay. I couldn't do what she had done, but I was doing something.

Not a good metaphor, though. It would be truer to say that I myself was reassured by her unawareness of anything that I might be doing on my own. It would have been unbearable if she had shown her old friendly interest. Where work was concerned, we had always left each other alone, so that being cut off now about such things was positively welcome. The simpler and more primitive our needs and emotions now, like those of babies for their mothers, the more absolute they feel. The exasperation of being followed about the house now by Iris is as strong and genuine as is my absolute need for it. Were she to avoid me, or "tactfully" leave me alone, I would pursue her as anxiously, if not quite so obsessively, as she now pursues me. I don't feel any particular pleasure or emotion when her whole face lights up at the sight of me when I return to the car after ten minutes of shopping. But I remember it if I wake up in the night, and then I reach out to her. The "lion face" of Alzheimer's used to be transformed in that way when her mother saw daughter Iris. Not that Iris's face has grown as expressionless as her mother's used to be. Sitting waiting for me in the car, she looks quite alert and amiable, and passing strangers smile at her.

But thank goodness that the stage of that old despair on waking seems to be over. Now she makes a soft chuckling sound and looks at me like the Teletubby baby in the blue sky on TV. No anxious queries. We exchange a few of the old nonsense words before she goes to sleep again. As the condition gets worse, it also gets better. It seems to compensate each new impoverishment. Should be more thankful for that.

* * * * *

The agony of travel nowadays. Iris has always loved travelling, and she craves it now more compulsively than ever. I have always detested the business of leaving home, and I was so thankful in the old days to drive her to the station and wave her good-bye.

Now I have a fever of travel angst—taxis, tickets, train times. Iris never worried about all that. She used to arrive at the station like a Russian peasant and wait for the first train to arrive.

The worst of both worlds. Although Iris is compulsively eager to be "going"—somewhere, anywhere—she is in as much of a flap in her own way as I am. At the station, she keeps repeating, "Why didn't you tell me we were going?" I had told her many, many times. Now I tell her again sharply, and with her own degree of querulous repetition. People look round at us. I am fumbling in my wallet checking the tickets. They are hard to separate, and after shuffling them wildly again and again, I can still find only one return ticket. The whole system is absurd; why must they give us four separate tickets when two would do? It's definitely not there. I rush to the ticket office, where a queue is made to unwind in serpentine fashion between rope barriers. The ticket man has drawn his little curtain and gone off. The customer at the other guichet seems to want a round-the-world ticket, and to be in no hurry about getting it. He and the ticket clerk canvass the possibilities in leisurely fashion. Iris clutches me anxiously, urging us to run to a train which has just come in, the wrong train, I hope. At last, the ticket man is free. I produce the receipt and the delinquent tickets. No, he can do nothing—it wasn't his sale. I turn away in despair. Why can't we just go home?

Iris has not understood the problem and keeps urging me towards the wrong train. At that moment, a man comes up to us and holds out a ticket. It is the original ticket man himself, strangely naked and unrecognisable now he's not behind the counter. He doesn't explain what happened, but just gives me a small collusive smile and walks rapidly back to his place of work.

On the train, I keep counting the tickets. The elderly couple opposite look sympathetically at Iris. I am clearly the one who's become a problem.

Utterly exhausted and drenched in sweat. Vague heart sensations, too. And the whole thing so trivial. Alzheimer's obviously has me in its grip, and the ticket man, too. As well as Iris, and probably everyone else.

Does the care-giver involuntarily mimic the Alzheimer's condition? I'm sure I do.

Sitting exhaustedly in the train, I suddenly recall a droll moment at the time when Iris seemed more or less to have decided to marry me. She was going down to her old school—to give the prizes or something—and suggested I should accompany her. After her business there was over, she wanted to call on the retired headmistress, a famous old white-haired lady who lived in a flat on the school premises. In her bleak way, the headmistress had been very kind, regarding schoolgirl Iris as the jewel in her crown. I was introduced, and after a few minutes I managed to slip away, leaving the pair of them together. When Iris came out, she was looking much amused. "Do you want to know what BMB thought about you?" she asked. I expressed a natural curiosity. "Well," said Iris, "she just said, 'He doesn't look very strong.'"

I didn't bother about being strong in those days. Now I have to try, but I'm sure the attempt wouldn't deceive BMB.

Kind friends up our street are giving a Sunday-morning drinks party. I used to enjoy the quiet of Sunday mornings, the Sunday paper, leisurely breakfast, with Iris working upstairs, absence of morning anxiety about what I had to do that day. In those days, I should have made some excuse, Iris acquiescing. She wouldn't have minded going but knew I wouldn't want to. Now it offers a welcome distraction. I say nothing about it until eleven. If I did, she would panic, demand why I hadn't told her sooner. She does not distinguish now between what she wants to do and what is happening.

"Are we going to London?"

"No, just up the street. You'll know them when we get there. They're very nice. You'll like it."

I know this is true, but it produces a "trouser grimace," as I now call it in my mind. Every evening, we have the battle of the trousers. She wants to go to bed in them, and in everything else she is wearing, too. My resistance to this is halfhearted, compared with the determination she shows on the issue. Sometimes I win, more or less dragging them off. Iris gives up the struggle, but she produces a frightful grimace, an expression wholly new and different from anything her face ever did in the past. It always unnerves me, and it is becoming more frequent in other situations.

Not that I care about her trousers. Our habits have never been exactly hygienic; and yet distinguishing day from night now seems vital to our saving routines. Twice in the day, at ten in the morning and five in the evening, panic and emptiness descend, not because there is something we have to do, but because there isn't. Routine has no suggestions to make. All I can do then is promise the next thing soon: a drink, lunch, or supper.

Iris's fear of other people if I'm not there is so piteous that I cannot bring myself to arrange for care-givers to "keep her company," or to take her to the age therapy unit. All that will have to come. Meanwhile, I am ruthless about getting her ready for the party, confident that she will enjoy it when she gets there, as they used to tell us in childhood.

She does. It is a nice party. I marvel, as I have often done before, at the way in which guests enjoy being guests. Standing opposite someone and keeping going, holding eye contact in the same practised, precarious way that one holds glass and canapé. Like a naval battle in Nelson's times: ship to ship, yardarm to yardarm. Sometimes another ship looms up through the noise of battle. Should I switch targets, or redouble broadsides against the present opponent? There is something remorseless about the concentration required. No one wants to be drifting aimlessly through the battle, guns silent, disengaged. . . .

The extraordinary thing is that Iris can serve her guns and return fire, as it were, just like everybody else. I wouldn't have brought her if I hadn't known it would be so. Her face becomes animated—no trace of trouser grimace; she is playing her part just like the rest of us. Mustn't this be good therapy? I should like to think so, but exercise in that sense would imply improvement, recovery. This happy distraction can be only for the moment. I close cautiously on the stern (still automatically Nelsonian) of the guest who is talking to Iris. He is giving a tremendous impression of being good at his work, and happy at it. Half-listening, while at the same time engaging my own opponent closely, I overhear a lively account of the way things are done in an insurance adjustment office. Smiling, Iris listens closely—her attention must be flattering. Then I hear her say, "What do you do?" From the face opposite her, it is evident that the question has been repeated several times in the last few minutes. Undiscouraged, he begins all over again.

Some people might actually find it more restful at a party to talk to someone more or less with Iris's condition. I think I should myself. Apart from making you feel you are performing a service to the community, it is also in the short run less demanding and taxing than the conventional art of party intercourse.

Coming up to me, the hostess says, "Isn't Iris wonderful?" She sounds surprised, perhaps thankful that there is no squeaking or gibbering going on. I am conscious of a base sense of annoyance, even exasperation. People who see Iris on such occasions assume there must be nothing much to worry about. Suppose I were to say to our hostess, "You should see how things are at home." Thank goodness one cannot or does not say things like that at parties.

When we get home, I try to keep Iris interested in the party, saying how much people had liked seeing her. In retrospect, the party does seem to have been a happy time; I am already looking back on it with nostalgia. But it is not remembered. Iris begins to say anxiously, "When do we go?" I wonder how many times she asked the insurance man what it was that he did.

MAY 10, 1997

I am continually surprised by the way in which the most unexpected people look a little embarrassed if I make some flippant remark about the caring services, the welfare ethic, even "lone" mothers (previously single mothers). Can it be that nice people don't mock such things, even as a joke? No one needs to be nice about sex anymore, or religion. But the modern feeling about social or state "compassion" is uncannily like the old silence about sex, or the reverence about religious beliefs. It's puritanical, too, blasphemy not now recognised as a part of faith, as it was in the older religions.

"Niceness" is always with us, and a good thing, too, but it shifts its ground, even though still clinging precariously to its ambiguities of meaning. Iris's novel *The Nice and the Good* implied these in a masterly way, with as much humour as precision. Does that novel—her others, too—nonetheless demonstrate in some way the inescapability of innocence, perhaps arising from a secure and happy childhood? Iris was both a nice child and a good one, and her parents were the same. None of the three had religion; all were, in the theological sense, naturally Christian souls. Like many philosophers, Iris is impatient with wickedness, its commonplaceness, its knowing conceit. The bad despise the good, confident, and with some justification, that the hapless good may think they "understand" the bad, but in fact can have no true awareness of them. In the characters of her novels, Iris substitutes the desire for power, which fascinates her, for commonplace, disgusting wickedness, which she is neither fascinated by nor understands. To understand wickedness, you must resemble it, at least possess some of its knowing conceit and its inherent dullness. You must be, as Isaiah Berlin said of Dostoevsky, "not a very nice man."

An argument with Iris once about that—or rather, about the good man, Alyosha Karamazov. A projection of the author's will, I said, whereas Dostoevsky's Underground Man slides effortlessly and absolutely into existence. Why? Because Dostoevsky was as boringly familiar with his Underground Man as he was with himself, while Alyosha is basically an idea, a good idea, of course. Iris objected that great novelists were explorers as well as natural knowers. Wasn't Dostoevsky going to send Alyosha into the pit of hell in a later volume, make him commit all the sins of man? Not real sins, I objected, because they wouldn't have been dull enough, nor conceited enough. Not *natural.* They would have been sins in the author's will, not in the book's reality.

I said this, as it made a reasonably smart point, but I knew my position was undermined by Iris's quiet good sense, by her niceness, in fact. I was point-scoring, something she never did in her novels, nor in her daily life. At the same time, I think one reason we fell in love, and got on so well, is that both of us have always been naive and innocent, at some deep healing level. Finding it in each other, but not saying so, or even knowing so. Iris is good. I'm not good inside, but I can get by on being nice. A wit remarked of Cyril Connolly, from whose features amiability did not exactly shine, that he was "not so nice as he looked." Iris is just as nice as she looks; indeed, in her case, the feeble though necessary little word acquires an almost transcendental meaning, a different and higher meaning than any of its common and more or less ambiguous ones.

Knowingness. Have got it in my head today, instead of "learning." Peter Conradi told me that the French word for it is *déniaiserie.* Fear of being naive?

And that awkward word, which I can hardly believe really exists, reminds me in some Proustian way of a disgustingly knowing boy at school. Haven't thought about him for years, if at all. One Sunday, his eye lit up with malicious glee when the lesson was read in school chapel. I couldn't help being curious, and he was delighted to tell me why. It was the story of the woman who anointed Jesus' feet with a precious ointment. "Jesus was awfully pleased with himself. When they said the ointment should have been sold and the money given to the poor, he said, 'Bugger that for a lark—I'm the one who matters, not the poor.' I'm going to take the piss out of God Clark about that."

"God" Clark was the chaplain. When I enquired how, as I was meant to, he said he'd do it in the Divinity Essay we had to write at half term. He did, too. But he failed to get a rise out of the chaplain. All too knowing about the ways of boys, the chaplain returned the essay without comment, merely congratulating the crestfallen youth on the fact that it was "well written."

"God" Clark, a saintly-looking old fellow with white hair, had a dark-haired young assistant chaplain with saturnine good looks, who was know as "Jesus" Steed.

Now why should I have remembered that? Having done so, I would once have rushed to tell Iris, sure that the story would amuse her. Now it wouldn't, alas. I can see her face if I were to tell her, with its bothered and confused look. We can still have jokes, but only very simple ones. Not anecdotes. Least of all anecdotes about "knowingness."

Iris once told me she had no "stream of consciousness." She did not talk to herself. She did not say to herself (I had said that I did), I am doing this—and then I must do that. Sainsbury's—the clouds—the trees are looking nice.

No trivial play with inner words? Did all once go into the world of creation, which lived inside her?

They say people with a strong sense of identity become the worst Alzheimer's patients. They cannot share with others what they still formulate inside themselves. Does Iris speak, inside herself, of what is happening? How can I know? What is left is the terrible expectancy. "When?" and "I want."

Is she still saying inside herself, like the blind man in Faulkner's *Soldiers' Pay*: "When are they going to let me out?"

Escape. The word hovers, though she never utters it.

Home is the worst place. As if something should happen here for her, which never does. Anxiety pushing behind at every second. Picking up things, as if to ward it off. Holding them in her hands like words. Wild wish to shout in her ear, "It's worse for me. *It's much worse!*"

This after the TV breaks down. It is I who miss it more obviously than Iris does, but in its absence she becomes increasingly restless. The recommended sedative seems not to help.

When are they going to let *me* out?

JUNE 4, 1997

Nightmare recollection of a day in the hot summer last year, just before or after our only swim in the Thames. What provoked the trouble, apart from the heat and a drink or two I had at lunch (when I normally try not to drink, Iris has her few drops of white wine with orangeade)? I must have been feeling unusually low. Rows like that are unpredictable, blowing up like squalls out of nowhere and subsiding as quickly. Then the sun is out, the water calm. One can even forget it is going to happen again. Quite soon.

The cause, though? The reason? There must be one. I remember being struck once, when reading Tolstoy, by his description of anger and emotion, a description which resembles the one theorised about by William James, the novelist's philosopher brother. According to James, at least as I recall, the anger or fear or pity is itself its own cause. I doubt this means much, but in Tolstoy, the notion becomes extraordinarily graphic: as when the movement of the tiny wrinkled fingers of Anna's baby are imitated involuntarily by Karenin's own fingers and face. His pity, even love, for this child of another man by his unfaithful wife existed purely in physical terms.

Was it for me some memory of the smell of Iris's mother when she was daft and elderly, arising now from Iris herself in the muggy heat, which expressed itself not in love and pity but in repulsion and disgust? Smell, as Proust knew, can certainly coincide with pleasure and relaxation, and become identified with those things. Or with their opposites? Iris is not responsive to subtle smells, but I have a very acute sense of them. Perhaps that divides us. I like almost all smells that one becomes conscious of without having to sniff at them, or recoil from them. All our houses have had their different smells, neither good nor bad in the obvious sense, but characteristic—that of Hartley Road, ironically enough, was especially memorable and attractive.

To me, the smell of Iris's mother's flat, though quite faint, was appalling. I had to nerve myself to enter; but Jack, who for quite a while looked after the old lady, never seemed to notice it; nor did Iris herself. The ghost of that smell certainly comes now from Iris from time to time: a familiar odour and a haunting of mortality. But it wasn't that which caused the row I made, although if William James was anything near right, physical causes are too wrapped up in their emotional results to be disentangled.

The trouble was, or seemed to be, my rage over the indoor plants. There are several of them along the drawing-room windowsill—cyclamen, spider plant, tiger plant, as we called a spotty one—to which I had become rather attached. I cared for them and watered them at the right intervals. Unfortunately, they had also entered the orbit of Iris's obsession with her small objects, things she has picked up in the street and brought into the house. She began to water them compulsively. I was continually finding her with a jug in her hand, and the windowsill and the floor below it slopping over with stagnant water. I urged her repeatedly not to do it, pointing out—which was certainly true—that the plants, the cyclamen in particular, were beginning to wilt and die under this treatment. She seemed to grasp the point, but I soon found her again with a jug or glass in her hand, pouring her water. Like Danaids, those sad daughters in Greek mythology, condemned forever to fill their sieves with water, punishment for having killed their bridegrooms on their wedding night.

I was not put out at the time: I was fascinated. I took to coming very quietly through the door to try to surprise Iris in the act, and I frequently did. Once when her great friend and fellow philosopher Philippa Foot (her mother, born in the White House, daughter of President Grover Cleveland) had come to see her, I found them both leaning thoughtfully over the plants, Iris performing her hopeless destructive ritual, Philippa looking on with her quizzically precise, polite attention, as if assessing what moral or ethical problem might be supposed by this task. I was also reminded of their colleague Elizabeth Anscombe, absently bringing up her immense brood of children, and once amusing her audience at some philosophical gathering with a sentence to illustrate some subtle linguistic distinction. "If you break that plate, I shall give you a tin one."

Whether or not the fate of the plants, or the ghost of an odour, had anything to do with it, that day I went suddenly berserk. Astonishing how a rage produces another person, who repels one, from whom one turns away in incredulous disgust at the very moment one has become him and is speaking with his voice. The rage was instant and total, seeming to come out of nowhere. "I told you not to! *I told you not to!*" In those moments of savagery, neither of us has the slightest idea to what I am referring. But the person who is speaking soon becomes more coherent. Cold, too, and deadly. "You're mad. You're dotty. You don't know anything, remember anything, care about anything." This is accompanied by furious aggressive gestures. Iris trembles violently. "Well," she says—that banal prelude to an apparently reasoned comment, often heard in that tone on BBC discussions, usually followed by some disingenuous patter that does not answer the question. Iris's "Well" relapses into something about "when he comes," or "must for other person do it now," or "dropping good to borrow when." I find myself looking in a mirror at the man who has been speaking. A horrid face, plum colour.

While I go on doing horrible things, as if kicking a child or a lamb, I suddenly think of the bursar of St. Catherine's College, a charming scholarly man, a financial wizard, a Parsee, who was telling me about his little son Minoo, a year or two old. "He's very tiresome. He's always breaking things. But it's not possible to be angry with him."

The bursar looked surprised and interested by his own reaction. I wonder briefly, if we'd had a child, would I have learnt not to be angry with it? In which case, would I not be angry with Iris now?

NOVEMBER 20,1997

Anger sometimes seems now to be a way of still refusing to admit that there is anything wrong. Like a sincere compliment. You are just the same as ever, bless you (or curse you), and so shall I be. I wouldn't insult you by pretending otherwise.

A happy stay, with our friend Audi in her little house in the middle of Lanzarote. Getting there is an ordeal, the charter flight always packed to the doors with holidaymakers. I am reminded of the old joke about Gericault's painting *The Raft of the Medusa,* with stricken castaways clinging on at all angles in the last stages of exposure and thirst. Reproduced with a holiday brochure caption: "Getting there is half the fun." But Peter and Jim come with us and look after us, so the whole ordeal is almost pleasurable.

Return a fortnight later. I have a heavy cold and feel unnaturally tired, although the journey up to this point could not have been easier. Peter puts us on the bus for Oxford. I sink back thankfully. Nearly home. The bus cruises steadily on through the dark, seeming to shrug off the rush-hour traffic on either side of it. The few passengers are asleep. But we have no sooner started than Iris is jumping up and down in agitation. "Where are we going? Where is the bus taking us?" She won't sit still, but rushes to the front and looks out anxiously ahead. I manage to get her sitting down. I say, "We're going back to Oxford. Back home." She replies, "No! No home. Why travelling like this? He doesn't know."

Before I can stop her, she is speaking agitatedly to the bus driver. She has caught hold of one of the bags, whose contents begin to spill on the gangway. I pick the things up, then push Iris into a seat opposite a sleeping woman. I apologize to the driver, who remains ominously silent. When I get back, the woman, a nice-looking person, is awake, and distraught, desperately trying to regain the handbag and other possessions which had been on the seat beside her. I take them from Iris and put them back, apologising again in a whisper. Iris says, "So sorry," and gives the woman her beautiful smile. I get Iris into another seat and give her a surreptitious violent punch on the arm by which I am holding her.

Gatwick to Oxford in the late Friday rush hour is a long way, every second of it occupied by tormented squirrel-like movements and mutterings. Iris grips the seat in front and stares ahead. A feeling of general distraction and unease eddies through the calm of the darkened bus. I can make out faces now alert and fixed resentfully. As the bus at last nears Oxford, I try to point out things she might recognise, but the agitation gets worse.

Clumsy escape from the stares of the passengers. Only one ancient taxi left, driven by a villainous-looking Indian with a gentle cultured voice. He starts to go the wrong way half-way up Banbury Road, and I distractedly put him right. He says, "Oh, no, I should know better, really. Very sorry about that." I give him a ten-pound note through the wire grille and get very little change, but I can't be bothered about that. I give some of it back as a tip and he says nothing. Open the door. Get inside the gate. The house feels deathly cold. I find Iris looking at me in a wonderful way, just as she used to do when we returned home together from some trying outing. I ignore her look, rush to the central-heating switch. Then I come back and say in a cold, furious voice, "You behaved disgracefully on the bus. I felt ashamed of you."

She looks surprised but then reassured, as if recalling an old cue. She would just be defending her corner by the kind old method—that is to say, not defending it. Leaving me to work out my nastiness, as if I were a child. "Well," she says. Her equivalent now of what might once have been a soothing "So sorry." I have lost my voice, can't hear, and am drowning in a cold that seems more ominous than an ordinary cold, as the bus driver's silence seemed more ominous than words. My chest hurts when I cough. After a few more ugly words, I say that I've probably got pneumonia. Hasn't she noticed I'm ill? She looks uncomprehending again. The moment of realisation and reassurance has gone with my own fit of cold fury, which brought them on. My appeal for sympathy leaves her lost and bewildered.

What'll she do if I die? If I'm ill and have to go to hospital. If I have to stay in bed—what'll she do then? Still exasperated by the bus business, I make these demands with increasing hostility and violence. I am furious to see my words are getting nowhere, and yet relieved, too, by this, so that I can continue to indulge my fury. She knows none of these things can or will happen. While I am still screaming at her, she says, "Let's go. There now. Bed." She says this quite coherently. We squeeze together up the stairs, huddle under the cold duvet, and clutch each other into warmth. In the morning, I feel a lot better.

Iris, I think, has never felt bad. She never caught my cold, as if the Alzheimer's is a charm against mere mundane and quotidian ailments. Jim washed and cut her hair in Lanzarote; Audi gave her a shower and a bath. She said to Audi as they stood together in the shower, "I see an angel. I think it's you." Having caught my cold, poor angel was in fact suffering from asthma and a serious chest infection, for which she had to start taking tetracycline, fortunately available over the counter on the island. How sensible, because Audi has never found a proper doctor there, though she has lived on the island on and off for years. Her temperature went up to nearly 103 degrees, but then came down quickly, much to our relief. I think we were all grateful in some way that Iris knew nothing about it. She reassured us by not knowing of troubles, and the tears of things.

Or rather, troubles touch her heart in invisible and mysterious ways. To Audi's cats, which she was once very fond of, she now seems almost indifferent. She strokes them absently. Peter and Jim's dog, Cloudy, whom she once loved to make much of, now seems to have, for her, the distance and impersonality of an angel. When she sheds tears softly and for short periods, she hides them with an embarrassment which she no longer feels about any other physical side of herself.

In the old days, she used to weep quite openly, as if it were a form of demonstrable and demonstrated warmth and kindness. Now I find her doing it as if ashamedly, stopping as soon as she sees I have noticed. This is so unlike the past; it is disturbing, too, in another way. It makes me feel she is secretly but fully conscious of what has happened to her and wants to conceal it from me. Can she want to protect me from it? I remember as a child finding my mother crying, and she stopped hastily, and looked annoyed. In Proust, the grandmother has a slight stroke while taking little Marcel for a walk in the park, and she turns her face away so that he should not see it all puckered and distorted.

There are so many doubts and illusions and concealments in any close relationship. Even in our present situation, they can come as an unexpected shock. Iris's tears sometimes seem to signify a whole inner world which she is determined to keep from me and shield me from. There is something ghastly in the feeling of relief that this can't be so; and yet the illusion of such an inner world still there—if it is an illusion—can't help haunting me from time to time. There are moments when I almost welcome it. Iris has always had—must have had—so vast and rich and complex an inner world, which it used to give me immense pleasure not to know anything about. Like looking at a map of South America as a child and wondering about the sources of the Amazon, and what unknown cities might be hidden there in the jungle. Have any of those hidden places survived in her?

Showing me a tracing from the most elaborate of the brain scans Iris underwent a year or so ago, the doctor indicated the area of atrophy at the top. The doctors were pleased by the clearness of the indication. I thought then—the old foolish romantic idea of the Amazon—that her brain world had lost its unknown mysteries, all the hidden life that had gone on in it. It had been there, physically and geographically *there.* And now it was proved to be empty. The grey substance that sustained its mysteries had ceased to function, whatever a "function," in there, can possibly mean.

Twice, Iris has said to Peter Conradi that she now feels that she is "sailing into the darkness." It was when he asked her, gently, about her writing. Such a phrase might be said to indicate the sort of inner knowledge that I had in mind. It seems to convey a terrible lucidity about what is going on. But can one be lucid in such a way without possessing the consciousness that can produce such language? And if consciousness can go on producing such words, why not many more, equally lucid?

Were I an expert on the brain, I should find it hard to believe in such flashes of lucidity revealing, as it were, a whole silent but conscious and watching world. It would be as if—to use a clumsy analogy from my hidden city in the jungle—a flash of lightning were to reveal its existence, and then the explorers found that it didn't exist after all. The words which Iris used with such naturalness and brilliance cannot be stacked there silently, sending out an occasional signal. Or can they? I notice that the eerie felicities which Iris has sometime produced, such as "sailing into the darkness" or "I see an angel," seem to come with a little help from her friends. They are like the things a young child suddenly comes out with, to the delight and amusement of parents and friends. But it was the friends or parents who unconsciously did the suggesting. Must have been.

Iris has heard nothing from a great friend, a novelist whom she had once befriended and inspired, counselled and consoled. Had this now famous friend left her, abandoned in her silence: Was it in resignation or in bitterness of spirit that she spoke those words? Sailing alone into the dark. . . .

In my own daily intercourse with Iris, words don't seem to be necessary, hardly appear to be uttered. Because we don't talk coherently, and because we talk without seeming to ourselves to be talking, nothing meaningful gets said. The clear things Iris does sometimes come out with are intended for public consumption. They are social statements. They have the air of last remarks before all the lights go out.

NOVEMBER 30, 1997

I always liked Sunday mornings, but Iris never noticed them. She still doesn't, but now I find TV a great help. Looking in on her as I potter about, I am relieved to see her sitting intently, like a good child, watching the Sunday-morning service. Later, she is still there; the service has changed to an animated cartoon featuring Bible history, Roman soldiers, and so on, in which she is equally engrossed. Thank goodness for Sunday-morning TV.

There are occasions when I have such a strong wish to remind Iris of something we did or saw that I find myself describing it hopefully, in great detail. I don't say, "You probably don't remember, but . . ." Instead, I now have the feeling that she is trying to follow something I am creating for her. Spring is more vivid when you talk about it in winter, and I find myself telling her about one of our visits with Peter and Jim to Cascob, in Wales, at the end of last May. The small schoolhouse, where twenty or thirty children were once taught, lies on a rising knoll at the end of a steep and narrow valley. It is an old place, a single large high-roofed room. Adjacent to it is the schoolmistress's house, one room up and one down. Although they were once separate buildings, Peter and Jim have joined the two and made some alterations, but the basic structure remains intact. The crown of the hillock on which their home stands slopes sharply down to their pond, with a little island in the middle, thick with alder and willow and with flowers in summer. Just beside the school is an extremely old church, half-buried in green turf nearly up to the window openings on one side, so that the sheep can look in. An immense yew tree, much older even than the church, makes a kind of jungle beside it, dark red with shadows.

On that visit to this enchanting place, we soon found a special routine. A pair of redstarts were nesting just above the back doorway. If we sat motionless in the little courtyard, or looked out of the schoolhouse window, we could see them come and go: small flamelike birds, looking much too exotic to be seen in the British Isles. The breast and tail (steort means "tail" in Old English) were bright cinnamon red, the head jet black, with a white ring on the neck. When they hovered near the nest, wary of a possible watcher, they were as jewel-like as hummingbirds.

After watching the redstarts, our ritual was to go round to the churchyard, where we could have quite a different experience. Jim had fixed a nesting box on a great ash tree where the graveyard bordered their copse. He told us a pair of pied flycatchers were nesting there. A flycatcher is a little bird, even more rare than the redstart, a migrant who now only comes back to the borders of south and central Wales. We stood by a gravestone, watching. Nothing happened for a long time. Suddenly and soundlessly, a neat little apparition in black and pure white appeared by the hole in the nesting box. It was motionless for a moment and then vanished inside. We looked at one another, hardly believing we had really seen it. It seemed like a pure speck of antiquity, robed in the hues of the old religion, almost as if a ghostly emanation from the church itself.

After this, we could not keep away from the grave mound by the edge of the copse, a vantage point only a few feet away from the nest on the ash tree. The little birds seemed unaware of us, just as ghosts would have been. Their busy movements had a soft spirit-like silentness. Peter and Jim told us they did have a small song, but we never heard them make a sound. Although we saw both birds, and identified the male and the female, we could not really believe in their physical existence at all. Like the ghosts in *Macbeth,* they came like shadows, so departed.

In the winter, I find myself telling all this, and she listens with a kind of bemused pleasure and toleration, as if I were making up a fairy story. She doesn't believe it, but she likes to hear it. I myself find that these bird memories, and the whole memory pattern of summer sunshine and green leaves, become subtly different from what it was like at the time. It really is as if I were making the whole thing up.

I remembered that Kilvert, the Victorian parson who once lived not far off in the same part of Wales and had so much loved writing his diary about his days, his walks, and his priestly duties, had once confided to it that what he wrote down was more real to him than what he had actually seen that day or the one before and was now writing about. Only memory holds reality. At least this seems to have been his experience, and that of a lot of other writers, too—romantic souls who, like Wordsworth (worshipped by Kilvert), made the discovery that for them to remember and to write was to create their lives, and their sense of living things. The actual experience was nothing beside it, a mere blur always on the move, always disappearing. Proust or D. H. Lawrence must have felt the same, however much Lawrence himself might protest about "Life—Life" being the great thing. Wordworth only *really* saw his daffodils when he lay on his couch and viewed them with his inward eye.

Iris's genius as a writer is rather different, I think, more comprehensive. Nor does one think of Shakespeare as creating this wonderful vision after the event. It seems to be a Romantic discovery, this sense that all depends on memory. But like all such generalisations, this is not altogether true: Some writers or artists—Vermeer for instance—create such vanished moments but without bothering to make a song and dance about it.

As I create, or re-create, those birds for Iris, I wonder what is going on in her head. Is she cognisant of an invention, a fairy tale instead of a memory? For a writer of her scale and depth, the power of creation seems so much more important than memory, almost as if it could now continue independent of it. And yet the one seems to depend on the other. So what are we remembering when we invent?

The main thing is, she likes to hear me talk about the birds. They must be just a part, a coming-and-going part, of the me she is always with. Once I was outside her, a reality quite separate from herself, her mind, her powers of being and creating. Not now.

Now I feel us fused together. It appalls me sometimes, but it also seems comforting and reassuring and normal.

Reminded of *The Girl with the Red Hat,* the Vermeer portrait that for me haunted our short but happy stay at The Hague. When we were there, I at once began to have that fantasy about it, which I told to Audi and Iris, separately I think. For Audi, I wanted it to be comic, a comical adventure fantasy, with sinister overtones, which we could laugh at together. Could it be that for Iris I instinctively tried to make it sound a bit like something in her own novels? As if I were trying to remind or inspire, or even carry on the torch by a kind of imitation? However that was, the story I wrote about it does not sound in the least like Iris, except perhaps to me. It came out much more like the fantasy I told Audi, who kindly said she enjoyed it when the book appeared a year later.

Life is no longer bringing the pair of us "closer and closer apart," in the poet's tenderly ambiguous words. Every day we move closer and closer together. We could not do otherwise. There is a certain comic irony—happily, not darkly comic—that after more than forty years of taking marriage for granted, marriage has decided it is tired of this, and is taking a hand in the game. Purposefully, persistently, involuntarily, our marriage is now getting somewhere. It is giving us no choice—and I am glad of that.

Every day, we are physically closer; and Iris's little "mouse cry," as I think of it, signifying loneliness in the next room, the wish to be back beside me, seems less and less forlorn, more simple, more natural. She is not sailing into the dark: The voyage is over, and under the dark escort of Alzheimer's, she has arrived somewhere. So have I.

This new marriage has designed itself, as Darwin once speculated that fish perhaps designed their own eyes, to bring to an end her fearful anxieties of apartness—that happy apartness which marriage had once taken wholly for granted. This new marriage needs us absolutely, just as we need it. To that extent, it is still a question of "taking it for granted."

The phrase "taking for granted" was in my head because I had just received a letter from the Japanese psychologist Takeo Doi. Admiring Iris's novels, he had once corresponded with her, and his ideas had interested her. As pen pals, they had got on, and the three of us had once met in Tokyo. He had read a piece of mine on marriage which had been commissioned by *The Times.* The paper had naturally wanted it to be about Iris's Alzheimer's, but I had also made our old point about taking marriage for granted, quoting Iris's character in *A Severed Head* who had lamented that her marriage "wasn't getting anywhere." This had struck the distinguished psychologist, the explorer of *amae,* the taken-for-granted bond which supplies the social cohesion of the Japanese people, and he had titled the essay which he now sent me "Taking for Granted." Japanese husbands and wives, he said, do not make a fuss about marriage, as in the Western style, but take it for granted. I wrote thanking him for the piece, and remarked that marriage was now taking us for granted, rather than we it.

As in the old days, nothing needs to be done. Helplessness is all. Yet it's amusing to contemplate "new marriage." Like New Labour, the New Deal, and so on? Not quite like that. Hard, though, to contemplate one's arrangements without their becoming, at least to oneself, a private form of public relations. I need our closeness now as much as Iris does, but I don't feel I need to cherish it. It has simply arrived, like the Alzheimer's. The best as well as the fullest consciousness of it comes in the early morning, when I am beside Iris in bed, tapping on my typewriter, and feel her hearing it in her doze, and being reassured by it.

In the past, she would have been up and in her study, in her own world. I am in mine, but it seems to be hers, too, because of proximity. She murmurs, more or less asleep, and her hand comes out from under the quilt. I put mine on it and stroke her fingernails for a moment, noticing how long they are, and how dirty. I must cut them and clean them again this morning. They seem to grow faster by the month, and I suppose mine do the same.

DECEMBER 14, 1997

As I am sitting in the kitchen, trying to read something, Iris makes her mouse noise at the door. She is carrying a Coca-Cola tin picked up in the street, a rusty spanner—where on earth did she get that?—and a single shoe.

Single shoes lie about the house as if deposited by a flash flood. Never a matching pair. Things in odd corners—old newspapers, bottles covered in dust. A mound of clothing on the floor of the room upstairs where she used to write. Dried-out capless plastic pens crunch underfoot. A piece of paper in her handwriting of several years ago with "Dear Penny" on it.

Rubbish becomes relaxing if there is no will to disturb it. It will see out our time. I think of the autumn in Keats's poem "Hyperion": "But where the dead leaf fell, there did it rest."

An odd parallel between the rubbish on the floor and the words that fly about the house all day. Words the equivalent of that single shoe.

Tone is what matters. All is okay with a child or cat or gunga exclamation. "The bad cat: What are we going to do with her?" I stroke her back or pull her backwards and forwards till she starts laughing. I imitate the fond way her father used to say in his mock-exasperated Belfast accent (she told me this long ago), "Have you got no sense at all?" Iris's face always softens if I mention her father in this way. Instead of crying, she starts to smile.

I rely on the bad-child ploy, which can easily sustain some degree of frenzy. "You bad animal! Can't you leave me alone *just for one minute!*" Or sometimes I sound to myself like Hedda Gabler needling her lover. But if I give it the tone of our child talk, Iris always beams back at me.

She never showed any interest in children before. Now she loves them, on television or in real life. It seems almost too appropriate. I tell her she is nearly four years old now—isn't that wonderful?

* * * * *

The Christmas business, it's all come around again. Iris has always enjoyed Christmas, and the socialising that goes with it. The festive season always makes me feel glum, though I go through the motions. Why not get away from it all? In the old days Iris wouldn't have liked that. Now I am not so sure. Change in one sense means little to her, yet a different scene of any sort can cause her to look around in astonished wonder, like Sleeping Beauty who when she stirred among the cobwebs saw—must have seen, surely—spiders and rats and mice running away in alarm. (I am assuming that the prince who woke her would have stepped tactfully back into the shadows.)

Wonder on the edge of fear. That shows in Iris's face if we go anywhere unfamiliar to her. A momentary relief from the daily pucker of blank anxiety. A change only relieves that anxiety for a few minutes, often only seconds. Then anxiety returns with new vigour. The calmness of routine has more to recommend it. But no choice really—Hobson's choice. Routine needs a change, and change finds some relief again in routine, like the people in Dante's hell who kept being hustled from fire into the ice bucket, then back again.

Well, not as bad as that. The point about Christmas could be that it combines a change with a routine, a routine of custom and ceremony that has at least the merit of a special occasion, of coming but once a year. Years ago, our friend Brigid Brophy and her husband decided to go to Istanbul for Christmas. "To eat our turkey in Turkey," as they explained. Iris then laughed politely, but she was not amused. Indeed, I am not sure she was not really rather shocked. Christmas to her was not exactly holy, but it meant something more important than the opportunity for a witticism about turkey in Turkey.

I think she welcomed at that time the idea of inevitability—something that has to happen. Mary and Joseph in the stable could do nothing about it—why should we need to?

Now I must encourage that instinct towards passivity, taking refuge in blest, or at least time-honoured, routines. No point in getting away from it all, nowhere to get away to. Alzheimer's will meet you there, like death at Samarra.

So we'll go to London as usual, visit my brother Michael, have Christmas dinner with him. We'll do all the usual things.

DECEMBER 25, 1997

It's Christmas morning. And we are doing all the usual things. Routine is a substitute for memory. Iris is not asking the usual anxious questions: "Where are we? What are we doing? Who is coming?"

Someone, or something, is coming. The silence it brings makes no demands. London is uncannily silent on Christmas morning. Nobody seems to be about. If there are churchgoers and church bells, we see none, hear none. The silence and the emptiness seem all the better.

We walk to Kensington Gardens up the deserted street, between the tall stucco façades falling into Edwardian decay, but still handsome. Henry James lived on the left here; Browning farther up on the right. We pass their blue plaques set in the white wall. A few yards back, we passed the great gloomy redbrick mansions where T. S. Eliot had a flat for many years. His widow must be in church now.

Our route on Christmas morning is always the same. We have been doing this for years. As we pass their spectral houses, I now utter a little bit of patter like a guide.

Henry James, Robert Browning, T. S. Eliot. On former mornings like these, we used to gaze up at their windows, talk a bit about them. Now I just mention the names. Does Iris remember them? She smiles a little. They are still familiar, those names, as familiar as this unique morning silence. Just for this morning, those writers have laid their pens down, as Iris herself has done, and are taking a well-earned rest, looking forward to their dinners. Thackeray, the gourmet, whose house is just round the corner, would have looked forward to his with special keenness.

Now we can see the park, and beyond it the handsome Williamite façade of Kensington Palace. When Princess Diana died, the whole green here was a mass of cellophane, wrapping withered flowers. And the crowds were silent, too. As quiet, the media said in an awed way, as it is in this morning's calm. The grievers were like good children at bedtime, folding their hands in ritual prayer. It was a tranquil ceremony, like our Christmas, as we wander now vaguely over the deserted road, usually a mass of traffic, and up the expanse of the Broad Walk.

A few dogs here, unimpressed by Christmas, but seeming merrier than usual in contrast with the silence. There is one bell now, tolling somewhere on a sweet high note.

Up in the sky, the jet trails move serenely on, seeming more noiseless than usual, their murmur fainter when it comes. Christmas morning in London is always calm and mild and bright. I can remember one time when it rained, even snowed a bit. I ask Iris if she can remember that Christmas. She smiles. No need to remember, as this ritual that has replaced memory goes on.

The Round Pond. Canada geese standing meditative, for once making no demands. The same path as usual, downwards, to the Serpentine. Nobody round the Peter Pan statue. Not even a Japanese couple with a camera. One Christmas, we met two middle-aged ladies from New Zealand here, who told us this statue was the one thing they really wanted to see in London.

Young Pan himself, bronze fingers delicately crooked, his double pipe to his lips, has the sublimely sinister indifference of childhood. Captain Hook, his great enemy, was always made nervous by that pose. He considered Peter to have Good Form without knowing it, which is, of course, the best Form of all. Poor Hook was in despair about this. It made Iris laugh when I told her, years ago, before we were married. I read a bit of the book to her (the book is much better, and funnier, than the pantomime play). Iris, I recall, was so amused that she later put the "good form" business into one of her own novels.

Iris's amusement may even have been shared, in a quiet way, by the sculptor himself, who covered the base of the group with elves and rabbits and snails in the Victorian fairy-tale tradition. But at the top, he put the elegant figure of a much more worldly young woman, scrambling determinedly over the plinth to proposition Peter, giving the bystander an agreeable view of her polished bronze derriere. It is clad in a modishly draped and close-fitting Edwardian skirt, and she looks much too old for Peter anyway. Could it be that Sir George Frampton, as well as being an excellent artist and sculptor, had a sense of humour about these matters? It certainly looks like it, on such a quiet, sunny Christmas morning, with real squirrels hopping about all round the statue, vainly soliciting the nuts which the fat little beasts have no trouble in getting from tourists on ordinary, busier days.

As we walk round and admire, I tell Iris that my mother assured me that if I looked hard enough over the railings, into the private dells where the bluebells and daffodils come up in spring, I might see fairies, perhaps even Peter Pan himself. I believed her. I could almost believe her now, with the tranquil sunshine in the park making a midwinter spring, full of the illusion of flowers and fairies as well as real birdsong.

Iris is listening, which she rarely does, and smiling, too. There have been no anxious pleas this morning, no tears, none of those broken sentences whose only meaning is the dread in her voice and the demand for reassurance. Something or someone this morning has reassured her, given for an hour or two what the prayer book calls "that peace which the world cannot give."

Perhaps it is the Christmas ritual. It is going somewhere, but it is also a routine, even though a rare one. It is both. And now it will go on. We shall return to my brother, who has attended matins this morning at Chelsea Old Church, where Sir Thomas More once used to worship. We shall eat sardines and sausages and scrambled eggs together, with a bottle or two of a Bulgarian red wine which goes with everything. The sort of Christmas dinner we all three enjoy, and the only time of the year Michael permits a little cookery to be done in his immaculate and sterile little kitchen. The sardines are routine for him, but the eggs and sausages represent a real concession. I shall do them, with Iris standing beside me, and we shall bring the wine.

A snooze then. Iris will sleep deeply. Later, we listen to carols and Christmas music. And I have the illusion, which fortunate Alzheimer's partners must feel at such times, that life is just the same, has never changed. I cannot imagine Iris any different. Her loss of memory becomes, in a sense my own. In a muzzy way—the Bulgarian wine, no doubt—I find myself thinking of the Christmas birth, and also of Wittgenstein's comment that death is not a human experience. We are born to live only from day to day. "Take short views of human life—never further than dinner to tea." The Reverend Sydney Smith's advice is most easily taken during these ritualised days. The ancient saving routine of Christmas, which for us today has been twice blessed.

CASE HISTORY

DANNIE ABSE

'Most Welshmen are worthless,
an inferior breed, doctor.'
He did not know I was Welsh.
Then he praised the architects
of the German death-camps—
did not know I was a Jew.
He called liberals, 'White blacks',
and continued to invent curses.

When I palpated his liver
I felt the soft liver of Goering;
when I lifted my stethoscope
I heard the heartbeats of Himmler;
when I read his encephalograph
I thought, *'Sieg heil, mein Führer.'*

In the clinic's dispensary
red berry of black bryony,
cowbane, deadly nightshade, deathcap.
Yet I prescribed for him
as if he were my brother.

Later that night I must have slept
on my arm: momentarily
my right hand lost its cunning.

TEN PATIENTS AND ANOTHER

RAPHAEL CAMPO

1. Mrs. G.

The patient is a sixty-odd-year-old
White female, who presents with fever, cough,
And shaking chills. No further history
Could be elicited; she doesn't speak.
The patient's social history was non-
Contributory: Someone left her here.
The intern on the case heard crackles in
Both lungs. An EKG was done, which showed
A heart was beating in the normal sinus
Rhythm, except for an occasional
Dropped beat. An intravenous line was placed.
The intern found a bruise behind her ear.
She then became quite agitated, and
Began to sob without producing tears.
We think she's dry. She's resting quietly
On Haldol, waiting for a bed upstairs.

2. Jamal

The patient is a three-year-old black male,
The full-term product of a pregnancy
That was, according to his grandmother,
Unplanned and maybe complicated by
Prenatal alcohol exposure. Did
OK, developmentally delayed
But normal weights and heights, until last week
When he ingested what's turned out to be
Cocaine, according to the lab results;
His grandmother had said she'd seen him with
Some baby powder on his face and hands
Before he started seizing and they brought
Him in. The vital signs have stabilized.
The nurse is getting D.S.S. involved.
The mom? She left it on the kitchen table.
That's her—the one who sings to him all night.

3. H. K.

The patient is a twenty-nine-year-old
Black man who lives in Dorchester. Upon
Returning from his shift—the patient is
A night nurse at a local hospital—
He was attacked by two assailants. Males,
White, late teens, shouting threats and epithets.
He thinks they followed him from work. He turned,
Attempting to respond, when he was struck
With two blunt objects in succession. One
Was glass; we know because some fragments were
Extracted from the wounds. He'd bled to a crit
Of twenty, which required stat transfusions.
The surgeons didn't want to operate
Until they had more information. CT scans
Revealed free blood inside the abdomen.
What's scary is he isn't even gay.

4. Kelly

The patient is a twelve-year-old white female.
She's gravida zero, no STD's.
She'd never even had a pelvic. One
Month nausea and vomiting. No change
In bowel habits. No fever, chills, malaise.
Her school performance has been worsening.
She states that things at home are fine.
On physical exam, she cried but was
Cooperative. Her abdomen was soft,
With normal bowel sounds and question of
A suprapubic mass, which was non tender.
Her pelvic was remarkable for scars
At six o-clock, no hymen visible,
Some uterine enlargement. Pregnancy
Tests positive times two. She says it was
Her dad. He's sitting in the waiting room.

5. John Doe

An elderly white male, unresponsive.
Looks homeless. Maybe he's been here before:
No chart. No history. His vital signs
Were barely present, temperature was down
Near ninety, pressure ninety over palp;
The pulse was forty, best as they could tell.
They'll hook him into a monitor before
They warm him up. I didn't listen to
His lungs—I bet I'd hear a symphony
In there. I couldn't check his pupils since
His lids were frozen shut, but there were no
External signs of trauma to the head.
They found this picture of a woman with
Two tiny kids still pinned inside his coat.
It's only three A.M. The night's young. If
He's lucky, by tomorrow he'll be dead.

6. S. W.

Extending from her left ear down her jaw,
The lac was seven centimeters long.
She told me that she slipped and struck her face
Against the kitchen floor. The floor was wet
Because she had been mopping. I guessed
She'd had to wait for many hours since
The clock read nearly midnight; who mops floors
So late? Her little girl kept screaming in
Her husband's thick, impatient arms: he knocked
Three times, each time to ask when we'd be done.
I infiltrated first with lidocaine.
She barely winced, and didn't start to cry
Until the sixteenth stitch went in and we
Were almost through. I thought my handiwork
Was admirable. I yawned, then offered her
Instructions on the care of wounds. She left.

7. Manuel

In Trauma 1, a gay Latino kid—
I think he's seventeen—is being tubed
For respiratory failure. "Sleeping pills
And Tylenol," I translated for him
As he was wheeled in. His *novio*
Explained that when he'd told his folks about
It all, they threw him out. Like trash. They lived
Together underneath the overpass
Of Highway 101 for seven weeks,
The stars obstructed from their view. For cash,
They sucked off older men in Cadillacs;
A *viejita* from the neighborhood
Brought *tacos* to them secretly. Last night,
With eighteen-wheelers roaring overhead,
He whispered that he'd lost the will to live.
He pawned his crucifix to get the pills.

8. F. P.

Another AIDS admission. This one's great:
They bring him in strapped down because he threw
His own infected shit at them—you better bring
Your goggles!—and a mask, we think he's got
TB. He's pissed as hell. Apparently,
He wants to die at home but somebody
Keeps calling 911. A relative
Back home in Iowa, or some damn place.
Just keep him snowed with Ativan—believe
You me, you do not want to get to know
This fucker. Kaposi's all over, stinks
Like shit—incontinent, of course. How long
Before you get down here? Because his nurse
Is driving me insane. Of course we got
Blood cultures . . . yeah, a gas—OK, I'll stick
Him one more time. The things you do for love.

9. Tommy

A twenty-one-year-old white man brought in
By ambulance—in hypotensive shock,
Shot in the back while buying drugs from three
Black men. The cord must be involved:
His legs are paralyzed, his penis is
Erect, and all sensation from below
The level of the entry site is lost.
They left him in the street for dead; I heard
Them say an alley dog was lapping up
His blood like milk when he was found. Before
He goes to surgery, he has to give
Informed consent, which he's refused to do
Thus far. He states he'd rather die than be
Dependent on his family for care.
They're questioning his competence, of course.
They're waiting on his folks. His wife just stares.

10. Maria

This G_2 P1 gives us a confusing
History. It sounds like she's been pregnant
Approximately thirty weeks, although
She can't recall her LMP. No pain,
But bleeding for about two days. Of course
She hasn't had prenatal care, and God
Only knows where the father is. She works
Two jobs that keep her on her feet all day.
She's been in the United States six months,
And doesn't speak a word of English. Bet
You she's illegal. Cervical exam
Is unremarkable, the os is closed.
I think we need an ultrasound to tell
Us more. Besides a look at the placenta,
We need some confirmation of her dates.
Her uterus can tell us more than she can.

11. Jane Doe #2

They found her unresponsive in the street
Beneath a lamplight I imagined made
Her seem angelic, regal even, clean.
She must have been around sixteen. She died
Who knows how many hours earlier
That day, the heroin inside her like
A vengeful dream about to be fulfilled.
Her hands were crossed about her chest, as though
Raised up in self-defense; I tried to pry
Them open to confirm the absence of
A heartbeat, but in death she was so strong,
As resolute as she was beautiful.
I traced the track marks on her arms instead,
Then pressed my thumb against her bloodless lips,
So urgent was my need to know. I felt
The quiet left by a departing soul.

THE 10,000TH AIDS DEATH IN SAN FRANCISCO

RAPHAEL CAMPO

January 1993

A woman hurried past me in the street
Today, reminding me it's not a dream:
While eating an expensive lunch in some
Expensive Caribbean restaurant
I keep imagining is Cuban-owned,
I notice that I keep imagining
The AIDS ward where I saw a man my age
Die yesterday. I can't say why, but when
He looked at me I wanted him to kiss
My face. I wanted him to live with me
And tell me stories, stories seventeen
Or eighteen hours long, involving sex
Beneath the stars, or with celebrities
Beneath some perfect, countless stars, about
The days before the epidemic killed
So many thousand people. Wanting him
To live, I stood erect beside his bed,
Wanting him. The sex itself was great,
I'm sure, but what I'd really like to know
Was how it felt to know that after lunch
In some expensive restaurant, your friends
Would be alive. Your friends would be alive—

To know no friend would die like that,
Of cryptococcal meningitis, or
Another kind of meningitis, or
A lung infection so severe it makes
A kiss impossible because the need
To breathe is even greater. Hurriedly,
I pay the bill, because I need to breathe
And suddenly I'm seeing stars, I see
Myself outside some Cuban restaurant.
A woman hurries past me, frowning, far.

ON HIS BLINDNESS

JOHN MILTON

When I consider how my light is spent
Ere half my days, in this dark world and wide,
And that one talent which is death to hide
Lodged with me useless, though my soul more bent
To serve therewith my Maker, and present
My true account, lest he returning chide;
"Doth God exact day-labour, light denied?"
I fondly ask; but Patience, to prevent
That murmur, soon replies, "God doth not need
Either man's work or his own gifts; who best
Bear his mild yoke, they serve him best. His state
Is kingly. Thousands at his bidding speed
And post o'er land and ocean without rest:
They also serve who only stand and wait."

John Milton probably wrote this sonnet between 1652, at the onset of his total blindness, and 1655; it was given the title "On His Blindness" in an eighteenth-century edition by Thomas Newton. This edition is from *The Norton Anthology of English Literature*, M. H. Abrams, general editor. 5th ed. (New York: Norton, 1986).

SUGGESTED LONGER READINGS

Some works resist excerpting or anthologizing; they are so crafted that they must be read in their entirety. For reading groups such as those devoted to literature and medicine, the process of reading and thinking about a long literary work may in itself be instructive. For those reasons and others, I recommend some essential texts which support and even underlie the works I have selected for this anthology. Some works, such as Chekhov's *Ward Number Six* and Tolstoy's *The Death of Ivan Ilich,* are readily available but too long to be included in the list of selections. They continue to be of lasting importance to any consideration of illness and its treatment in our world. The list of readings which follows includes many works which have proved themselves indispensable to individuals and reading groups dedicated to bringing the humanities and medicine into a lasting partnership. Each of the following selections is invaluable, but each is also particularly relevant to one or more of the thematic organizations of this anthology, and is so identified.

Some long works supply theoretical grounding for the issues and dilemmas of contemporary medicine. Susan Sontag wrote two philosophical essays now published under one title, *Illness as Metaphor,* essays which are crucial for people willing to consider the ways in which our culture names and frames serious illnesses such as cancer, tuberculosis, and AIDS. Sontag's project is to demystify, and to liberate us from conceptual frameworks of illness that limit our ability to conquer it when we can, and to live with intelligent dignity when we cannot. Sontag's death from cancer, and her insistence on participating in a debilitating course of treatments, including an unsuccessful bone-marrow transplant, may enlarge the discussion. Recently published photographs by Sontag's companion, Annie Leibowitz, also testify to Sontag's unflinching candor as she fought what she termed "obliteration." **Section One: The Experience of Illness.**

Robert Murphy, who was a distinguished cultural anthropologist, takes up where Sontag leaves off in his autobiographical work *The Body Silent.* Unlike Sontag, who did not make her own cancer the centerpiece of her literary investigation, Murphy examines his paralysis and approaching death from a benign but inoperable tumor wrapped around his spinal column. Using his professional skills, Murphy describes himself as an observer-participant in the world of the disabled, and provides an intimate and lucid account of the profound losses and equally profound insights offered by chronic illness and disability. Murphy's insistence on maintaining a level tone and emphasizing his identity as a "talking head" evokes complex responses from readers; it may literally take years before a participant brings the discussion back to this text to allow others to acknowledge the effects that unspoken fear had on the original discussion. A long-time clinician confessed that until the conversation based on *The*

Body Silent, she had never spoken to any of the patients she happened to walk by who were in Murphy's condition. At the time of his death, Murphy and his equally distinguished cultural anthropologist wife, Yolanda Murphy, were about to embark on a funded study of people who, reduced to immobility by profound disability, continued to choose life. **Section One: The Experience of Illness; Section Four: Coming to Terms.**

Marianne A. Paget's book, *A Complex Sorrow,* edited by one of her close friends, Marjorie L. DeVault, has been universally praised by those working in the field of humanities and health care. Though we have excerpted one section, the whole book rewards all readers interested in issues of communication, and as well, in the work of the spirit. Paget's letters and the reminiscences of her friends who accompanied her in the last stages of her experience of mis-diagnosis, cancer, treatment, and death are intertwined in this remarkable book. **Section One: The Experience of Illness; Section Five: Healing Costs.**

Annie Ernaux's slim book, *Happening,* works like a depth charge. Published in 2000, *Happening* is based on the journals Ernaux kept in 1963 when she became pregnant and decided to have an abortion. A Michel Leiris epigraph that Ernaux chose for the book reads: I wish for two things: that happening turn to writing. And that writing be happening. The book is a rare fusion of immediacy and distance, experience and reflection. As charged as the practice of abortion is to medicine and culture in our time, this book allows for an intense and yet mediated account of the experience itself. The prose is immediate and transparent in an excellent translation from the original French. Ernaux's book would be especially effective in conjunction with Gwendolyn Brooks's short but large-spirited poem, "the mother." **Section One: The Experience of Illness; Section Four: Coming to Terms.**

There is also Andrew Solomon's indispensable book about depression, *The Noonday Demon: An Atlas of Depression.* As its title indicates, Solomon's book is an extraordinarily readable account not only of his own experience, but of depression's history, treatments, and persistence in human history itself. Solomon read and traveled widely for this book and for his own journey into the sources of his depression–which persists. He provides fascinating and moving accounts of individuals as well as an exhaustive bibliography of resources. The real appeal of this book, however, is its immediacy, the sense of Solomon's experience and personality speaking with scrupulous fidelity to the sources, whether personal or literary, that he has explored on his own behalf and on behalf of all those who have been touched—and scarred—by depression. **Section One: The Experience of Illness; Section Five: Healing Costs.**

Sophocles, one of the three great Greek tragedians whose works have come down to us in many translations, left several plays which are enthralling studies of issues central to humanities at the heart of medicine. The concluding play of the Oedipus trilogy, *Oedipus at Colonus,* presents a remarkable picture of Oedipus in his old age. Sophocles, who himself lived to a very old age, presents Oedipus, old and blind, seeing into the deepest realities of the human condition, meditating upon the meaning of his tempestuous life and of life itself. **Section Two: Beginnings and Endings.**

King Lear, one of Shakespeare's darkest and richest tragedies, rewards reading and discussion in the light of the extended span of years now provided in the Western world. The play is rich in its study of generations, its presentation of daughters and sons confronted by the tragic incursions of age, frailty, dementia, and wisdom entwined with loss. There are rewards associated with the excursion into Shakespeare's most difficult plays. The rich humanity of the aging Lear along with his contemporary, Gloucester, and their difficult relations with their children, ring with authenticity across hundreds of years. While it would seem that the primary discussion focus would be upon gerontology, those discussing the text may well identify with the daughters and sons, using the discussion as an opportunity to air their own grievances and disappointments. Such a discussion can offer a great opportunity to consider the subjectivity that medical practitioners bring to their work, providing for unexpected richness in the work of the reading group. As a drama, Shakespeare's play allows consideration of the differing perspectives brought by family members, whose experiences go back to act one, and clinicians who enter at act four or five of a history. **Section Two: Beginnings and Endings.**

The interrelationship between individual illness and community experience is at the heart of Terry Tempest Williams' haunting book, *Refuge.* Williams chronicles the cycle of flood and recovery of the Great Salt Lake at the same time that she chronicles the deaths from cancer of her mother and grandmother, members of a prosperous and loving Mormon family. The book offers a gripping and slowly evolving portrait of the complex interrelationship between nature and culture, between the health of the land and the health of those who live on it. Sharp disagreement between practitioners concerned with environmental issues and those more focused on genetic disposition may emerge when Williams' book is the text everyone has in common. **Section Two: Beginnings and Endings; Section Five: Healing Costs**.

Pat Barker's fictional trilogy, *Regeneration, The Eye in the Door,* and *Ghost Road* follows the career of a great psychiatrist, William Rivers, and his patients both real and fictional, through the course of the First World War. Barker's novels rely heavily on documentary materials, which underpin her portrait of Rivers, an anthropologist and pioneering psychiatrist in the treatment of what came to be known as "shell shock." The ethical dimensions of practicing medicine designed to restore soldiers to health so that they can return to the front lines has never been better portrayed. At the same time, Barker grounds her characters in the historical moment. In the end, it is Rivers as anthropologist who provides the wide lens that gives universal context to the unique particulars of his practice and his patients' lives and deaths. **Section Three: Trauma and Recovery; Section Five: Healing Costs.**

Philoctetes, another tragedy by Sophocles, is less well-known than the Oedipus plays, but it is in some ways more central to the concerns of medicine, focusing as it does upon the incurable wound and the challenge to social and political identity that such a wound represents. Illnesses which were once fatal may now be lived with; the rewards of life, however, may be tempered by stigma along with depression and despair. In his play about Philoctetes, the wounded warrior whose wound never ceases to fester, Sophocles considers the implications of chronic illness deeply and imaginatively. This play offers a rich subject for contemplation and discussion. **Section Four: Coming to Terms.**

Mark Salzman, who has published beautiful and fascinating work in poetry and prose, wrote a short novel called *Lying Awake,* the story of a nun whose poetic visions ultimately are revealed to result from a form of epilepsy which may be cured by a relatively simple surgical procedure. The intersection of body and soul is beautifully presented in this work, which deeply involves readers in the joys and ultimate challenges of the religious life. **Section Four: Coming to Terms.**

In her acclaimed work *The Spirit Catches You and You Fall Down,* Anne Fadiman vividly evokes one of the dilemmas at the heart of contemporary medicine: cross-cultural misunderstanding. Though Fadiman looks at a particular community in California where Hmong families make up a significant segment of the population, and depend on the local medical facilities staffed by practitioners proficient in high-tech Western medicine, the cultural perils have wide application. Fadiman's book is distinguished by the willing participation of both Hmong community members and thoughtful medical practitioners willing to reflect on their own frustrating and difficult experiences. One literature and medicine participant, a member of the medical community and his hospital's governing board, successfully pressed for an improved translator's program after reading Fadiman's book. Another incorporated Arthur Kleinman's questioning techniques into his treatment of his poor elderly patients from rural Maine. **Section Five: Healing Costs.**

Though there are many long works to add to this brief list, *The Iliad* and *The Odyssey* must be included. There is a choice of translations: for speed and immediacy, there are prose translations by Rouse, while Robert Fagles's magnificent poetic renderings offer a more compelling but more time-consuming experience. Especially when read and discussed in conjunction with all of Jonathan Shay's work with Viet Nam veterans, the masterpieces by Homer demonstrate the lasting aftermath of war. At a time when terms such as heroism, nation, and glory are bitterly contested, Homer's evenhanded and unflinching presentation of physical and moral casualties opens the way to new understanding of the costs of a warrior culture. One of the most poignant moments in a hospital-based discussion group turned on the definition of the word "heroism," when a doctor faced the reality of a mentor choosing not to engage in a debilitating fight against his own encroaching cancer. It was by remembering Patroclos, a compassionate warrior who wept as he consoled the wounded and the dying, that the group came to a redefinition of healer. **Section Five: Healing Costs.**

The choice of deep, challenging, and sometimes lengthy works of literature lifts the tone of a reading and discussion group. Long after a discussion has receded into the past, it may affect individual lives and even change a hospital culture in small but perceptible ways. Participants also register pride in reading and thinking about great works, some of which they were required to read in school, many years before these works took on the resonance that comes with the context of literature considered during a career and within the culture of medicine. People who experience illness as well as those living with its effects on friends and family can enrich their experience through these and other full-length works of fiction, non-fiction, and drama.

NOTES ON AUTHORS AND SELECTIONS

Dannie Abse "The smile was" 235
"Case History" 624

"The smile was" by Dannie Abse virtually expresses the rhythms and pauses of the labor of childbirth. As a poet and practicing doctor, Abse has never flinched from empathy or introspection. The difficult physical labor towards childbirth, and its long-awaited conclusion, are given from the perspective of the absorbed practitioner. Like Dylan Thomas, Abse was born in Wales—in Cardiff, in 1923. Also like Thomas, Abse has published in many genres, though he is most widely recognized for his poetry. Having earlier maintained a separation between his work as a doctor and as a poet, Abse came to regard the two parts of his life as inseparable, and his poetry has grown stronger and deeper over time.

As "Case History" makes clear, Dannie Abse brought to the practice of medicine his full identity as a Jew, a Welshman, and a physician. His willingness to reflect on his duty to consider the welfare of his patient while acknowledging his barely contained fury is wonderfully expressed in the physical and historical details that fuse during his examination of the patient. In its tight construction and brevity, this poem celebrates and illustrates the integrated personality; its concluding image condenses thousands of years of recorded biblical language in the wry account of physical sensation.

Felicia Nimue Ackerman "Applicants" 25

Eligibility for expensive and technically sophisticated transplant surgery rests on many factors. Felicia Nimue Ackerman's incisive short story explores some of the criteria not always understood, including the presumed value of a close relationship with a potential caregiver. From the perspective of the applicant, the cost of receiving care may not be quantifiable using conventional means. In this story, Ackerman, who teaches philosophy at Brown University, examines the emotional calculations that may determine the fate of a desperately ill patient.

Conrad Aiken "Silent Snow, Secret Snow" 78

In "Silent Snow, Secret Snow," Conrad Aiken presents a compelling account of the onset of mental illness in an adolescent. The relentless advance of alienation from reality, and the retreat into an interior landscape of snow, achieve the hallucinatory effect of the breakdown experience. Born in Savannah, Georgia, in 1889, Aiken suffered acute trauma in his own early life, when he discovered the bodies of his parents: his father had killed Aiken's mother and then himself. Aiken was raised by an aunt and educated at Harvard. In later life, he was a highly productive writer of poetry and prose, and an important early advocate for the work of Emily Dickinson. Here Aiken employs the short story, his favorite form, to project the consuming effects of the illness which overwhelms the boy's personality and family ties. Conrad Aiken died in 1973.

Edward Albee *The Sandbox* 152

Edward Albee's short play, The Sandbox, *was published and first performed in 1959. It is funny, mordant, and begs to be read aloud. Its subtitle, "A Brief Play, in Memory of my Grandmother (1876–1959)," suggests that memory and affection will permeate the work. Given the seemingly affectionate subtitle, audiences and readers alike must experience a jolt of confusion, even alarm, at the literal sandbox setting and the emotionless generic characters of Mommy, Daddy, Grandma, and The Young Man, who act out Albee's vision of contemporary America's take on family, aging, and death. Born in 1928 in Washington, D.C., Albee was adopted shortly afterwards by a couple from the wealthy suburb of Larchmont, New York. Exposed to the theater from a young age, in all his theatrical works Albee has embedded a caustic view of familial relationships. He has gone on to write numerous full-length plays that have enthralled audiences over the decades since* The Sandbox *first burst on the scene.*

Louisa May Alcott "A Night," from *Hospital Sketches* 556

Alcott, who brought the Civil War into her most famous book, Little Women, *served as a nurse during the war, and published* Hospital Sketches *as a recollection of that experience. Alcott's life was shorter than Whitman's (she lived from 1832 to 1888), but the war was just as significant for her. In Chapter IV of* Hospital Sketches *Alcott describes her promotion to the position of Night Nurse. Her tone, rich with common sense and a deliberately low level of intensity, contrasts with that of "The Wound-Dresser." Alcott is equally unblinking in the face of horror, but consistently looks towards the natural night world outside the locked hospital windows for solace and peace of mind.*

Jean Améry "Torture," from *At the Mind's Limits* 357

Jean Améry, like his admirer, the more famous Primo Levi, was a survivor of Auschwitz. Born in Austria in 1912, to a Roman Catholic mother and a non-practicing Jewish father, Améry came to his identity as a Jew not by practice but according to the legalities of his time. In this essay, he describes his experience at the hands of his captors, with a lucidity that was at once his greatest strength as a writer and philosopher, and his enduring vulnerability as a survivor. The violation of the physical boundary of the self that Amery presents in "Torture" has resonance for survivors of invasive surgery and of the many forms of torture that persist in our time, as almost every urban center now provides refuge to survivors of wars and torture. A reviewer noted that Améry's texts are "notoriously intransigent," but this essay, like all those he wrote reflecting on his experiences, is compellingly readable.

Anonymous Patient "Let Us Have Medicos of Our Own Maturity" 206

This brief and memorable poem appeared anonymously in a collection of poetry and prose entitled Fevers and Frets *published in 1989. The poem expresses in pithy terms a desire often felt and not so often candidly expressed for a sense of generational parity between patients and practitioners.*

Donald Antrim "Black Mountain, 1977" 203

Donald Antrim's brief memory piece, "Black Mountain, 1977," transforms decades of experience into an extraordinarily compressed and evocative meditation on a family's sorrow and survival. Alcoholism, abuse, and mental illness are all in focus, at the same time that the writer evokes the fragile yet enduring bonds that allow compassion and understanding to grow along the vines of affection across generations. Antrim, who was born in 1958, has had an important and influential career as a fiction writer.

W. H. Auden "Musée des Beaux Arts" 7

Wystan Hugh Auden, born in Birmingham, England in 1907, was trained as a physician; that training served him throughout his poetic life. He was a master of calculated flat affect. With scrupulous understatement, in this famous poem he evokes the life of art facing up to and inscribing life. The Breughel painting posing as the subject of Auden's meditation is itself the retelling of a myth. The rich realism of the Dutch master becomes emblematic of an attitude towards human experience and suffering that is both unflinching and illuminating. The detachment Auden praises in Breughel is a prescription for a form of compassion. This poem is positioned as a kind of epigraph for all that follows. Auden emigrated to the United States in 1939, and died as a US citizen in 1973. He was the pre-eminent Anglo-American poet of the twentieth century.

Peter Baida "A Nurse's Story" 568

"A Nurse's Story" won First Prize at the 1999 O'Henry Awards; its author, Peter Baida, died shortly before the award was bestowed. Focusing on a recognizable and dedicated nurse in her last days, Baida's story makes tangible the particular stresses and rewards of nursing in the late twentieth-century. His hospital and its administrators, as well as the nurse's colleagues, are believable and complex. At the same time, without preaching, Baida conveys the enduring appeal and moral grandeur of the nurse's life. Baida was only forty nine when he died.

Henri Barbusse "The Eleventh" 495

Long before the advent of Managed Care, in a terse and beautiful parable originally written in French, Henri Barbusse contemplated the spiritual costs of care that is rationed. "The Eleventh" evokes all the dimensions of suffering in a world ruled by the unequal distribution of scarce resources. Ordinarily when we consider Managed Care, we focus on the needs and frustrations of the ill and those who represent them. As if writing in a timeless world, Barbusse shows the moral devastation of those who carry out the rules of scarcity; he provides a measure of the real costs to a whole culture in which not enough care can be given. Barbusse, who lived from 1873 to 1935, wrote the best-known and most influential anti-war novel in France, Le Feu, *published in 1916. He wrote deliberately throughout his life to improve the lives of common people.*

John Bayley *Elegy for Iris* 600

Dementia and Alzheimer's Disease haunt the contemporary imagination. When philosopher and novelist Iris Murdoch began to disappear into the ravages of Alzheimer's, her husband not only cared for her, but began his memoir, Elegy for Iris. *This excerpt illustrates Bayley's strategy for remaining sane while tending to the real Iris and to the person who was vanishing. Bayley's work is touching, evocative, and useful in its demonstration of the resources of memory for the caretaker towards the end of a beloved partner's existence. Bayley was born in 1923 and has had a long and distinguished career as a writer, teacher, and critic.*

Sallie Bingham "Mending" 348

Sallie Bingham's "Mending" offers the perspective of a woman who describes herself as a professional patient. In a story whose slow, persistent cadences mirror the seemingly glacial process of therapeutic recovery, Bingham draws readers into the search for an integrated self in a person deeply fragmented by a tormented childhood, adolescence, and young adulthood. "I was still, and always would be, one of the walking wounded," the narrator says, using timeworn language appropriate for those wounded in the everyday skirmishes of life. Now living in New Mexico, Sallie Bingham has had a rich and varied career as a writer and activist. She was born in 1937 in Louisville, Kentucky into a prominent family. A prolific writer, she continues to devote energy to writing and to creating archives of women's experience.

Arna Bontemps "A Summer Tragedy" 220

Arna Bontemps was born in Alexandria, Louisiana in 1902, and died in 1973, after a long and varied career that included active participation in the Harlem Renaissance. The pressing physical and financial realities of aging, in both rural and urban settings, were apparent to him as an African-American writer who moved in wide circles. Long-term care remains a vexed and vexing concern in contemporary life; as life expectancy increases and families fracture and reform, we face persistent questions about self-reliance and reliance upon others for the care of our elders. Published decades ago, "A Summer Tragedy" offers a clear-eyed and compassionate glimpse of the considered choice of one old and devoted couple whose lives are no longer "useful."

Gwendolyn Brooks "the mother" 407

Gwendolyn Brooks was born in 1917, and died in 2000. She was a figure of great prestige and accomplishment, winning the Pulitzer Prize for her poetry, as well as lifetime achievement awards from the National Endowment for the Arts and from the National Book Foundation. This much-anthologized and deservedly famous poem carries the full weight of abortion and its aftermath—the heaviness of irrevocable loss, the insistent grappling with multiple levels of truth and responsibility. Brooks compresses imaginary futures and the denial of life, giving full weight to choice and all its consequences. The emotional territory of abortion has rarely been so clearly outlined or so lovingly defined.

Jeanne Bryner "This Red Oozing" 276

In "This Red Oozing," the poet, writing from her perspective as a nurse, marvelously fuses compassion, empathy, and necessary detachment to reveal the immediate and lasting effects of rape. "Doctors in the ER speak like priests," she writes, acknowledging the desires and limits of medicine to heal and to cure what may never be healed, never cured. Jeanne Bryner was born in Appalachia in 1951, and reflects in her work a profound understanding of the lives of working people. Her well-received book, Tenderly Lift Me, *contains biographical sketches of nurses, along with poems and photographs. She continues to integrate her poetic skill and her understanding of and respect for the nurses with whom she practices.*

Mikhail Bulgakov "The Steel Windpipe" 269
"Baptism by Rotation" 498

Mikhail Bulgakov, born in the Ukraine in 1891, lived to 1940, through some of the most difficult and transformative years in Russia's history. Originally trained as a physician, Bulgakov only practiced for a few years, but he mined his experience in A Country Doctor's Notebook *from which these two selections are taken. Bulgakov portrays the experience of a doctor new to his practice and to the community he serves; each vignette is carefully constructed to give the reader a sense of immediacy and urgency as the doctor undergoes a sometimes traumatic immersion into the lives and deaths of his peasant patients. "The Steel Windpipe," whose effect is similar to that of the well-known short piece by William Carlos Williams, "The Use of Force," shows the emergency treatment of diptheria to be as much the doctor's trauma as the child's, whom he succeeds in treating.*

In "Baptism by Rotation," *Bulgakov examines one of the thorniest issues in the shared world of patients and caregivers: learning on the job. As the young doctor hesitates in the face of a horribly difficult delivery, his instructions come not from his medical education but from the experienced nurse at his side. The creation of an empathetic relationship, Bulgakov indicates in this brief tale, should include the delicate relations between and among caregivers—indeed it must, if inexperienced practitioners are to follow a cardinal principle of the Hippocratic Oath: First, do no harm. Bulgakov soon gave up the practice of medicine to follow a career of journalistic and dramatic writing.*

Raphael Campo "Ten Patients and Another"
and "The 10,000th AIDS Death in San Francisco" 625

Campo, who was born in 1964, writes as a gay man, a doctor who practiced throughout the most devastating years of the AIDS deaths in the heart of San Francisco. He writes with clinical intensity of his patients, noting their individuality even as he is overwhelmed by their numbers. Campo makes himself a recording angel, evoking the specificity of each patient, in a series of lines as intimate and assured as a contour drawing made without lifting the pencil from the pad. Campo's career as a poet has been marked by a number of awards, including the William Carlos Williams award, especially fitting since it recalls Williams's excellence as both physician and writer.

Raymond Carver "Cathedral" 417

Born in 1938, Raymond Carver died in 1988, ending the career of a writer who brought new attention to the short story, earning him among other honors, the Mildred and Harold Strauss Living Award. Like many of Carver's intense and polished narratives, the stunning short story "Cathedral" can evoke strong responses. Written in Carver's much-studied low affect, conversational style, the story seems to be about "this blind guy." The narrative proceeds slowly, irritatingly slowly, apparently without promise. Eventually, the narrator, after some resistance, agrees to help the blind man visualize a cathedral. "Well, it's a strange life," the blind man says, resting his hand on the hand of the narrator. Empathy, when it arrives, provides the underpinning to a life as firmly as a flying buttress.

Marion Deutsche Cohen "A Separate Species: Relationships with the World and with Ourselves" 591

Marion Deutsche Cohen, born in 1943, is a mathematician, poet, mother, and professor. But for the purposes of her intensely written book, her primary identity is that of the "well spouse." And in several lacerating chapters, the author provides the kinds of details not usually revealed about the effects of long-term and chronic illness upon those who provide care at home. Cohen's description of the cost is complex and layered, taking into full account the physical toll (exhaustion from lack of sleep being primary). But the most important cost, detailed in the chapter excerpted here, is the changed or "spoiled" identity of the caregiver.

Samuel Taylor Coleridge "Dejection: An Ode" 42

Samuel Taylor Coleridge (1772–1834) is probably best known for his long narrative poem, "The Rime of the Ancient Mariner," and for his poetic fragment "Kubla Khan," the miraculous result of an interrupted, opium-induced dream. With his close friend William Wordsworth, Coleridge was a major force in the creation of English Romanticism as both critic and poet. He suffered from numerous physical and emotional ailments, including depression. "Dejection: An Ode" illustrates Coleridge's extraordinary ability to fuse classical learning and psychological immediacy in the gripping account of the uniquely debilitating experience of depression.

William Cowper "The Cast-Away" 39

English poet and hymn writer William Cowper, who lived from 1731 to 1800, was a lifelong sufferer from depression. A devout Methodist in the early years of Methodism in England, he was saved from suicide by devoted religious friends, who made him part of their household and gave him poetic tasks which occupied his mind and heart. He was also enraptured by the natural world, whose imagery pervades his poems and hymns. "The Cast-Away" uses a narrative verse form and vivid natural images to communicate in metaphorical form the urgent nature of the suicidal yearning that may characterize acute depression.

Cortney Davis "What the Nurse Likes" 506

Cortney Davis has done invaluable work as a nurse, a poet, and an anthologist; she illustrates and integrates experience and the representation of experience, giving voice to the world of medicine and its practitioners. In "What the Nurse Likes," Davis writes in a confessional and yet dispassionate tone of the world of the nurse's experience, revealing the delights and the costs in the same spare, honest cadences. Having lived briefly in Texas, Davis, born in 1945, is a long-time resident of Connecticut, where she continues to work and to write. She is especially interested in the writings of caregivers who record their everyday experiences.

Jan de Hartog *The Hospital* 509

In 1962, Jan de Hartog and his wife, Marjorie, part of a small group of Quakers in Houston, Texas, began to volunteer at a hospital which served a population of poor black residents; the hospital was dangerously under-funded and ill-maintained. In The Hospital, *de Hartog tells the luminous and gritty story of the transformation of the hospital and the volunteers. As a tugboat captain who worked for the Resistance in Holland during the Second World War, de Hartog was no stranger to hardship and danger. He went on to write, among other notable books, a two-volume fictionalized account of the rise of Quakerism. Jan de Hartog was born in 1914 and died in 2002. He and his wife Marjorie were eventually honored by the city of Houston, and lived there again at the end of de Hartog's life.*

Theodore Deppe "Admission, Children's Unit" 493

At once intimately observed and universal, "Admission, Children's Unit" brings the reader very close to the moment at which the professional caregiver encounters sin in the form of child abuse. But the poem also looks into the heart of the caregiver who, like St. Lawrence, investigates his own heart and soul, and finds a new fragrance, "never before smelled on earth." Judgment and empathy, the poet suggests, may not always exist in the same heart. Theodore Deppe was born in Duluth, Minnesota in 1950. He is a graduate of Vermont College's MFA in Writing Program, and holds degrees from Earlham and Berea Colleges. The author of Children of the Air *(1990) and* The Wanderer King *(1996), both from Alice James Books, and* Cape Clear: New and Selected Poems *(Salmon Books, 2002), Deppe has been awarded a Pushcart Prize, two NEA grants, and fellowships from the Massachusetts Cultural Commission and the Connecticut Commission for the Arts. He is presently writer-in-residence at Phillips Academy.*

Toi Derricotte "Delivery" 241

In a variety of genres, over decades, Toi Derricotte has given voice to the experiences of African-American women, especially those, like herself, who live in a borderland of racial difference and complexity. Born in 1941 in Detroit, Michigan, Derricotte has been a successful teacher and lecturer, taking her poetry and other writing to campuses across the country. Derricotte's poem about birth, part of a book-length exploration of childbearing, conveys unmistakably the experience of the body as a battleground. The baby fighting to be born, and the mother fighting to accomplish the birth and find her connection to this emerging life, provide the intense rhythm and images that drive this poem.

Emma Donoghue "What Remains" 211

Emma Donoghue often grounds her fiction in documented history. The lives of the two elderly artists who are at the center of "What Remains" did indeed follow the trajectory described in the story. But, as is true so often in Donoghue's work, it is the imaginative entry into the specific details of the nursing home existence that allows the reader to experience the transcendent survival of unique selves in the disguises of age. Emma Donoghue was born in Dublin, Ireland, in 1969. With a PhD from Cambridge University, Donoghue moved to Canada, where she has lived for some years. She continues to publish widely.

Florence Elon "Premature Elegy" 448

Seven poems make up the sequence Florence Elon has titled "Premature Elegy"; they provide a scaffolding of sorts for an extended meditation on the still-living but now dying parent. Scrupulously, the poet documents the moment and the memories, giving voice to the patient and to those who crowd around the bedside. The poems convey the energies of illness, recollection, and the artifacts of personality, as the living person takes charge in the slow march towards death. Florence Elon was born in New York City in 1939; she now lives and works as a poet and editor in Berkeley, California.

Anita Endrezze "Ponies Gathering in the Dark" 413

"Ponies Gathering in the Dark" immerses the reader in the experience of a Native American healing tradition. The pace of this brief story remarkably conveys the immensely long and deep natural tradition that underlies the life work of one aging healer. The story conveys, as well, the changes in the world that will render his healing obsolete. Anita Endrezze was born in 1925. She works as a poet and as a short story writer; recognition for her work has come in the form of such honors as the Weyerhauser/Bumbershot Award in 1992 and the Washington Governor's Writers Award in 1993.

Susan Glaspell "A Jury of Her Peers" 278

"A Jury of Her Peers" is a touchstone in the literature of domestic abuse. A conspiracy of silence among the women who meet in the home of Minnie Foster crowns the long, unintentional conspiracy of silence that allowed a woman to be brutalized within a marriage that a whole community saw and none acknowledged. Domestic violence has long been both visible and invisible; the scrupulous fidelity to detail in Susan Glaspell's story locates it within the long history of that community. Born in 1876, Glaspell was not primarily a writer of short stories, but is better known as a Pulitzer Prize-winning playwright—her first rendition of this story was as the much-produced play Trifles*—and cofounder with her first husband of the Provincetown Players. Glaspell died in 1948.*

Donald Hall "Without" 404

Donald Hall was a well-regarded and widely published teacher, poet, and essayist long before his wife, the poet Jane Kenyon, contracted cancer. Recognition for his work includes the Caldecott Medal and his appointment as Poet Laureate of the United States. The poems Hall wrote during Kenyon's illness and after her death testify to an astonishing fusion of emotion, experience, and deeply refined technical skill. Poems from his collection Without, *including the title poem included in this section, describe the difficult personal journey into a life changed by illness and loss. Donald Hall was born in 1928, and continues to write poetry that reflects his thoughtful and illuminating experiences.*

Joy Harjo "Three Generations of Native American Women's Birth Experience" 126

When she writes of the births of her two children, Native American writer and activist Joy Harjo, born in 1956, soberly contrasts the experiences: one, when she was barely sixteen, and the other, four years later. She further embeds each experience in the history of her family and her tribe, and implicitly in the experience of childbirth in a world divided by race and generation. Harjo walks between and within these worlds, allowing the reader to share a series of complex birth stories whose meaning is still evolving. Educated at the University of New Mexico, and with an MFA from the University of Iowa, Harjo has won recognition as a poet as well as a writer of fiction and memoir.

Nathaniel Hawthorne "Rappaccini's Daughter" 181

In our time, educated parental decision-making about the lives of children is a subject for scrutiny and some concern. In this early American short story, Hawthorne presents the ultimate ethical implications of parental control over a child's physical and emotional life. Written long before the era of genetic testing and counseling, Hawthorne's story posits the case of a scientist father who designs the life of his daughter as a life-long experiment. Hawthorne was born in 1804 in Salem, Massachusetts, and died in 1864. He wrote deeply affecting and sometimes searing works of fiction that both exemplified and questioned the New England beliefs that shaped his consciousness and America itself.

Jack Hodgins "Astonishing the Blind" 460

"Astonishing the Blind" by Jack Hodgins is the final story in his collection entitled Damage Done by the Storm. *The story seems to come to us from a great distance; the narrator writes as an observer, one in whom the springs of feeling have dried. The caregiving in this story is observed rather than felt by the narrator, and it is through the eyes of the deliberately detached, gifted woman pianist that we come to understand what can be seen and what can only be felt. Continuing to care for one who is absent, through death, dementia, or infidelity, may be understood as a chore, a blessing, even a gift. The quiet conclusion of this story offers hope in a small, closely observed change of behavior; it is a momentary victory over the entropy of feeling. Jack Hodgins, who was born in 1938, is an admired Canadian writer whose work includes many short stories and novels.*

Molly Holden "Hospital" 108

Molly Holden's poem, "Hospital," uses the most ordinary language to offer a remarkable and penetrating glimpse of the uneasy spiritual territory occupied by a determinedly secular person with a serious illness. Born in 1927, Holden contracted MS in 1964, the same year in which her remarkable first book of poetry was published in England. Her long experience with a debilitating illness infuses her poetry, which is in the tradition of the work of Thomas Hardy. In six brief and neatly turned stanzas, Holden provides a penetrating awareness of the struggle for spiritual grace outside of traditional and well-organized religious consolations for illness and mortality. Holden's Selected Poems, *from which this work is taken, was published in 1987.*

Juliet S. Kono "Homeless," "Son, After the Attempt," "The First Time," "Royally Pissed," "Nest," "The Struggle," "The Permission," "In a Rush," and "The Way" 251

Juliet S. Kono was born in 1943; she grew up in Hilo, Hawai'i and now lives in Honolulu. These nine poems are taken from a series describing the mental illness, suicide attempt, and eventual loss of a son that appeared in 1995 in Tsunami Years, *a special double issue of* Bamboo Ridge, *the Hawai'i Writers' Quarterly. In addition to this stunning work, Kono has published another collection of poems* (Hilo Rains, *1988) and a short story collection. In 2005, Kono was awarded the Hawai'i Award for Literature.*

Leonard Kriegel "In Kafka's House" 56

Born in New York in 1933, writer and retired City University of New York Professor of English Leonard Kriegel is self-described as a "cripple," an identity he first experienced at the age of eleven when he contracted polio. "In Kafka's House" is the final essay in a collection published in 1991. Dense and beautifully written, it leaps immediately into the territory of a dream, fusing physical reality (the paralysis resulting from childhood polio) and metaphor (Kafka's immense short story "Metamorphosis"), and immersing the reader in the struggle of the self to remain intact within the weakened body.

Maxine Kumin "Hello, Hello Henry" and "The Last Words of Henry Manley" 207
"On Being Asked to Write a Poem in Memory of Anne Sexton"
and "October, Yellowstone Park" 409

Poems by Maxine Kumin, inspired by her neighbor, Henry Manley, have been appearing over the years; they chart the experience of aging in place, which is what so many desire for themselves and those they love. An award-winning poet (including the Pulitzer Prize for Poetry in 1973), Kumin lives, works, and writes on a farm in Northern New England. Her close relationship to the natural world, especially her horses, contributes to the effectiveness of her observant and measured style. Born in 1925, Kumin was badly injured in an accident involving one of her beloved horses; she describes her recovery in Inside the Halo and Beyond: The Anatomy of a Recovery, *published in 2000.*

Kumin's poetry is remarkable for its technical accomplishment and its emotional accessibility. The range of her work is tremendous, from intensely observed poetry of the natural world to the probing of internal wounds and raptures. Kumin's friendship with Anne Sexton was legendary, and is reflected in the numerous poems Kumin wrote in the months and years after Sexton's suicide. Individual poems trace the unique and implacable course of grief, and its slow transformation into reflection after such a loss.

Jane Lazarre "A Sense of Threat" 92

Jane Lazarre's journey through breast cancer and treatment, recounted in Wet Earth and Dreams: A Narrative of Grief and Recovery, *follows the course of her illness, including its deep association with her mother's early death from breast cancer. Lazarre's book is especially effective because of her established success as a truthful chronicler—in prose and poetry—of her journey into interracial marriage and motherhood. Born in 1943, Lazarre has been a long-time faculty member of the Eugene Lang College of the New School University in New York City, and has been writing with deep political and social engagement for decades. Ambivalence and uneasiness are familiar subjects for Lazarre, and in this excerpt she provides especially valuable insight into the depersonalizing nature of chemotherapy, and the slow development of community among sufferers.*

Robert Lipsyte "Innocents Abroad" 17

Robert Lipsyte brought to his experience of testicular cancer a unique capacity for observation and description. His long and successful career as a sports writer and journalist provided not only the ability to recognize the similarities to other arenas of struggle, but also the discipline to capture the experience in pithy and gripping prose. Born in 1938, Lipsyte began his career at the New York Times *at the age of nineteen, and enjoyed success not only as a sports journalist, but also as a novelist and memoirist. He describes* In the Country of Illness *as "mortality confronted with hard-earned outrage." The opening chapter reprinted here is just the kind of candid reporting that provides reassurance through wry and self-revealing details.*

John Milton "On His Blindness" 633

John Milton's great sonnet, "On His Blindness," demonstrates in its very construction the difficult process through which the great poet found sense in his affliction. The literary giant of seventeenth-century Britain, Milton is best known for his monumental poems Paradise Lost, Paradise Regained, *and* Samson Agonistes. *A devout and passionate Christian and advocate for intellectual freedom, he brought to bear on the "problem" of his blindness the full arsenal of his powers as a poet. In effect, in this poem, Milton wrestles with his angel and emerges exhausted but triumphant, having constructed the meaning of his blindness in accordance with his faith and his mission as a poet.*

Michel de Montaigne "Of Training" 8

Born into the beginnings of the Renaissance in France, Michel de Montaigne lived from 1533 to 1592. Living on his land, as both a devout Catholic and a pragmatic thinker, he virtually invented the personal essay. Like so many that he wrote hundreds of years ago, this essay speaks to us with the full force of his personality and his distilled introspection. Montaigne examined himself with a combined rigor and affection, believing, as he notes in this essay, that what he learned about himself would tell him about others. His essays are introspective without being self-absorbed; this one, stemming from an almost-fatal accident, provides us with living testimony about a near-death experience. As Montaigne wrote: "It is not my deed that I write about; it is my essence." Reading Montaigne, we learn about ourselves.

Lorrie Moore "People Like That Are The Only People Here: Canonical Babbling in Peed Onk" 466

"What is the story?" the narrator asks early on in this rich account of a baby's brush with mortality. Lorrie Moore's powerful short story, "People Like That Are the Only People Here," wrestles from beginning to end with the necessary and seemingly impossible task of giving form and meaning to the inexplicable appearance of suffering and death in the lives of small children. The reduction of each complex individual to a title (Mother, Baby, Doctor, Surgeon) both mocks and salutes the habits of the chart and the practitioners, at the same time that the narrative inspects the most minute bits of language for clues to the possibility of meaning behind the meaninglessness that must torment every parent. Born in 1957, Moore has had a distinguished career as a writer of short stories and novels. She is Professor of English at the University of Wisconsin, Madison.

Ruth Nadelhaft "Labors of Love" 131
"Ashes to Ashes to Ashes" 429

"Labors of Love" might be subtitled "Ideology and Childbirth," for it is as much about prevailing attitudes towards labor and delivery as it is a personal recollection of three generations of childbirth experiences. Born in 1938 to a mother born in 1910, Nadelhaft intimately experienced changing fashions in labor and delivery. Amid medical and statistical studies of maternal and infant mortality, rates of caesarean sections, and uses of various forms of anaesthesia, there is still a need for honest firsthand recollections of individual women's experiences within the contexts of medical traditions that may determine what might appear to be personal choices. Educated in New York City and Madison, Wisconsin, residing in New York and upstate Maine, the author recalls regional practices through time and both inner and outer spaces.

In "Ashes to Ashes to Ashes," Nadelhaft describes the slow and unique process of apprehending loss; despite scrupulous attempts to prepare for the decline and death of parents, the experience itself is surprising and complex. The physical remains after cremation, an increasingly common choice in contemporary Western cultures, oblige mourners to consider their emotional futures through the choices they make to keep, to bury, or to dispose of the ashes. Nadelhaft's parents, who celebrated their sixtieth wedding anniversary just weeks before the death of her father, died within months of one another at the end of 1993 and the beginning of 1994.

Leslie Nyman "Wisteria" 443

Being present at the death of a patient remains one of the greatest challenges and rewards of giving care. Leslie Nyman, born in 1949, was a registered nurse for fifteen years, and her short story comes to us from that perspective. "Wisteria" evokes memory and nostalgia, which in a patient, who drifts in and out of reality, frightens a young and inexperienced nurse. By the end of the story, having understood and even accepted death's welcomed presence, the nurse is able to smell the perfume of her co-workers. Nyman now writes and gardens in western Massachusetts.

Flannery O'Connor "The Enduring Chill" 161

Flannery O'Connor was born in 1925 in Savannah, Georgia; she died in August 1954, having suffered from Lupus, which killed her beloved father at an early age as well. O'Connor's mordant humor, which infuses all her remarkable fiction, seems to have been essential to her character (she achieved a brief notoriety as a young child for teaching a chicken to walk backwards). All of her fiction offers a kind of layered reality. A searing study of generations, love, resentment, and an inexplicable illness, "The Enduring Chill" makes use of themes familiar to much of O'Connor's remarkable body of work. The familial antagonisms, unexpected humor, deep patterns of rural Southern life, and a son's frantic attempts to escape those constraints illuminate this study of disease. Simultaneously, the redeeming power of grace, always a possibility in O'Connor's contemplation of soul-sickness, enters the sick room.

Marianne A. Paget "The Work of Talk" 375

Marianne (Tracy) Paget was born in 1940 and died—after an abbreviated life—in 1989. She was a sociologist investigating the contexts for medical mistakes, and in the course of her work she suffered a missed diagnosis, which led to her untimely death. Determined to dramatize the communication errors which she saw at the heart of much medical practice, she constructed a unique amalgam of medical science and gripping drama, presenting tortuous (tape recorded and transcribed) dialogues between patients and doctors woven together with anguished commentary from an imaginary chorus. This chapter, from her posthumously published collection of letters and essays, presents part of the dramatic text and Paget's own analysis of her intentions and the play's effect. Single, with a network of devoted friends, Paget convinced her doctors that her complicated treatments could be accomplished with the cooperation of her friends, out of hospital. Her writing and her life make a substantial contribution to medical practices.

Katherine Philips "Orinda Upon Little Hector Philips" 406

Katherine Philips was English; she was born in 1631 into a prosperous merchant family, and died in 1664. In a time when women poets were rare, and published women poets even rarer, Philips was well known and highly regarded. In her brief life, she became a mother twice. "Orinda Upon Little Hector Philips" is a concise and formal expression of her intense grief after the loss of her son, who was, according to the poem, little more than a month old when he died. Through the work's tight and formally ordered construction, the grief of the young mother speaks poignantly across the generations. "Scarce forty days" has the same literary effect as that of the very well-known construction: "Fourscore and seven years ago."

Eileen Pollack "Milk" 111

Eileen Pollack was born in 1956; her short story, "Milk," was published in the Spring, 1994 issue of Ploughshares. *Pollack has published widely, including a book of short fiction, and has held visiting professorships as well as a long-term appointment at the University of Michigan. "Milk" offers an intimate experience of the first difficult days after delivery for two women of differing race and class. The vagaries of hospital care seem to speak for themselves, as physicians, nurses, and medical students move in and out of the room shared by the two women. In understated prose, Pollack provides a sobering portrait of communication failures that signal an absence of empathy that has serious medical consequences for one woman and her baby.*

Rachel Naomi Remen "Mystery and Awe" 534

Kitchen Table Wisdom *is composed of a series of brief and evocative essays that focus on the emotional demands of practicing medicine. Remen, herself a practicing medical doctor, works as a therapist with doctors whose lives seem especially vulnerable to the demands of their practices. Born in 1938, Remen valiantly discloses her own vulnerabilities; living with Krohn's Disease for decades, she is especially sensitive to the long-term and familial sources of both pain and hard-won insights. She is willing to disclose both her love of medicine and her own lapses in empathy and understanding—her search for what she calls loving kindness for herself and for her patients and colleagues.*

Susan Fromberg Schaeffer "Homage to Isaac Bashevis Singer" 70

Susan Fromberg Schaeffer is the author of several novels, a collection of short stories, and five books of poetry. Born in Brooklyn in 1941, Schaeffer received a PhD in Literature from the University of Chicago, and was appointed to a named professorship at Brooklyn College in 1985. This short story testifies to her long involvement with the work of Singer, and with the experience of the Holocaust and its aftermath. Faced with overwhelming events whose meaning appears indeterminate, Singer and many other post-Holocaust writers turned to narrative, as does Mrs. Klopstock, the protagonist of Schaeffer's short story. It is through narrative that Mrs. Klopstock wrests control of her illness from uncomprehending doctors and frightened family members.

Anne Sexton "Doctors," "The Wall," and "The Poet of Ignorance" 47

In many of her poems, Anne Sexton articulated the intense and unending attempt to make sense and give poetic structure to her experiences of madness and depression. Terse and propulsive, like the three gathered here, Sexton's poems allow us to grasp the force of the struggle in which she was engaged. Adding a powerful dimension to her work is the charged nature of her religious belief, which is as alive in the poems as the madness she fought. Born in 1928, Sexton's life included marriage, motherhood, teaching, and hospitalizations. She committed suicide in 1974, an act whose profound reverberations are reflected in the work of her great friend and fellow poet Maxine Kumin.

Jonathan Shay "Betrayal of 'What's Right'" 295

Born in 1942, Jonathan Shay, MD, PhD, has now written two books about his work with traumatized veterans of the Viet Nam war; this excerpt is from the first. (His more recent book, Odysseus in America: Combat Trauma and the Trials of Homecoming, *brings the story home, with Odysseus.) Shay treats and studies trauma in the context of the Trojan War, as reported by Homer in the two great epics that have survived many centuries and many wars. The juxtaposition of ancient literature and contemporary suffering serves both to enlarge and to deepen the veterans' and the reader's understanding of the immediate and long-term consequences of physical and emotional trauma. Shay came to his remarkable calling as a result of his own traumatic experience, a stroke that put an end to his first career as a researcher. Returning to his earlier study of Greek literature, he developed a theory about trauma and recovery—that all trauma has recognizable biological and psychological consequences—which has led to his decades of work with veterans, and which informs his practice as a psychiatrist.*

Marisa Silver "What I Saw from Where I Stood" 336

Marisa Silver was born in 1960, and grew up in Shaker Heights, New Jersey. She is a successful director of films and documentaries, as well as a writer of short stories. "What I Saw from Where I Stood" draws readers towards the traumatic past, which darkens and informs the present: the story which unfolds. The accident and its aftermath recreate the terror and uncertainty of the stillbirth that haunts this couple a year after the event. Living with loss poses different challenges to each of the characters, and every new danger offers another glimpse back to the first breach of their imagined safety. "We can't live like this," the narrator says, but coming back to life is a slow and uncertain journey, traced in the final pages of this acclaimed piece. (After its initial publication in The New Yorker, *the work was selected for* Best American Short Stories 2001*).*

Pat Staten "The Day My Father Tried to Kill Us" 311

Pat Staten was born in Topeka, Kansas in 1945. A playwright and author, in her short story, "The Day My Father Tried to Kill Us," she shows the traumatic effects of combat on a veteran and his family—but the war is the Second World War, the "good war" whose veterans lived out the consequences of their wartime experiences individually, and usually without the help of veterans' support groups such as those Jonathan Shay still leads decades after the conclusion of the Viet Nam war. Staten's story, told in several tenses, reflects the fragmented and painful recollection of memory from the several points of view of one daughter: the frightened five-year old; the furious fifteen-year old; and the puzzled and still mending twenty-five year old who tells the story which will always seem incomplete.

Wislawa Szymborska "Report from the Hospital," "The Suicide's Room," and "In Praise of Feeling Bad About Yourself" 456

Wislawa Szymborska's poetry, composed in Polish, comes to us in translation, so there may be additional richness and depth not available to us even in loving translation. Born in 1923, Szymborska won the Nobel Prize for literature in 1996. Her poems are so immediate and engaging that they speak to us as if in a language we recognize by its penetrating truthfulness. In "Report from the Hospital," for example, Szymborska tells us what it is like to be delegated to visit a dying friend in the hospital. Coming to terms does not appeal to everyone; the poet opens her heart and allows her readers to see into their own.

Dylan Thomas "Elegy," "Do Not Go Gentle Into That Good Night," "And Death Shall Have No Dominion," and "A Refusal to Mourn the Death, by Fire, of a Child in London" 228

The great Welsh poet Dylan Thomas wrote several poems which memorialize the passage of generations. From his collected poems, these four exemplify the poet's intense focus on the connections between individuals and generations. The demand the poet makes upon his dying father, "Do not go gentle," is balanced by the equally stern injunction of "A Refusal to Mourn," with its stunning final line: "After the first death, there is no other." Thomas, who was born in Wales in 1914, was memorialized primarily as a poet, though he wrote and published widely in many genres. In his last years, especially during his travels in America, Thomas became notorious, especially on college campuses, as a hard-drinking figure of Dionysian inspiration. He died in 1953 of pneumonia and acute alcoholism.

Frank T. Vertosick, Jr. "A Woman's War" 521

Why We Hurt: The Natural History of Pain *is primarily Frank T. Vertosick's attempt as a physician to explain to lay readers the functions of pain in human existence. His attempt falters, however, as he confesses, when he confronts the childbirth pain of his own wife. Vertosick's willingness to engage with and then reveal his own discomfort is instructive for health care practitioners and lay readers alike. Vertosick is also the author of numerous technical articles and a study of intelligence.*

Fred W. Voget, with Mary K. Mee "I'm Born a Crow Indian" 144

The collaboration between Fred W. Voget and Mary K. Mee produced the book from which this excerpt is taken. Born in 1913, Voget married Mee, his assistant, in 1942. They worked together as anthropologists, preserving and filtering the experiences of their subjects, such as Agnes Yellowtail Deernose. The birth and early childhood customs that Agnes describes provide a secure foundation for her memory, allowing her to construct the narrative of her book, and to juxtapose her Crow origins against the culture of the White people who gradually surrounded her but never obliterated her Crow beginnings.

Darcy Wakefield "Cleaning" 53

"Cleaning," from Darcy Wakefield's collected short essays chronicling her experience of ALS (from which she died in December 2005, some two years after being diagnosed), reveals her extraordinary determination to retain her perspective in the midst of a consuming and debilitating illness. Born in 1970 in Maine, where she lived and worked throughout her brief life, Wakefield wrote for National Public Radio, and taught at the University of Southern Maine. Her personality emerges clearly in this chapter, as in the rest of her memoir, which was collected and published in 2005.

Walt Whitman "The Wound-Dresser" 553

During the Civil War, Walt Whitman served as a volunteer nurse, working part-time as a clerk in the Office of the Army Paymaster (and in other Army offices as well), to support himself. Whitman was born in 1819 and lived until 1892. His experience of the Civil War and its aftermath profoundly informed his poetry. In this monumental poem, Whitman suggests that scenes of the wounded and dying return to him in dreams even as the world turns away from the memory of the terrible war and its losses. The poem, in the relentless present tense, contains details as harrowing as any found in clinical accounts of war-inflicted injuries. Yet Whitman's tender regard for his patients, his willingness to enter imaginatively into their agony, makes this suffering as readable as it is indelible.

INDEX OF AUTHORS AND SELECTIONS

BIOGRAPHY MONOGRAPHS

The Center for Biographical Research at the University of Hawai'i at Mānoa is dedicated to the interdisciplinary and multicultural study of life writing through teaching, publication, and outreach activities.

In addition to *Biography: An Interdisciplinary Quarterly,* published since 1978, the Center sponsors the University of Hawai'i Press Biography Monograph series, designed to further the study and practice of life writing in all its forms. A chronological list of previous monographs follows:

Anthony Friedson, ed. *New Directions in Biography* (1981)

Gloria Fromm, ed. *Essaying Biography: A Celebration for Leon Edel* (1986)

Frank Novak, Jr. *The Autobiographical Writings of Lewis Mumford: A Study in Literary Audacity* (1988)

Mari Matsuda, ed. *Called from Within: Early Women Lawyers of Hawaii* (1992)

Alice M. Beechert and Edward D. Beechert, eds. *John Reinecke: The Autobiography of a Gentle Activist* (1993)

Koji Ariyoshi. *From Kona to Yenan: The Political Memoirs of Koji Ariyoshi,* edited by Alice M. Beechert and Edward D. Beechert (2000).

Leon Edel. *The Visitable Past: A Wartime Memoir* (2001).

For further information about the Center or its publications, contact the Center f Biographical Research, University of Hawai'i at Mānoa, Honolulu, Hawai'i 968 USA; telephone/fax: (808) 956-3774; biograph@hawaii.edu; www.hawaii.edu ograph.

or
22
/bi-